Human Anatomy and Physiology

Theory and Practicals

Questions and Answers

for Paramedical and Allied Health Sciences Students

As per the latest Competency-based Education Guidelines

- Question–Answer Format
- Multiple Choice Questions
- *Viva Voce*
- Short and Long Answer Questions
- Match the Columns
- Draw Labelled Diagrams
- Case Studies
- 16 Chapters
- 21 Practicals

Goal

The main goal of learning anatomy and physiology is to derive comprehensive knowledge of gross structures, and microscopic anatomical structures, related functions, developments of human body parts and their correlation with various clinical conditions and diseases.

Mission

At the end of anatomy studies, a student should be able to:

1. Comprehend the normal body structures, clinically relevant inter-relationships, functional and cross-sectional anatomy of the various structures of the body and related functions.
2. Identify the microscopic structures of tissues and organs and correlation of their functions in normal state and in pathological conditions.
3. Demonstrate knowledge of basic principles involved in the sequential development of normal body parts and effects of genetic variations, pathogens and common teratogens on the growth of the body.
4. Explain horizontal correlation of anatomy and physiology aspects with premedical subjects (medical biochemistry, nutrition), vertical integration with paramedical subjects (medical microbiology, pharmacology, preventive medicine, hematology, pathology) and vertical integration with medical subjects (pediatrics, gynecology, obstetrics, and ophthalmology).

Skills

At the end of the course, the students should be able to:

1. Identify and locate all the structures of the body and describe the related specific features.
2. Explain various normal functions and disturbed functions in the pathological conditions.
3. Identify the microscopic structures of various types of normal tissues and affected tissues in various pathological conditions.
4. Identify gross congenital anomalies.
5. Safely perform the following techniques: Blood collection (venipuncture), intramuscular and intravenous injections, lumber puncture, CSF collection, arterial blood collection, determination of blood pressure, use of spirometer, oximeter, microscopy and basic hematology practicals.

Human Anatomy and Physiology

Theory and Practicals

Questions and Answers

for Paramedical and Allied Health Sciences Students

Praful B Godkar PhD

Former

Pool Officer, Department of Biochemistry, Haffkine Institute, Mumbai, Maharashtra, India
Biochemist and Scientific Officer, Hospitals of Municipal Corporation of Greater Mumbai, Maharashtra, India
Head, Department of DMLT, Founder and Head, Department of Clinical Laboratory Science (CLS)
SNDT University, Mumbai, Maharashtra, India
Research Guide, Department of Health Sciences, Symbiosis International University, Pune, Maharashtra
National Research Council (NRC) Fellow, Walter Reed Army Institute of Research, Silver Spring, MD, USA

Author of renowned textbooks on medical laboratory technology, medical biochemistry and medical microbiology, immunology, parasitology

Darshan Praful Godkar MD FACC FAHA FASE FASNC

President and Chairman, Advanced Cardiology LLC, Morris, Union, Sussex and Warren Counties over 6 Offices
Interventional and Structural Cardiologist, Saint Barnabas Medical Center, NJ, USA
Director, Radial Interventions, Cooperman Barnabas Medical Center, NJ, USA
Director, Radial program, Saint Barnabas Medical Center, NJ, USA

CBSPD

CBS Publishers & Distributors Pvt Ltd

New Delhi • Bengaluru • Chennai • Kochi • Kolkata • Lucknow • Mumbai
Gujarat • Hyderabad • Jharkhand • Nagpur • Patna • Pune • Uttarakhand

Disclaimer

Science and technology are constantly changing fields. New research and experience broaden the scope of information and knowledge. The authors have tried their best in giving information available to them while preparing the material for this book. Although all efforts have been made to ensure optimum accuracy of the material, yet it is quite possible some errors might have been left uncorrected. The publisher, the printer and the authors will not be held responsible for any inadvertent errors, omissions or inaccuracies.

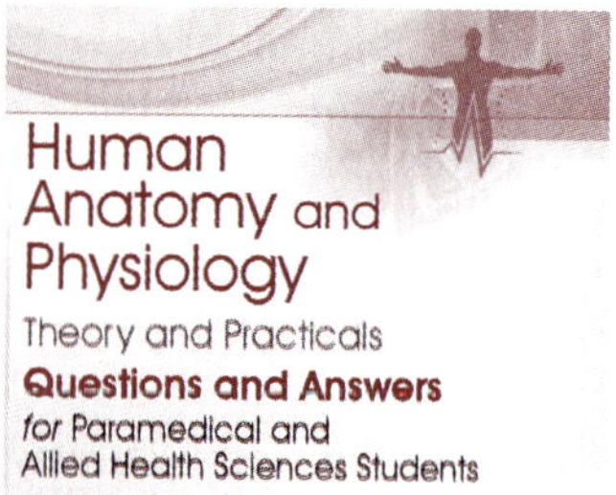

ISBN: 978-93-49057-97-5

First Edition 2025

Published by Satish Kumar Jain and produced by Varun Jain for

CBS Publishers & Distributors Pvt Ltd

4819/XI Prahlad Street, 24 Ansari Road, Daryaganj, New Delhi 110 092, India

Ph: 011-23289259, 23266838 Fax: 011-23243014
Website: www.cbspd.com e-mail: delhi@cbspd.com

Corporate Office: 204 FIE, Industrial Area, Patparganj, Delhi 110 092, India
Ph: 011-49344934 Fax: 011-49344935
e-mail: publishing@cbspd.com; publicity@cbspd.com

Branches

- Bengaluru: Seema House 2975, 17th Cross, KR Road, Banasankari 2nd Stage, Bengaluru 560 070, Karnataka, India
  Ph: +91-80-26771678/79 Fax: +91-80-26771680 e-mail: bangalore@cbspd.com
- Chennai: 18/8B, Subbarayan Street, Shenoy Nagar, Chennai 600 030, Tamil Nadu, India
  Ph: +91-44-42032115, 26681266 e-mail: chennai@cbspd.com
- Kochi: 42/1325, 1326, Power House Road, Opposite KSEB, Power House, Ernakulum 682018, Kochi, Kerala, India
  Ph: +91-484-4059061–67 Fax: +91-484-4059065 e-mail: kochi@cbspd.com
- Kolkata: 147, Hind Ceramics Compound, 1st Floor, Nilgunj Road, Belghoria, Kolkata 700056, West Bengal, India
  Ph: +91-33-25330055/56 e-mail: kolkata@cbspd.com
- Lucknow: Basement, Khushuma Complex, 7 Meerabai Marg (behind Jawahar Bhawan), Lucknow 226001, UP, India
  Ph: +91-522-4000032 e-mail: tiwari.lucknow@cbspd.com
- Mumbai: PWD Shed, Gala No. 25/26, Ramchandra Bhatt Marg, Next JJ Hospital Gate No. 2, Opp. Union Bank of India, Noorbaug, Mumbai 400009, Maharashtra, India
  Ph: +91-22-66661880/89 e-mail: mumbai@cbspd.com

Representatives

- **Gujarat** 0-9879558667
- **Hyderabad** 0-9885175004
- **Jharkhand** 0-9811541605
- **Nagpur** 0-8692091830
- **Patna** 0-9334159340
- **Pune** 0-9664372571
- **Uttarakhand** 0-9716462459

Printed at: Sri Prints, Delhi, India

to

All the paramedical staff members and practitioners
who take great care of our healthcare systems

Preface

You have brains in your head. You have feet in your shoes. You can steer yourself any direction you choose

—*Dr Seuss*

It gives us a great pleasure to introduce a book *Human Anatomy and Physiology, Theory and Practicals: Questions and Answers for Paramedical and Allied Science Students*. This was a long-standing request from the students, during our recent educational sessions. This book includes basic anatomy and physiology theory and practicals, according to the latest complete syllabi suggested by all the paramedical courses and the undergraduate Competency-based Medical Education (CBME) concept suggested by National Medical Commission of India (NMC), 2024.

The layout of this textbook has been organized by keeping in mind the following main objectives: (1) To provide comprehensive knowledge to the students of the gross and microscopic structure and development of the human body and (2) to provide a basis for understanding the clinical correlation of organ structures, and related various parts with various clinical conditions and diseases.

Our introduction to Competency-based Medical Education (CBME) concept in this textbook will be useful for the students to integrate knowledge of anatomy and physiology with other premedical subjects such as medical biochemistry and nutrition, with paramedical subjects such as general medicine, microbiology, pharmacology and also with case studies related to ophthalmology, pediatrics, gynecology and obstetrics.

This textbook contains 16 chapters and 21 practicals, with the following various types of questions and related answers: MCQs, match the columns, long answer, short answer, table viva voce, practical viva voce, labeled diagrams and questions based on pathophysiology–anatomy corelations.

We have presented this textbook in two colors. It contains 608 colored illustrations and important tables; which will be useful in learning and understanding the subject matter very well.

In Chapter, 16 we have included the practicals prescribed by all the paramedical subject councils. This chapter covers the hematology practicals that includes: Basic reagents, glassware, equipment, instruments, various types of techniques, standard operation procedures (SOPs), laboratory mathematics and laboratory safety.

Hematology practicals are covered with information on: Instructions given to the patient, specimen types and collection methods, clinical significance, normal ranges (reference ranges), with SOPs, safety and quality control (QC) measures. These experiments are safe and used in current laboratory practice. SOPs are based on manual as well as semi-automated methods and presented with standard compositions of the reagents. Students and teachers will be able to perform practicals, easily and quickly by referring to the SOPs.

On the basis of information given in this book, students will be able to adapt to safety precautions right from the first day of working in a hematology laboratory. Students will be able to select appropriate requirements by referring to SOPs. Students will also be able to understand principles of various conventional techniques and use of routine and specialized hematology laboratory tests and basic instrumentation.

Introduction of theory and practicals together will be useful for the students to prepare various research-based projects in the final semester. Project presentations will give boost to the various abilities of students such as thinking, innovation and creativity.

This textbook will be useful as a standard guide book for the preparation of qualifying competitive examinations required to apply for jobs or to pursue higher education in gulf countries and in English-speaking countries such as USA, UK, Canada, New Zealand and Australia.

This textbook will be useful as a standard book of anatomy and physiology in question–answer format for the students of paramedical subjects such as medical laboratory technology (MLT), clinical laboratory science (CLS), dentistry, optometry, biomedical sciences, physiotherapy, biotechnology, graduate and postgraduate students of life sciences, biochemistry, microbiology, zoology, botony, etc. This book will also be useful for the students of medicine to get basic information on anatomy and physiology.

We look forward to suggestions from students and teachers for further updating this book.

Praful B Godkar
Darshan Praful Godkar

Acknowledgments

It is with deep gratitude and sincere appreciation, we acknowledge the opportunity given to us to present this book *Human Anatomy and Physiology, Theory and Practicals: Questions and Answers for Paramedical and Allied Health Sciences Students* by Mr Satish Kumar Jain, President and Managing Director of CBS Publishers & Distributors Pvt Ltd, New Delhi.

We acknowledge with great appreciation, the continued guidelines provided by Mr YN Arjuna (Senior Vice President—Publishing, Editorial and Publicity) and Ms Ritu Chawla (GM—Production), CBS Publishers & Distributors Pvt Ltd, during the making of this book.

We deeply thank Editor and Content Development incharge Dr Ashu Singh, Mr Neeraj Sharma, Ms Jyoti Kaur and Mr Parmod Kumar for the excellent layout, presentation of figures and fine editing of this book.

Our thanks are due to Mr Vineet Agarwal for the effective communication done between us and CBS Publishers & Distributors Pvt Ltd, New Delhi, during the publication process.

We are thankful to Ms Radha Darshan Godkar, NREMT, for writing the basic script and MCQs for Chapter 1.

Praful B Godkar
Darshan Praful Godkar

Contents

Human Anatomy and Physiology

Theory and Practicals

Questions and Answers

for Paramedical and Allied Health Sciences Students

As per the latest Competency-based Education Guidelines

- Question–Answer Format
- Multiple Choice Questions
- *Viva Voce*
- Short and Long Answer Questions
- Match the Columns
- Draw Labelled Diagrams
- Case Studies
- 16 Chapters
- 21 Practicals

Goal

The main goal of learning anatomy and physiology is to derive comprehensive knowledge of gross structures, and microscopic anatomical structures, related functions, developments of human body parts and their correlation with various clinical conditions and diseases.

Mission

At the end of anatomy studies, a student should be able to:

1. Comprehend the normal body structures, clinically relevant inter-relationships, functional and cross-sectional anatomy of the various structures of the body and related functions.
2. Identify the microscopic structures of tissues and organs and correlation of their functions in normal state and in pathological conditions.
3. Demonstrate knowledge of basic principles involved in the sequential development of normal body parts and effects of genetic variations, pathogens and common teratogens on the growth of the body.
4. Explain horizontal correlation of anatomy and physiology aspects with premedical subjects (medical biochemistry, nutrition), vertical integration with paramedical subjects (medical microbiology, pharmacology, preventive medicine, hematology, pathology) and vertical integration with medical subjects (pediatrics, gynecology, obstetrics, and ophthalmology).

Skills

At the end of the course, the students should be able to:

1. Identify and locate all the structures of the body and describe the related specific features.
2. Explain various normal functions and disturbed functions in the pathological conditions.
3. Identify the microscopic structures of various types of normal tissues and affected tissues in various pathological conditions.
4. Identify gross congenital anomalies.
5. Safely perform the following techniques: Blood collection (venipuncture), intramuscular and intravenous injections, lumber puncture, CSF collection, arterial blood collection, determination of blood pressure, use of spirometer, oximeter, microscopy and basic hematology practicals.

CHAPTER

1

Introduction to the Human Body

SAQ: Short answer question: Marks: 2
BAQ: Brief answer question: Marks: 4 or 5
LAQ: Long answer question: Marks: 9 or 10

MCQs: Multiple choice questions: Marks: 0.5 each
Match the columns: Marks: 0.5 each
Draw a labelled diagram: Marks: 5

Objective: To describe the branches of academic study, "anatomy and physiology" and their relation.

INTRODUCTION

The anatomy and physiology subjects are very important to understand the basic framework of body parts, the location of various organs, knowledge regarding various body systems such as the skeletal system, circulatory system, respiratory system, digestive system, nervous system, reproductive system, etc., the location of cells, tissues, various bones, joints, and their related functions. Anatomy and physiology subjects help to get knowledge of human development and to understand how the body grows and changes during a lifetime.

Anatomy and physiology are the fundamental subjects to study in courses related to paramedical and medical subjects. The study of these subjects is important to get basic information on the health status of an individual body and is also extremely useful to pursue a career in the health professions. Mastery of anatomy and physiology subjects is necessary to understand and arrive at the right diagnosis; while examining a patient and also understanding related clinical reports and then taking appropriate action to treat the diseases. Good knowledge of anatomy and physiology is also useful for understanding the effects of nutrition, infections, genetic errors and effects of medicines on the human body and also for understanding the use of medical devices and procedures during the treatment of a disease.

Objective: To describe important terms related to anatomy and physiology.

IMPORTANT TERMS

SAQ: Define the following terms.

Ans: (Each term-related answer is equivalent to one SAQ.)

- *Human anatomy:* It is the study of body structure and its relationship with related body structures.
- *Human physiology:* It is the study of the functions of the body parts.
- *Human anatomy branches:* Include gross anatomy, microscopic anatomy, developmental anatomy and pathological anatomy.
- *Gross anatomy:* It is the observation of body structure with unaided eyes.
- *Microscopic anatomy:* It is the observation of the body structure using a microscope.
- *Developmental anatomy:* It is the study of the structure of the body from conception to birth.
- *Pathological anatomy:* It is the study of structural changes caused by a specific disease.
- *Human physiology branches:* Include cellular physiology, developmental physiology, and pathological physiology.
- *Cellular physiology:* It is the study of various components of cells.
- *Developmental physiology:* It is the study of cells as an organism grows.
- *Pathological physiology:* It is the study of functional changes that occur in an organism in a disease.
- *Histology:* It deals with the microscopic examination of a tissue.
- *Histopathology:* It deals with the study of diseased tissue.

ANATOMY AND PHYSIOLOGY SUBJECTS ARE STUDIED TOGETHER

LAQ: Why are anatomy and physiology subjects studied together?

Ans: Anatomy and physiology are subdivisions of biology. These subjects are always related together and studied together. The various parts of the human body form very well-organized units. Each of these body units functions to make the body operate as a complete unit. A specific structure of the body determines what specific functions could take place by that structural unit. Anatomy and physiology provide basic knowledge about the human body and various functions performed by the human body.

A normal person is usually good in health. Subclinical conditions do not show specific signs and symptoms. Adverse changes in the anatomy of the body affect the related physiology. The changes in anatomy and physiology lead to the presence of clinical conditions. A clinical condition means the presence of recognizable clinical signs and symptoms, due to a specific disorder or disease. A disorder leads to disturbed normal functioning of the body and its cause may not be known. When the cause of a disorder is determined, the diagnosis of a disease is confirmed.

The following are some examples of gross anatomical and physiological changes in a patient, which could be seen by eyes: A specific rash on the face and other parts of the body, swellings on the face and feet, excessive loss of hair, bleeding from any external parts of the body, difficulty in breathing, etc. Microanatomical changes caused by disorders and diseases could be seen by studying stained tissue sections, blood and other body fluid smears on glass slides, using a microscope. Good knowledge of anatomy and physiology helps to find out which part of the body is affected by a specific disease; and with proper identification and treatment, a patient can make full recovery.

A medical team is comprised of general physicians, specialists, surgeons, laboratory technicians, X-ray technicians, biochemists, microbiologists, pharmacists, nurses, dentists, physiotherapists, and nutritionists. Each category of this team requires good knowledge of anatomy and physiology subjects to perform individual duties very well.

Objective: To describe human beings concerning a classification scheme.

CLASSIFICATION OF HUMAN BEINGS

SAQ: Why classification of human beings is important?

Ans: The classification is useful to know the origin and evolution of human beings. The classification of human beings is important since it easily facilitates the study of a wide variety of organisms. The classification is useful to understand and study the similarities, features, and differences between different living organisms. The classification also helps to understand how organisms are grouped under different categories.

BAQ: Classify human beings using taxonomic classification.

Ans: The following is the classification of human beings based on taxonomic classification (Table 1.1).

Table 1.1: Classification of human beings

Taxon	*Grouping*	*Characteristics*
Kingdom	Animalia	Cells with defined internal components
Phylum	Chordata	Dorsal hollow nerve cord, pharyngeal pouches, and notochord (a cartilaginous skeletal rod supporting the body)
Subphylum	Vertebrata	Vertebral column, bony endoskeleton
Class	Mammalia	Mammary glands, three auditory ossicles, attached placenta, hair, muscular diaphragm
Order	Primates	Large brain, prehensile hands, modified digits for grasping
Family	Hominidae	Flattened face, well-developed vocal structure
Genus	Homo	Well-developed and large cerebellum, bipedal
Species	Sapiens	Posture and locomotion, opposable thumb

Note: Prehensile means part of an animal's body that can hold things.

Objective: To describe levels of the organization of the human body.

LEVELS OF BODY ORGANIZATION (Fig. 1.1)

SAQ: Describe the various levels of body organization.

Ans: The basic levels of organization in the body are:
1. Microscopic forms such as atoms, molecules and
2. Macroscopic forms such as cells, tissues, organs, organ systems, and the human organism.

LAQ: Describe the various levels of body macroscopic organization.

Ans: The macroscopic organization of the body is formed of cells, tissues, organs and organ systems (Fig. 1.1).

Cell

A cell is defined as the basic and the smallest functioning unit of the body.

Tissue

A tissue is formed when the cells are spaced uniformly and bind together.

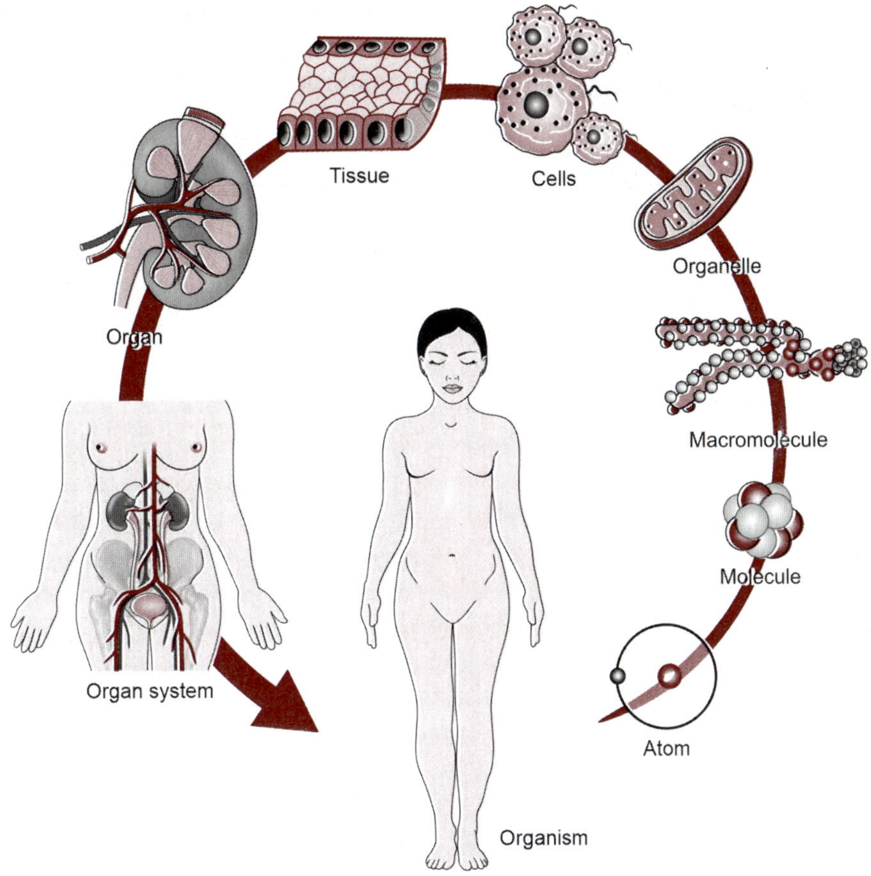

Fig. 1.1: Levels of the body organization

Matrix

The cells are bound together by a matrix, which is a non-living matter secreted by the cells. The matrix may be present in liquid, semisolid or solid form and may vary in composition from one tissue to another tissue. For example, blood tissue has a liquid matrix and bone tissues are bound by a solid matrix.

Organ

An organ is composed of several integrated tissue types that perform a specific function. For example, the femur is an organ. The components of the femur are bone tissue, nervous tissue, blood (vascular) tissue, and cartilaginous tissue. The femur helps to maintain body support and muscular support and helps the circulatory system by providing bone marrow cells (Fig. 1.2).

The organs are the functional elements in the body and often; they are physically distinct. The following are the various examples of organs: Kidneys, lungs, liver, heart, stomach, gastrointestinal tract, pancreas, blood, blood cells, hair, teeth, nerves, etc. All these organs are defined by a shape and a location in the body and they perform specific functions.

System (Fig. 1.2)

A system is an organization of two or more organs and structures associated with them, working as a unit to perform a common function or set of functions.

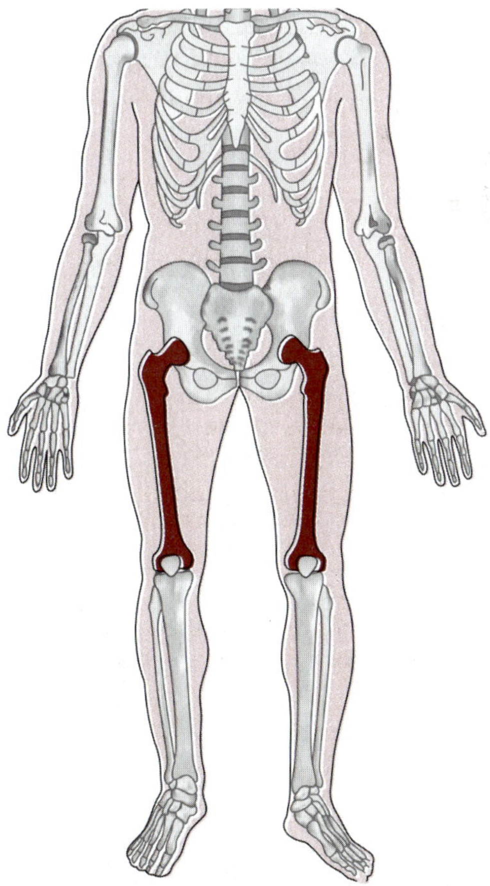

Fig. 1.2: An example of organ—femur

Organ Systems (Fig. 1.3)

Although each organ has its specific functions, these also function together in groups, called organ systems. Doctors categorize disorders and their own medical specialities according to the organ systems. The following are the various organ systems:

- Skeletal system
- Integumentary system
- Muscular system
- Nervous system
- Cardiovascular system
- Lymphatic system
- Respiratory system
- Digestive system
- Urinary system
- Endocrine system
- Reproductive system

Body (Fig. 1.3)

A body is the physical structure of a person that includes various organ systems.

Objective: To describe the various basic organ systems.

LAQ: Briefly describe the various organ systems and their respective functions.

Ans: The following are the various organ systems (Fig. 1.3):

Skeletal system, integumentary system, muscular system, nervous system, cardiovascular system, lymphatic system, respiratory system, digestive (gastrointestinal) system, urinary system, endocrine system, and reproductive system.

DESCRIPTION AND FUNCTIONS OF ORGAN SYSTEMS

Digestive (gastrointestinal) system (Fig. 1.3): It extends from the mouth to the anus. This system includes the mouth, the oesophagus, the stomach, the small intestine, and the large intestine. The digestive system also includes the associated organs such as the pancreas, the liver, and the gallbladder.

Functions: The digestive system produces digestive substances and enzymes for the breakdown of complex food components. It facilitates the digestion of food and absorption of digested microproducts, which can be used by the body cells for their metabolic reactions. The digestive system also facilitates the movement of food materials in the gastrointestinal tract.

Integumentary system (Fig. 1.3): Includes the epidermis, dermis, hypodermis, the glands associated with the integumentary system, hair, and nails.

Functions: The integumentary system forms a physical barrier between the external environment and the internal environment and plays a very important role in maintaining and protecting the body.

Nervous system (Fig. 1.3): It is comprised of the central nervous system, which is made up of the brain and the spinal cord and the peripheral nervous system, which is made up of the nerves that form branches from the spinal cord and spread to all the parts of the body.

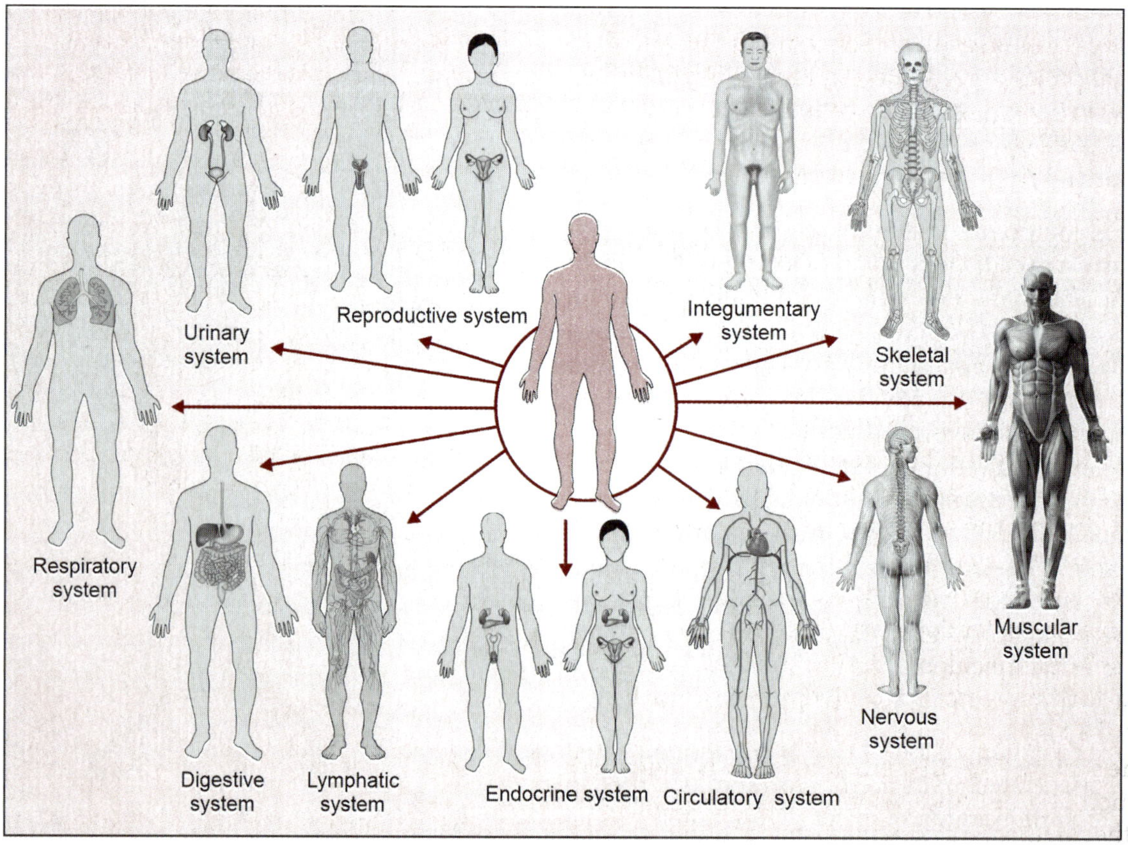

Fig. 1.3: Various organ systems

Functions: The main function of the nervous system is to send messages from the various parts of the body to the brain, and from the brain back to the body to perform related specific functions.

Circulatory system (Fig. 1.3): It is made up of blood vessels, such as arteries and veins.

Functions: The arteries carry pure, oxygenated blood away from the heart and the veins carry impure deoxygenated blood to the heart, and then to the lungs. The circulatory system carries oxygen, various nutrients, and hormones to the cells, and helps in the process of removal of waste products from the body; such as carbon dioxide, urea, creatinine, etc.

Cardiovascular system (Fig. 1.3): Includes the heart (cardio) and the blood vessels (vascular).

Functions: The cardiovascular system is responsible for pumping and circulating the blood to the various organs and the cells to provide oxygen and nutrients and back to the lungs to expel carbon dioxide and capture oxygen using the haemoglobin in the red blood cells.

Lymphatic system (Fig. 1.3): It is a part of the circulatory system and the immune system. It includes spleen, thymus gland, lymph nodes and lymph.

Functions: It protects body from the foreign invaders like microorganisms and maintains normal body fluid levels. It also plays an important role in the absorption of fats in the digestive tract and the removal of cellular waste products. The lymphatic system also plays an important role in controlling the number of blood cells in circulation and training the lymphocytes to perform normal functions.

Immune system (Fig. 1.3): Contains the important primary lymphoid organs that include the thymus and the bone marrow (which produce red and white blood cells) and secondary lymphoid tissue, which contains the spleen, tonsils, lymph nodes, lymph vessels, adenoids, the skin and the liver.

Function: The immune system provides the body with a defence system, which protects against microorganisms and other foreign substances.

Respiratory system (Fig. 1.3): Contains nostrils, pharynx, larynx, trachea and two lungs.

Functions: The respiratory system provides oxygen to the cells of the body for their normal functions; during the inspiration process and removes the carbon dioxide produced during the cellular activities, during the expiration process.

Musculoskeletal system (Fig. 1.3): Includes the bones, muscles, ligaments, tendons, and joints.

Functions: The musculoskeletal system supports the body and facilitates normal movements of the body parts and the body.

Endocrine system (Fig. 1.3): Includes various endocrine glands such as the hypothalamus, the pituitary, the thyroid, the pancreatic alpha and beta cells, the adrenal gland, etc.

Functions: The endocrine system secretes hormones, which are added directly to the general blood circulation. The hormones maintain the normal functioning of the body by controlling homeostasis.

Urinary system (Fig. 1.3): Contains two kidneys, the renal pelvis, ureters, the bladder and the urethra.

Functions: The urinary system plays an important role in the regulation of the composition of extracellular fluid by controlling the excretion of water, salts and waste products through the formation and excretion of urine. By performing these functions, the urinary system plays an important role in maintaining blood volume and blood pressure.

Reproductive system (Fig. 1.3): Includes the male reproductive system and the female reproductive system. The male reproductive system includes the external genitals (the penis, testes and scrotum) and the internal parts include the prostate gland, vas deferens and urethra. The female reproductive system includes the external part and the internal organs such as the uterus, ovaries, Fallopian tubes, cervix and vagina.

Functions: The parts of the male and female reproductive systems play important roles in processes such as reproduction (production of offspring), fertility (ability of a person to conceive children), and sex.

The male reproductive system produces the sperm, and the female reproductive system produces the egg cells. The reproductive system of the female protects and nourishes the fetus until birth.

Note:

1. All of the organs, except the reproductive system that are parts of the body system are formed within the six-week embryonic period of prenatal development. Many organs and body systems also become functional during this time.
2. Prenatal development is the process in which the development of a baby takes place from a single cell after conception and then into a zygote, an embryo and later on into a fetus (Fig. 1.4). A zygote is formed by a fertilization event between two gametes, one belonging to a male and another to a female.
3. The organs of the reproductive system are formed between 10 and 12 weeks of conception and become functional when a person attains puberty at the age of 12–13 years.
4. The process of prenatal development takes place in three main stages. The first two weeks after conception are known as the germinal stage (zygote formation). From the third week up to the eighth week is known as the embryonic period (embryo formation). The period from the ninth week up to birth is known as the fetal period (fetus formation) (Figs 1.4 and 1.5).

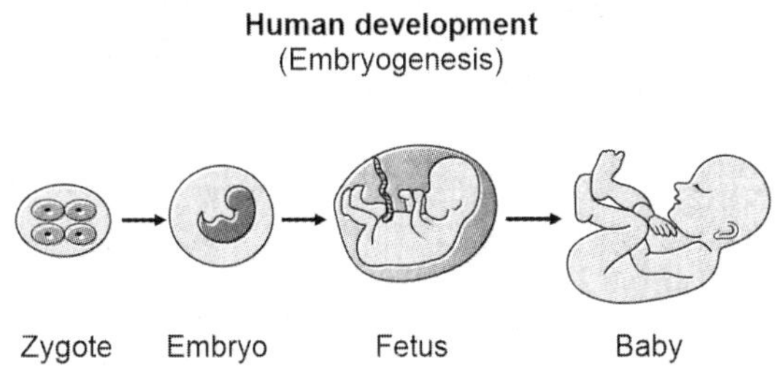

Fig. 1.4: Process of prenatal development

Objective: To describe the regional anatomy and anatomical positions.

REGIONAL ANATOMY AND ANATOMICAL POSITIONS

SAQ: What is the regional anatomy?

Ans: Regional anatomy is the study of the interrelationships of all of the structures in a specific body region. The human body can be roughly divided into the following five regions: Head, neck, torso or trunk (part of body except head, arms and legs), upper extremity and lower extremity (Fig. 1.5). Torso can be divided into thorax and abdomen (Fig. 1.6).

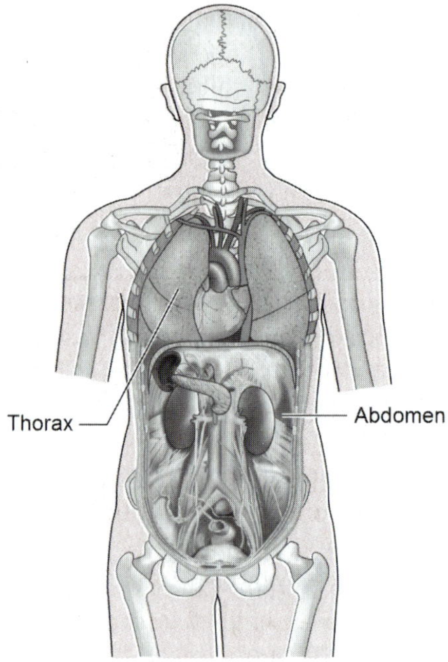

Fig. 1.6: Thorax and abdomen

BODY PARTS

BAQ: Label the body parts of male and female.

Ans: Figure 1.7A indicates the main body parts of male and female:

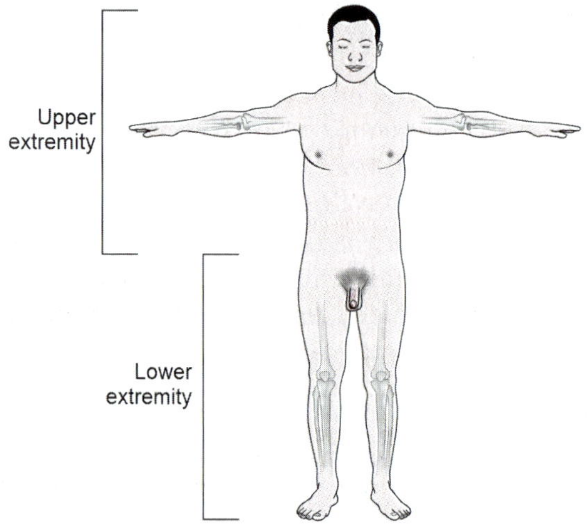

Fig. 1.5: Main human body divisions

Objective: To identify and locate principal body regions.

BODY REGIONS (Figs 1.7B and 1.8A–D)

BAQ: What are body regions? Give four examples.

Ans: Each main area of the body (such as the head, neck, thorax, abdomen, and upper, and lower extremities) area contains specific smaller regions (Fig. 1.8B). The following are some examples of the smaller regions of the body parts:

- The cubital fossa is an area of transition between the arm and the forearm. It is located in a depression on the anterior surface of the elbow joint (Fig. 1.8A).

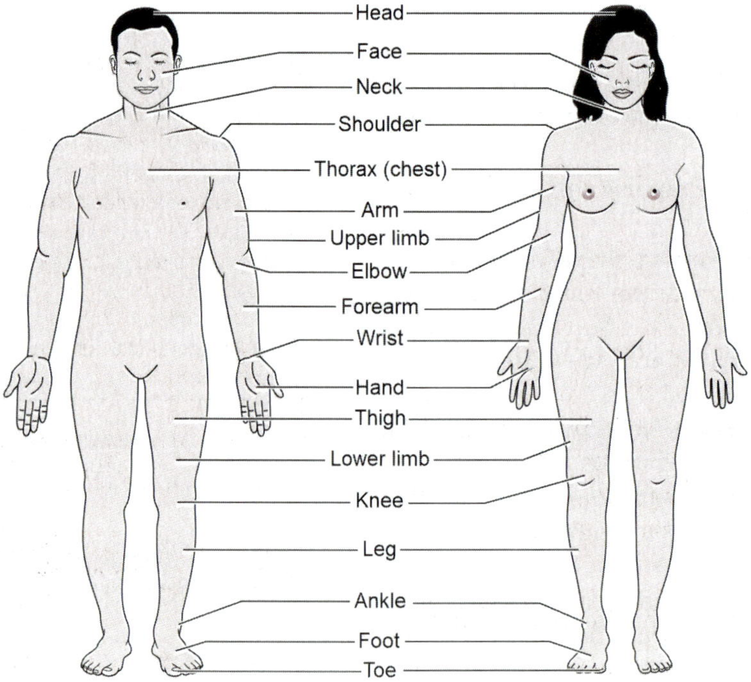

Fig. 1.7A: Male and female body parts

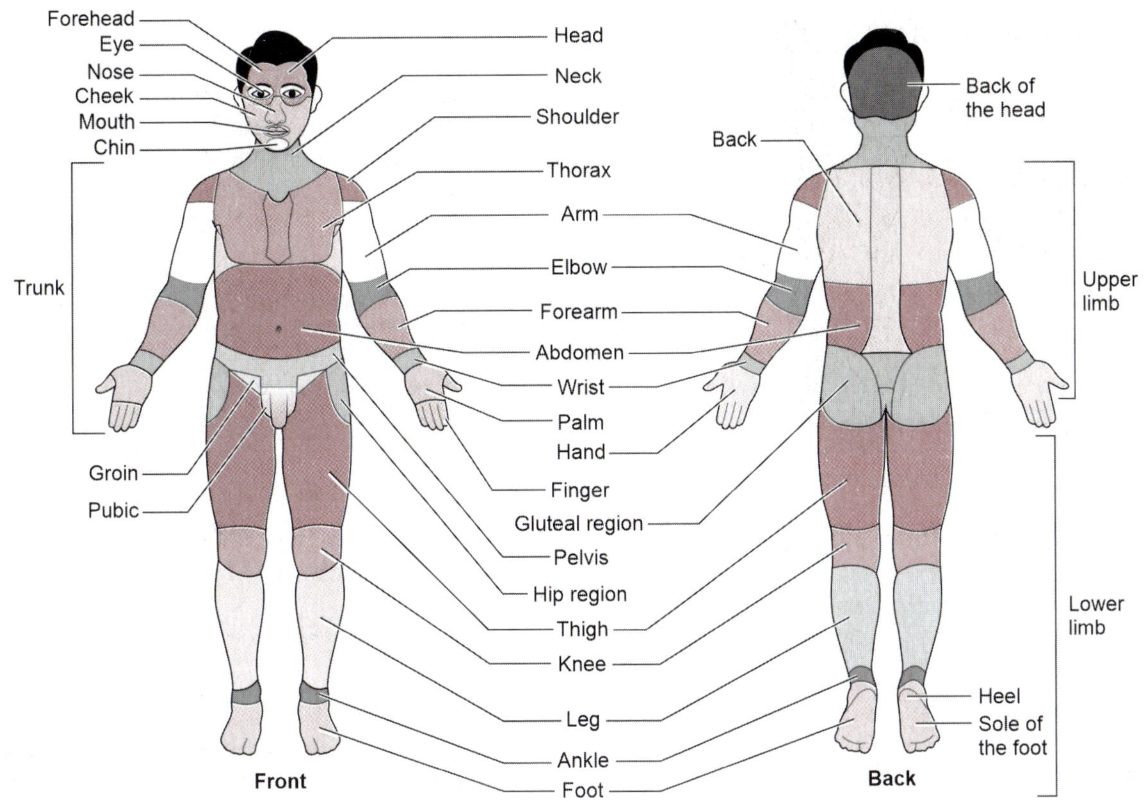

Fig. 1.7B: Various regions of the body

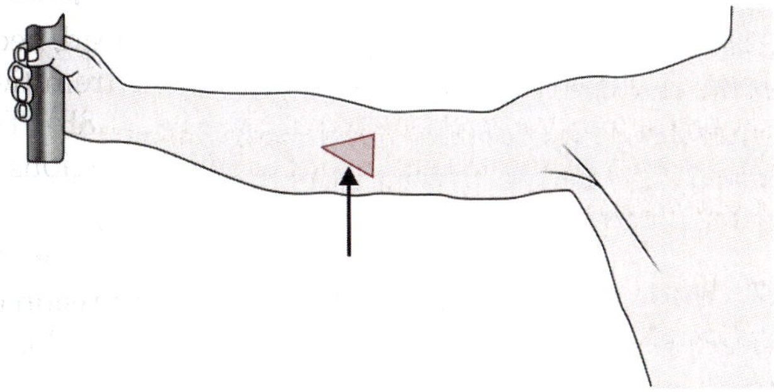

Fig. 1.8A: Cubital fossa region

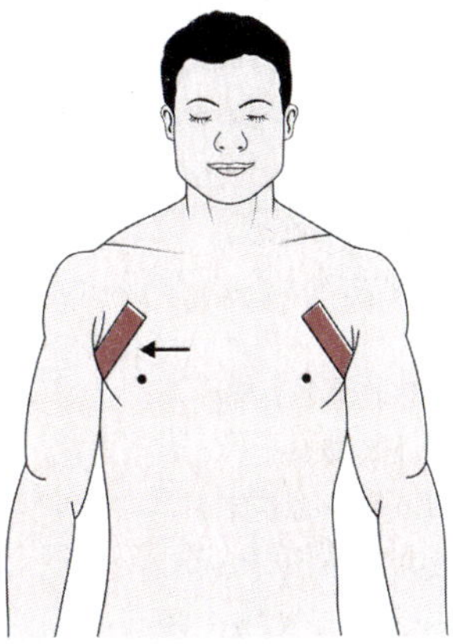

Fig. 1.8B: Axilla region

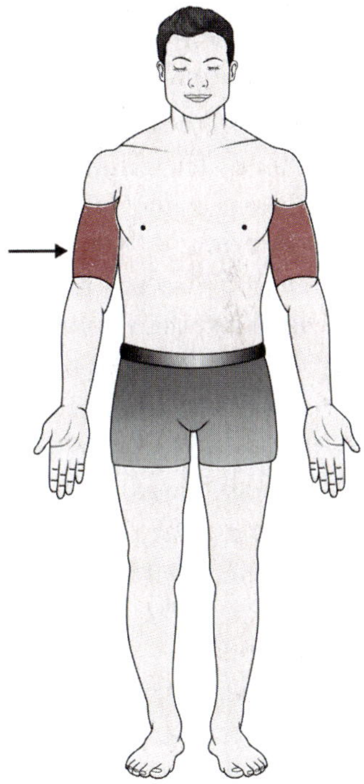

Fig. 1.8C: Brachium region

- The axilla is an anatomical region under the shoulder joint where the arm connects to the shoulder (Fig. 1.8B).
- The brachium is the part of the arm from the shoulder to the elbow (Fig. 1.8C).
- The popliteal fossa is a diamond-shaped space behind the knee joint (Fig. 1.8D).

SAQ: Why study of the regional anatomy is important?

Ans: Study of regional anatomy is useful for understanding the inter-relationships of body structures. The study of regional anatomy is useful to understand, how cells, muscles, nerves, blood vessels, and other parts of body structures work together to serve a particular body region.

BAQ: Draw labelled figures of the following parts:

(A) Cubital fossa
(B) Axilla
(C) Brachium
(D) Popliteal fossa

Ans: Refer to Figs 1.8A to D.

Objective: To describe the descriptive and directional terms related to the anatomical structures.

IMPORTANT DIRECTIONAL TERMS

SAQ: Define the following terms.

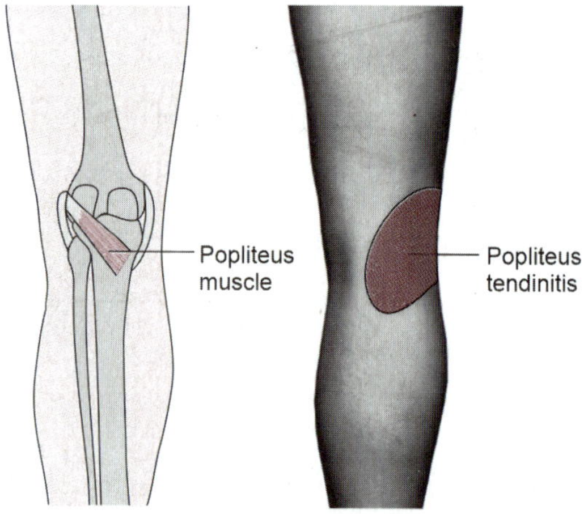

Fig. 1.8D: Popliteus region

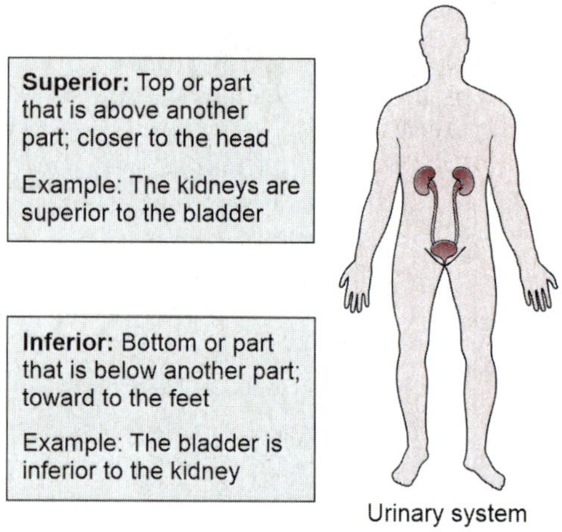

Fig. 1.9: Superior and inferior positions

Ans: (Each term-related answer is equivalent to one SAQ)

- ***Anterior or ventral:*** Towards the front.
  Example: The knee cap is located on the anterior side of the leg.
- ***Distal:*** Away from the main mass of the body.
  Example: The thumb is distal to the wrist.
- ***Proximal:*** Towards the main point of origin of a part or mass of the body.
  Examples: The knee is proximal to the foot. The proximal end of the femur joins with the pelvic bone.
- ***Posterior or dorsal:*** Towards the back.
  Example: The kidneys are posterior to the intestines.
- ***Medial:*** Towards the middle line of the body.
  Example: The chest is medial to the arms.
- ***Inferior or caudal:*** Away from the head and towards the bottom.
  Example: The legs are inferior to the trunk.
- ***Lateral:*** Towards the side of the body.
  Example: The arms are lateral to the chest.
- ***Internal:*** Away from the surface of the body.
  Examples: The brain is internal to the cranium.
- ***External:*** Towards the surface of the body.
  Examples: The skin is external to the muscles.
- ***Visceral:*** Related to internal organs.
  Examples: The visceral organs are wrapped in the peritoneum.
- ***Parietal:*** Related to the body walls.
  Examples: Parietal cells of the stomach secret hydrochloric acid.

SAQ: What are the anatomical positions? Give examples.

Ans: The anatomical position means the positioning of the body when the body is standing upright and facing forward with each arm hanging on either side of the body, and the palms facing forward. The legs are parallel, and the feet are flat on the floor and facing forward (Fig. 1.9).

The main directions for parts of the body are, superior, inferior, anterior, posterior, medial, and lateral.

Figure 1.10 indicates, how the terms proximal and distal are used for describing positions of the limbs.

Objectives: To identify different body planes

BODY PLANES (Fig. 1.11)

BAQ: What are the important body planes? What is the importance of understanding the various body planes?

Ans: The body planes can be used to identify and locate the positions of the internal organs of a person. Individual body organs can also be divided by planes to identify smaller structures within that organ.

The following set of three flat surfaces passing through the body is used to project structural arrangement: Sagittal plane, coronal plane and transverse plane.

SAQ: What are the sagittal, parasagittal and mid-sagittal planes?

Ans: The sagittal plane, also referred to parasagittal plane; divides the body into unequal right and left portions. The midsagittal plane divides the body into equal right and left portions. Sagittal planes (parasagittal planes) run parallel to the midsagittal plane (Figs 1.11 and 1.12).

SAQ: What is the coronal plane?

Ans: The coronal plane divides the body into front and back portions (Fig. 1.12).

SAQ: What is the transverse plane?

Ans: The transverse plane divides the body into superior (upper) and inferior portions (Fig. 1.12).

BAQ: Draw labelled figures of various body planes.

Ans: Refer to Fig. 11.12.

SAQ: What are the advantages of computerized tomography (CT), magnetic resonance imaging (MRI), and positron emission tomography imaging (PET) scans over X-ray examinations of body parts?

Ans: In X-ray examination, only vertical plane images could be studied. While by computerized tomography

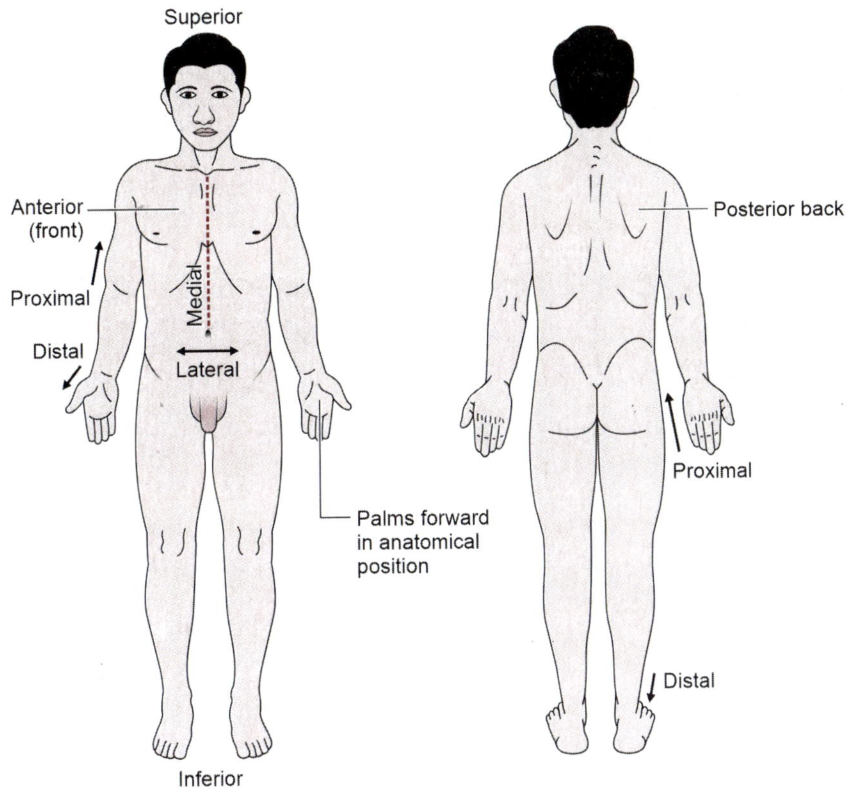

Fig. 1.10: Main anatomical positions

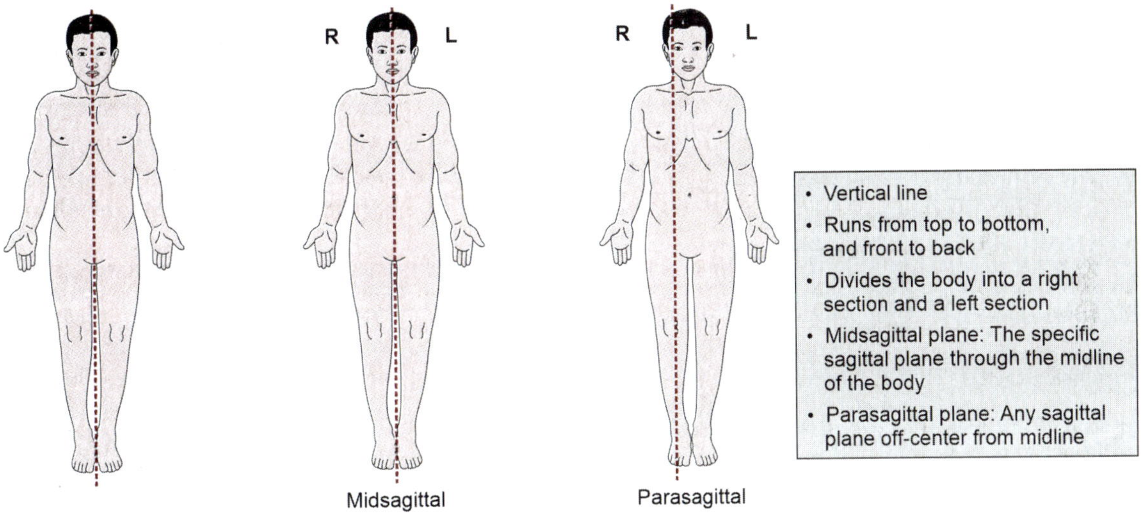

Fig. 1.11: Sagittal planes

(CT scan), magnetic resonance imaging (MRI), positron emission tomography imaging (PET scan) and ultrasound examination (sonography), along with vertical plane images of the body, transverse and sagittal plane images also could be seen and studied.

Objective: To identify the body cavities and the organs within them.

BODY CAVITIES (Table 1.2 and Fig. 1.13)

BAQ: What are various body cavities and their respective importance?

Ans: The body cavities contain delicate internal organs (Fig. 1.13). These protect delicate internal organs. A specific body cavity is useful for the internal organs to grow and move independently of the outer body wall.

Table 1.2: Human body cavities and membranes

	Name of cavity	*Membranous lining*
Dorsal body cavity	Vertebral canal	Meninges
Ventral body cavity	Thoracic cavity	Pericardium pleural cavity
	Abdominopelvic cavity	Peritoneum

The main prominent body cavities are: (1) Dorsal (posterior) cavity and (2) ventral (anterior) cavity.

The dorsal body cavity further contains the following cavities: (1) Cranial cavity, enclosed by the skull and

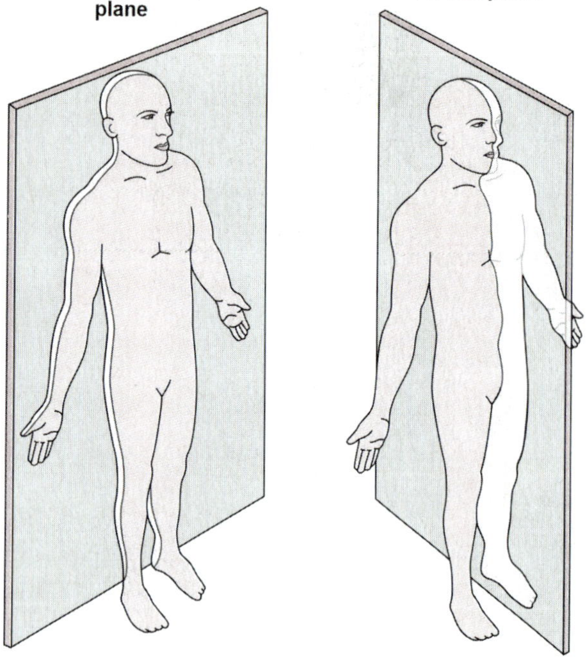

Fig. 1.12: Various body planes

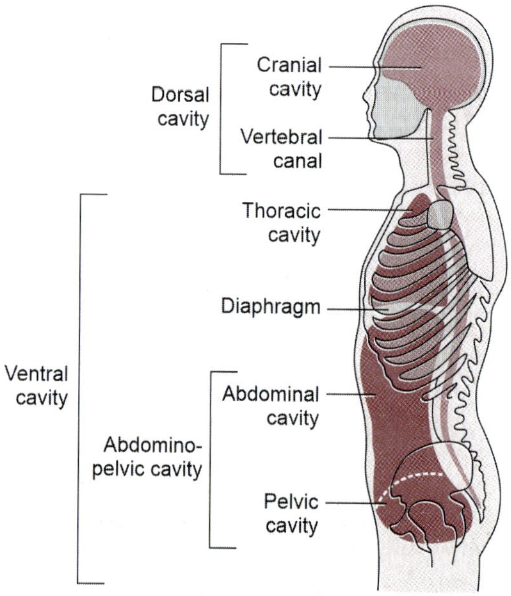

Fig. 1.13: Various body cavities (Lateral view)

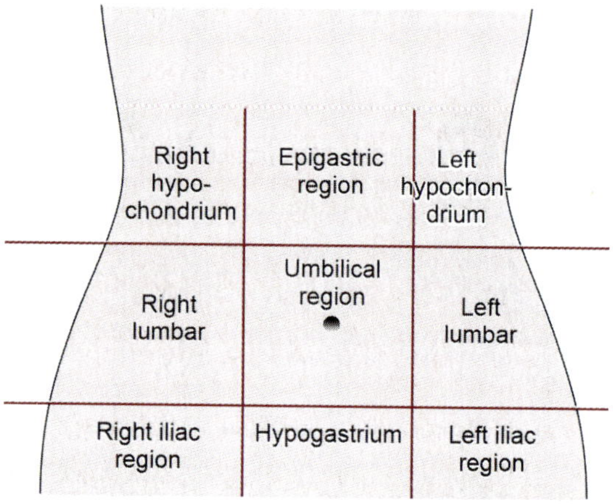

Fig. 1.14: Regions of the abdominal cavity

contains the brain, and (2) Spinal cavity is enclosed by the spine and contains the spinal cord (Fig. 1.13).

The ventral body cavity further contains the following cavities: (1) Thoracic cavity, enclosed by the ribcage and contains the lungs and heart; and (2) abdominopelvic cavity. Abdominopelvic cavity can be further divided into A. Abdominal cavity is enclosed by the ribcage and pelvis and contains the kidneys, ureters, stomach, intestines, liver, gallbladder, and pancreas; and B. Pelvic cavity, which is enclosed by the pelvis and contains bladder, anus and reproductive system.

SAQ: What are the various regions of the abdominal cavity?

Ans: Various regions of the abdominal cavity are shown in Fig. 1.14.

Objective: To describe the various body membranes and their functions.

BODY MEMBRANES (Figs 1.16–1.21)

SAQ: What are the various body membranes and their main functions?

Ans: Body membranes are thin layers of epithelial tissue (Fig 1.15). It is generally bound to an underlying layer of connective tissue. Following are the four types of membranes:

1. Cutaneous membranes
2. Serous membranes
3. Mucous membranes
4. Synovial membranes.

Main function: The main function of the body membranes is to cover, protect, and separate other structures or tissues in the body.

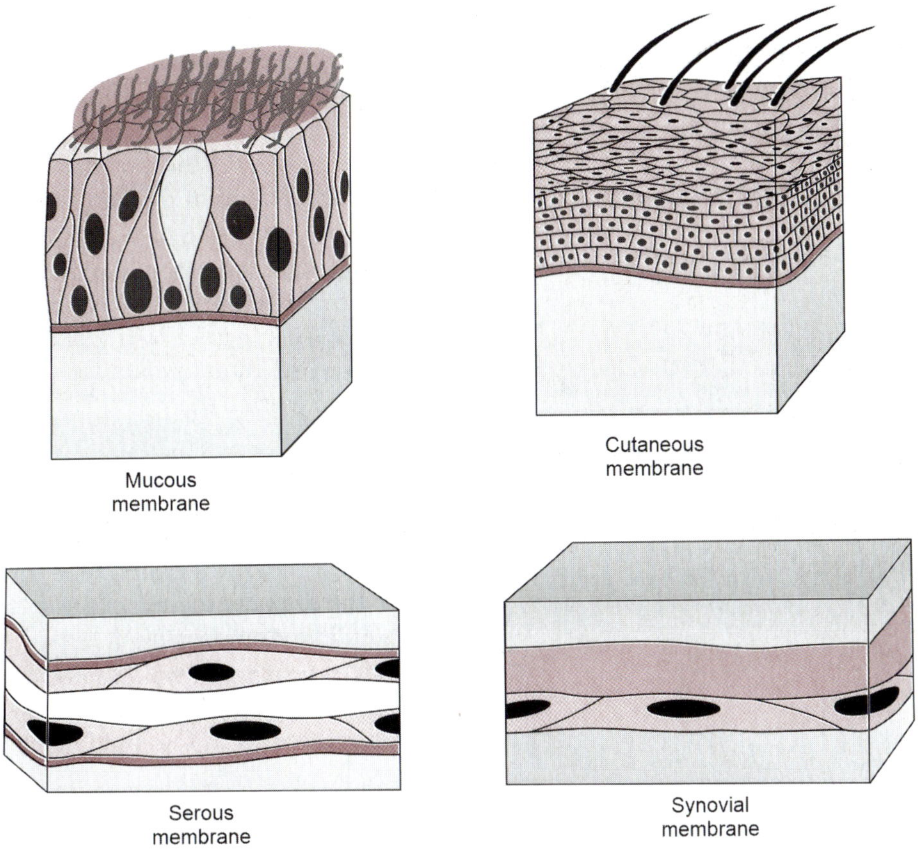

Fig. 1.15: Body membranes

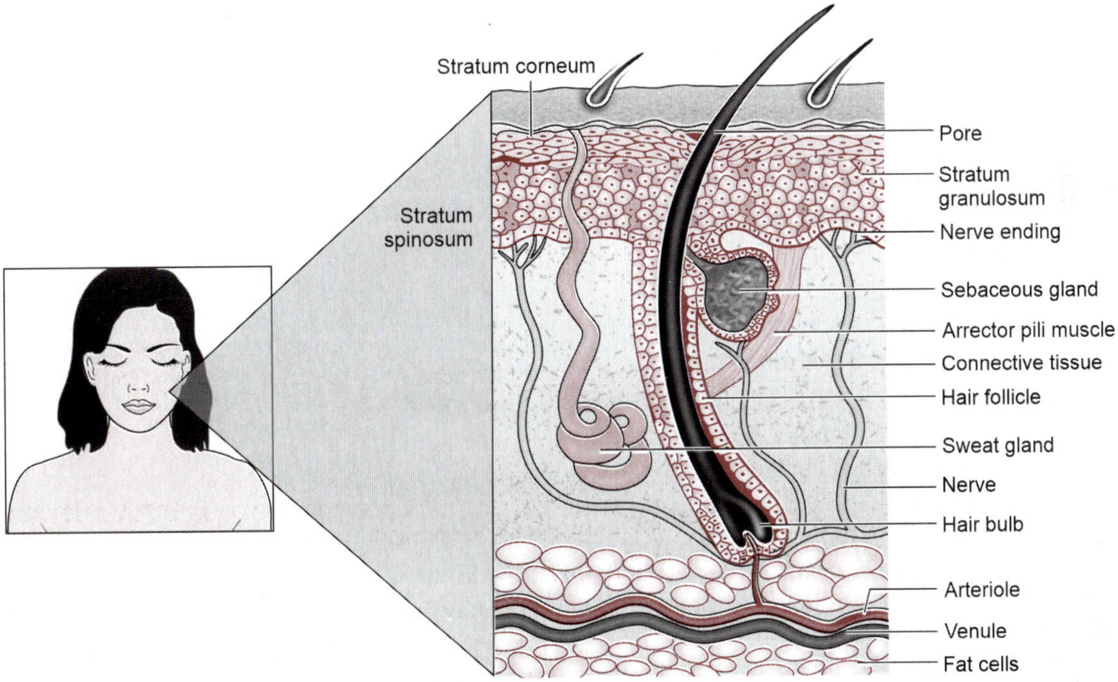

Fig. 1.16: Cutaneous membrane

Cutaneous Membrane (Fig. 1.16)

SAQ: Write a note on the cutaneous membrane.

Ans: The cutaneous membrane is the technical term for the skin. The primary role of the skin is to protect the rest of the tissues of the body and organs from physical damage such as abrasions, damage from chemicals, and microorganisms.

Serous Membrane (Figs 1.17 and 1.18)

SAQ: Write a note on the serous membrane.

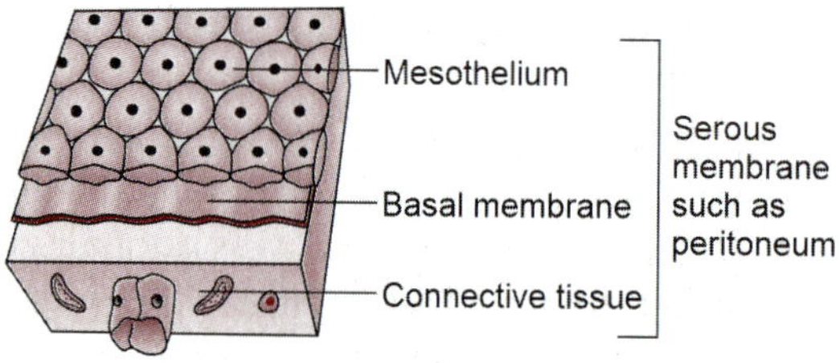

Fig. 1.17: Serous membrane

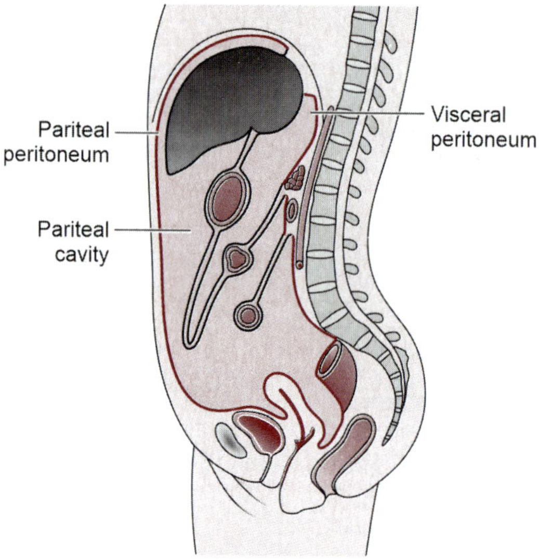

Fig. 1.18: Peritoneum

Ans: The serous membrane is a smooth tissue membrane that lines the contents and inner wall of body cavities. These body cavities secret serous fluid, which facilitates lubricated sliding movements between opposing surfaces. The pericardial cavity membrane (surrounding the heart), pleural cavity membrane (surrounding the lungs) and peritoneal cavity membrane (surrounding most organs of the abdomen) are the three serous cavities within the human body.

Mucous Membrane (Fig. 1.19)

SAQ: Write a note on the mucous membrane.

Ans: Mucous membranes line various structures of the body such as the mouth, nose, eyelids, trachea, lungs, stomach, intestines, ureters, urethra, urinary bladder, etc.

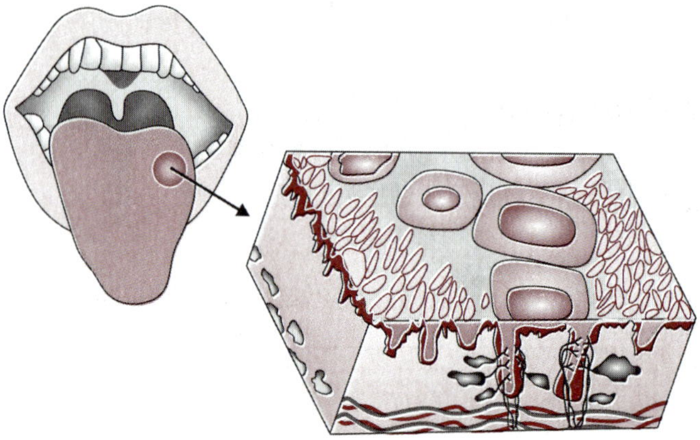
Fig. 1.19: Tongue—mucous membrane

Mucous membranes form a surface layer of epithelial cells over a deeper layer of connective tissue.

The epithelial layer of the membrane consists of either stratified squamous epithelium (multiple layers of epithelial cells), with the top flat layer or simple columnar epithelium (a layer of column-shaped epithelial cells).

Mucous membranes are tough. These are able to resist abrasion and other forms of wear associated with exposure to external substances like food particles. They contain cells specifically adapted for absorption and secretion. The main substance secreted from mucous membranes is mucus.

Synovial Membrane (Fig. 1.20)

SAQ: Write a note on the synovial membrane.

Ans: The synovial membrane is a specific connective tissue that lines the inner surface of capsules of synovial joints and tendon sheath.

The synovial membrane secretes synovial fluid which serves a lubricating function, that allows joint surfaces to smoothly move across each other.

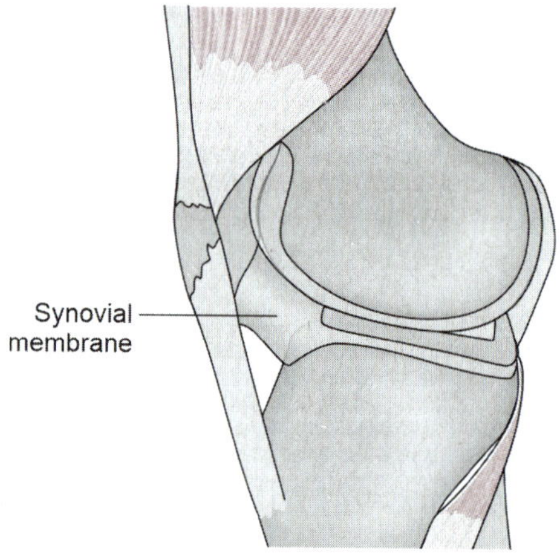

Fig. 1.20: Synovial membrane

Objective: To identify various visceral organs and study the composition and properties of various fluids within the visceral membranes.

VISCERAL ORGANS (VISCERA)

SAQ: What are visceral organs?

Ans: Visceral organs are located within the anterior body cavity. The viscera of the thoracic cavity contains the heart and lungs (Figs 1.22A and B) and the viscera of the abdominal cavity contains the stomach, small intestine, large intestine, liver, gallbladder and spleen (Fig. 1.21).

Organs in Thoracic Cavity and Pericardial Cavity

SAQ: What organs are present in the thoracic cavity and the pericardial cavity, respectively?

Ans: The thoracic cavity is divided into two pleural cavities, one each for lungs. The area between the two

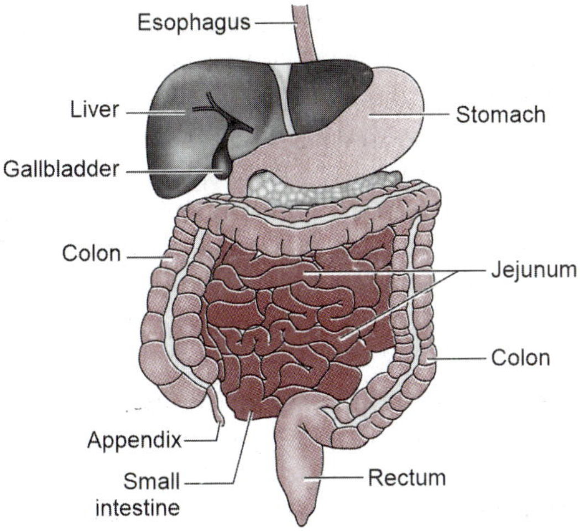

Fig. 1.21: Organs in the abdominal cavity

lungs is known as the mediastinum (Figs 1.22A and B). Pericardial cavity contains the heart.

SAQ: Why thoracic organs are placed in separate compartments?

Ans: Each thoracic organ is placed into separate compartments. In case of any traumatic situation, trauma is minimized and the risk of disease spreading from one organ to another organ is decreased. For example, if one lung collapses due to trauma, the other lung continues to function normally.

Pleural Fluid (Fig. 1.23)

SAQ: Write information on the plural fluid along with the functions and related clinical condition.

Ans: Pleural fluid is located between the layers of the pleura. The pleura is a two-layer membrane that covers the lungs and lines the chest cavity.

Functions: Pleural fluid keeps the pleura moist and reduces friction between the membranes during breathing.

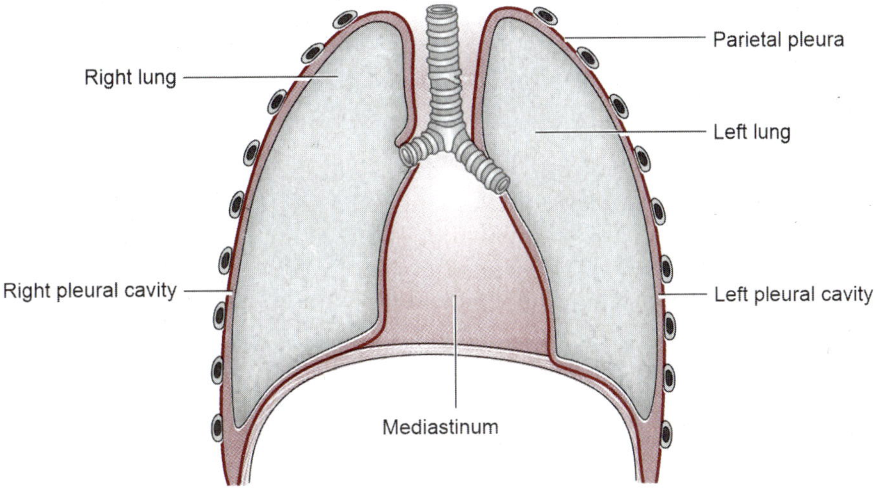

Fig. 1.22A: Mediastinum and pleural cavities containing lungs

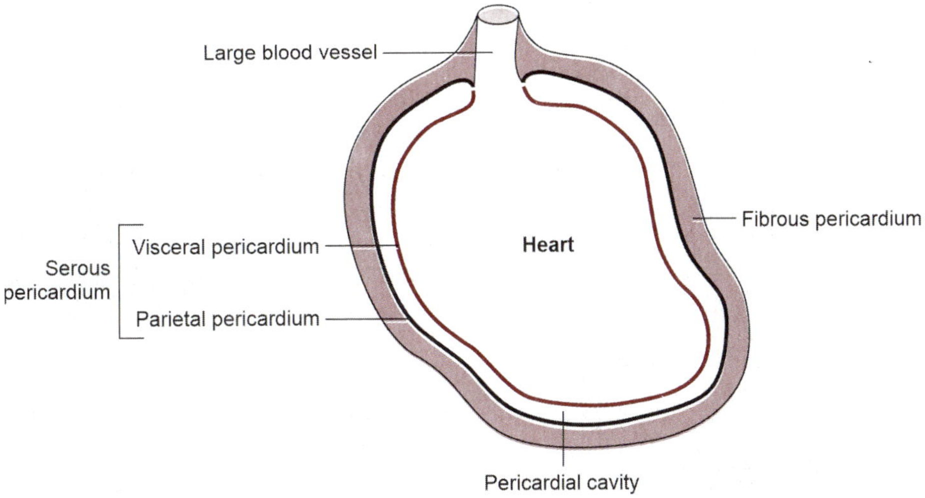

Fig. 1.22B: Pericardial cavity and pericardium

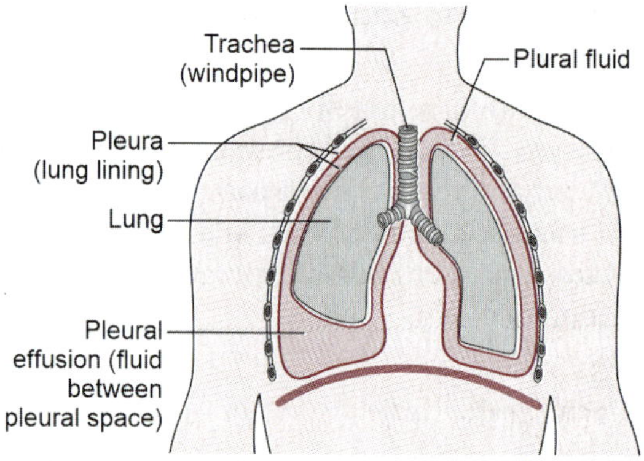

Fig. 1.23: Pleural fluid

Clinical condition: An increase in pleural fluid quantity (Fig. 1.23: Plural effusion) and change in normal composition indicates specific clinical conditions related to lungs.

Pericardial Fluid (Figs 1.24A and B)

SAQ: Write information on the pericardial fluid along with the functions and related clinical condition.

Ans: The inner layer of the pericardium is attached to heart muscle. Small amount of pericardial fluid is present in the pericardial sac (Fig. 1.24A).

Function: Pericardial fluid is used to decrease friction between the pericardial layers. It also facilitates smooth heart movements during the heartbeats.

Clinical condition: Increase in the pericardial fluid quantity and change in normal composition indicates specific clinical conditions related to the heart (Fig. 1.24 B).

Peritoneal Fluid (Figs 1.25 and 1.26)

SAQ: Write information on the peritoneal fluid along with the functions and related clinical condition.

Ans: Peritoneal fluid is a serous fluid made by the peritoneum in the abdominal cavity.

Functions: Peritoneal fluid lubricates the surface of tissue that lines the abdominal wall and pelvic cavity. Peritoneal fluid covers most of the organs in the abdomen.

Clinical condition: An increased volume of peritoneal fluid is called ascites. Increase in the pleural fluid quantity and change in normal composition indicates specific clinical conditions related to abdominal cavity (Fig. 1.26).

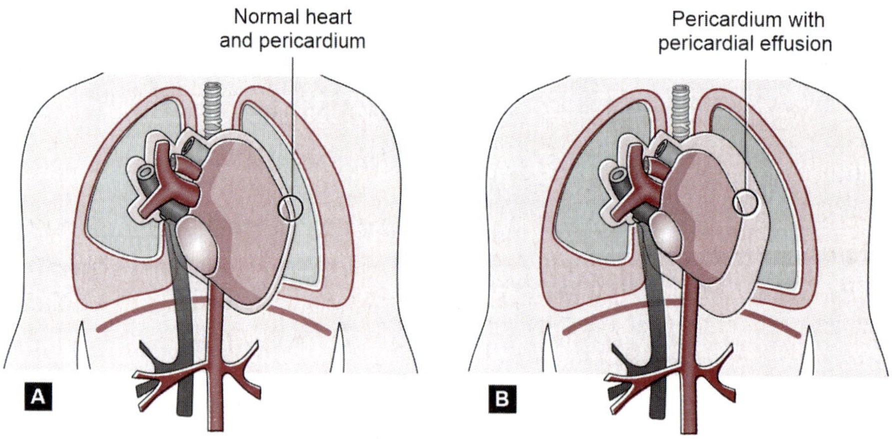

Fig. 1.24: Pericardial fluid: (A) normal and (B) increased

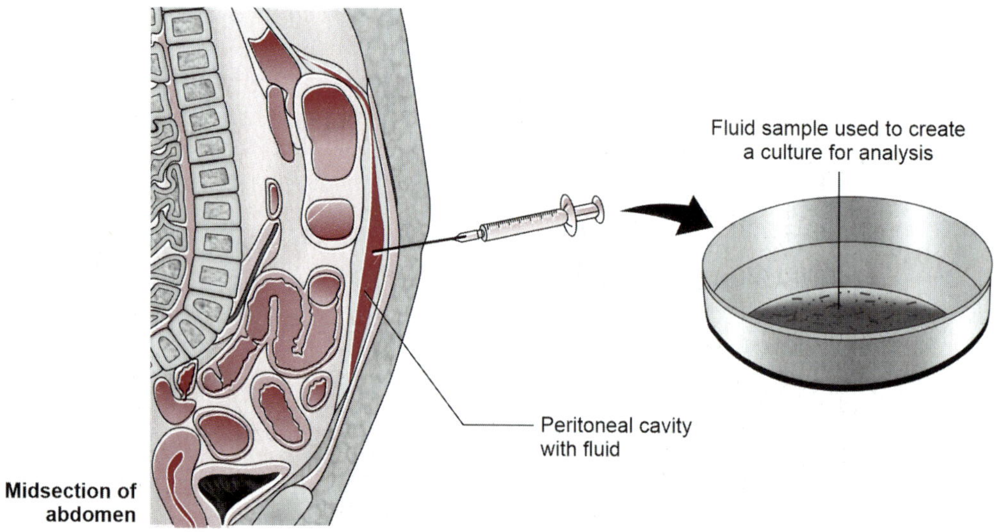

Fig. 1.25: Peritoneal fluid

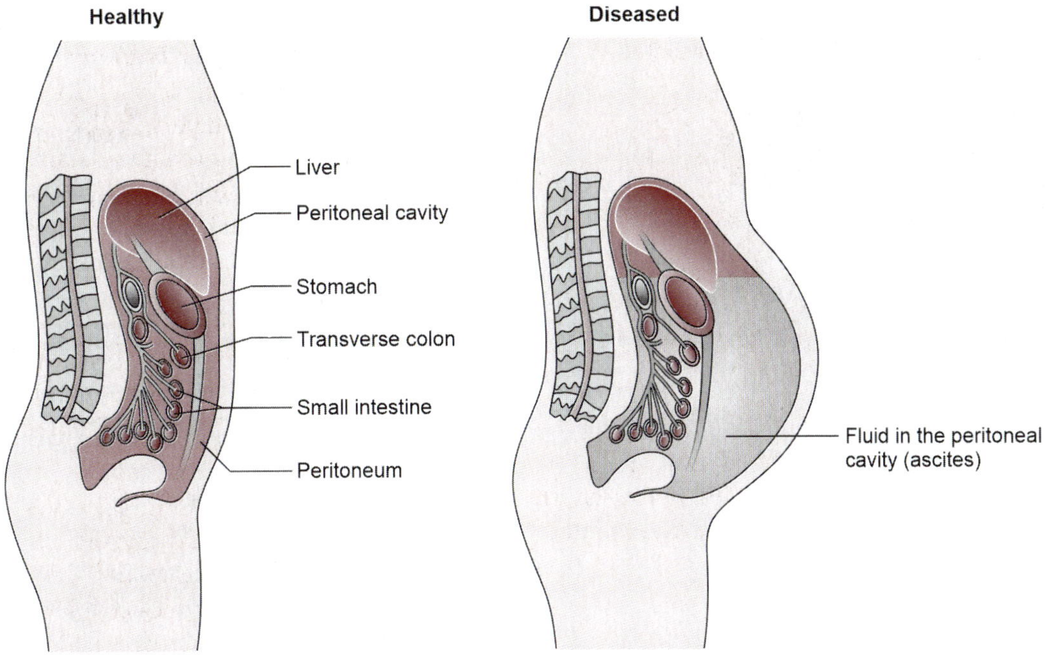

Fig. 1.26: Increased peritoneal fluid (ascites)

Cerebrospinal Fluid (CSF) (Figs 1.27A and B)

SAQ: Write information on the cerebrospinal fluid (CSF) along with the functions and related clinical conditions.

Ans: Cerebrospinal fluid (CSF) is a clear and colourless body fluid present within the tissue that surrounds the brain and spinal cord (Figs 1.27A and B).

Function: CSF protects the brain and spinal cord by action like a cushion against sudden impact or injury. CSF also plays an important role in removing waste products produced in the central nervous system.

Clinical condition: Normal cerebrospinal fluid (CSF) composition changes in clinical conditions that affect the brain and the spinal cord.

MESENTERY (Fig. 1.28)

SAQ: What is the mesentery and its function?

Ans: Mesentery is a fold of membrane that attaches the intestine to the abdominal wall. It holds the intestine in a specific place.

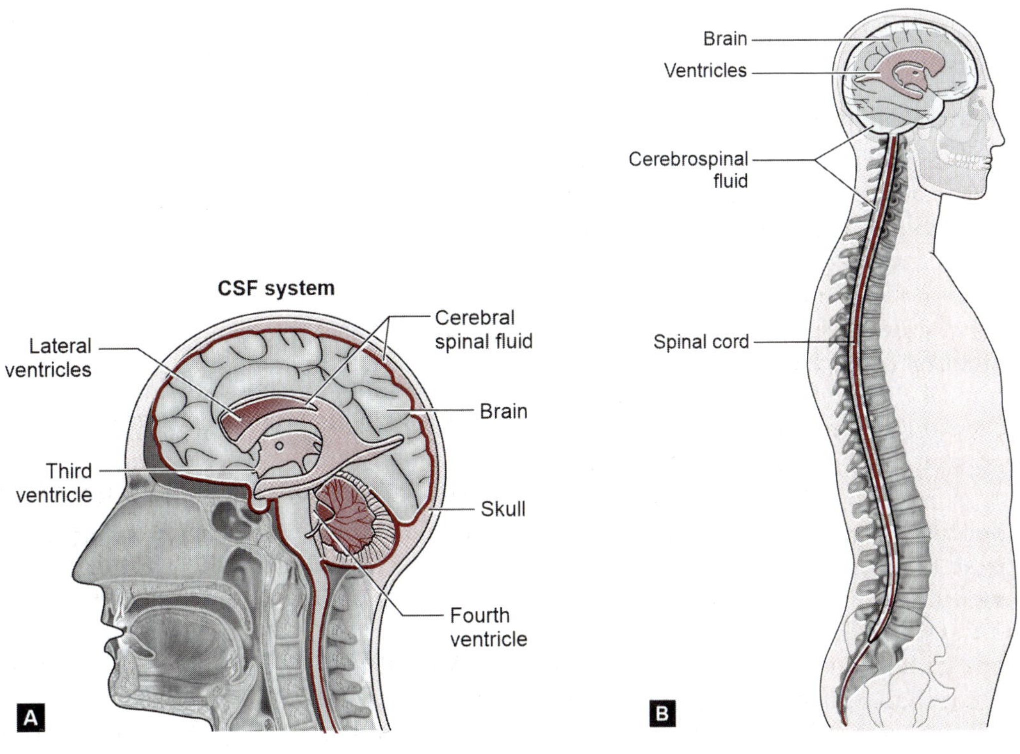

Figs 1.27A and B: Cerebrospinal fluid

Introduction to the Human Body

1

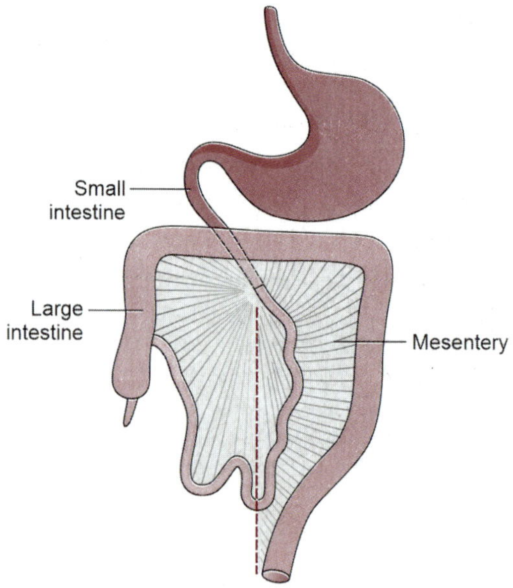

Fig. 1.28: Mesentery

Objective: To describe homeostasis and feedback mechanisms.

HOMEOSTASIS

BAQ: Write a note on homeostasis.

Ans: Homeostasis means the maintenance of a state of steady internal physical and chemical conditions in the case of a living person. Homeostasis includes maintenance of normal body temperature and body fluid balance. All the organs and tissues of the body perform various functions and maintain homeostasis by maintaining normal constituents of extracellular and intracellular fluids relatively constant.

The human body possesses many control systems to maintain homeostasis. Negative feedback systems and positive feedback systems work appropriately to maintain homeostasis.

BAQ: Write a note on the feedback mechanism.

Ans: The feedback mechanism is a physiological regulation system in a living body that works to return the body to homeostasis. A negative feedback loop and a positive feedback loop manage to maintain homeostasis.

When a person suffers from a disease or injury, homeostasis gets disturbed. For example, raised fever and disturbed internal body fluid balance in microbial infections is an indications of disturbed homeostasis. Similarly, excessive loss of blood by internal and external bleeding due to any accident will lead to disturbed homeostasis.

A negative feedback loop is a self-regulating type of system. In a negative feedback loop, increased output from the system inhibits future production of related products by the system. The body reduces its own manufacturing of certain proteins or hormones when their levels get too high. For example, when thyroid hormones are required, the body will stimulate thyroid stimulating hormone (THS), which stimulates the

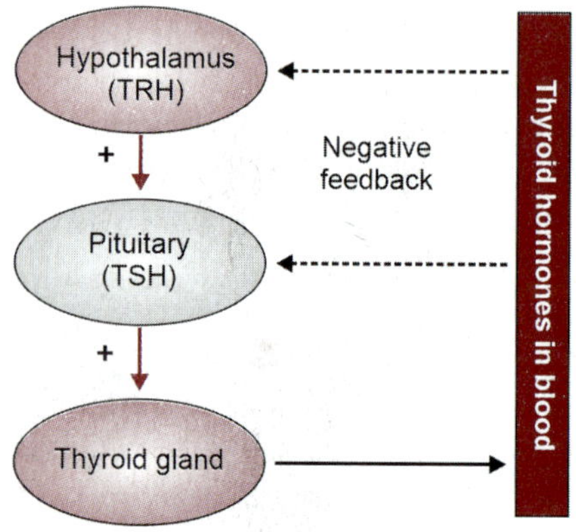

Fig.1.29A: Negative feedback mechanism

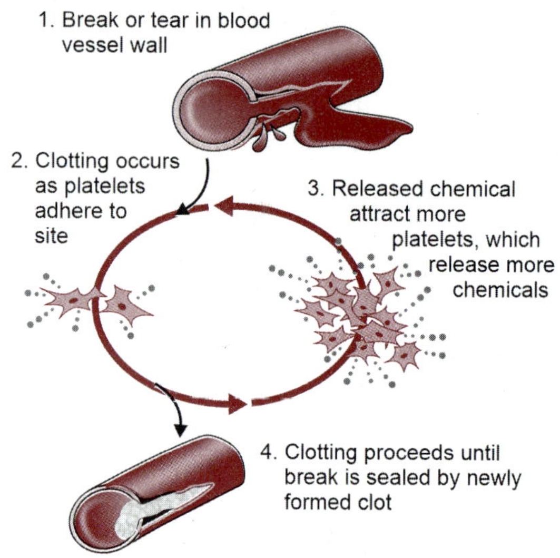

Fig. 1.29B: Positive feedback mechanism

thyroid gland to stimulate thyroid hormones. Once a normal level of thyroid hormone is reached, the blood levels of these hormones inhibit secretion of TSH and then no more increase in thyroid hormones takes place (Fig. 1.29A).

In a positive feedback system, the end-products formed in a chemical reaction increase the speed of that chemical reaction. For example, when bleeding takes place, a large number of platelets gather there and a fibrin clot forms at the site of bleeding. The clotting will continue till the damaged part of the body gets sealed (Fig. 1.29B).

Objective: To describe the clinical conditions related to the disturbed homeostasis and related terms.

SAQ: Write a note on the disturbed homeostasis.

Ans: When the cells in the body are not able to function normally, homeostatic balance is disrupted. Disturbed homeostatic imbalance leads to a state of disease.

BAQ: Define the following terms: Disease, illness, disorder, and syndrome.

Ans: Disease is a condition in which a disturbed structural and functional state of an organ system or many organ systems is observed. A specific disease is associated with specific signs and symptoms. A disease is distinct and measurable using various diagnostic tests. For example, liver disease can be diagnosed by signs and symptoms of jaundice and also by correlating symptoms with laboratory tests.

Ill means a person is not in good health and illness is the state of being mentally and physically ill.

A disorder indicates that a specific disease may be present, however, sufficient evidence may not be there for diagnosis purposes. Examples of disorders are anxiety, depression, stress, etc. Diagnosis of these disorders may be nonconclusive by diagnostic tests.

A syndrome is a set of medical signs and symptoms of a specific disease or disorder, which are correlated with each other. Examples are nephrotic syndrome (related to kidney disease), acquired immunodeficiency syndrome (AIDS), Down syndrome, etc.

> *Note:*
> 1. Morbidity means a diseased condition.
> 2. A medical condition or a health condition includes all diseases, disorders and also conditions like pregnancy and childbirth; that normally receive medical treatment.

> **Objective:** To describe the major factors that cause diseases.

MAJOR FACTORS THAT CAUSE DISEASES

BAQ: What are the major factors that cause diseases?

Ans: According to the definition of the World Health Organization (WHO), health is a state of complete mental, physical, and social well-being. Abnormalities in the chemical constituents and with the rate of reactions in the living cells are exhibited by various diseases. The following are the major factors responsible for causing diseases in humans:

- Biological agents such as bacteria, fungi, viruses and other parasites
- Certain toxic chemicals and drugs
- Endocrine imbalance leading either to hormonal excesses or deficiencies
- Autoimmune diseases involving immunological reactions
- Nutritional imbalances caused by nutritional excess and deficiencies
- Genetic disorders
- Oxygen deficiency caused by loss of blood and by pathological conditions leading to a considerable decrease in circulating red blood cells which result in depletion of oxygen-carrying capacity.
- Physical agents such as radiation, atmospheric pressure, electric shock and sudden change in temperature.

> **Objective:** To describe the terms—pathophysiology and pathology.

PATHOPHYSIOLOGY AND PATHOLOGY

SAQ: Write a brief note on pathophysiology and pathology.

Ans: Pathophysiology is the study of the disturbed physiological processes that are associated with a disease or injury.

Pathology is a branch of biological science that deals with the nature of a disease through a study of its causes, its process and its effects with associated structural and functional alterations. A clinical laboratory makes use of principles of pathology by using test reports of blood, urine, CSF, sputum, tissues, etc.

> **Objective:** To describe the importance of radiology.

RADIOLOGY

BAQ: Write a note on radiology.

Ans: Radiology is a field of medicine that uses medical imaging to diagnose and treat diseases within the body of a person. Various imaging techniques such as X-ray radiography, computed tomography (CT), and nuclear medicine including positron emission tomography (PET), magnetic resonance imaging (MRI) and ultrasound tests are used to diagnose diseases.

> *Note:* Clinical laboratory tests and radiology tests are useful to:
> 1. Reveal the causes of the diseases
> 2. Screen easy diagnosis
> 3. Suggest effective treatment
> 4. Assist in monitoring the progress of a pathological condition
> 5. Help in assessing response to therapy

> **Objective:** To describe the terms horizontal and vertical integration of premedical subjects (anatomy, physiology and nutrition) paramedical subjects (microbiology and pharmacology) and medical subjects (paediatrics, orthopaedic, obstetrics and gynaecology) as a part of competency-based education.

HORIZONTAL INTEGRATION OF THE PREMEDICAL SUBJECTS

BAQ: What is the meaning of horizontal integration of a specific event related to "anatomy" with other pre-medical subjects such as physiology, biochemistry and nutrition? Give examples.

Ans: Horizontal integration of a specific event related to "anatomy" with other pre-medical subjects is useful to understand the effects of specific anatomical changes on physiologic and biochemical aspects of an individual and support nutrition to control and get rid of the anatomical change.

- For example, when a person suffers from severe kidney disease,

- The related anatomical change is a significant decrease in the functional micro units (nephrons).
- The related physiologic change is a decrease in the rate of blood filtration at the kidneys.
- The related biochemical change is an increase in the excretory substances such as urea, creatinine, uric acid, etc., in the blood circulation.
- The related nutritional support is: To keep moderate amounts of protein and salt in the diet to decrease the workload on the kidneys.

BAQ: What is the meaning of vertical integration of the above-mentioned case (patient suffering from kidney disease) with other paramedical subjects such as microbiology and pharmacology? Give examples.

Ans: The correlation of the paramedical subjects in this case is useful as follows:

Microbiology: To identify microorganisms, that may cause kidney disease.

Pharmacology: To select an effective drug to treat microbial infection.

BIBLIOGRAPHY

1. "Anatomy of the Human Body". 42nd Edition. Henry Gray, Editor-in-chief: Susan Standring, Elsevier (2020)
2. Ross and Wilson Anatomy and Physiology in Health and Illness, 13th Edition, by Allison Wynn Grant, Anne Waugh, and Kathleen J. W. Wilson (2018).
3. Medical Biochemistry, Theory and Practicals, 1st Edition. Praful B. Godkar, Darshan P. Godkar, CBS Publishers and Distributors (2024).

MULTIPLE CHOICE QUESTIONS (MCQs)

Q.A. Select the correct option.

1. The thyroid gland belongs to this body system:

(A) Skeletal
(B) Integumentary
(C) Lymphatic
(D) Endocrine system

2. The hair belongs to this body system:

(A) Skeletal
(B) Integumentary
(C) Lymphatic
(D) Endocrine system

3. The anatomical position of the ear is:

(A) Medial
(B) Lateral
(C) Superficial
(D) Proximal

4. The ventral body does not contain:

(A) The spinal cavity
(B) The thoracic cavity
(C) The abdominal cavity
(D) Both (A) and (B)

5. The axilla region is:

(A) The chest area
(B) The armpit
(C) The forearm
(D) The shoulder region

6. The popliteal fossa is:

(A) The chest area
(B) The armpit
(C) The forearm
(D) The area behind the knee joint

7. This term defines the position of the knee relative to the hip:

(A) Medial (B) Distal
(C) Lateral (D) Proximal

8. This part separates the thoracic cavity from the abdominal cavity:

(A) The abdominal septum
(B) The sternum
(C) The diaphragm
(D) The abdominal wall

9. This organ is present in the thoracic cavity:

(A) Heart (B) Stomach
(C) Liver (D) Pancreas

10. This plane divides the body into upper and lower portions:

(A) Midsagittal (B) Transverse
(C) Coronal (D) Sagittal

11. This plane divides the body into the left and right half of the body:

(A) Midsagittal (B) Transverse
(C) Coronal (D) Sagittal

12. This fluid is a serous fluid, which lubricates the surface of tissue that lines the abdominal wall and pelvic cavity:

(A) Pericardial fluid
(B) CSF
(C) Peritoneal fluid
(D) Synovial fluid

13. This fluid is a serous fluid, that lubricates the surface of the brain and spinal cord:

(A) Pericardial fluid
(B) CSF
(C) Peritoneal fluid
(D) Synovial fluid

14. The term parietal refers to:

(A) Forming part of cell wall
(B) Forming part of a cavity wall
(C) Internal body organ
(D) A and B

15. The term visceral refers to:

(A) Forming part of cell wall
(B) Forming part of a cavity wall
(C) Internal body organ
(D) Both (A) and (B)

ANSWERS

1. D 2. B 3. B 4. A 5. B 6. D 7. B
8. C 9. A 10. B 11. A 12. C 13. B 14. D
15. C

Q.B. Label the main anatomical positions.

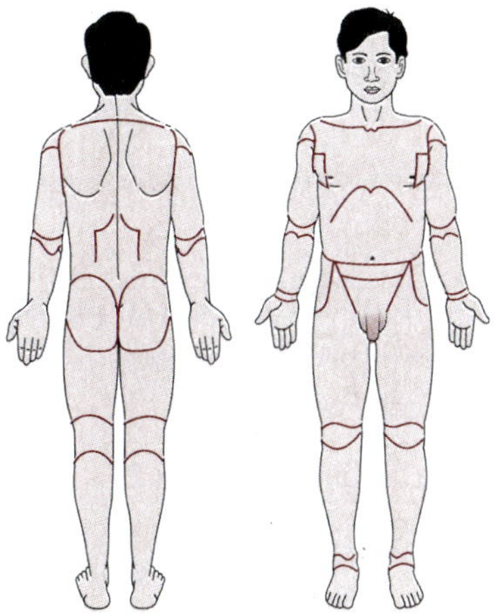

ANSWER:

Refer to page 9, Fig. 1.10

Q.C. Write the principal organs and functions of the following systems:

1. Respiratory system
2. Urinary system
3. Nervous system
4. Reproductive system
5. Digestive system

MATCH THE COLUMNS

I	II
1. Epithelial tissue	A. Medial
2. Toward the feet	B. Posterior
3. Mesentery	C. Facilitate movements of body parts
4. Connective tissue	D. Covers organs and body surfaces
5. Toward the back	E. Nerve impulse transmission
6. Muscle tissue	F. Binds, supports and protects body parts
7. Toward the head	G. Supports abdominopelvic viscera
8. Nervous tissue	H. Inferior or caudal
9. Upper surface of the body	I. Superior
10. Toward the midsagittal plane	J. Dorsal

ANSWERS

1. D 2. H 3. G 4. F 5. B 6. C 7. I
8. E 9. J 10. A

CHAPTER

2

Cell Structure, Functions and Tissues

SAQ: Short answer question: Marks: 2
BAQ: Brief answer question: Marks: 4 or 5
LAQ: Long answer question: Marks: 9 or 10
MCQs: Multiple choice questions: Marks: 0.5 each
Match the columns: Marks: 0.5 each
Draw a labelled diagram: Marks: 5

Objective: To describe the human cell and distinguish between eukaryotic cells and prokaryotic cells.

CELL (Fig. 2.1)

Introduction

SAQ: What is a cell?

Ans: The cell is the smallest unit of the human body. It is the basic unit of the various tissues of the body. The cell is the unit of which larger body masses are built. A cell cannot be further divided without losing its identity. The cell is composed of a nucleus surrounded by cytoplasm, which contains various cell organelles such as mitochondria, endoplasmic reticulum, Golgi apparatus, peroxisome, etc. Each of these cells is enclosed by a cell membrane. The human body is composed of trillions of cells.

SAQ: What is a tissue and what are fibers?

Ans: Each tissue is composed of cells (living matter) and fibers (non-living matter). Although the cells have certain common characteristics, they are specialized and are of various types. The specialized cell differs from other specialized ones in shape, size and functions. The type of arrangement of cells and fibers enables to recognition of the various tissues.

SAQ: How does a living human cell survive and carry out different functions?

Ans: The human cell takes nutrients from blood that circulates them by blood capillaries and converts those nutrients into energy in the form of adenosine triphosphate (ATP) molecules. This energy, cells use to carry out specialized functions, required for survival. The cells also contain the hereditary material of the body in the nucleus in the form of DNA and can make identical copies of themselves.

Objective: To describe the basic components (organelles) of a human cell and their respective functions.

EUKARYOTIC CELL (Figs 2.1 and 2.2)

SAQ: What is a eukaryotic cell?

Ans: A eukaryotic cell contains cytoplasm and various organelles (functioning components) enclosed by a membrane, known as a plasma membrane. In the nucleus of a eukaryotic cell genetic material is present, which can be differentiated into the chromosomes.

Cytoplasm

BAQ: Write a note on the cytoplasm of a human cell.

Ans: The cytoplasm of a human cell is a watery and homogeneous gel-like solution of protein, sugars and various salts. It is basic in nature. The cytoplasmic fluid has an osmotic pressure equal to 0.9 g/dl sodium chloride (normal saline). It contains (1) cytoplasmic (endoplasmic) reticulum, (2) Golgi apparatus, (3) mitochondria, (4) centrosome, (5) lysosome and (6) cytoplasmic inclusions.

The cytoplasm is made up of about 80% water and cytosol. It is a medium of the cells in which various organelles, meaning functioning units of the cell can operate within the cell. All of the functions of a cell related to growth and replication are carried out in the cytoplasm of a cell.

The cytosol is the material (matrix) of the cytoplasm. It forms about 70% of the cell volume. The cytosol is a complex mixture of microscopic cytoskeleton filaments, dissolved organic and inorganic molecules, and water. The cytoskeleton of the cytosol is made up of protein microfilaments (actin filaments) and microtubules. The cytoskeleton performs several important functions, including participation in cell division, and allows the cells to assume specific shape and movement. It also provides a specific track for the movement of organelles and the movement of micronutrients within the cells.

The cytosol can be divided into two parts: Endoplasm and ectoplasm. The endoplasm is the inner more dense fluid portion of the cytoplasm and the ectoplasm is the outer layer of the cytoplasm, which is a less dense, watery part of cytosol and is immediately adjacent to the cytoplasmic membrane (plasma membrane).

SAQ: What is the difference between cytoplasm and protoplasm?

Ans: The cytoplasm is present surrounding the nucleus in a cell. The protoplasm contains cytoplasm and the nucleus.

Cytoplasmic Membrane

BAQ: Describe the cytoplasmic membrane and its functions.

Ans: The cell membrane is a biological membrane. It is approximately 100 Å thick, double-layered, semipermeable membrane. It is made up of protein and lipid components. The cell membrane surrounds the protoplasm of a cell and separates the interior of all cells from the outside environment.

The cell membrane consists of the phospholipid bilayer with embedded proteins and glycoproteins. The cell membrane is involved in a variety of cellular processes such as cell signalling, cell adhesion, and ion conductivity. The cell membrane also plays a role in anchoring the cytoskeleton to provide shape to the cell, and in attaching to the extracellular matrix and other cells to form tissues.

The cell membrane is selectively permeable to ions and organic molecules. It controls the movement of substances in and out of the cell. It conducts the exchange of food and secretory products in the following ways: (1) Passive transport: When the movement of substances is under the influence of osmotic pressure. (2) Active transport: When the movement of substances is under the influence of chemical interactions and electrical changes. The cytoplasmic membrane also plays an important role in pinocytosis (cell drinking) and phagocytosis (cell eating).

SAQ: What is the difference between a eukaryotic cell and a prokaryotic cell?

Ans: The eukaryotic cell has a complex cell structure with a well-defined cell membrane, well-organised membrane-bound organelles and nuclear material in the form of chromosomes present in the nucleus (Fig. 2.2). The eukaryotic cell multiplies by mitosis. While a prokaryotic cell has a simple cell structure. The cell organelles are not bound by specific membranes and the genetic material is present as a single piece of DNA (Fig. 2.1). Prokaryotic cells multiply by binary fission (separation of a parent cell into two daughter cells).

CELL ORGANELLES (Fig. 2.2)

Each organelle of a cell is composed of a specific structure and each organelle performs individual specific functions. The human cells contain the following various organelles: The nucleus, the rough and smooth endoplasmic reticulum, ribosomes, the Golgi apparatus, lysosomes, centrioles, etc.

Nucleus (Fig. 2.2)

BAQ: Write a note on the nucleus of a cell.

Ans: The nucleus of a cell contains a colloidal solution of proteins with various salts, called nucleoplasm. It contains the important nucleic acid, deoxyribonucleic acid (DNA). Most of the protein is bound to DNA and it stains intensely with basic dyes due to the acidic nature of nucleoproteins. DNA plays a very important role in cell division and transmission of hereditary characters. With the help of ribonucleic acid (RNA), nucleus also plays an important role in the synthesis of various proteins.

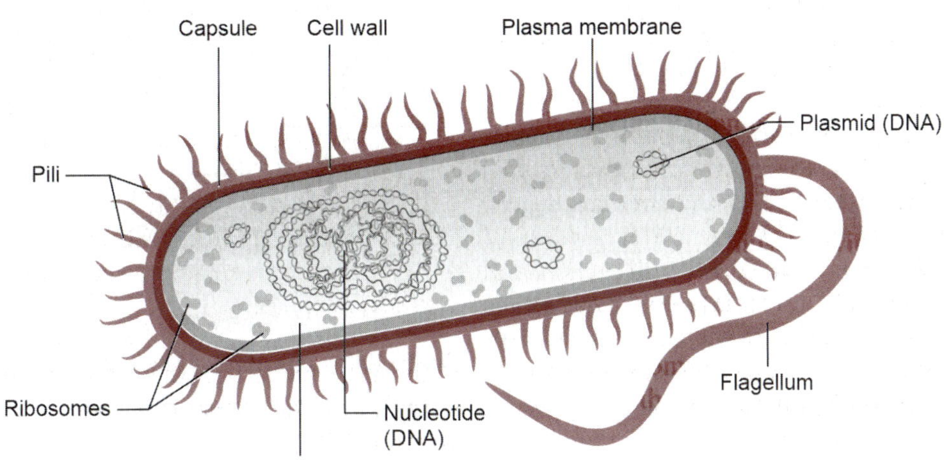

Fig 2.1: Prokaryotic cell

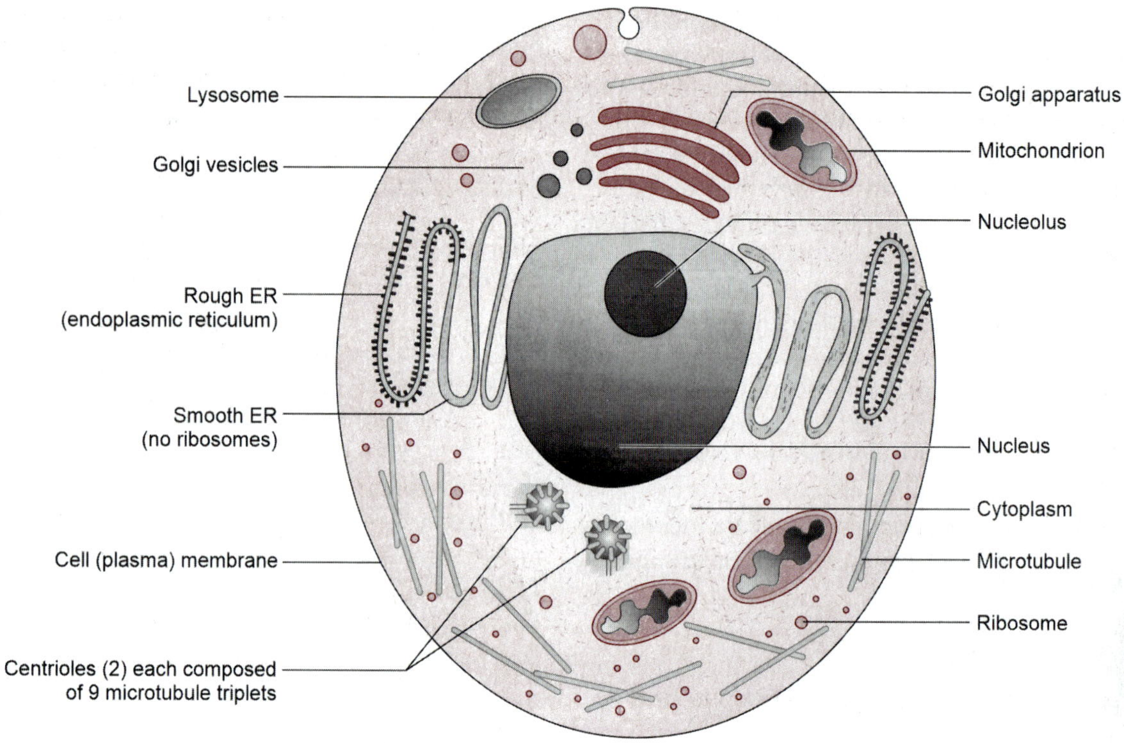

Fig. 2.2: Human cell

The nucleus generally contains one or two refractile particles called nucleoli. They are rich in RNA and these are active in the synthesis of proteins.

The nucleus is surrounded by a nuclear membrane. It comprises a double membrane. The outer membrane exhibits nuclear pores which are open to the cytoplasm. Through these pores, contact with the cytoplasmic (or endoplasmic) reticulum is made.

Endoplasmic Reticulum (Figs 2.2 and 2.3)

BAQ: Write a note on the endoplasmic reticulum.

Ans: The endoplasmic reticulum (ER) is made up of two subunits: (1) Rough endoplasmic reticulum (RER) and (2) smooth endoplasmic reticulum (SER).

Rough endoplasmic reticulum (RER), is a series of connected flattened sacs (Fig. 2.2). It is known as a rough endoplasmic reticulum (RER) due to the appearance of its outer surface, in which ribosomes are present. Ribosomes play a very important role in the synthesis of various proteins required for the body. Synthesized proteins are then packaged into vesicles and transported to the Golgi apparatus organelle for further processing. Vesicles in the cytoplasm are tiny sacs that transport synthesized material within or outside the cell (Figs 2.3 and 2.4).

Smooth endoplasmic reticulum (SER) does not contain ribosomes and it is involved in the synthesis of lipids and supply of calcium ions for various functions of the cell. The free ribosomes in the cytoplasm are involved in the synthesis of protein, necessary for the cell itself.

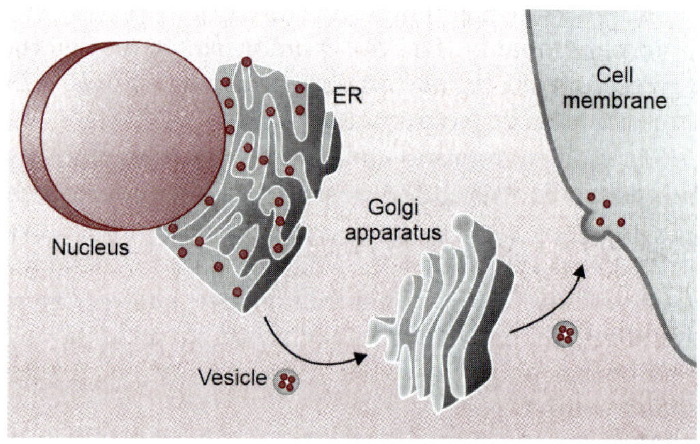

Fig. 2.3: ER and vesicle transport

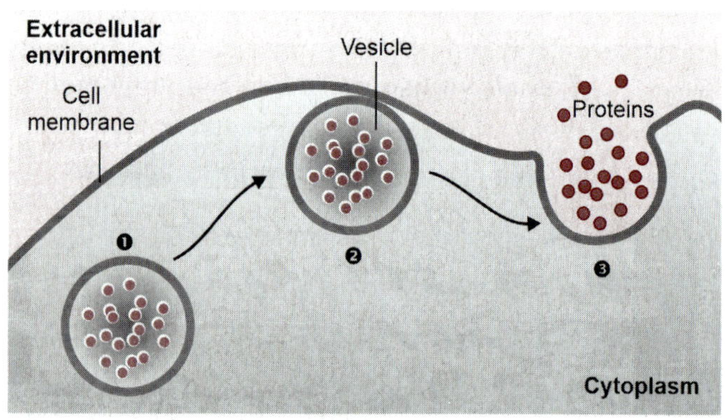

Fig. 2.4: Exocytosis

Golgi Apparatus (Figs 2.2 and 2.5)

BAQ: Write a note on the Golgi apparatus.

Ans: The Golgi apparatus forms a part of the cellular endomembrane system. It is composed of stacks of membrane-bound structures known as cisternae. A human cell contains approximately 40–100 such stacks. Each cisterna appears like a flat disc enclosed by a membrane. It primarily modifies proteins delivered from the rough endoplasmic reticulum (Fig. 2.5). It is also involved in the transport of lipids around the cell and the creation of lysosomes. The cisterna contains special Golgi enzymes which modify proteins that travel through it. Modified proteins are then transported to various parts of the body according to their specific requirements.

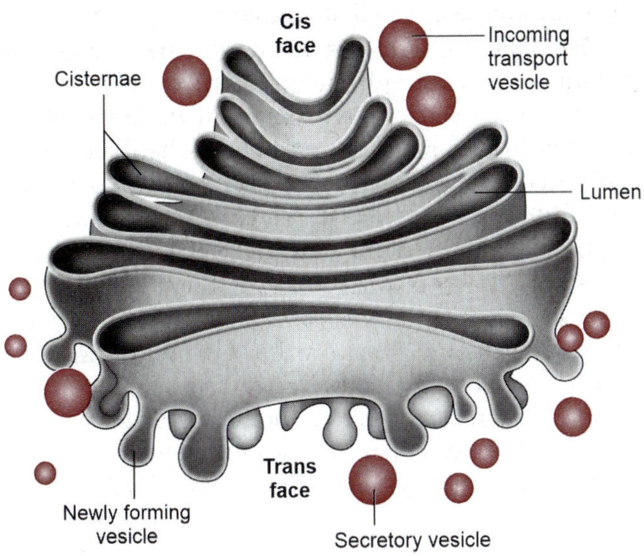

Fig. 2.5: Golgi apparatus

Mitochondria (Figs 2.2 and 2.6)

BAQ: Write a note on the mitochondria.

Ans: The mitochondria are fluid-filled vessels, enclosed by inner involuted membrane folds (cristae) and an outer single layer made up of proteins. These are minute bodies scattered throughout the cytoplasm. The internal chamber of mitochondria (matrix) contains various enzymes that participate in the metabolism of amino acids, lipids and carbohydrates. The mitochondrial matrix also contains a circular double-stranded DNA, RNA and ribosome, which are responsible for the synthesis of mitochondrial protein.

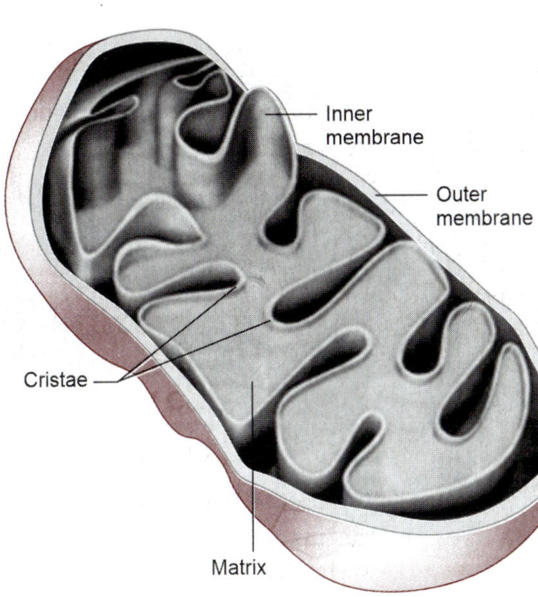

Fig. 2.6: Mitochondrion

The mitochondria are the powerhouses that manufacture and supply energy for the metabolic reactions of body cells in the form of ATP.

Centrosome (Centriole) Bodies (Figs 2.2 and 2.7)

BAQ: Write a note on the centrosome (centriole) bodies.

Ans: The centrosomes are small refractile bodies (one or two) found near the nucleus of the living cells. During mitosis, the two centrioles move to the opposite poles of the cell and support a skin of fine protoplasmic rays. Along this spindle, the chromosomes arrange themselves after their division.

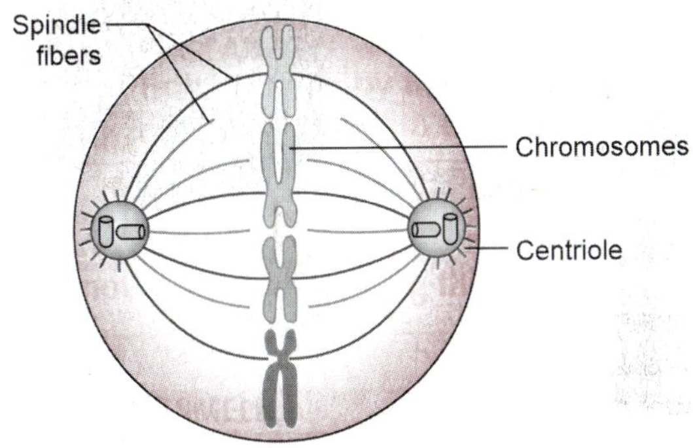

Fig. 2.7: Centrosome

Lysosome (Fig. 2.8)

BAQ: Write a note on the lysosome.

Ans: The lysosome is a membrane-bound cell organelle. It contains many digestive enzymes, which act in an acidic medium. The cells use lysosomes to destroy invading viruses and bacteria by using lysosome enzymes. The lysosomes also play an important role in the degrading and recycling of cellular waste after the cellular destruction caused by invading viruses and bacteria. If the cell is damaged beyond repair, lysosomes play an important role in the self-destruction process of the cell called programmed cell death, or apoptosis.

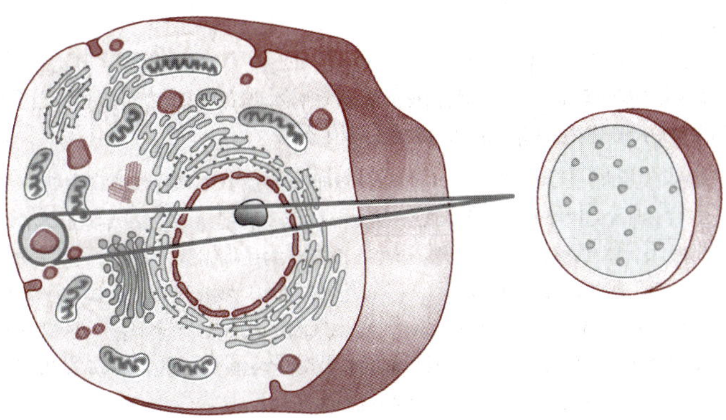

Fig. 2.8: Lysosome

Peroxisomes (Fig. 2.9)

BAQ: Write a note on the peroxisomes.

Ans: The peroxisomes are spherical or oval single-membrane cellular organelles. They contain oxidative enzymes in the crystalline core (Fig. 2.9), such as urate oxidase, amino acid oxidase, lactate oxidase, etc. The catalase enzyme present in the peroxisome protects the cell from toxic substances such as hydrogen peroxide produced during oxidative metabolic reactions. An oxidative metabolic reaction is a chemical reaction in which oxygen is used by cells to make energy from sugars (aerobic respiration or cell respiration).

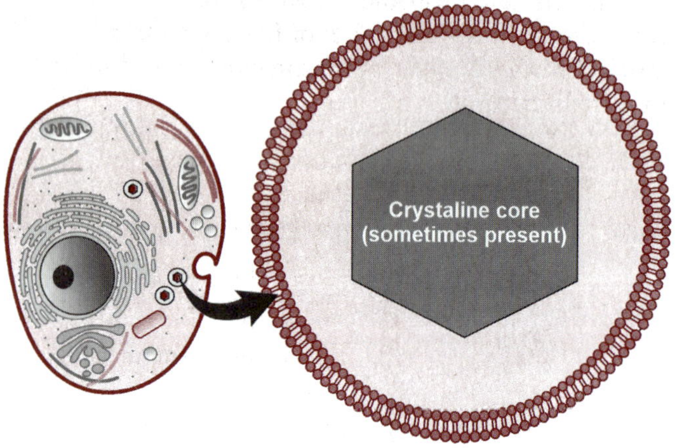

Fig. 2.9: Peroxisomes in a human cell

Cytoplasmic Inclusions

SAQ: What are cytoplasmic inclusions?

Ans: The cytoplasmic inclusions are non-protoplasmic, inert substances found within the cytoplasm. These may be produced due to cell activity or may be taken up from the surrounding medium. Following are some of the important cytoplasmic inclusions: Glycogen, fat globules, mucin granules, and remaining components of ingested material.

BAQ: Draw a labelled diagram of eukaryotic cells.

Ans: Refer to Fig. 2.2.

CELL COMPONENTS INVOLVED IN PROTEIN SYNTHESIS AND TRANSMISSION OF HEREDITARY CHARACTERS

Deoxyribonucleic Acid (DNA) and Ribonucleic Acid (RNA) (Figs 2.10 and 2.11)

BAQ: Write a note on the deoxyribonucleic acid (DNA) and the ribonucleic acid (RNA).

Ans: The DNA is a double-stranded molecule present in the nucleus of a eukaryotic cell and it is also found in the mitochondria. DNA is a polymer composed of basic units, deoxynucleotides, which are made up of purine bases such as adenine and guanine, deoxyribose (pentose sugar), and phosphoric acid. The basic units of DNA are deoxyadenosine monophosphate dAMP, deoxyguanine monophosphate (dGMP), deoxycytosine monophosphate (dCMP) and deoxythymine monophosphate (dTMP). The RNA is also made up of nucleotide units. However, it contains; pyrimidine bases such as uracil (U), cytosine (C) and thymine (T).

In DNA and RNA, the bases form hydrogen bonds with their complementary purines and pyrimidines, respectively. Thus, the purines adenine (A) and guanine (G) pair up with the pyrimidines thymine (T) and cytosine (C), respectively (Fig. 2.9). In the case of RNA, the complement of A is U instead of T and the pairs that form are adenine : uracil and guanine : cytosine.

The DNA is a right-handed double helix. It consists of two antiparallel right-handed double helix in which one strand runs in a 5′-to-3′ direction while the other in a 3′-to-5′ direction. The two strands are held together by hydrogen bonds formed by complementary base pairs (Fig. 2.9). In a human cell, there are 46 chromosomes (23 pairs) which contain about 100,000 genes.

DNA is the chemical basis of heredity and it is considered as the reserve source of genetic information. DNA is exclusively responsible for maintaining the identity of different species of organisms. Every aspect of the cellular function is under the control of DNA. A gene is a unit of heredity and it does not have independent existence but it is a stretch of DNA (Fig. 2.10).

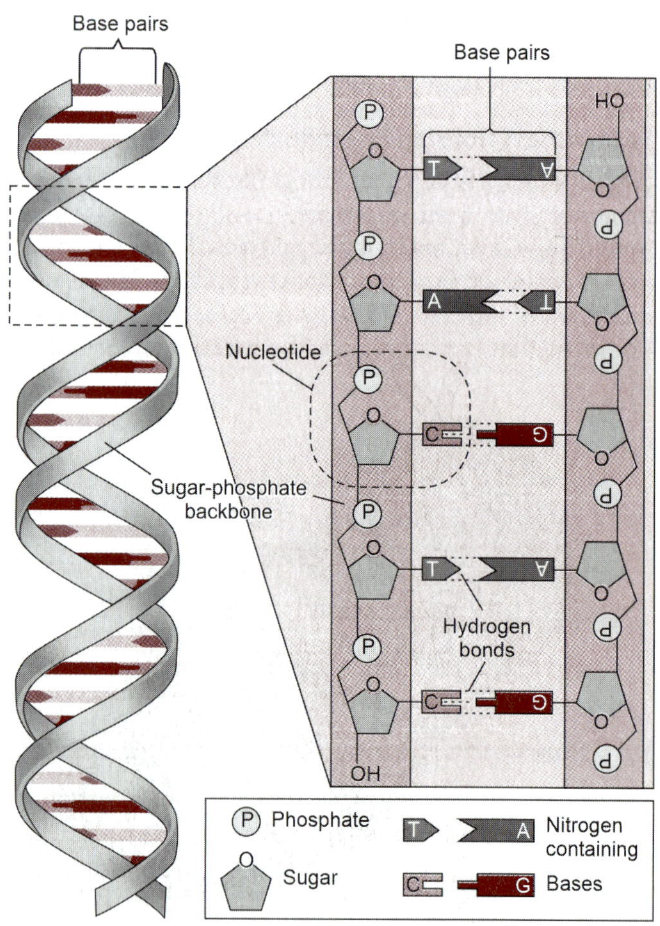

Fig. 2.10: Deoxyribonucleic acid

The following different types of RNAs are present in the nucleus and cytoplasm (Fig. 2.11):

1. **Messenger RNA (mRNA):** It specifies the sequence of amino acids in the protein synthesis (translation procedure).

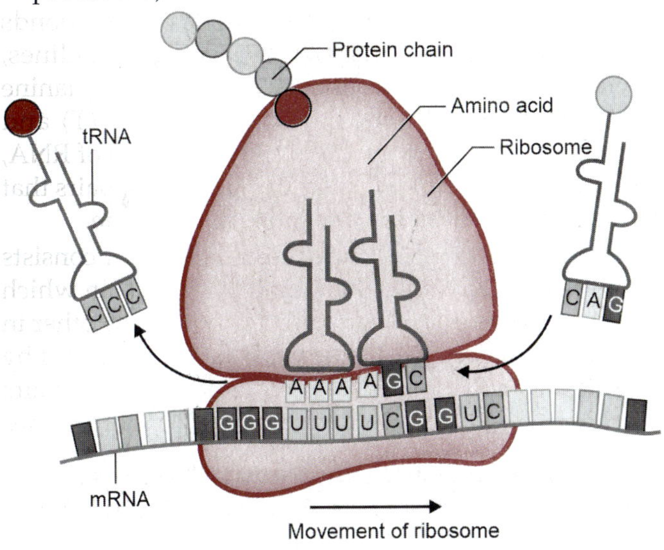

Fig. 2.11: mRNA, ribosome and t-RNA

2. **Ribosomal RNA (rRNA):** Ribosome is comprised of about 60% rRNA and 40% protein by weight. The ribosomal RNA are the main sites of protein synthesis. rRNA plays a significant role in the binding of mRNA to ribosomes and protein synthesis.
3. **Transfer RNA (tRNA):** It plays an important role in protein synthesis. tRNAs decode a specific codon of mRNA, using their anticodons, and transfer a specific amino acid to the end of a polypeptide chain in the protein synthesis.

Chromosomes (Figs 2.12–2.14)

BAQ: What are chromosomes?

Ans: In the eukaryotic cell, the extremely long DNA molecule maintains orderly and compact three-dimensional structures in the form of chromosomes. Each diploid human cell contains two full complements of the human genome, which means the complete set of genes. Each copy of the genome consists of 3.2 billion nucleotides. This genetic material is organized into 23 homologous chromosome pairs, including one pair of sex chromosomes. Each pair is contributed by

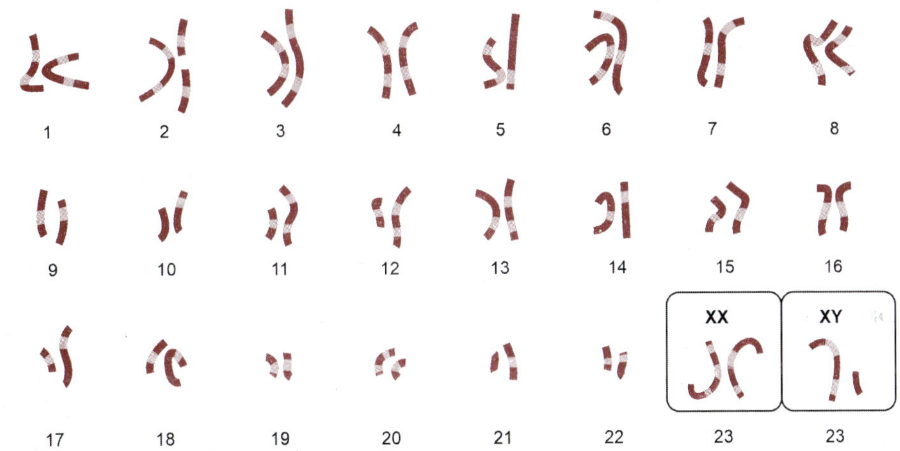

Fig. 2.12: Normal chromosomes

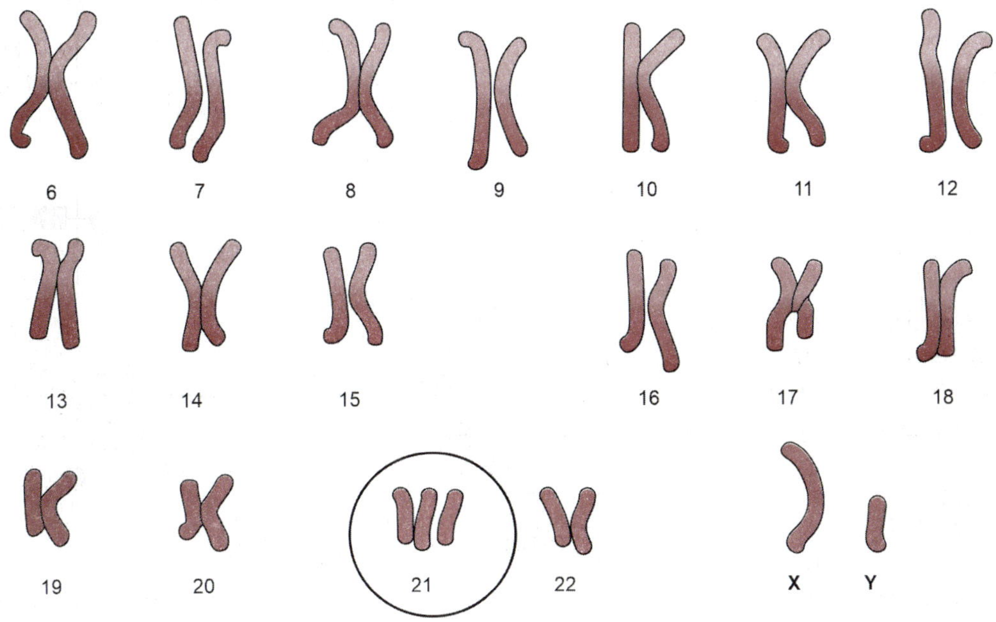

Fig. 2.13: Extra chromosome 21 in Down syndrome

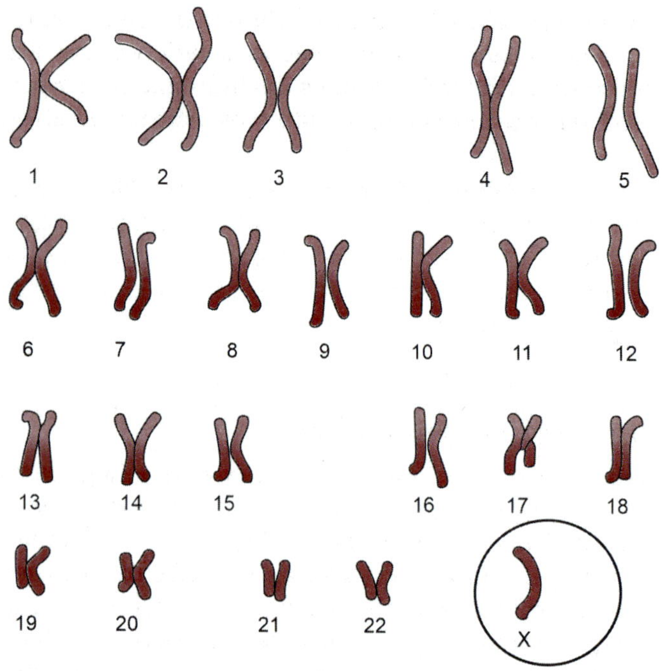

Fig. 2.14: Deletion of one X-chromosome in Turner syndrome

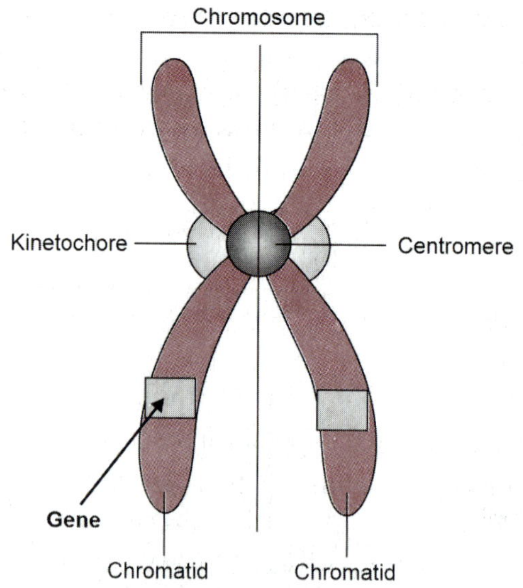

Fig. 2.15: Normal chromosome structure

a specific form combined with maternal origin and paternal origin. Each chromosome is a highly-ordered structure of a single double-stranded dsDNA molecule and is present in a compact form due to DNA-binding proteins. Aberrations in chromosome numbers can lead to various syndromes and diseases. Such genetic abnormalities often result in developmental and health issues, as seen in conditions like Down syndrome and Turner syndrome (Figs 2.13 and 2.14). These disorders arise from an atypical number of chromosomes, either extra or missing.

A single chromosome is composed of two double helices of DNA. Each double helix is termed a chromatid and the two chromatids are held together by the centromere, which is an unreplicated region of DNA. The centromere divides the chromosome into two arms. The shorter arm is known as the p-arm and the longer arm is known as the q-arm (Fig. 2.15).

The structural organization of the human genome is intimately related to the control of DNA transcription, replication, recombination and repair. The genes control the protein synthesis by following two procedures: (1) Transcription and (2) translation.

BAQ: Draw a labelled diagram of normal chromosome structure.

Ans: Refer to Fig. 2.15.

> **Objective:** To describe the basic concepts, "central dogma, "hereditary transmission" and "protein synthesis".

SAQ: What is transcription?

Ans: Transcription is the process of formation of an RNA copy of a specific gene sequence. This copy is called a messenger RNA (mRNA). mRNA leaves the cell nucleus and enters the cytoplasm and it combines with sRNA and directs the synthesis of a specific protein (Fig. 2.16).

SAQ: What is translation?

Ans: Translation is the process in which the ribosomes in the cytoplasm synthesize proteins as directed by mRNA with the help of various tRNA molecules (Fig. 2.11).

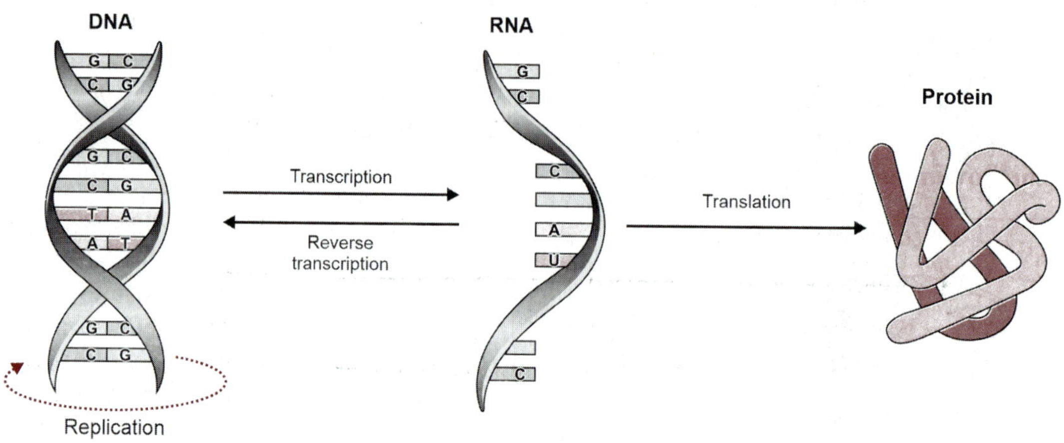

Fig. 2.16: Central dogma

SAQ: What is the central dogma?

Ans: The central dogma (Fig. 2.16) of molecular biology means the flow of genetic information, from DNA to RNA, to synthesize a specific protein. That means, once this information goes from DNA into the protein, it cannot get out of the protein and go back in the reverse direction.

Objective: To describe the basic chromosomal disorders.

Chromosomal Disorders (Figs 2.17 and 2.18)

SAQ: Write a note on the chromosomal disorders.

Ans: The chromosomal disorders take place; when there is a change in the number of chromosomes or the structure of chromosomes. The well-known condition is Down syndrome (trisomy 21), in which a person has an extra chromosome (Fig. 2.13). Down syndrome leads to specific facial appearance (Fig. 2.17), developmental delays and intellectual disability. Down syndrome persons have some of the following physical characteristics: Smallmouth, protruding large tongue, small chin, flat nasal bridge, slanted eyes, poor muscle tone, etc.

In the case of Turner syndrome (Fig. 2.18), one of the X chromosomes (sex chromosomes) is missing or partially missing (Fig. 2.14). Only females are affected by Turner syndrome, which leads to a variety of medical and developmental problems; including short height, heart defects and failure of the development of ovaries.

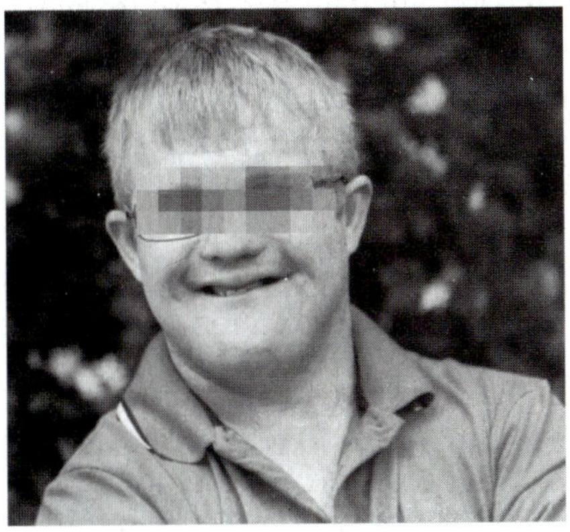

Fig. 2.17: Image of a person with Down syndrome

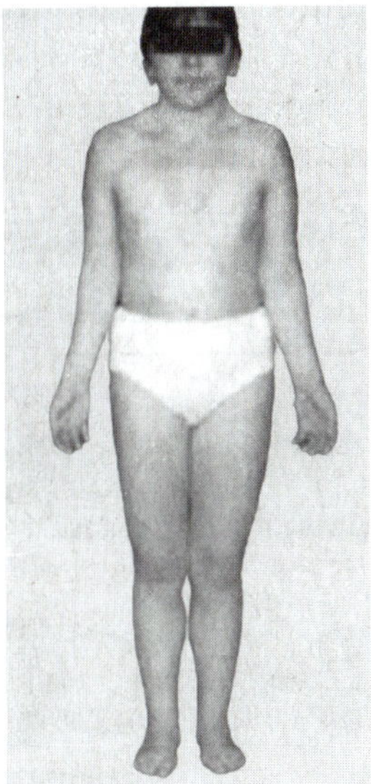

Fig. 2.18: A girl suffering from Turner syndrome

Objective: To describe mitosis and meiosis and the importance of these events.

CELL DIVISION

BAQ: Write a note on the cell division.

Ans: The cell division is the most important event in life and it goes on from time to time in the body. When cells divide, they make new cells. A single cell divides to make two daughter cells and these two cells then divide to make four cells, and this process of cell division is continuous in a living individual.

Cells regulate their division by using specific proteins called cyclins for cell-to-cell communication. Cyclin signals act to communicate to cells when to start dividing and later on when to stop dividing. Cells need to stop dividing at the right time. If a cell fails to stop dividing at the right time, tissues grow abnormally leading to the formation of a tumor.

The following are two ways of cell division: (1) Mitosis and (2) meiosis.

1. **Mitosis:** Leads to a division of a single cell, which divides into two cells that are replicas of each other and have the same number of chromosomes. This type of cell division takes place for the basic growth of the body cells, and also for the repair, and maintenance purposes of tissues.
2. **Meiosis:** It is necessary for sexual reproduction. Meiosis leads to a cell division into four cells that have half the number of chromosomes. Reduction of the number of chromosomes by half is important for sexual reproduction and it is necessary for genetic diversity.

MITOSIS (Fig. 2.19)

BAQ: Write a note on mitosis.

Ans: Mitosis leads to a division of a single cell, which divides into two cells that are replicas of each other and have the same number of chromosomes. Mitosis takes place through the following stages: Interphase, prophase, metaphase, anaphase and telophase.

- ***Interphase:*** In the interphase, the cell gets ready for mitosis.
- ***Prophase:*** It is the first stage of the cell division. In the early part of prophase, the centrosome is duplicated and the separated parts of chromosomes take their positions at opposite poles. Later on, the two centrosomes, which migrate to the opposite poles of the cell, remain attached by fine spindle-like threads. The chromatin becomes concentrated and forms rod-shaped chromosomes. Nucleoli disappear at this stage.

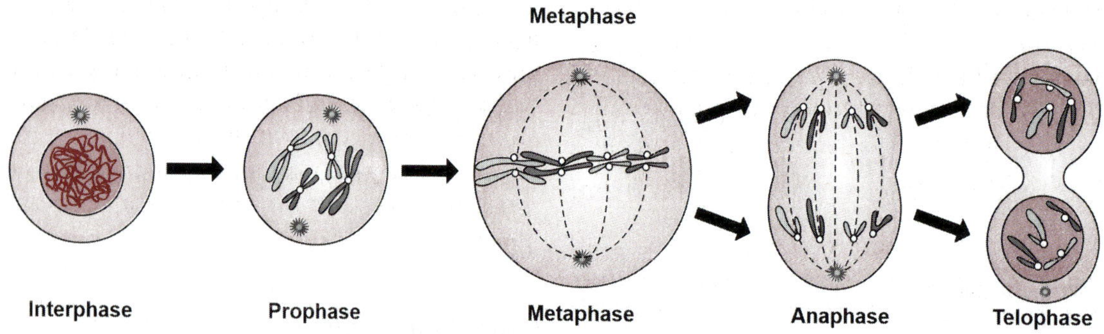

Fig. 2.19: Various stages of mitosis

- ***Metaphase:*** In metaphase the nuclear membrane disappears. Chromosomes arrange themselves around the centre of the cell and appear to be attached to the spindle of the centrosome.
- ***Anaphase:*** In anaphase the chromosomes replicate and two groups of sister chromatids form. The two groups of chromosomes then begin to move away from each other. They arrange themselves around the centrosome and the spindle breaks.
- ***Telophase:*** In this phase, a constriction appears around the centre of the cell body. The nuclear membrane reappears and the spindle disappears. The constriction of the cytoplasm increases until the cell is divided. The chromosomes disappear thread-like chromatin reappears and the two new cells formed are known as the daughter cells. These cells grow and reproduce further by mitosis.

Meiosis

BAQ: Write a note on meiosis.

Ans: Meiosis is cell division in sexually reproducing organisms. Meiosis reduces the number of chromosomes in the gametes (sperm or egg). Meiosis comprises two successive nuclear divisions with only one round of DNA replication.

Meiosis includes the stages of meiosis I (prophase I, metaphase I, anaphase I, telophase I), and meiosis II (prophase II, metaphase II, anaphase II, telophase II).

Meiosis I

The following are the various stages of meiosis I:

Prophase I: During prophase I, DNA is exchanged between homologous chromosomes in a process called homologous recombination. This process results in chromosomal crossover. The paired and replicated chromosomes are called bivalents (tetrads), which have two chromosomes and four chromatids, with one chromosome coming from each parent (Fig. 2.20).

Metaphase I: In metaphase I, the nuclear membrane disappears and a spindle forms. The homologous pairs move together along the metaphase plate and the homologous chromosomes align along an equatorial plane that bisects the spindle (Fig. 2.19).

Anaphase I: In anaphase I, the homologous chromosomes separate and one of each pair travels to each of the two poles of the cell. In this process, the chromosome number reduces from $2n$ to $1n$ (Fig. 2.20).

Telophase I: Two daughter cells are formed during telophase I. The 23 chromosomes at each pole remain double-stranded and are called dyads. A nuclear membrane is formed around each group of 23 dyads. These usually go immediately into the second cell division (meiosis II) to separate the sister chromatids.

Meiosis II

The four main steps of meiosis II are, prophase II, metaphase II, anaphase II, and telophase II.

Prophase II: In prophase II, the nucleoli and the nuclear envelope disappear. Centrioles move to the polar regions and arrange spindle fibers for the second meiotic division.

Metaphase II: In metaphase II, the centromeres of the paired chromatids align along the equatorial plate. The

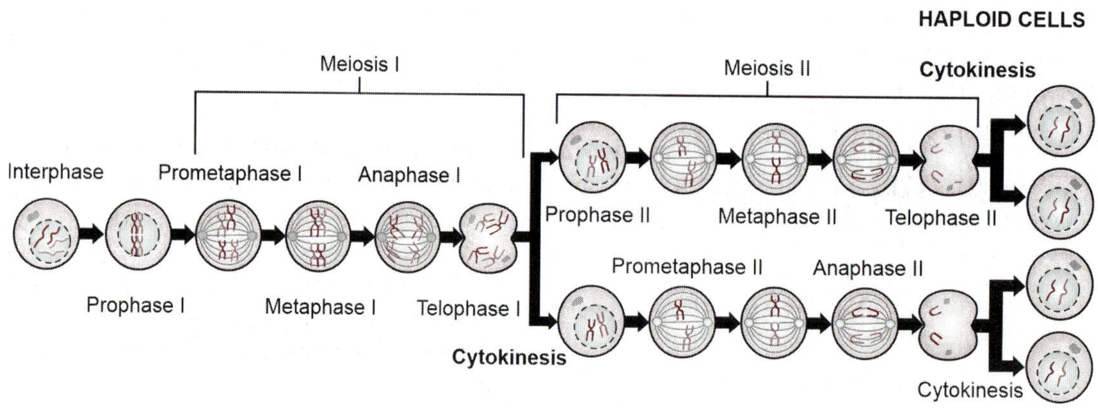

Fig. 2.20: Various stages of meiosis

centromeres contain two kinetochores that attach to spindle fibers from the centrosomes at each pole.

Anaphase II: In anaphase II, the centromeres are cleaved and the sister chromatids move toward opposing poles.

Telophase II: Telophase II is similar to telophase I. It is marked by uncoiling an increase in the size of chromosomes and the disappearance of the spindle. Nuclear envelope reform and cleavage or cell wall formation eventually produce a total of four daughter cells, each with a haploid set of chromosomes. Meiosis is now complete and ends up with four new daughter cells.

Objective: To describe cellular injury and death of cells.

CELLULAR INJURY AND DEATH OF CELLS

BAQ: Write a note on cellular injury and death of cells.

Ans: Normal cellular function requires a balance between the physiological demands of a cell and its metabolic capability, which maintains a state of homeostasis, which means maintenance of a stable and constant condition of properties like temperature and pH. The cells can alter their functional state in response to any stress to maintain homeostasis by undergoing hypertrophy (increase in mass) or hypotrophy (decrease in mass). Cell injury can be averted if any situation that leads to stress is controlled. Irreversible injury to the cells can lead to pathological changes leading to cellular death. Cellular injury can be caused by the following factors: Nutritional imbalances (related to deficient proteins, carbohydrates, lipids, vitamins, etc.), infectious agents, (e.g. bacteria, viruses), chemical agents (drugs and nontherapeutic agents), physical agents (radiations, electric shock, trauma, heat, cold, etc.), adverse immunological reactions, genetic derangements, and oxygen deprivation. There are following two morphological patterns of cellular death: (1) Necrosis and (2) apoptosis.

Necrosis

Necrosis is a type of cellular death caused by excessive cell swelling and denaturation of proteins leading to cellular rupture.

Apoptosis

Apoptosis occurs when a cell dies as an internal program organized to eliminate unwanted cells produced during embryogenesis and pathological conditions, without disrupting a normal tissue.

Objective: To describe the process and importance of the transport of substances across the cell membrane.

TRANSPORT OF SUBSTANCES ACROSS THE CELL MEMBRANE

Transport across the plasma membrane is essential to the life of a cell. Certain substances must move into the cell to support metabolic reactions necessary for its survival. Some substances produced by the cell for export, which should pass out to reach specific areas of the body and cellular waste materials produced in metabolic reactions should move out of a cell; otherwise, accumulation of waste products could be toxic to the cell. The following are various ways of transport of substances across a cell membrane:

Passive Transport (Figs 2.21–2.24)

SAQ: What is passive transport?

Ans: Passive transport means moving biochemicals and other atomic or molecular substances across the cell membranes. Passive transport is dependent on the permeability of the cell membrane. The four main kinds of passive transport are diffusion, facilitated diffusion, filtration and osmosis.

BAQ: Write a note on diffusion.

Ans: Diffusion (Fig. 2.21) is the net movement of substances from an area of high concentration of that substance to an area with lower concentration. The difference in concentration between the two areas is often termed the concentration gradient, and diffusion

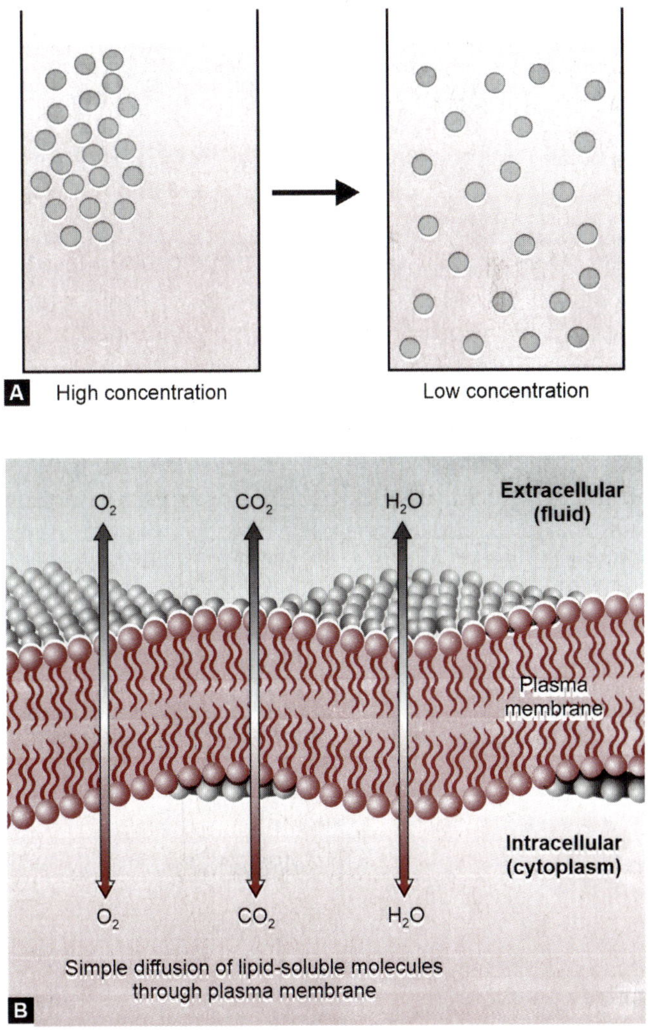

Figs 2.21A and B: Diffusion

will continue until this gradient has been eliminated. Since diffusion moves material from an area of higher concentration to the lower, it is described as moving solutes "down the concentration gradient" (when compared with active transport, which often moves material from an area of low concentration to an area of higher concentration). An example is the passage of water, carbon dioxide and oxygen through the plasma membrane of the cell.

BAQ: Write a note on filtration.

Ans: Filtration (Fig. 2.22) is the movement of water and solute molecules across the (cell) membrane due to hydrostatic pressure generated by a specific system. Depending on the size of the membrane pores, only solutes of a certain size may pass through it. For example, the membrane pores of the Bowman's capsule in the kidneys are very small. Water molecules of urine pass through the pores of the Bowman's capsule. However, large protein molecules like globulins and also blood cells cannot pass through glomerular wall of Bowman's capsule. Small protein molecule like albumin may get filtered through it. On the other hand, the membrane pores of liver cells are extremely large, which allows a variety of solutes to pass through and get metabolized.

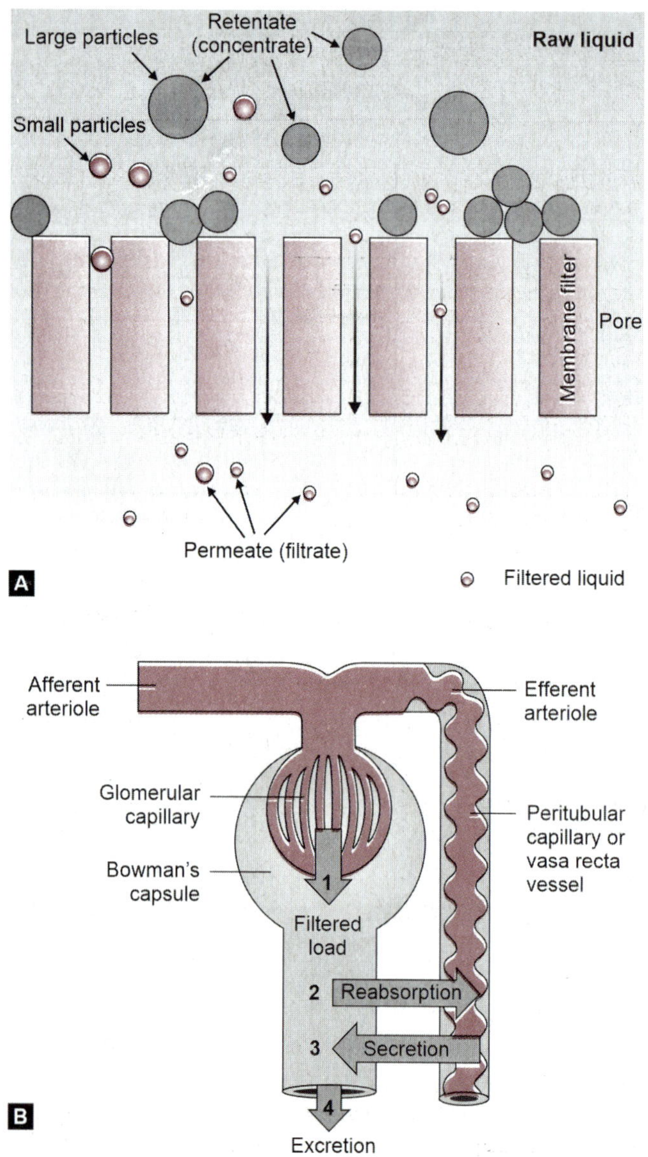

Figs 2.22A and B: Filtration

BAQ: Write a note on facilitated diffusion.

Ans: Facilitated diffusion (Fig. 2.23) is the movement of molecules across the cell membrane through special transport proteins that are present in the plasma membrane. Many large molecules, such as glucose, are insoluble in lipids (of the cell membrane) and too large to fit through the membrane pores. Therefore, it will bind with its specific carrier proteins, and the complex then binds to a receptor site and moves through the cellular membrane. Facilitated diffusion is a passive process, in which the solutes still move down the concentration gradient.

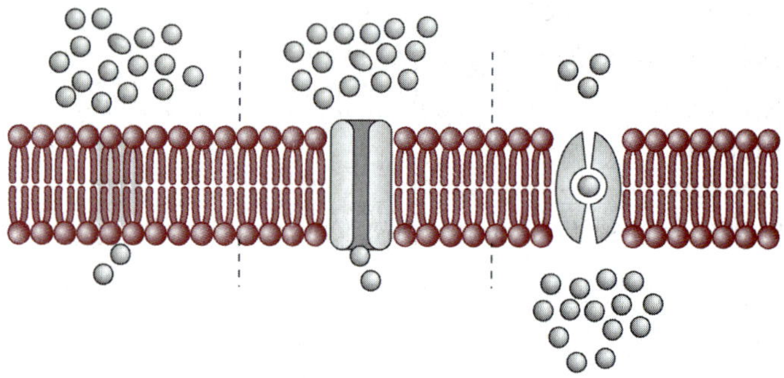

Fig. 2.23: Facilitated diffusion

BAQ: Write a note on osmosis.

Ans: Osmosis (Fig. 2.24) is the diffusion of water molecules across a selectively permeable membrane. The net movement of water molecules through a partially permeable membrane is from a solution of high water potential to an area of low water potential. Hence, when red blood cells are kept in a hypertonic solution, which has low water potential, water from red blood cells will move to the hypertonic solution and red blood cells will shrink. Similarly, when red blood cells are kept in pure water which has high water potential, water will move to red blood cells and red blood cells will swell and burst, leading to hemolysis. Hence, in a clinical laboratory,

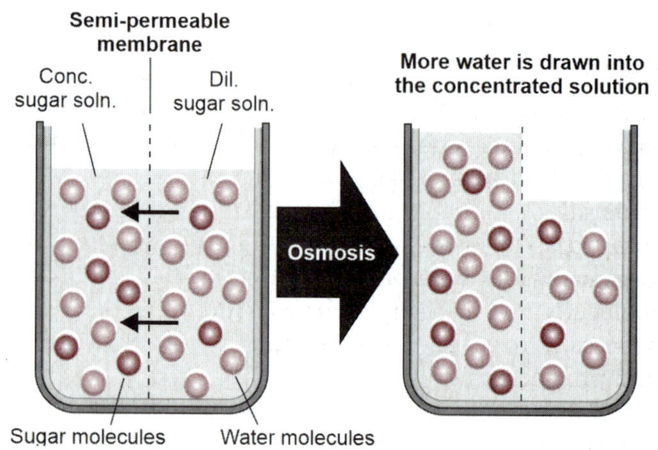

Fig. 2.24: Osmosis

for practicals related to experiments involving blood, normal saline (0.85%, isotonic solution) is used, which has the same water potential as red blood cell contents (Fig. 2.25).

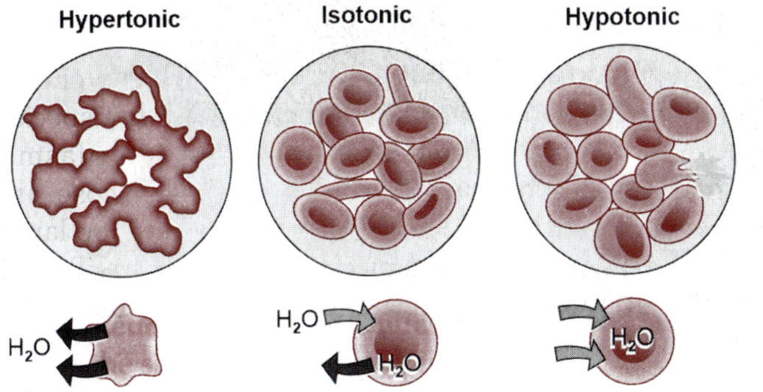

Fig. 2.25: Effect of hypertonic, hypotonic and isotonic solutions on red blood cells

Active Transport (Fig. 2.26)

BAQ: Write a note on active transport.

Ans: Active transport (Fig. 2.26) is the movement of a substance against its concentration gradient, i.e. from low concentration to high concentration by using ATP molecules. In all cells, this is usually required for the transportation of essential molecules such as glucose, amino acids, fatty acids and various ions required for cell metabolism. Active transport uses energy in the form of ATP molecules, unlike passive transport, which does not use any type of energy. Examples of active transport include the uptake of glucose in the intestinal cells.

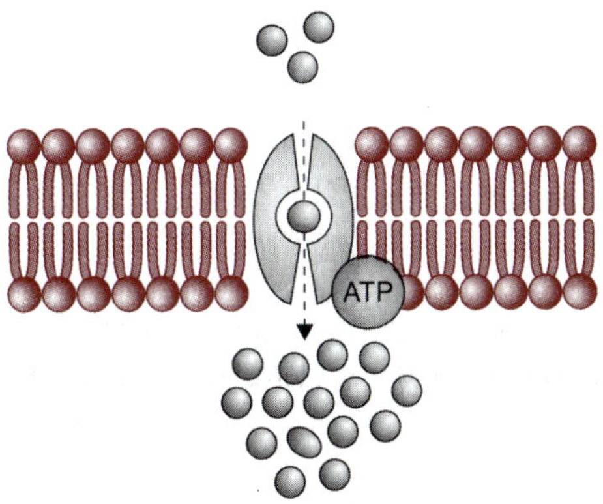

Fig. 2.26: Active transport

Endocytosis (Fig. 2.27)

BAQ: Write a note on endocytosis.

Ans: Endocytosis (Fig. 2.27) is a process by which cells take in various types of materials around them. In this process, the cellular membrane folds around the desired materials outside the cell. The ingested particle becomes trapped within a pouch, vacuole or inside the cytoplasm. Enzymes from lysosomes are then used to digest the molecules and these are then absorbed in the cell by this process. Two main types of endocytosis are pinocytosis and phagocytosis.

In pinocytosis, cells engulf liquid particles. In humans, this process occurs in the small intestine, where intestinal cells engulf fat droplets.

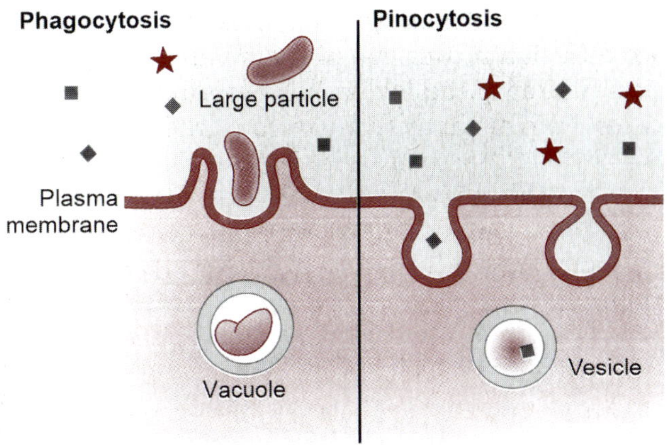

Fig. 2.27: Endocytosis: Phagocytosis and pinocytosis

In phagocytosis, cells engulf solid particles. It is the main mechanism used by immune cells to remove invading microorganisms and cell debris. The ingested material is then digested in the specific vacuoles known as phagosomes.

Exocytosis (Fig. 2.28)

BAQ: Write a note on exocytosis.

Ans: Exocytosis (Fig. 2.28) is the process by which cells excrete waste and other large molecules from the protoplasm.

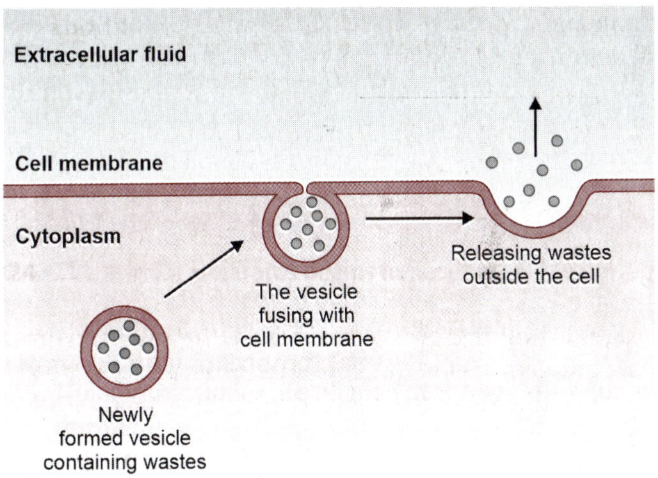

Fig. 2.28: Exocytosis

Objectives:
- To distinguish between four major tissues.
- To describe classification, various types, structure and location of various types of tissues.

TISSUES (Fig. 2.29)

Introduction

BAQ: What is a tissue?

Ans: A tissue is a group of cells found together in the body. The cells in a tissue share common characteristic features and embryonic origin. The cells are arranged in an organised pattern in a tissue to perform the specific functions of the tissue.

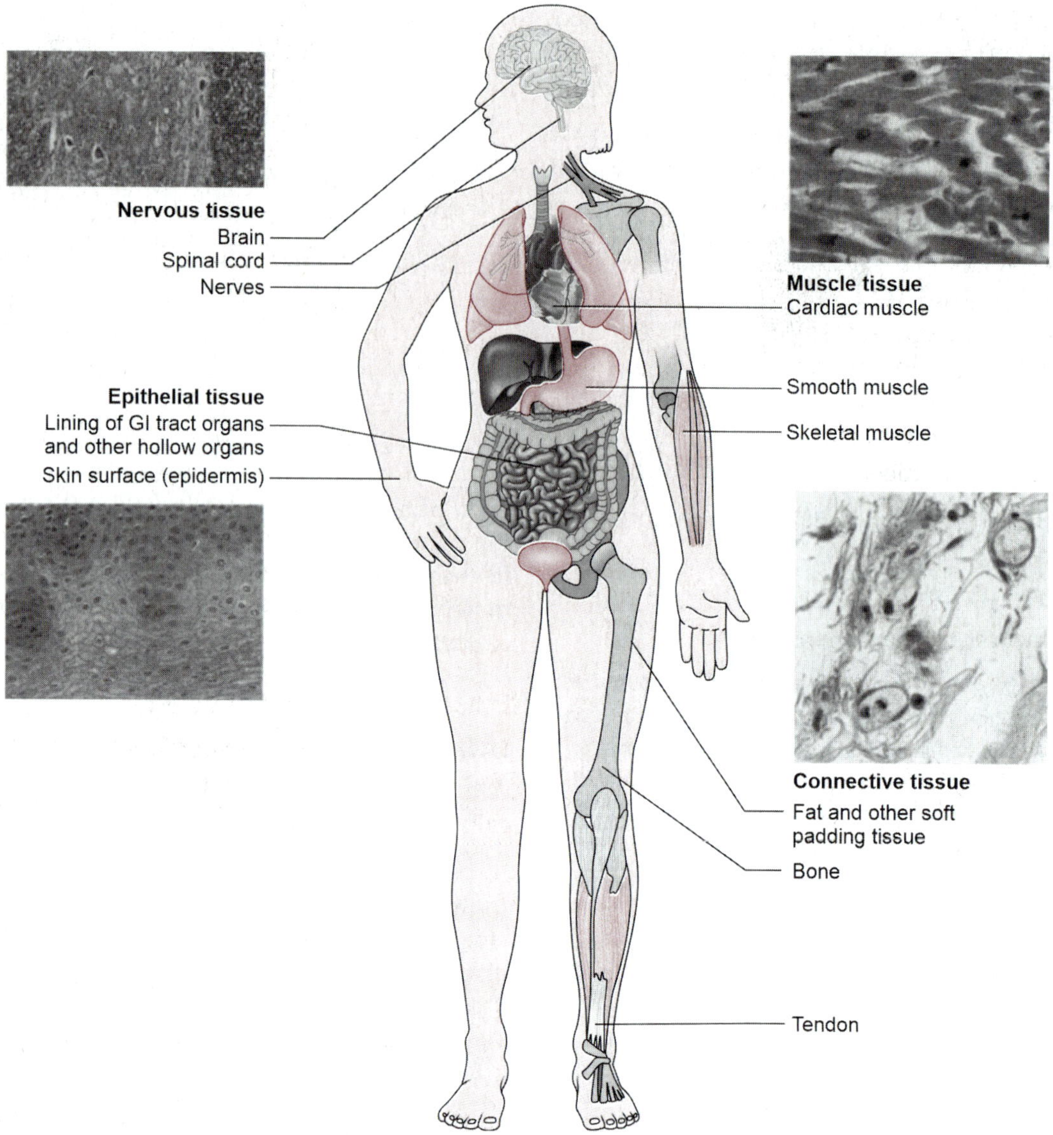

Fig. 2.29: Various types of tissues

The following are the four basic types of tissues: (1) Epithelial tissue, (2) connective tissue, (3) muscle tissue, and (4) nervous tissue (Fig. 2.29).

EPITHELIAL TISSUES (Figs 2.29 and 2.30)

LAQ: Write a note on epithelial tissues (epithelium).

Ans: Epithelial tissue (or epithelium) forms the covering of all body surfaces. It is a thin tissue that forms the outer layer of the body's surface and internal organs. Epithelial tissue covers body surfaces, cavities and hollow organs, and is the major tissue in various glands (Fig. 2.30). The epithelial tissues perform the following variety of functions:

- The epithelial tissues provide the first line of protection to the body from physical, chemical, and biological damage. Epithelium cells act as gatekeepers of the body and control the permeability of cells by allowing only selective transfer of materials across the cell surface. All substances that enter the body need to cross an epithelium tissue.

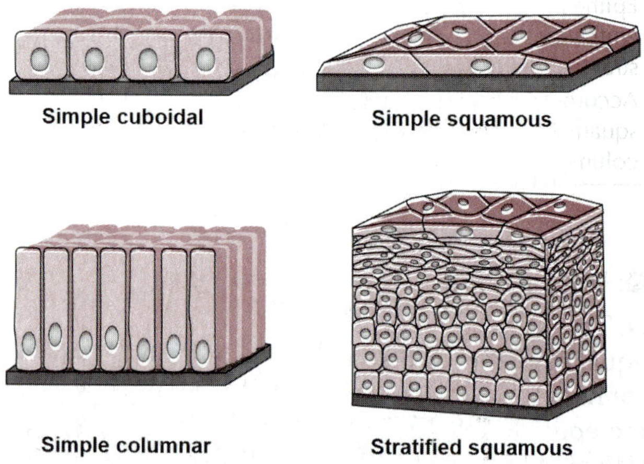

Fig. 2.30: Various types of epithelial tissues

- The epithelial cells secrete enzymes and hormones, which act as catalysts in metabolic reactions. The epithelial cells also secret mucus to facilitate important procedures in the body, and also secret the breast milk. They play an important role in cellular procedures involving absorption, excretion, filtration, diffusion, and sensory reception.

Formation of Epithelial Tissue

Epithelial tissue is derived from the following three major embryonic layers: Ectoderm, mesoderm and endoderm. The epithelial tissue made up of cutaneous membranes develops from the ectoderm. The epithelial tissue made up of most of the mucous membranes develops from the endoderm. The epithelial tissue that lines blood and lymph vessels and open spaces in the body is derived from mesoderm. The epithelial tissue that lines vessels in the cardiovascular and lymphatic systems is called endothelium and epithelial tissue in the form of the serous membranes lining of the true cavities is called mesothelium.

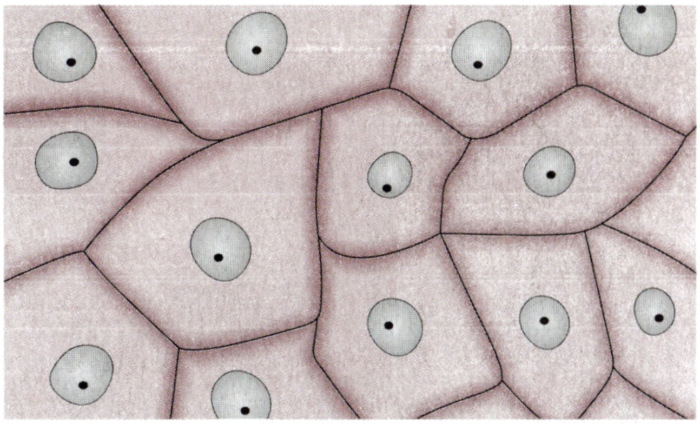

Fig. 2.31: Epithelial cells

Important Features of Epithelial Tissue

All epithelial tissues share the following important structural features:

1. Epithelial tissue is highly cellular. It does not contain significant extracellular material present between cells.
2. Adjoining cells of epithelial cells form specialized intercellular connections called cell junctions.
3. An epithelium is made up of one or more cellular layers. The outer surface of epithelium is either exposed to the outside of the body or a lumen or cavity inside a body. The deeper inner surface of epithelium is bound to a basement membrane of epithelium and underlined connective tissue.
4. Epithelial tissues are avascular means these are without blood vessels and composed of tightly packed cells.
5. Epithelial tissues are capable of replacing damaged and dead cells caused due to severe environmental factors.

> *Note:*
> 1. Epithelium made up of a single layer is called simple epithelium and epithelium made up of many layers is called stratified epithelium
> 2. According to the shape of the cells, the epithelium is called squamous (with flattened surface), cuboidal (cubic shape) or columnar (appear like columns) (Fig. 2.30).

Epithelial Cells (Figs 2.30 and 2.31)

BAQ: Write a note on the epithelial cells.

Ans: The epithelial cells (Fig. 2.31) are characterized by unequal distribution of organelles and membrane-bound proteins between their top (apical) and basal surfaces. Some epithelial cell structures are adapted to specific functions. For example, cilia are extensions of the apical cell membrane. These are supported by microtubules. These extensions beat in unison to facilitate the movement of fluids and particles along the surface. The ciliated epithelia line the ventricles of the brain. The ciliated epithelia line of the respiratory system is useful for sweeping dust particles and pathogens up and out of the respiratory tract. The ciliated epithelia are also useful in the circulation of the cerebrospinal fluid (CSF).

Classification of Simple Epithelial Tissue (Fig. 2.30)

BAQ: Write a note on the classification of simple epithelial tissue.

Ans: The following are five types of simple epithelial cells (Fig. 2.30):

1. **Simple squamous epithelium:** These epithelia are single-layered, tightly bound flattened cells. These cells play an important role in blood filtration at the kidneys and the diffusion of gases in the lungs. These epithelia are present in capillary walls, the lining of alveoli of the lungs, linings of body cavities and visceral organs.
2. **Simple cuboid epithelium:** These epithelia are single-layered cube-shaped cells. These epithelia play an important role in body processes like secretion, excretion and absorption. These epithelia form covering the surface of ovaries, lining of nephron, tubules, salivary ducts and pancreatic ducts.
3. **Simple columnar epithelium:** These epithelia are made up of non-ciliated column-shaped cells. These epithelia play an important role in the processes such as absorption, secretion and protection. These epithelia are present in the linings of the digestive tract, the gallbladder and the excretory ducts of some glands.
4. **Simple ciliated columnar epithelium:** These epithelia are made up of a single layer of ciliated-column-shaped cells. These epithelia play an important role in the transportation of micromolecules by ciliary motion. These epithelia are present in the lining of Fallopian tubes and certain areas of the respiratory tract.
5. **Pseudostratified ciliated columnar epithelium:** These epithelia are made up of a single layer of ciliated irregularly-shaped cells (Fig. 2.32). These epithelia play an important role in ciliary motion, secretion and protection. These epithelia are present in the lining of respiratory passages and auditory (Eustachian) tubes.

> *Note:* Epithelial cells in close contact with the underlying connective tissues secrete glycoproteins and collagen from their basal surface which forms the basal lamina. The basal lamina interacts with the reticular lamina secreted by the underlying connective tissue, forming a basement membrane that helps to anchor the layers together.

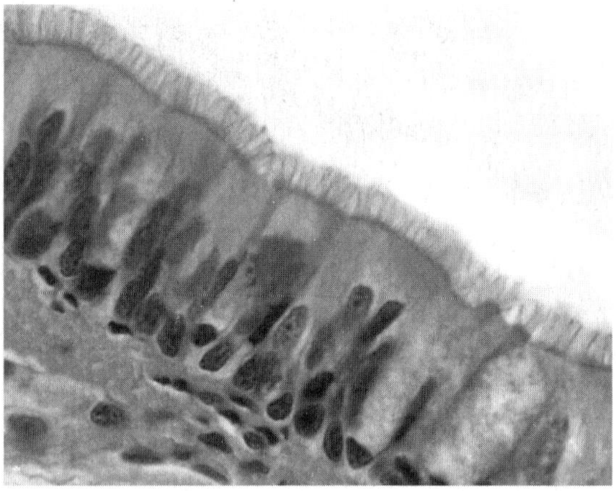

Fig. 2.32: Pseudostratified ciliated columnar epithelium

SAQ: Enumerate the names of various types of epithelial tissues.

Ans: The following are the names of various types of epithelial cells:

1. Simple squamous epithelium
2. Simple cuboid epithelium
3. Simple columnar epithelium
4. Simple ciliated columnar epithelium
5. Pseudostratified ciliated columnar epithelium

SAQ: Enumerate the functions of the epithelial tissue.

Ans: The following are the various functions of epithelial tissue:

1. Protection of the internal and external body parts.
2. Facilitation of various processes such as filtration, absorption and secretion functions.
3. Facilitation of detection of outside sensory stimuli, with the help of the sensory nerve endings embedded inside it.
4. Absorption of digested micronutrients in the gastrointestinal tract.
5. Exchange of respiratory gases in the cells of the tissues and in the lungs.
6. Facilitation of movement of food particles on their surface with the help of cilia on the surface of the gastrointestinal tract.
7. Excretion of compounds like creatinine and cations like potassium in the nephrons of kidneys.
8. Secretion of sweat, saliva, digestive enzymes, milk, etc., by the glandular epithelial cells.

Stratified Epithelium Tissue (Fig. 2.30)

BAQ: Write a note on the stratified epithelial tissue.

Ans: A stratified epithelium is a type of epithelial tissue that is composed of more than one layer of epithelial cells. The stratified epithelium can be classified as follows:

1. **Stratified squamous epithelial tissue (keratinized):** These epithelia are the outermost flattened layers. These are multilayered and contain keratin protein and dead cells. The function of these epithelia is to provide protection to the internal layers of an organ. Stratified squamous epithelial tissue (keratinized) is present in the epidermis of the skin.
2. **Stratified squamous epithelial tissue (non-keratinized):** These epithelia are multilayered and do not contain keratin. The cells in these epithelia are alive and provide flexibility and protection to the organ. Stratified squamous epithelial tissue (non-keratinized) is present in the oral and nasal cavities, oesophagus, vagina, and anal canal.
3. **Stratified cuboidal epithelium:** These epithelia usually contain two layers of cube-shaped cells. These epithelia provide strength to luminal walls, present in tubular structures like vessels and intestines. Stratified cuboidal epithelium is present in the ducts of larger sweat glands, salivary glands and the pancreas.
4. **Transitional epithelium:** These epithelia contain many layers of rounded non-keratinized cells. These epithelia are able to swell if internal pressure increases. Transitional epithelium is present in the lining of the urinary bladder and in specific parts of the ureters and urethra.

SAQ: Enumerate the names of various types of stratified epithelial tissues.

Ans: The following are the names of various types of stratified epithelial cells:

1. Stratified squamous epithelial tissue (keratinized skin)
2. Stratified squamous epithelial tissue (non-keratinized
3. Stratified cuboidal epithelium
4. Transitional epithelium

Glands

LAQ: Write a note on the glands.

Ans: The glands are groups of epithelial cells that secret specialised secretions. The glands are of two types: (1) Exocrine glands and (2) endocrine glands.

Exocrine Glands

Certain epithelial cells invade the underlying connective tissue, during prenatal development and form exocrine glands. Exocrine glands are specialized secretory glands. These are of two types: Simple exocrine glands and compound exocrine glands.

Simple Exocrine Glands

These have a single, unbranched duct. Simple exocrine glands are of the following types:

a. Simple unicellular glands: Secretions of these cells protect and lubricate the surrounding area.
   Examples: Goblet cells in the nasal mucosa (Fig. 2.33).
b. Simple tubular glands: Secretions of these glands help in the digestion.
   Examples: Intestinal glands.
c. Simple branched tubular glands: Secretions of these glands protect and help digestion.
   Examples: Gastric glands and uterine glands (Fig. 2.34)

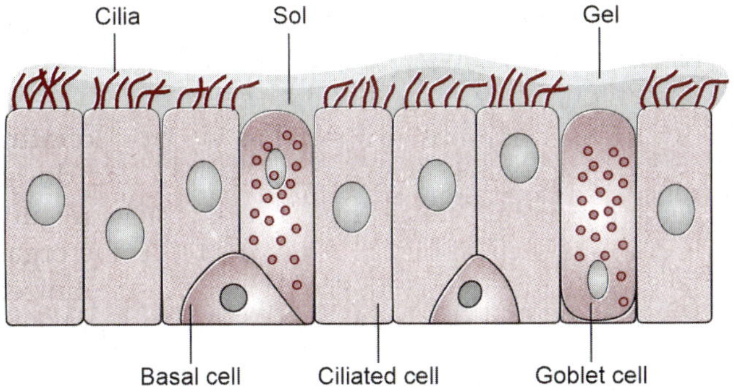

Fig. 2.33: Globlet cells in the nasal mucosa

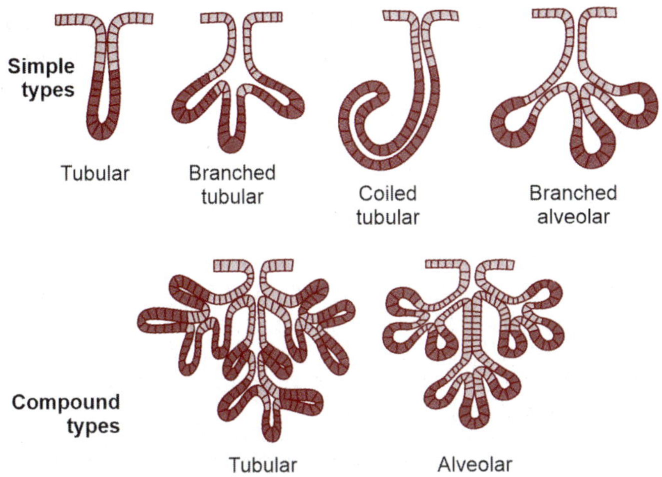

Fig. 2.34: Various types of exocrine glands

d. Simple coiled tubular glands: Secretions of these glands regulate temperature.
Examples: Eccrine sweat glands (Fig. 2.34).

e. Simple acinar glands: Secretions of these glands provide additional components to spermatozoa functions.
Examples: Seminal vesicle (Fig. 2.34).

Compound Exocrine Glands

These have branched duct systems (Fig. 2.34). These can be subclassified as follows:

Compound tubular glands: Secretions of these glands in the intestine lubricate and help in digestion and kidneys, and lubricate the male urethra. *Examples:* Liver and bulbourethral glands (Fig. 2.34).

Compound acinar glands: These provide infant nutrition and help in the digestion process. *Examples:* Salivary glands and mammary glands (Fig. 2.34).

Compound tubuloacinar glands: Secretions of these glands help in digestion. *Examples:* Pancreatic gland and salivary gland (parotid) (Fig. 2.35).

Compound branched acinar cells: Secretions of these cells condition the skin. *Examples:* Sebaceous cells (Fig. 2.36).

> *Note:* Acinar means related to a small sac-like cavity in a gland.

BAQ: Draw a labelled diagram of various types of exocrine glands.

Ans: Refer to Fig. 2.34.

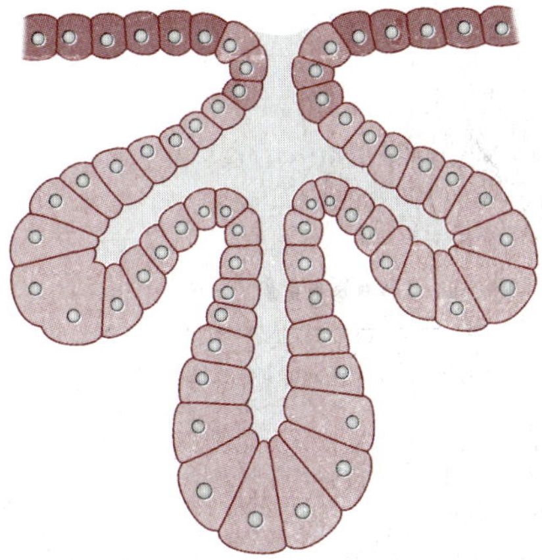

Fig. 2.35: Simple branched acinar gland

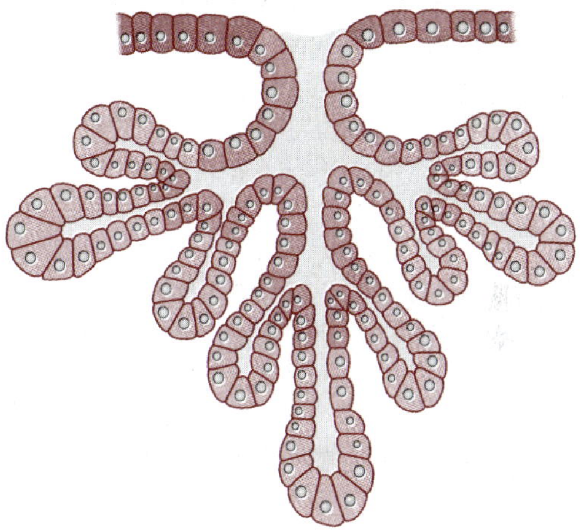

Fig. 2.36: Compound tubular acinar glands

SAQ: What is the difference between the exocrine glands and the endocrine glands?

Ans: The following is the main important difference between the exocrine glands and endocrine glands: Exocrine glands secrete substances into a ductal system to an epithelial surface, and endocrine glands secrete hormones directly into the bloodstream (Fig. 2.37).

Secretory Classification of Exocrine Glands (Fig. 2.38)

BAQ: Describe the exocrine glands on the basis of the secretory classification.

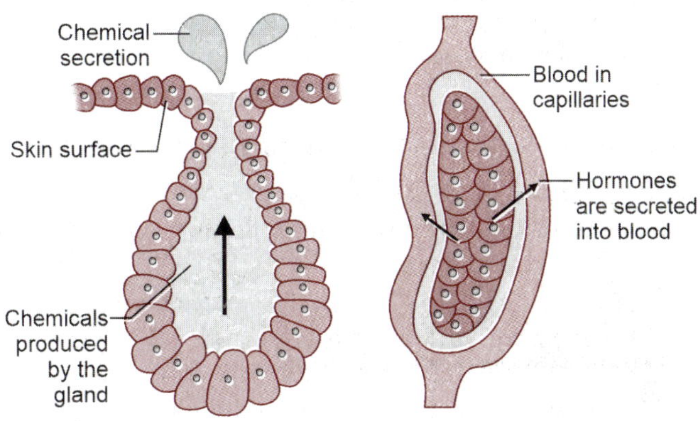

Fig. 2.37: Exocrine gland and endocrine gland

Ans: On the basis of secretory classification, the exocrine glands are of the following three types: (1) Merocrine, (2) apocrine and (3) holocrine (Fig. 2.38).

1. **Merocrine glands:** Merocrine glands are comprised of secretory cells that excrete products by secreting secretions into the ducts and then to internal space without causing any damage or loss in the secretory cell. Examples of merocrine glands are the pancreatic gland, salivary glands and eccrine sweat glands.
2. **Apocrine glands:** Secretory cells of these glands pass secretions through the cell membrane by forming elevations on the cell membrane and then pass outside the cell. Apocrine glands are found in the eyelid, ear, skin, and breast. Apocrine glands in the breast secrete fat droplets into breast milk and those in the ear form earwax. Apocrine glands in the skin and the eyelid are sweat glands. Most apocrine glands in the skin are in the following parts of the body: The groin, armpits, and the area around the nipples of the breast. Apocrine glands in the skin secrete secretions, which usually have an odour.
3. **Holocrine glands:** Secretions of these glands are produced in the cytoplasm of the cell and released by the rupture of the plasma membrane, which leads to the destruction of the cell and the secretion of the product is released into the lumen. This type of secretion is seen in sebaceous glands associated with hair follicles.

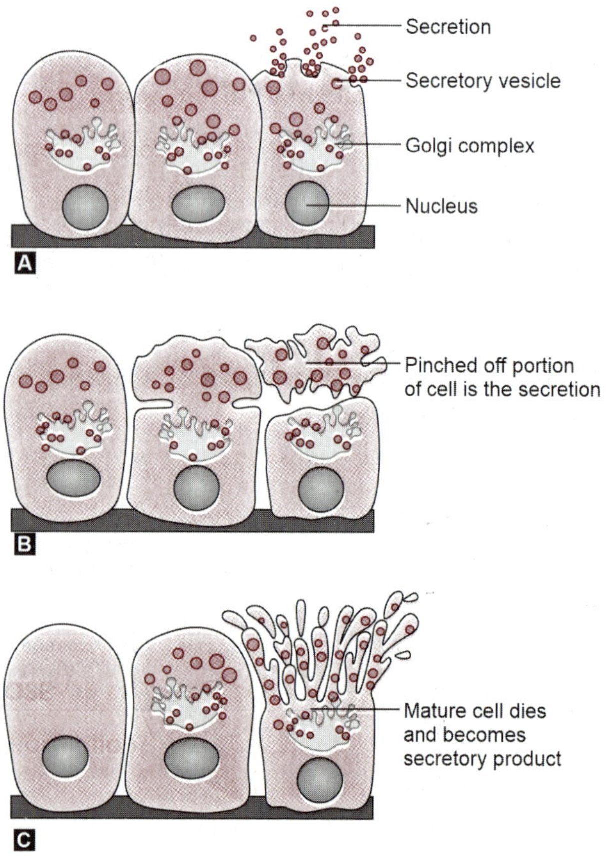

Fig. 2.38: Merocrine, apocrine and holocrine secretions

CONNECTIVE TISSUES (Fig. 2.39)

LAQ: Write a note on the connective tissues.

Ans: Connective tissues (Fig. 2.39) are present throughout the body. Connective tissues are characterized by the presence of a large amount of intercellular matrix with relatively few cells. The connective tissue cells are capable of reproducing at a slow rate. Most connective tissues get a good blood supply, however, some types of connective tissues do not get a blood supply. Connective tissues give support and provide structure, framework and protection to other tissues and organs in the body.

Various types of cells are present in the connective tissue. The following are three common types of connective tissue cells: (1) Fibroblasts, (2) macrophages, and (3) mast cells.

Unlike epithelial tissue, which is composed of closely packed cells with little or no extracellular space in between the cells, connective tissue cells are dispersed

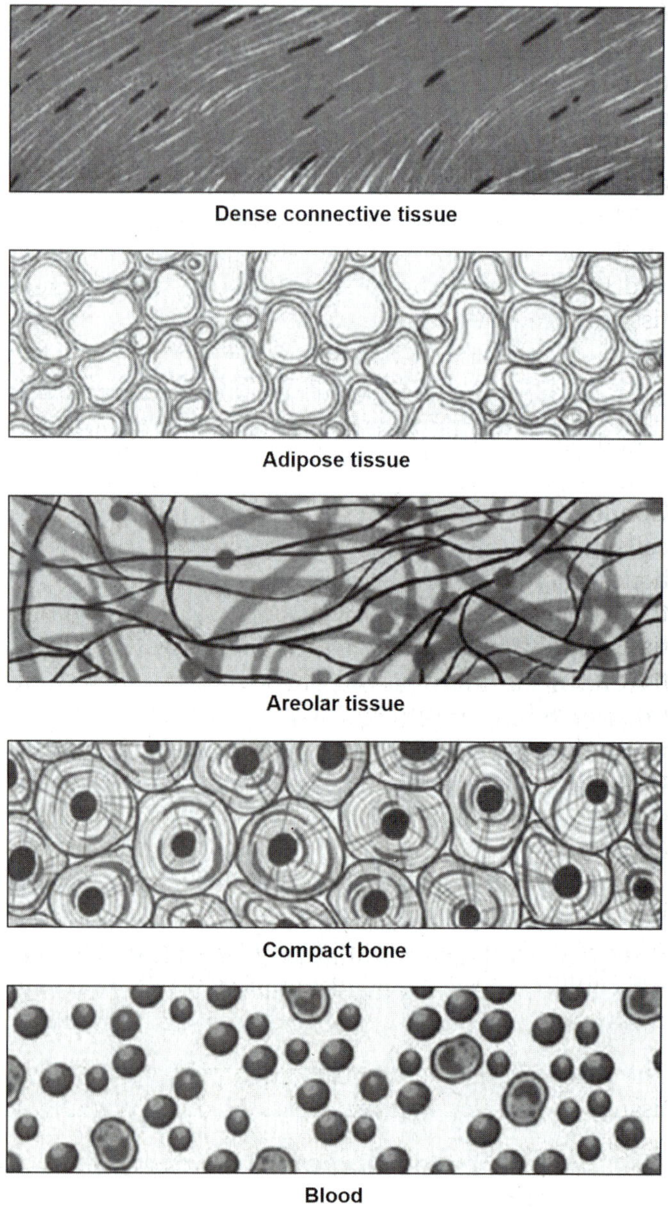

Fig. 2.39: Various types of connective tissues

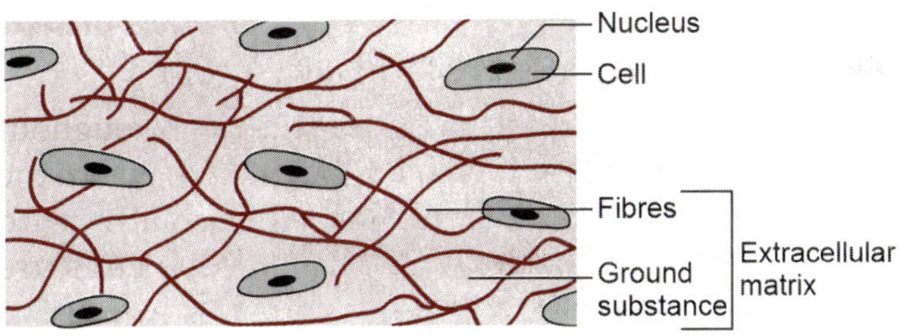

Fig. 2.40: Extracellular matrix, ground substance, fibers and cell of connective tissue

in a matrix. Usually, the matrix is a large amount of extracellular material produced by the connective tissue cells. The connective cells are embedded within the matrix. The matrix plays a very important role in the functioning of connective tissue. The amorphous ground substance of connective tissue is a transparent material, which has the properties of a viscous solution (hydrated thin gel). The main constituents of the amorphous ground substance are large complexes of protein and carbohydrate, called glycosaminoglycans (mucopolysaccharides).

The most common cell found within the connective tissue is the fibroblast. Fibroblasts secrete polysaccharides and fibrous proteins called collagen, which combine with extracellular fluids to form a viscous ground substance and form the extracellular matrix (Fig. 2.40).

The following are three main types of fibers secreted by the fibroblasts: (1) Collagen fibers, (2) elastic fibers, and (3) reticular fibers. These fibers hold connective tissues together.

Functions of Connective Tissues

Connective tissues perform the following various functions in the body: (1) In the form of connective tissue sheaths, they support and connect other tissues. Connective tissue sheath connects surrounding muscle cells, and then to the tendons that attach muscles to bones, and then connective tissues attach tothe skeleton that supports the positions of the body, (2) connective tissues protect the form of fibrous capsules and bones that protect delicate organs and the skeletal system, (3) connective tissue in the form of blood contains specialized cells such as white blood cells and macrophages in tissues that defend the body from the entry of microorganisms, (4) connective tissue in the form of blood and lymph, performs the following functions: Transport of fluids, nutrients, chemical messengers, waste products, etc. (5) connective tissue in the form of adipose cells stores excess energy in the form of fat and contributes to the thermal insulation of the body.

Classification of Connective Tissues (Figs 2.41–2.44)

The following are the various categories of connective tissue: (1) Loose connective tissue, (2) dense connective tissue, (3) cartilage, (4) bone and (5) blood.

Loose Connective Tissue

BAQ: Write a note on the loose connective tissue.

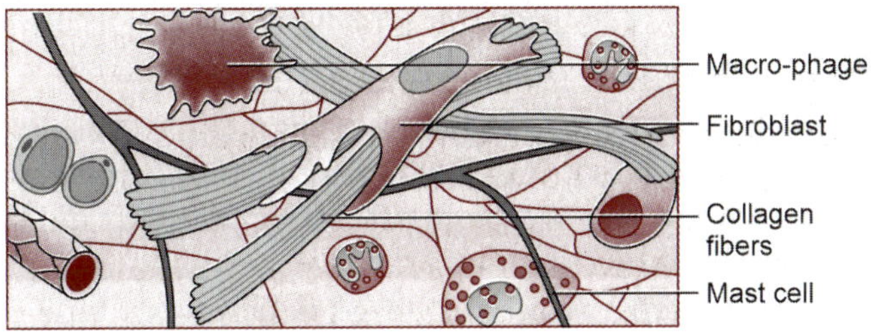

Fig. 2.41: Loose connective tissue

Ans: Loose connective tissue (Fig. 2.41): It contains large amounts of matrix and few fibers. Loose connective tissue is found between many organs where it acts both to absorb shock and bind tissues together. It allows water, salts, and various nutrients to diffuse through to adjacent or imbedded cells and tissues.

The following are the various types of loose connective tissues:

1. **Aerolar tissue:** It is loose connective tissue made up of collagen. It contains fibroblasts and mast cells. These are present deep in the skin and function as binding and protection to surrounding cells, vessels and organs.
2. **Adipose tissue:** It is a type of loose connective tissue. Adipose tissue contains adipocytes, that store lipids (fat) in the form of droplets. These droplets fill most of the cytoplasm. A large number of blood capillaries facilitate rapid storage and mobilization of lipid molecules to adipose tissue. Adipose tissue is located beneath the skin, around internal organs, and in bone marrow in the muscular system and the breast. Adipose tissue protects surrounding cells, vessels and organs from severe cold temperatures and acts as a reserve source of energy (in the form of ATP (Fig. 2.42).
3. **Reticular tissue:** It is made up of loose and thin reticular fibers. The cells that make the reticular fibers are called fibroblasts or reticular cells. Reticular connective tissue forms a protective covering for other cells in many organs, such as bone marrow and lymph nodes.

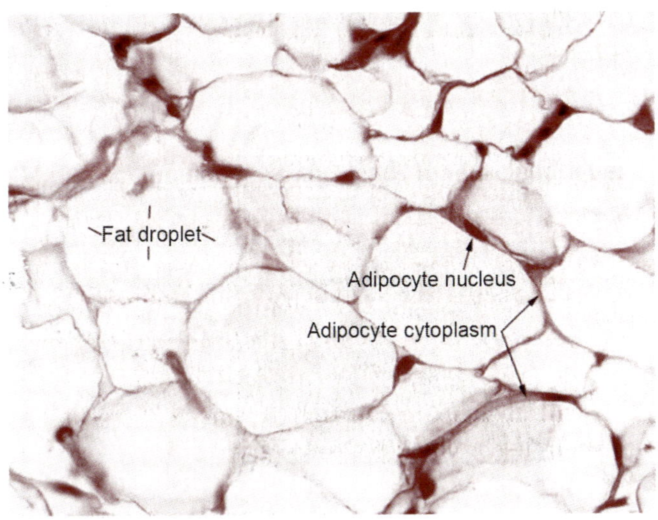

Fig. 2.42: Adipose tissue

Dense Connective Tissue (Figs 2.43–2.46)

BAQ: Write a note on dense connective tissue.

Ans: Dense connective tissue contains large amounts of fibers and less ground substance. Dense connective tissue can be: (A) Dense regular connective tissue or (B) dense irregular connective tissue.

(A) The dense regular connective tissue is a type of connective tissue that consists mainly of collagen fibers, which are densely packed, and arranged in parallel order (Fig. 2.47). Tendons and ligaments are examples of dense

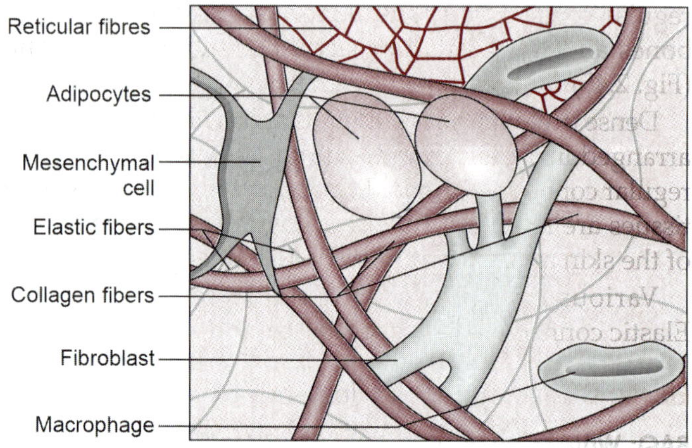

Fig. 2.44: Various components of connective tissue

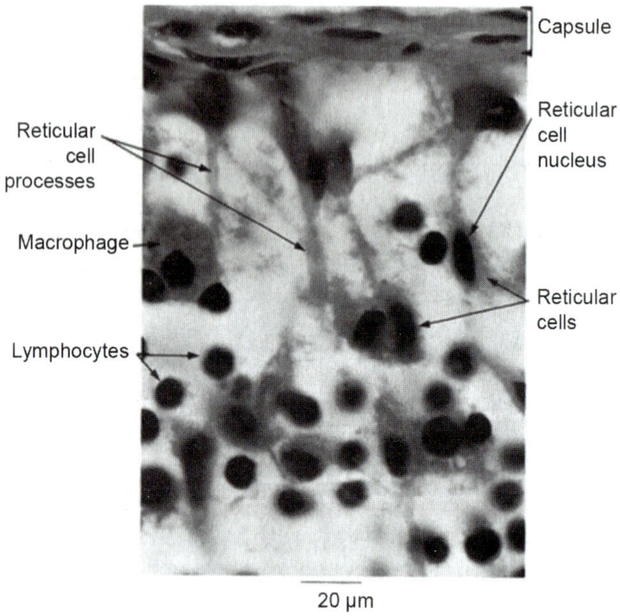

Fig. 2.43: Dense connective tissue

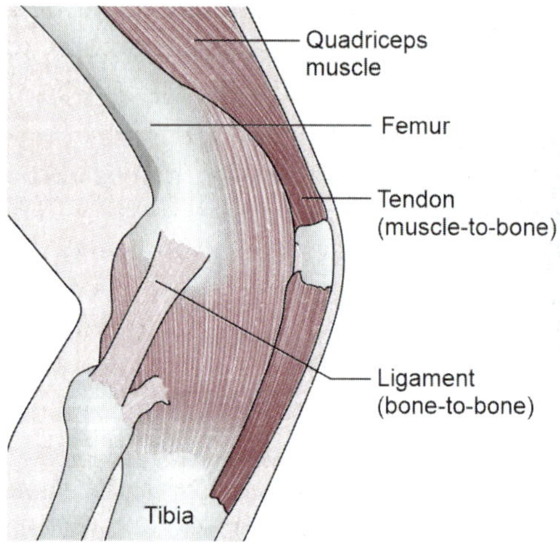

Fig. 2.45: Ligaments and tendons

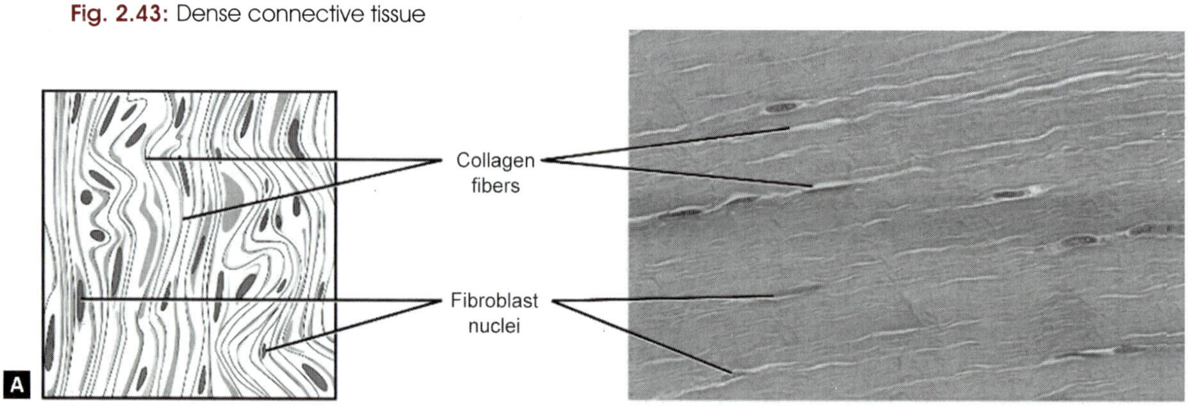

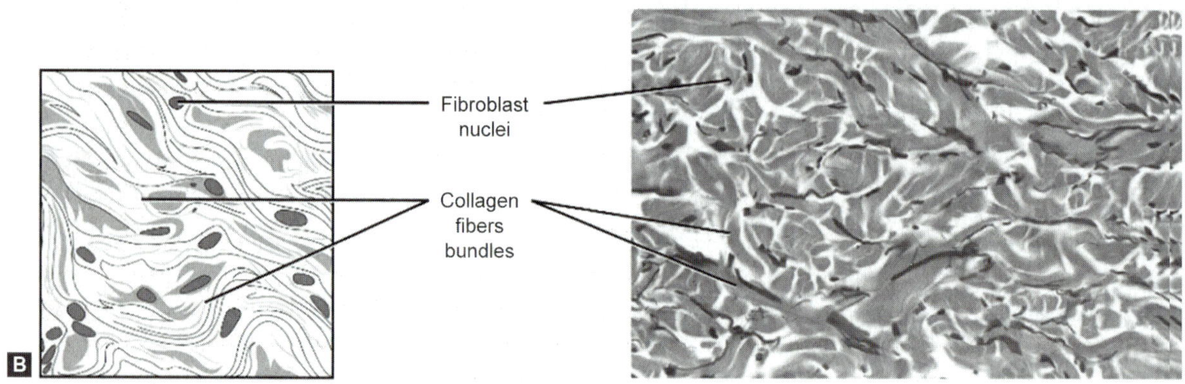

Figs 2.46A and B: (A) Regular and (B) irregular connective tissues

regular connective tissue. Tendons connect muscles to bones and ligaments connect a bone to another bone (Fig. 2.45).

Dense irregular connective tissue has fibers that are not arranged in parallel bundles (Fig. 2.46) as seen in dense regular connective tissue. The dense irregular connective tissues are found in the lower layers of the dermis part of the skin and the protective white layer of the eyeball.

Various examples of dense connective tissue are Elastic connective tissue, cartilage, and bone.

Elastic Connective Tissue (Fig. 2.47)

BAQ: Write a note on elastic connective tissue.

Ans: Elastic connective tissue is a dense connective tissue that contains a large number of elastic fibers in addition to collagen fibers. Elastic fibers allow the tissue to return to its original length after stretching. This type of connective tissue is present as an elastic layer in the wall of an artery.

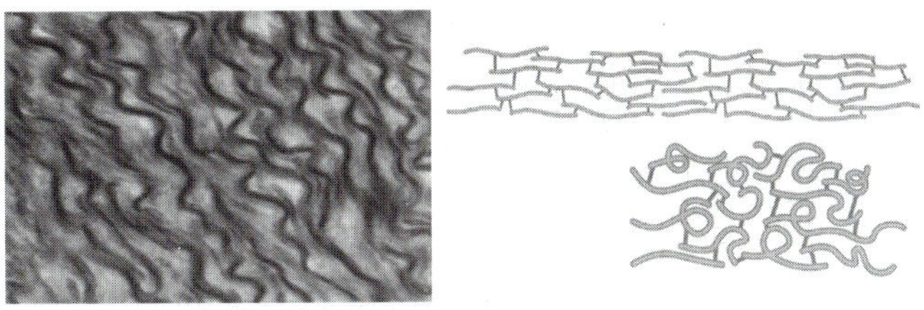

Fig. 2.47: Elastic connective tissue

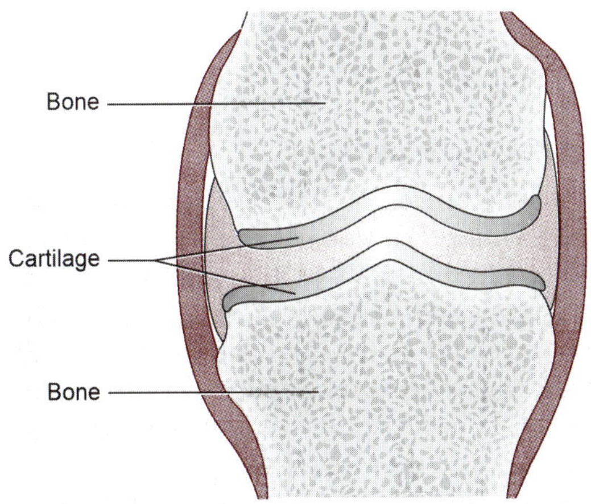

Fig. 2.48: Bone and cartilage difference

Cartilage (Figs 2.48 and 2.49)

BAQ: Write a note on cartilage.

Ans: Cartilage is a flexible dense connective tissue. It is avascular and contains specialized cells called chondrocytes, which are present within the matrix. The chondrocytes produce collagen and other specialized proteins, which stick together to form a gel-like, cartilaginous matrix. The cartilage provides shape to specific parts of the body and acts as a cushion between bones in joints (Fig. 2.48). The following are various examples of cartilage: Hyaline cartilage, elastic cartilage, fibrocartilage, etc.

Hyaline cartilage is found in the nose, larynx, trachea and ribs. It covers and protects bones (Fig. 2.49).

Elastic cartilage is found in the external ear, epiglottis and larynx. Elastic cartilage provides strength, and elasticity, and maintains the shape of certain organs such as the external ear (Fig. 2.49).

Fibrocartilage is found in ligaments, intervertebral discs, and joint capsules. Fibrocartilage provides tough material to the intervertebral discs and other parts in which it is present (Fig. 2.49).

Bone (Figs 2.50–2.52)

BAQ: Write a note on the bone.

Ans: Bone is the strongest dense connective tissue with a hard matrix of calcium and phosphorous. It contains specific bone cells known as osteoblasts and osteocytes.

The periosteum is the tough and thin outer membrane covering the bone. Muscles, ligaments, and tendons attach to the periosteum. The epiphyseal plate is a hyaline cartilage plate at each end of a long bone. Spongy bone is a porous type of bone (Fig 2.50). It contains a large number of blood capillaries and contains red bone marrow. Spongy bone is usually located at the ends of a long bone (the epiphyses), and surrounded by hard or compact bone. In the centre of a bone, the bone marrow is

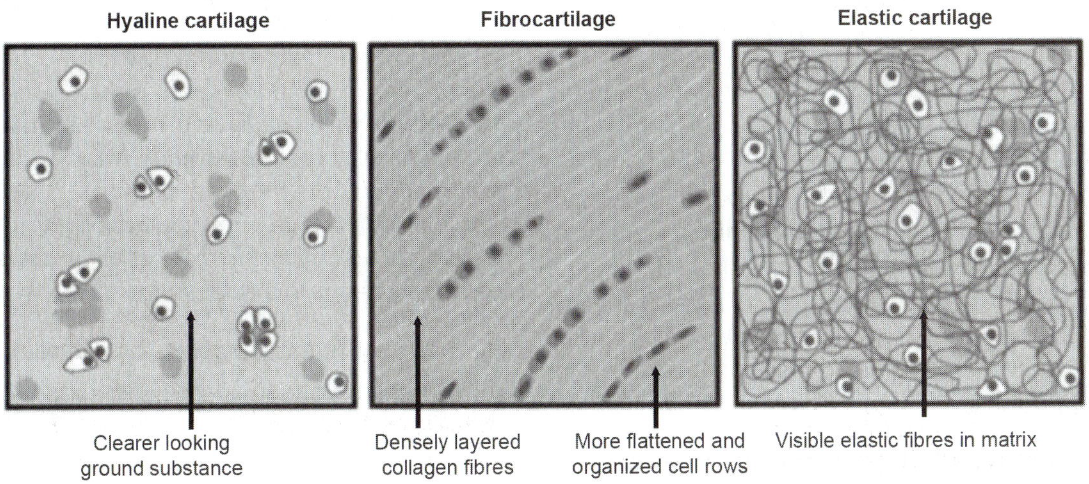

Fig. 2.49: Hyaline cartilage, fibrocartilage and elastic cartilage

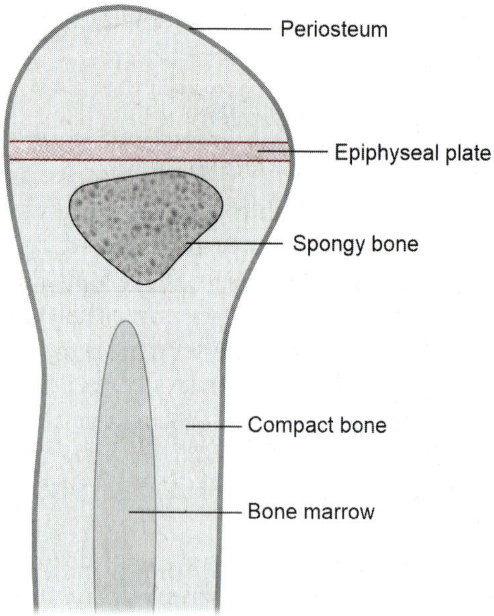

Fig. 2.50: Bone anatomy

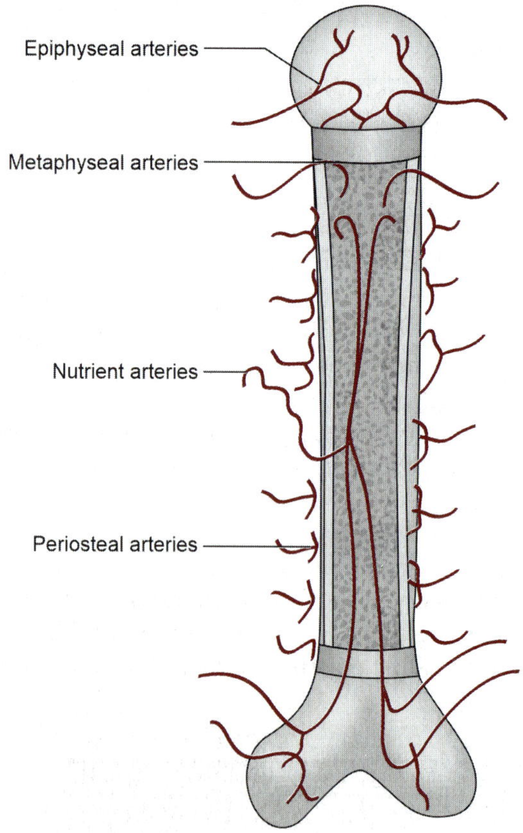

Fig. 2.51: Blood supply to bone

located. It is a spongy substance. Bone marrow produces bone marrow stem cells and other substances, which are capable of producing blood cells.

Beneath the hard outer shell of the periosteum tunnels and canals are present, through which blood and lymphatic vessels pass to carry nourishment for the bone cells (Fig. 2.51).

BAQ: Draw a labelled diagram of bone structure.

Ans: Refer to Fig. 2.52.

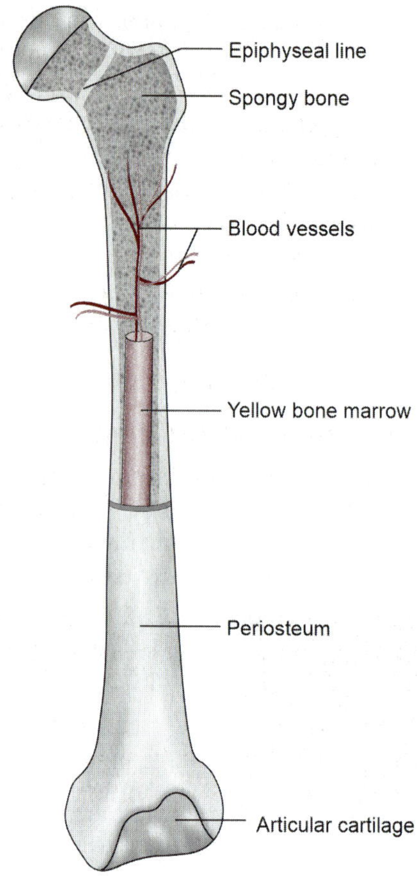

Fig. 2.52: Bone structure

Blood (Fig. 2.53)

BAQ: Write a note on blood.

Ans: Blood is a fluid connective tissue. An average of five litres of blood is present in the human body. Blood is made up of average 60–65% liquid and 35–40% solids. The liquid part is known as plasma, which contains about 90% water and 10% of solids. The solid is comprised of various proteins, enzymes, hormones and electrolytes and the solid part contains cells such as red blood cells, white blood cells, and platelets (Fig. 2.53).

The main function of the red blood cells (erythrocytes), is to carry oxygen from the lungs to the body tissues and carbon dioxide as a waste product, away from the tissues and back to the lungs, to expel in air.

White blood cells are part of the body's immune system. They help the body to fight against infectious organisms, cancer cells and other abnormal foreign components and protect the body from various diseases. Platelets are mainly responsible for the clotting of blood in the case of internal and external bleeding incidences and play a very important role in hemostasis (stopping bleeding from blood vessels).

SAQ: Enumerate the functions of connective tissues.

Ans: Connective tissues perform the following various functions in the body:

1. In the form of connective tissue sheaths, they support and connect other tissues.

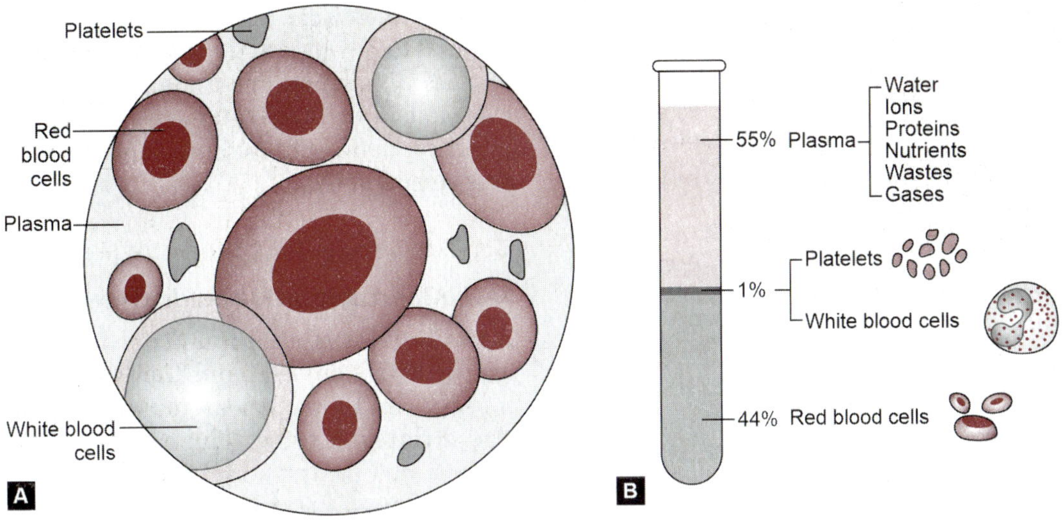

Figs 2.53A and B: Blood and blood components

2. Connective tissues protect the form of fibrous capsules and bones that protect delicate organs and the skeletal system.
3. Connective tissue in the form of blood contains specialized cells such as white blood cells and macrophages in tissues that defend the body from the entry of microorganisms.
4. Connective tissue in the form of blood and lymph, performs the following functions: Transport of fluids, nutrients, chemical messengers, waste products, etc.
5. Connective tissue in the form of adipose cells stores excess energy in the form of fat and contributes to the thermal insulation of the body.

MUSCLE TISSUE (Fig. 2.54)

SAQ: Write a note on muscle tissue.

Ans: Muscle tissue is composed of cells that have the unique ability to contract to facilitate movement of the body parts. The muscle tissue is highly cellular in nature and it is very well supplied with blood by blood vessels. Muscle tissue can be categorized into the following three types: (1) Skeletal muscle tissue, (2) smooth muscle tissue, and (3) cardiac muscle tissue.

Skeletal Muscle (Figs 2.54 and 2.55)

SAQ: Write a note on skeletal muscle.

Ans: Skeletal muscle tissue is made up of fibers that are cylindrical, multi-nucleated, and striated (having long thin lines, and marks of strips of colour). The skeletal muscles are under voluntary control. These are attached to bones by tendons, and they produce various types of movements of the body parts concerning each other. Unlike smooth muscle and cardiac muscle, skeletal muscle is under voluntary control.

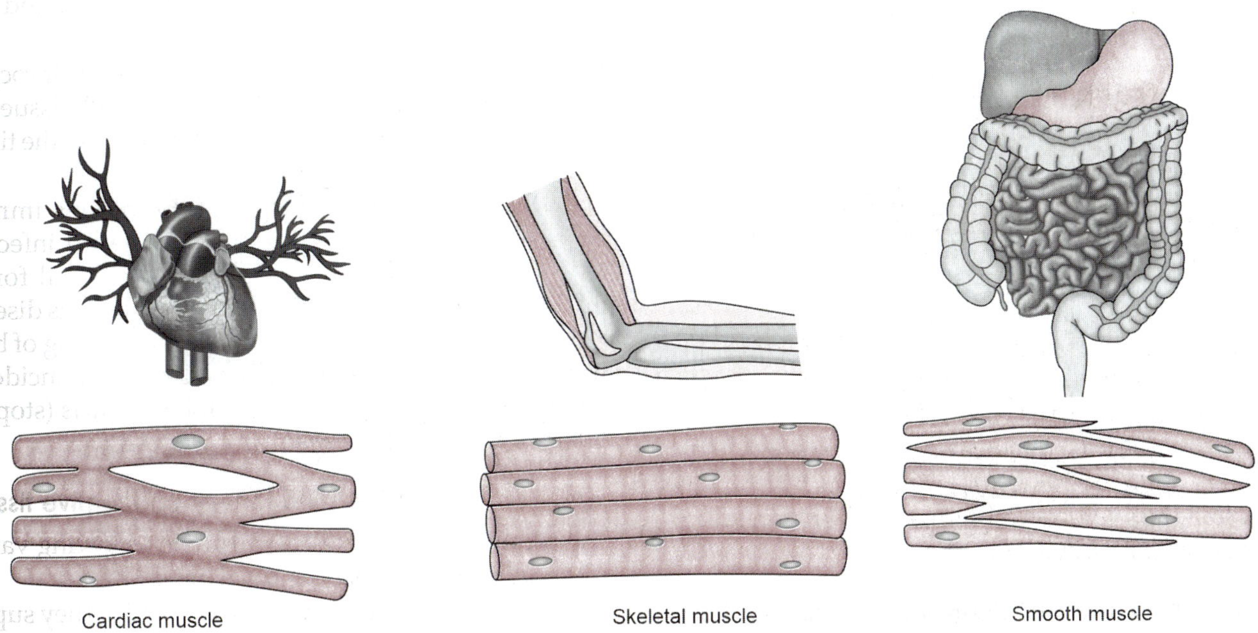

Fig. 2.54: Muscle tissues

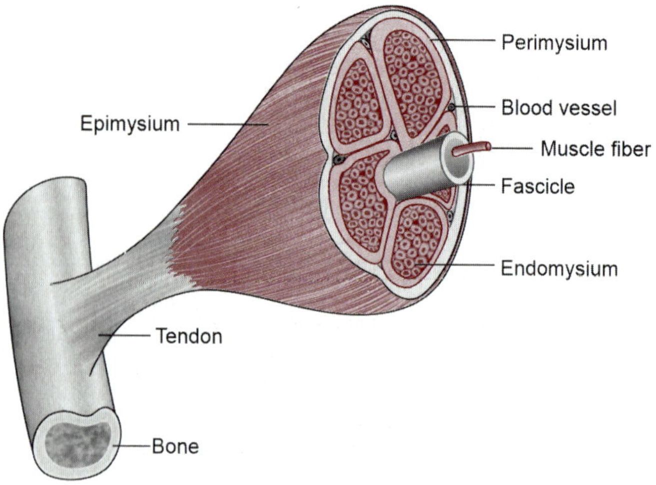

Fig. 2.55: Structure of skeletal muscle

Smooth Muscle (Fig. 2.56)

SAQ: Write a note on smooth muscle.

Ans: Smooth muscle is made up of spindle-shaped cells. The smooth muscle cell contains a centrally located, single nucleus. Smooth muscles lack striations. Smooth muscle is found in the walls of the respiratory tract, urinary tract, reproductive system, blood vessels, lymph vessels, and various hollow organs such as the uterus, stomach, intestines, and bladder.

Smooth muscle can be divided into the following two subgroups: (1) Single-unit smooth muscle and (2) Multi-unit smooth muscle.

Single-unit muscle cells are joined by intra-connections (gap junctions) so that the muscle contracts as a single unit. This type of smooth muscle is found in the walls of all visceral organs except the heart, which contains cardiac muscle in its walls.

Multi-unit smooth muscle is composed of cells that are mainly not interconnected. Hence, contraction does not spread from one cell to the next cell. Multiunit smooth muscle is found in airways leading to the lungs and also in large arteries.

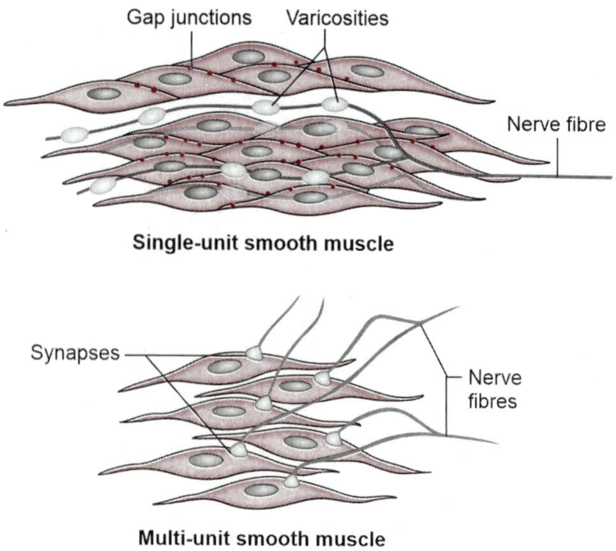

Fig. 2.56: Smooth muscle

Smooth muscle tissue contains special contractile proteins called actin and myosin. These proteins contract and relax to cause movement of the tissue. Smooth muscle contracts involuntarily, which means a reflex or action done without conscious control or will, like a sneeze or a yawn.

Cardiac Muscle (Myocardium) (Fig. 2.57)

SAQ: Write a note on the cardiac muscle (myocardium).

Ans: Cardiac muscle is found only in the heart wall. It is also known as myocardium. Cardiac muscle is contractile muscle, similar to skeletal muscle. It is an involuntary and striated muscle. The cardiac muscle performs coordinated contractions that allow the heart to pump blood through the circulatory system.

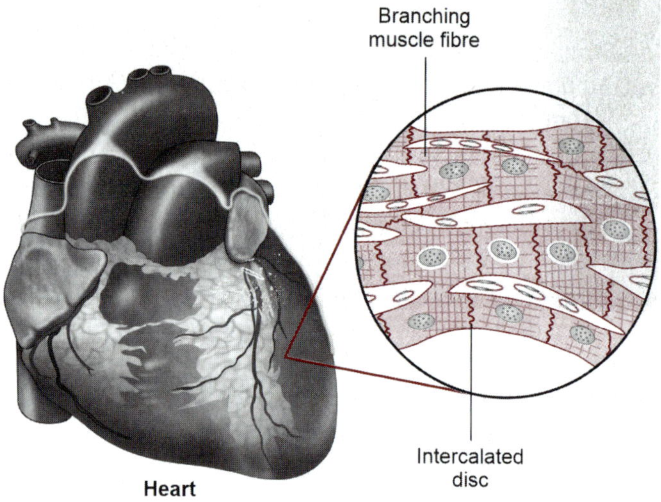

Fig. 2.57: Cardiac muscle

NERVOUS TISSUE (Figs 2.58–2.61)

SAQ: Write a note on nervous tissue.

Ans: Nervous tissue mainly consists of two types of cells, neurons and neuralgia. Nervous tissue is found in the brain, the spinal cord, and nerves. It is responsible for the coordination and control of many body activities. The basic unit of nervous tissue is a nerve cell. The nerve cells generate and conduct nerve impulses.

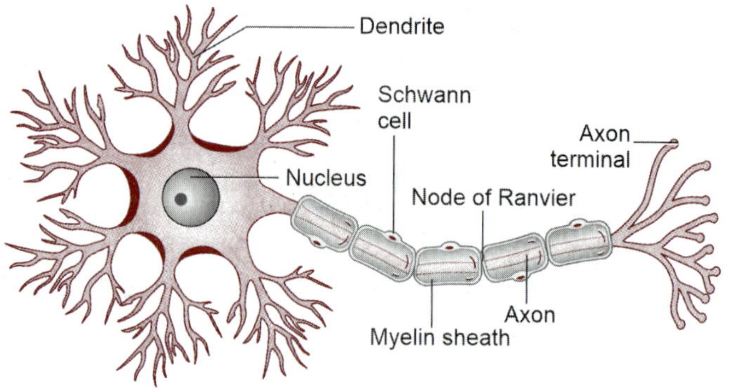

Fig. 2.58: Nerve cell (neuron)

SAQ: Write a note on the nerve cell (neuron).

Ans: The nerve cells (neurons) have three principal parts: Dendrites, cell body, and one axon. The basic structure of the neuron can be observed under a microscope. The basic structural components of an average neuron include the following components: Dendrite, cell body, nucleus, node of Ranvier, myelin sheath, Schwann cell, axon and axon terminal. The nerve cells in the nervous tissue generate and conduct nerve impulses (Figs 2.58 and 2.59).

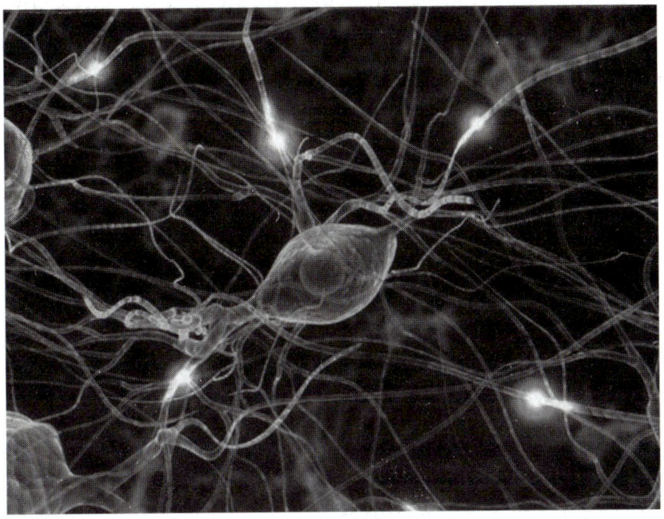

Fig. 2.59: Nerve impulses

BAQ: Draw a labelled diagram of nerve cells.

Ans: Refer to Figs 2.58 and 2.60.

The neuroglia (glial cell of glia) (Fig. 2.61)

BAQ: Write a note on the neuroglia (glial cells).

Ans: Based upon their appearance, function, and origin, the following four types of neuroglia cells have been identified in the central nervous system: (1) Astrocytes, (2) oligodendroglia, (3) ependymal cells, and (4) microglia. The neuroglia cell functions primarily to support neurons.

Astrocytes (Fig. 2.61)

Astrocytes are star-shaped cells with many connections. They are important components of the brain. They are closely associated with neuronal synapses. They play an important role in the transmission of electrical impulses within the brain.

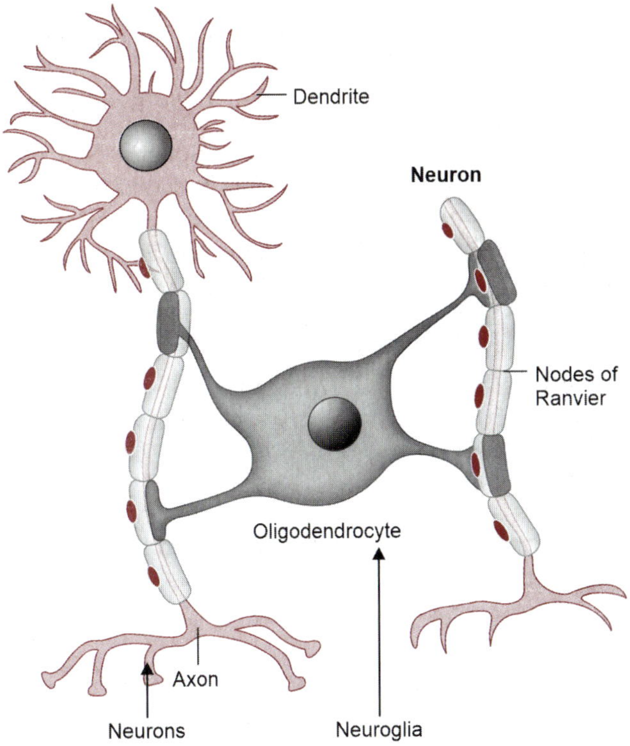

Fig. 2.60: Neurons and Neuroglia

Oligodendrocytes (Fig. 2.61)

Oligodendrocytes are similar to astrocytes. However, these have short and few connections. These cells form and modify myelin, a multilayered sheath of membrane, that is spirally wrapped around axon segments.

Microglia (Fig. 2.61)

Microglia are minute neuroglia cells that are located throughout the brain and spinal cord. They act as the first immune defence cells in the central nervous system and act by removing harmful microorganisms. These cells are also involved in the repair of damaged nerve tissue.

Ependymal Cells (Fig. 2.61)

Ependymal cells are simple columnar types of cells. These are important components of the epithelial lining of the cavities in the brain and the central canal of the spinal cord. Ependymal cells play an important role in the production and regulation of cerebrospinal fluid (CSF)

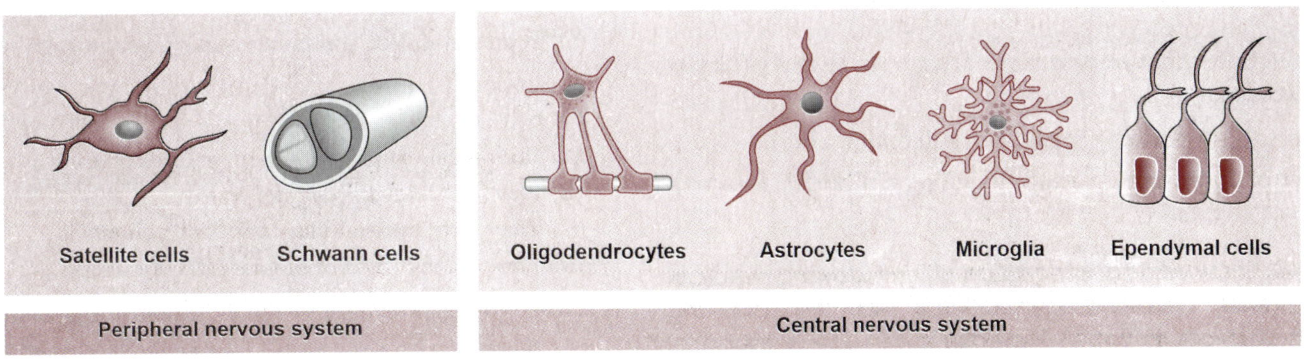

Fig. 2.61: Various types of neuroglia

Their top surfaces are covered by a layer of cilia, which circulate CSF around the central nervous system.

Schwann Cells (Fig. 2.61)

Schwann cells are the main glial cells in the peripheral nervous system. These cells play important roles in the development, maintenance, and regeneration of peripheral nerves. These cells form myelin sheaths and play an important role in the repair of damaged neurons.

Satellite Cells (Fig. 2.61)

Satellite cells are small, flattened cells found in the nerve cell bodies of the peripheral nervous system. These are responsible for regulating and stabilising the environment around nerve cell bodies.

BAQ: Draw a labelled diagram of various types of neuroglia.

Ans: Refer to Fig. 2.61.

> **Objective:** To understand and explain the central theme of competency-based medical and paramedical education (CBME): Horizontal and vertical integration of subjects.

BAQ: Show horizontal integration of paramedical subjects: Physiology and biochemistry, with the following anatomical change: Inflammation of mucosal cells of the pharynx (pharyngitis).

Ans:

Horizontal Integration with Physiology

Difficulty in the swallowing process of food through the oesophagus.

Horizontal Integration with Biochemistry

Initiation of inflammatory reactions that involve the production of prostaglandins, bradykinins, leukotrienes, etc., by the immune cells, at the site of inflammation.

BAQ: Show vertical integration of the paramedical subjects: microbiology, pharmacology and preventive medicine, with the following anatomical change: Inflammation of mucosal cells of the pharynx.

Ans:

Vertical Integration with Microbiology

Identification of infectious organisms.

Vertical Integration with Pharmacology

Selection of an appropriate drug to cure the pharynx infection.

Vertical Integration with Preventive Medicine

Use of appropriate vaccine to prevent microbial infection (pharyngitis).

BAQ: Show vertical integration of the following medical subjects: Obstetrics–gynecology with the following anatomical change: Increase in the size of mucosal cells of the pharynx (pharyngitis).

Ans:

Vertical Integration with Obstetrics and Gynecology

Complete cure of the throat infection for the normal course of pregnancy and to prevent the infection from passing to the fetus.

BIBLIOGRAPHY

1. Medical Biochemistry, 1st Edition (2023). Godkar PB, Godkar DP, CBS Publishers, New Delhi, India.
2. Textbook of Medical Laboratory Technology, 4th Edition, (2024). Godkar PB, Godkar DP, Bhalani Publishing House, Mumbai, India.
3. Anatomy of the Human Body. 42nd Edition. Henry Gray, Editor-in-chief: Susan Standring, Elsevier (2020).
4. Ross and Wilson Anatomy and Physiology in Health and Illness, 13th Edition, by Allison Wynn Grant, Anne Waugh, and Kathleen J. W. Wilson (2018).
5. Schaum's outline of theory and problems of Human Anatomy and Physiology, 2nd Edition (1997), Tata MaGraw-Hill Publishing Company Limited, New Delhi, India.

MULTIPLE CHOICE QUESTIONS (MCQs)

Select the correct option.

1. These are located in the mitochondria:

(A) Cytochrome oxidase (B) Succinate dehydrogenase
(C) Amylase (D) Both (A) and (B)

2. The most active site of protein synthesis:

(A) Nucleus (B) Ribosome
(C) Mitochondrion (D) Cell sap

3. Mitochondrial DNA is:

(A) Circular double-stranded
(B) Circular single-stranded
(C) Linear double helix
(D) None of these

4. These are cellular organelles called "suicide bags":

(A) Lysosomes (B) Ribosomes
(C) Nucleolus (D) Golgi bodies

5. The Golgi complex:

(A) Synthesizes proteins
(B) Produces ATP
(C) Provides a pathway for transporting chemicals
(D) Forms modified components like glycoproteins

6. The following points about microfilaments are true, *except*:

(A) They form cytoskeleton with microtubules
(B) They provide support and shape
(C) They form intracellular conducting channels
(D) They are involved in muscle cell contraction

7. The following substances are cell inclusions, *except*:

(A) Melanin (B) Glycogen
(C) Lipids (D) Vitamins

8. Enzymes catalyzing electron transport are present mainly in the:

(A) Ribosomes
(B) Endoplasmic reticulum
(C) Lysosomes
(D) Inner mitochondrial membrane

9. rRNA is produced mainly in the:

(A) Endoplasmic reticulum
(B) Ribosome
(C) Nucleolus
(D) Nucleus

10. Genetic information of nuclear DNA is transmitted to the site of protein synthesis by:

(A) rRNA (B) mRNA
(C) tRNA (D) Polysomes

11. The powerhouse of the cell is:

(A) Nucleus (B) Cell membrane
(C) Mitochondria (D) Lysosomes

12. The digestive enzymes of cellular compounds are confined to:

(A) Lysosomes (B) Ribosomes
(C) Peroxisomes (D) Polysomes

13. Which group is involved in manufacturing substances needed by the cell?

(A) Lysosome, vacuole, ribosome
(B) Ribosome, rough ER, smooth ER
(C) Vacuole, rough ER, smooth ER
(D) Smooth ER, ribosome, vacuole

14. Which of the following clues would tell you whether a cell is prokaryotic or eukaryotic?

(A) The presence or absence of a rigid cell wall
(B) Whether or not the cell is partitioned by internal membranes
(C) The presence or absence of ribosomes
(D) Whether or not the cell contains double-stranded DNA

15. When a cell undergoes mitosis:

(A) The daughter cells have identical genes.
(B) The amount of cytoplasm in the mother cell and in each of the daughter cells is equal.
(C) There is an exact duplication and division of all of the organelles between daughter cells.
(D) Both (A) and (B)

16. When a eukaryotic cell divides, the daughter cells:

(A) Manufacture all the organelles from material in the cytoplasm.
(B) Receive enough of the organelles to start up the new cells and produce additional organelles as needed.
(C) Produce individual organelles that attach to the spindle fibers and are distributed just like chromosomes.
(D) Produce an equal number of organelles distributed to each cell.

17. Mitosis and meiosis are divisions of the:

(A) Nucleus (B) Cytoplasm
(C) Chromosomes (D) Nucleus and chromosomes

18. Chromatids that are attached at the centromere are called:

(A) Mother chromatids
(B) Daughter chromatids
(C) Sister chromatids
(D) Either (A) or (B)

19. The number of DNA molecules present in a duplicated chromosome is:

(A) 1
(B) 4
(C) Half that of an unduplicated chromosome
(D) 2

20. In mitosis, if a parent cell has 16 chromosomes, each daughter cell will have:

(A) 64 chromosomes (B) 32 chromosomes
(C) 16 chromosomes (D) 8 chromosomes

21. Term used to describe cells with two of each kind of chromosome is:

(A) Polyploid (B) Diploid
(C) Triploid (D) Haploid

22. Chromosomes are duplicated during which portion of the cell cycle?

(A) M (B) G1
(C) G2 (D) S

23. The interval before the onset of DNA replication is:

(A) The G1 stage (B) The G2 stage
(C) The M stage (D) The S stage

24. The spindle apparatus begins to become visible during:

(A) Anaphase (B) Metaphase
(C) Interphase (D) Prophase

25. The chromosomes are aligned at the spindle equator during:

(A) Anaphase (B) Metaphase
(C) Interphase (D) Prophase

26. The nuclear membrane reforms during:

(A) Anaphase (B) Metaphase
(C) Interphase (D) Telophase

27. The distribution of cytoplasm to daughter cells is accomplished during:

(A) Prokaryotic fission (B) Mitosis
(C) Meiosis (D) Cytokinesis

28. If meiosis did not occur in sexually reproducing organisms:

(A) Growth of the zygote would be halted
(B) Eggs would be haploid, but sperm would be diploid
(C) Gametes would be haploid
(D) The chromosome number would double in each generation.

29. Sexual reproduction:

(A) Leads to uniform characteristics in a population
(B) Results in new combinations of genetic traits
(C) Produces genetic clones
(D) Either (B) or (C)

30. Employing meiosis:

(A) Alternate forms of genes are shuffled
(B) Parental DNA is divided and distributed to form gametes
(C) The diploid chromosome number is reduced to haploid
(D) All of the above

31. A group of cells similar in form, function and organ is known as:

(A) Simple tissue (B) Complex tissue
(C) Organ system (D) Organ

32. This is not a function of epithelial tissue:

(A) It covers the outer surface of the organ and lines the inner surface of cavities
(B) It produces immunoglobulins
(C) It protects the body from injury, chemicals and microbes
(D) It may be secretory in nature

33. Collagen is present in:

(A) Muscle fiber (B) White fiber
(C) Yellow fiber (D) Both (A) and (B)

34. Yellow fiber is made up of:

(A) Collagen (B) Reticulin
(C) Elastin (D) Both (A) and (C)

35. By these muscles are joined to the bones:

(A) Areolar tissue
(B) Ligament
(C) Membrane
(D) Both (A) and (B)

36. One bone is joined with another bone by this tissue:

(A) Tendon (B) Ligament
(C) Blood (D) All of these

37. These are cardiac muscles:

(A) Branched and with single nucleus
(B) Unbranched and multinucleated
(C) Uninucleate unstriated
(D) None of these

38. This one is the fat-storing tissue in the body:

(A) Areolar tissue (B) Muscles
(C) Adipose tissue (D) Cartilage

39. Cartilage has widely spaced cells and a solid matrix consists of:

(A) Fat globules and sugars
(B) Magnesium compounds
(C) Calcium and phosphate compounds
(D) Protein and sugars

40. The following tissue may secretary glands:

(A) Muscles (B) Areolar tissue
(C) Epithelial tissue (D) Connective tissue

41. One of the following is a connective tissue:

(A) Epithelial tissue (B) Blood
(C) Muscle (D) Nervous tissue

42. This type of tissue covers the external surface of the body and organs:

(A) Connective tissue (B) Epithelial tissue
(C) Muscle tissue (D) Nervous tissue

43. This type of tissue is responsible for voluntary movements in the human body:

(A) Muscle tissue (B) Epithelial tissue
(C) Nervous tissue (D) Connective tissue

44. The basement membrane is specifically present in:

(A) Nervous tissue (B) Connective tissue
(C) Muscle tissue (D) Epithelial tissue

45. Globlet cells are specifically present in:

(A) Unicellular gland (B) Intracellular gland
(C) Salivary gland (D) Multicellular gland

46. This is an example of a holocrine gland:

(A) Salivary gland (B) Sebaceous gland
(C) Sweat gland (D) Pancreatic gland

ANSWERS

1. D	2. B	3. A	4. A	5. D	6. C	7. D
8. D	9. C	10. B	11. C	12. A	13. B	14. D
15. A	16. B	17. D	18. C	19. D	20. C	21. B
22. D	23. A	24. D	25. B	26. D	27. D	28. D
29. B	30. D	31. A	32. B	33. B	34. C	35. B
36. B	37. A	38. C	39. D	40. C	41. B	42. B
43. A	44. D	45. A	46. B			

MATCH THE COLUMNS

I	II
1. Nucleus	A. Capillary walls
2. Smooth endoplasmic reticulum	B. Urinary bladder lining
3. Golgi apparatus	C. Urinary bladder lining
4. Lysosome	D. Cell control centre
5. Simple squamous epithelium	E. Seminal vesicle
6. Simple columnar epithelium	F. Detoxification and synthesis of steroids
7. Transitional epithelium	G. Intestinal gland
8. Simple acinar gland	H. Formation of lysosomes
9. Simple tubular gland	I. Intestinal wall
10. Compound tubular gland	J. Contain hydrolytic enzymes

ANSWERS

1. D	2. F	3. H	4. J	5. A	6. C	7. C
8. E	9. G	10. I				

CHAPTER

3

Integumentary System

SAQ: Short answer question: Marks: 2	**MCQs:** Multiple choice questions: Marks: 0.5 each
BAQ: Brief answer question: Marks: 4 or 5	**Match the columns:** Marks: 0.5 each
LAQ: Long answer question: Marks: 9 or 10	**Draw a labelled diagram:** Marks: 5

Objective: To enumerate and discuss the components of the integumentary system and their respective functions.

INTRODUCTION (Fig. 3.1)

BAQ: Write a short note on the integumentary system.

Ans: The integumentary system (Fig. 3.1) comprises the skin and its following appendages: The epidermis, dermis, hypodermis, hair, nails and exocrine glands associated with the skin. The skin is the largest organ in the body and the average thickness of human skin is about 1.5 millimeters. The average weight of skin is about 4.5 kg and it has a surface area of about 20 square feet.

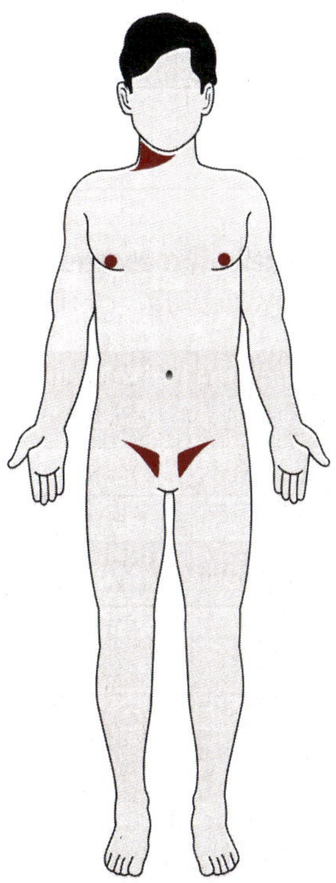

Fig. 3.1: Integumentary system

The integumentary system forms a physical barrier between the external environment and the internal environment and serves to protect the body from microorganisms, dehydration, ultraviolet light, and mechanical damage.

In addition to the barrier function, the integumentary system also performs other functions such as regulation of body temperature and cell fluid and synthesis of vitamin D. The integumentary system detects stimuli, and senses pain, temperature, touch, and deep pressure. In addition to secreting sweat to cool the body, the exocrine glands of the skin also excrete waste products out of the body.

SAQ: Why the skin is considered an organ?

Ans: The skin is considered an organ since it is comprised of several kinds of tissues that function together.

Objective: To describe the embryonic origin of the skin.

SAQ: What is the embryonic origin of the skin?

Ans: By the eleventh week of embryonic development the main layers of the skin are formed. The epidermis is derived from the ectoderm germ layer. The dermis and the hypodermis are derived from the mesoderm germ layer.

COMPONENTS OF THE INTEGUMENTARY SYSTEM

Objectives:
- To list and describe the layers of the integumentary system.
- To describe the structural layers and functions of the epidermis.

Epidermis (Figs 3.2 and 3.3)

BAQ: Write a note on the epidermis layer of the skin.

Ans: The epidermis is the most superficial layer of the skin and 90% of it is made up of keratinocyte cells (Fig. 3.2). It covers mostly the entire surface of the body. The epidermis covers and protects the thicker and deeper dermis layer (Figs 3.3A, B). The epidermis layer is an avascular region. It is about 0.1 mm thick and made of 40 to 50 rows of layered squamous epithelial cells. The cells of the epidermis receive all of their nutrients through the diffusion of fluids from the dermis layer.

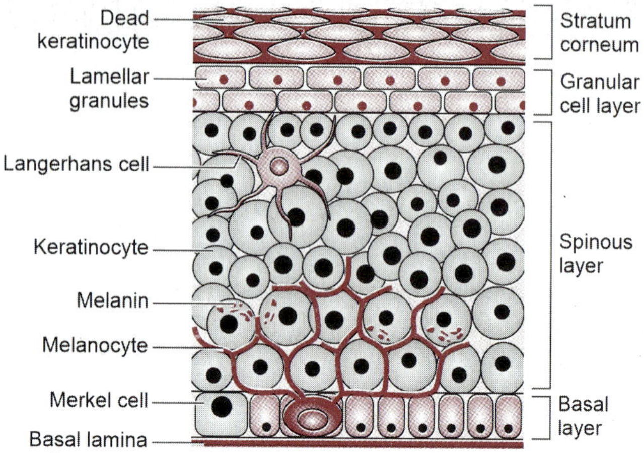

Fig. 3.2: Various cells of the epidermis

The deepest region of the epidermis is the stratum basale (SB). It contains stem cells, which are capable of reproducing all other cells of the epidermis. The cells of the stratum basale are cuboidal keratinocytes, melanocytes, and Merkel cells. Above the stratum basale is the stratum spinosum (SS) layer. In this layer, Langerhans cells are found along with many rows of spiny keratinocytes held together by desmosomes (Fig. 3.4).

The epidermis is made up of various cells such as keratinocytes (90%), melanocytes (8%), Langerhans cells (1%) and Merkel cells (1%).

Keratinocytes develop from stem cells at the base of the epidermis. Keratinocytes produce and store the keratin protein, which makes the keratinocytes tough, scaly and water-resistant. Melanocytes produce the pigment melanin, which protects the skin from ultraviolet radiation and sunburn. Langerhans cells are capable of detecting and fighting pathogens that may try to enter the body through the skin. Merkel cells have a very important ability to sense touch. Merkel cells are connected to nerve endings in the dermis to sense light touch.

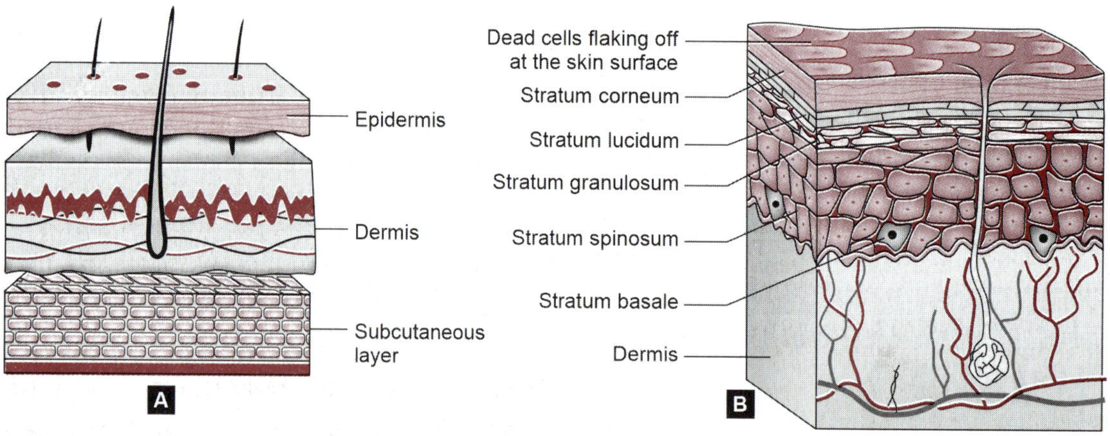

Fig. 3.3: (A) Main layers of skin, (B) anatomy of epidermis

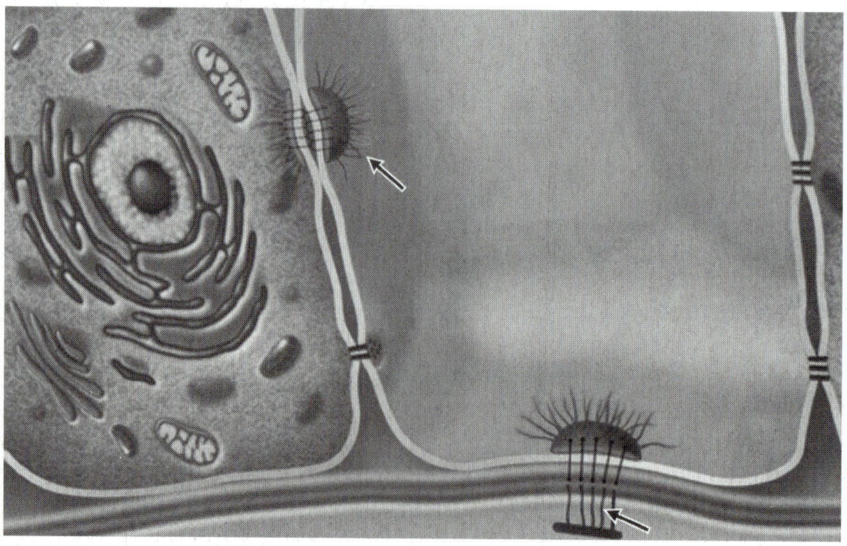
Fig. 3.4: Desmosomes holding the cells

SAQ: Name various cells of the epidermis and their functions.

Ans: Keratinocytes produce and store the keratin protein, which makes the keratinocytes tough, scaly and water-resistant. Melanocytes produce the pigment melanin, which protects the skin from ultraviolet radiation and sunburn. Langerhans cells are capable of detecting and fighting pathogens that may try to enter the body through the skin. Merkel cells have a very important ability to sense touch.

BAQ: Draw a labelled diagram of the anatomy of the epidermis.

Ans: Refer to Fig. 3.3B.

> *Note:* Cell division (mitosis) of skin cells occurs in the deep stratum basale and partly in the stratum spinosum since these layers are close to blood capillaries, which supply nutrients and oxygen to dividing cells. As the cells divide longitudinally, only about 50% of the cells remain in proximity to the dermis layer. Remaining cells are pushed away from the blood capillaries and cellular death occurs. As the keratinocytes degenerate, the keratinization process forms tough and waterproof keratin skin. When the cells move further, they become flattened and with a scale-like appearance which leads to cornification. The dead cells act as a buffer to the external environment.

SAQ: What is the eleidin protein of the skin?

Ans: The eleidin protein is present in the stratum lucidum layer of the epidermis. It is a transformation product of the amino acid complex keratohyalin, a lifeless matter deposited in the form of minute granules. The eleidin facilitates the protective and water-repellent function of the skin.

SAQ: What is a callus?

Ans: A callus (Fig. 3.5) is an overdevelopment of the stratum corneum of palms and soles due to pressure on the skin of the area. It protects against mechanical abrasion.

SAQ: What is a blister?

Ans: A blister (Fig. 3.6) is a vesicle of interstitial fluid seen between the stratum basale and the stratum spinosum layers. It develops in response to hard friction on the surface of the skin and serves as a cushion to protect the delicate stratum basale layer.

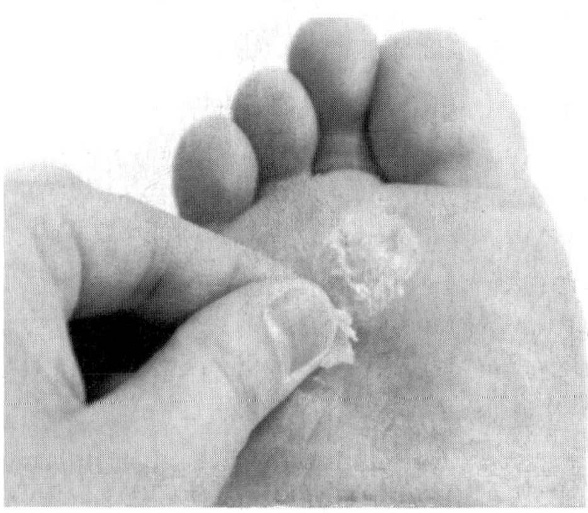

Fig. 3.5: Callus on the skin

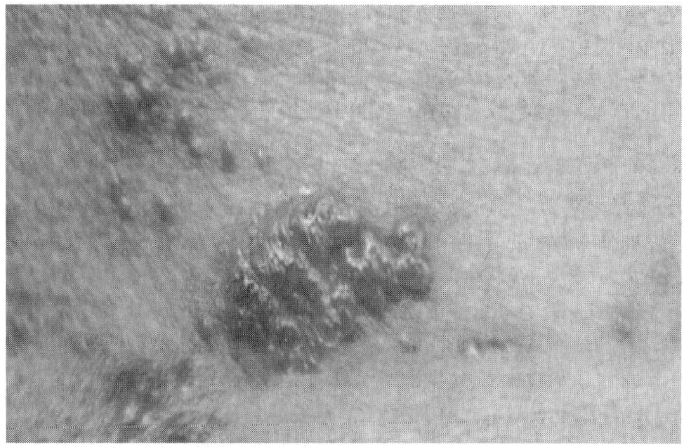

Fig. 3.6: Skin blisters

SAQ: What is a boil or furuncle?

Ans: A boil or furuncle (Fig. 3.7) is a localized bacterial infection originating in the hair follicle or skin gland. Carbuncle is similar to boil but involves a subcutaneous layer of skin (Fig. 3.8).

BAQ: Draw a labelled diagram of the epidermis.

Ans: Refer to Fig. 3.2.

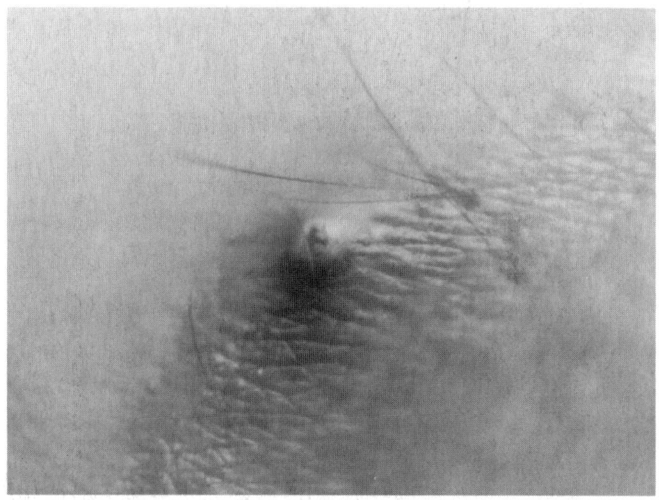

Fig. 3.7: Skin boil

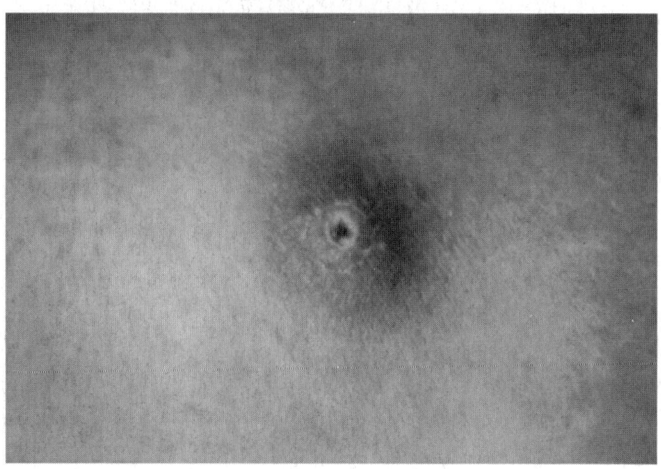

Fig. 3.8: Skin carbuncle

Objective: To describe the structural layers and functions of the dermis.

Dermis (Figs 3.9 and 3.10)

BAQ: Write a note on the anatomy of the dermis.

Ans: The dermis is a layer of the skin found below the epidermis (Fig. 3.9). The dermis is thicker than the epidermis and it gives strength and elasticity to the skin. It is mostly made of dense irregular connective tissue along with nervous tissue, blood, and blood vessels. The dermis contains two distinct regions: (1) The papillary layer and (2) the reticular layer (Fig. 3.10).

The papillary layer is the superficial layer of the dermis, which covers the epidermis. The papillary layer contains many finger-like extensions called dermal papillae which protrude towards the epidermis. The dermal papillae increase the surface area of the dermis and contain many blood vessels and nerves that are projected toward the surface of the skin. Nutrients and oxygen are provided by blood flowing through the dermal papillae for the cells of the epidermis. The nerves of the dermal papillae are responsible for feeling temperature, touch and pain through the cells of the epidermis.

The reticular layer is the thicker and tougher part of the dermis. It is the deeper layer of the dermis. The reticular layer is made of dense irregular connective tissue that contains collagen and elastin fibers, which provide strength and elasticity to the skin. The reticular layer also contains blood vessels to supply nutrients to the skin cells and nerve tissue to sense pain and pressure in the skin.

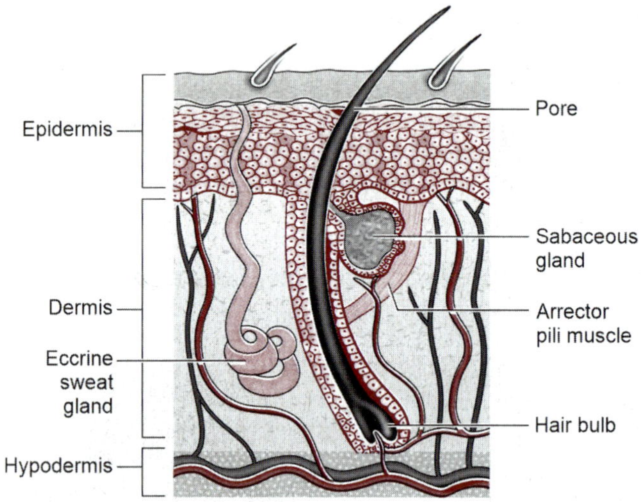

Fig. 3.9: Anatomy of dermis

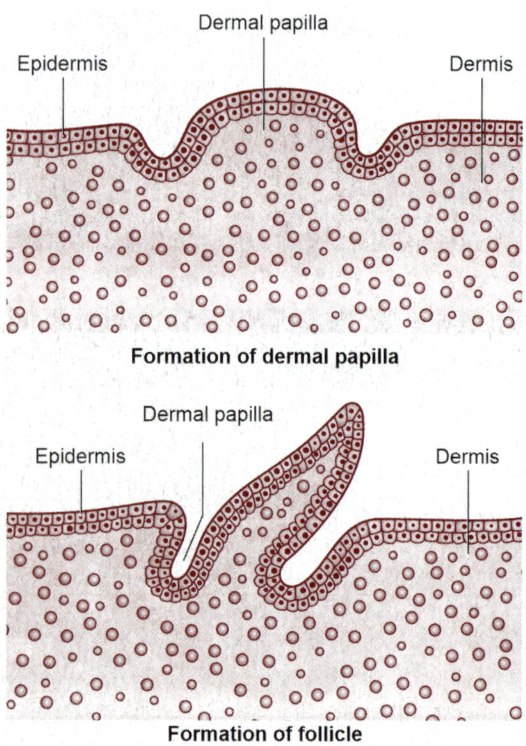

Fig. 3.10: Dermal papilla and follicle

Hypodermis (Fig. 3.11)

Objective: To describe the structural layers and functions of the hypodermis.

BAQ: Write a note on the anatomy of hypodermis.

Ans: Hypodermis is present deep inside the dermis (Fig. 3.11). The hypodermis is also known as subcutis or subcutaneous tissue. It is a layer of loose connective tissues. The hypodermis acts as the flexible connection between the skin, muscles below the skin, bones and adipose tissue. In the hypodermis, areolar connective tissue contains loosely arranged elastin and collagen fibres. Due to areolar connective tissue, the skin is able to stretch and move independently of its underlying structures. Hypodermis also contains adipose tissue containing triglycerides. Adipose tissue also acts as an insulator for the body. Females have thicker hypodermis compared to that of a males, due to the greater deposition of fats in this tissue.

BAQ: Draw a labelled diagram of hypodermis.

Ans: Refer to Fig. 3.11.

Objective: To describe the various skin disorders.

BAQ: What is the significance of discolouration of the skin?

Ans: The discolouration of the skin may indicate a specific dysfunction. For example, cyanosis is a bluish discolouration of skin that appears in persons with certain respiratory (carbon monoxide poisoning) or cardiovascular disease (Fig. 3.12). In jaundice, skin may appear yellowish (Fig. 3.13). Erythema is a redness of skin due to vascular trauma (Fig. 3.14).

Objective: To describe the various skin disorders.

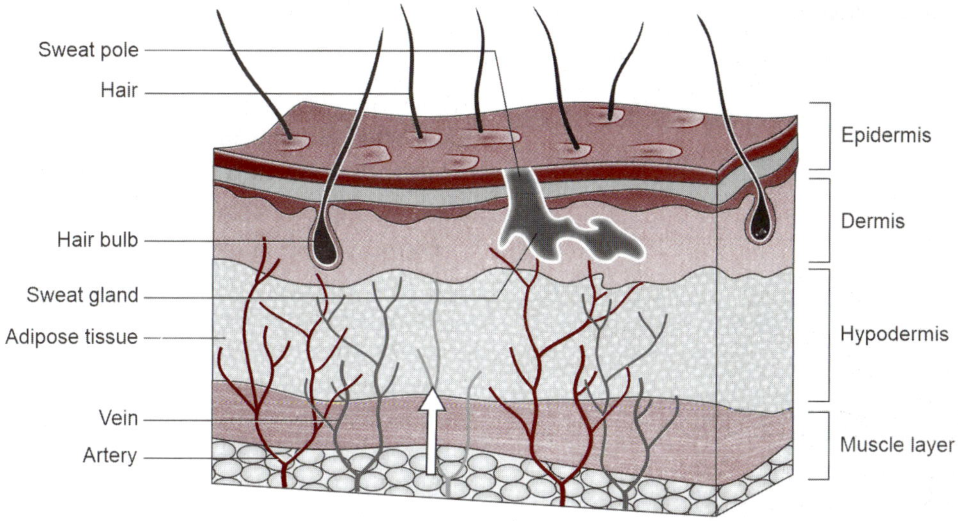

Fig. 3.11: Hypodermis (subcutaneous tissue) part of skin

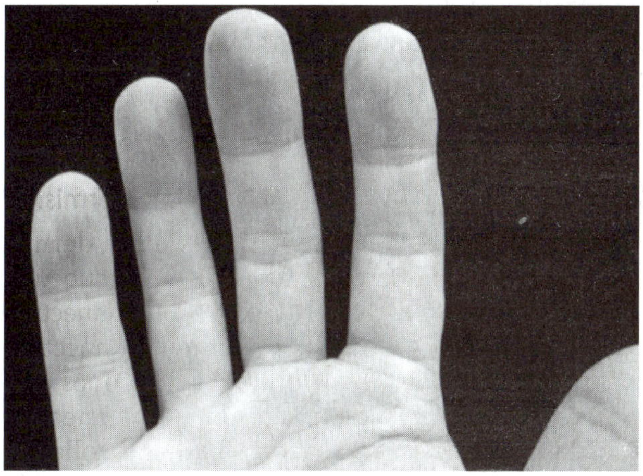

Fig. 3.12: Bluish skin in cyanosis

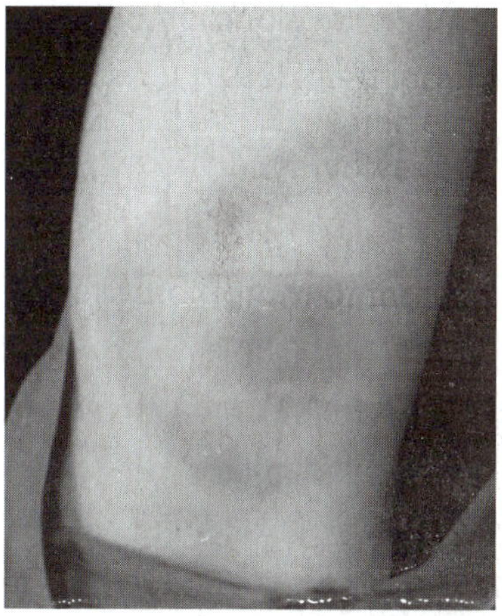

Fig. 3.14: Erythema

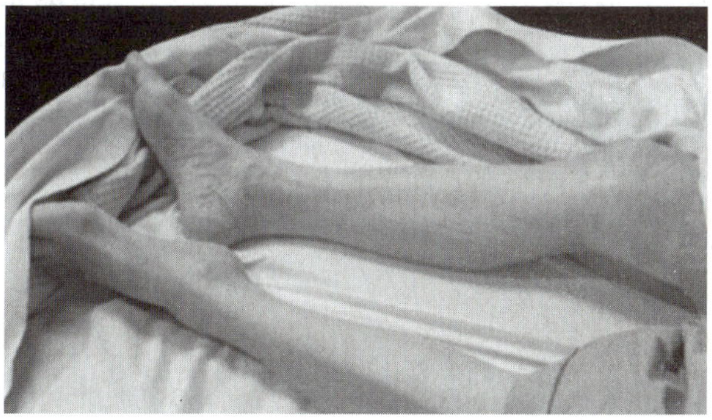

Fig. 3.13: Yellow skin in jaundice

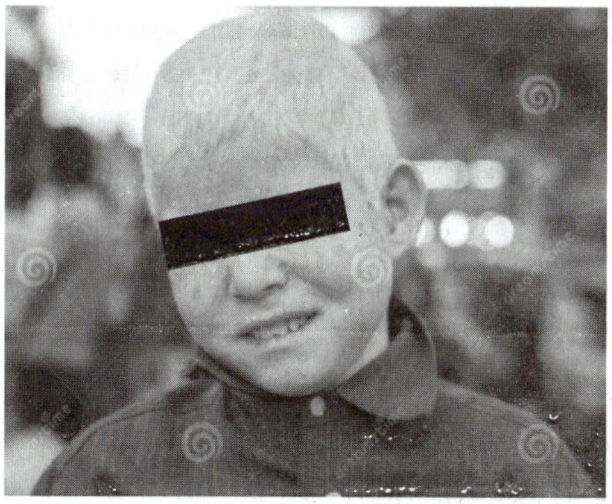

Fig. 3.15: White skin in albinism

SAQ: What is the importance of the physical examination of the skin by a physician?

Ans: The physical examination of the skin by a physician considers texture, colour and responsiveness. The physical examination provides useful information regarding the health of the skin and also the indication of certain clinical conditions. For example, the yellow colour of the skin (Fig. 3.13) indicates jaundice and the pale colour of the skin indicates anaemia. Similarly, the bluish colour of the skin indicates cyanosis (Fig. 3.12).

SAQ: What is albinism?

Ans: In albinism, the skin of the affected person appears white. The skin of a normal person contains normal melanocytes, which are capable of producing melanin, which imparts dark colour to the skin. However, in albinism, due to a genetic defect, there is a lack of enzyme tyrosinase, which converts the amino acid tyrosine to melanin. In the absence of tyrosinase, tyrosine is not converted to melanin and the skin of the affected person appears white (Fig. 3.15).

SAQ: What are friction ridges?

Ans: Friction ridges are unique to an individual. These are print patterns that occur on the anterior surface of the hands and the plantar surface of the feet. The friction ridges are prominent on the skin covering digits and are known as fingerprints (Fig. 3.16).

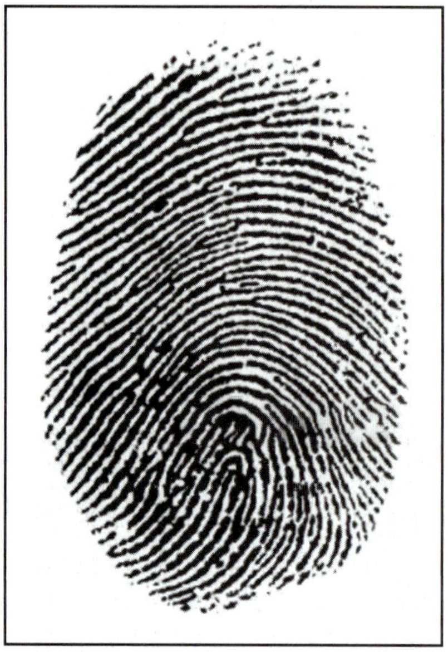

Fig. 3.16: Fingerprint

SAQ: What are bedsores?

Ans: Bedsores (decubitus ulcers) are ulcerated wounds that may occur in the case of weak and elderly patients, who lie in one position for very long periods of time.

A bedsore develops due to reduced blood supply to the skin for a longer phase. The skin dies and the bedsore first appears as a red and painful area. The colour of the bedsores, later on, becomes pale purple (Fig. 3.17). Eventually, the skin breaks open and the affected skin area becomes susceptible to infections.

In the case of a bed-ridden patient, the bedsores usually develop below the waist. However, bedsores can occur on the elbows, hips, knees, ankles, heels, shoulder blades, between fingers and toes, the base of the spine.

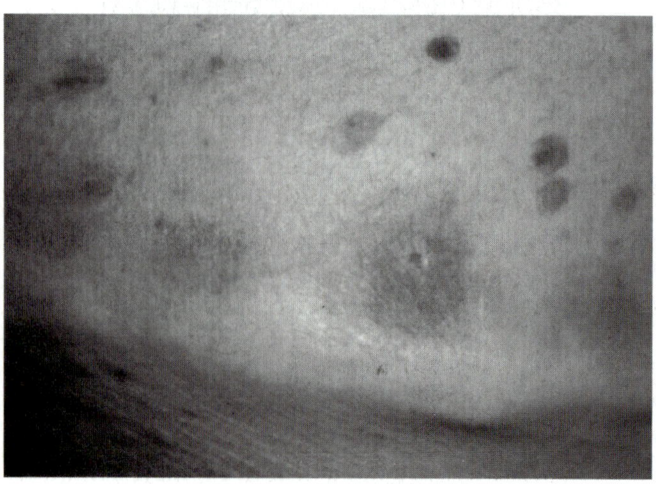

Fig. 3.17: Bedsores

Objective: To describe the structural layers and functions of hair.

HAIR (Figs 3.18 and 3.19)

BAQ: Write a note on hair under the following heads: (1) Introduction and (2) applied anatomy.

Ans:

1. **Introduction:** Hair is an accessory organ of the skin. Hair is derived from the epidermis, however grows its roots deep into the dermis. The arrector pili muscles in the dermis attach to hair follicles and help the shaft to stand and trap air close to the epidermis for temperature control. The hair structure divides into the externally visible hair shaft and the hair follicle within the skin (Fig. 3.18). It is made of tightly packed columns of dead keratinocytes. Three main parts of hair are the follicle, root, and shaft (Fig. 3.19). The hair follicle is present deep into the dermis as a depression of epidermal cells (Fig. 3.18). The hair follicles contain stem cells which reproduce to form the keratinocytes that form the hair (Fig. 3.18). Melanocytes produce melanin pigment which gives the hair a specific colour. The hair root is present within the follicles below the skin. The hair shaft is the part of the hair seen outside of the skin.

Hair Anatomy and Functions (Fig. 3.19)

2. **Applied anatomy**: The hair shaft and root are made up of three specific layers of the cells, cuticle, cortex,

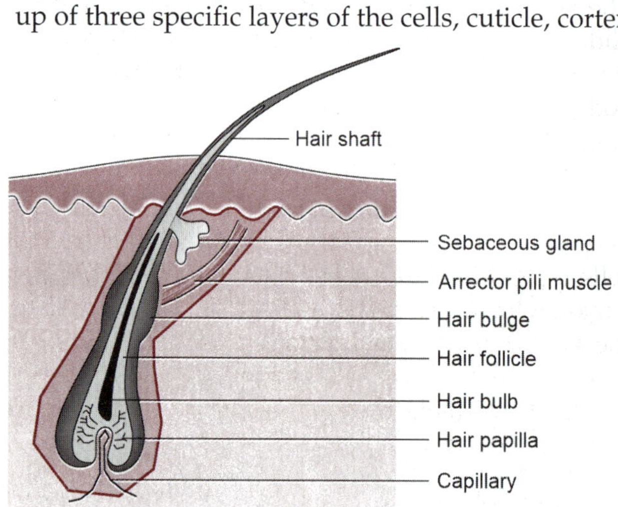

Fig. 3.18: Hair

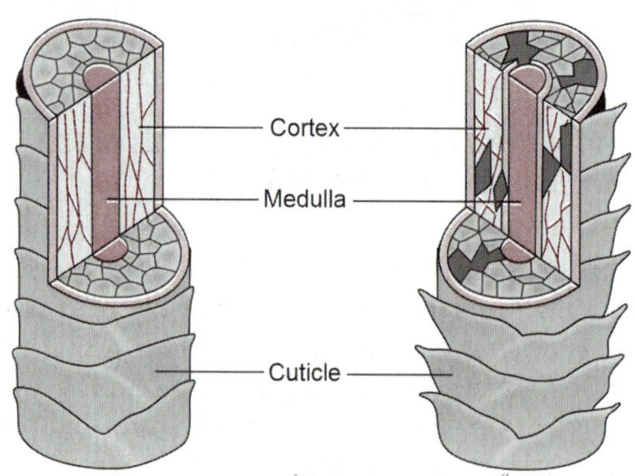

Fig. 3.19: Hair structure

and medulla (Fig. 3.19). The cuticle is the outermost layer made of keratinocytes. The cortex cells are present under the cuticle and are responsible for the width of the hair. The cortex cells contain pigments that impart colour to the hair. The medulla is not present in all hairs.

Body hair gives protection from UV radiation and also insulates the body by trapping warm air around the skin. Hair loss takes place naturally in men and women.

BAQ: Draw a labelled diagram of the anatomical features of hair.

Ans: Refer to Fig. 3.18.

> **Objective:** To describe the structural layers of nails and their functions.

NAILS (Fig. 3.20)

BAQ: Write a note on nails and nail anatomy.

Ans: Nails are accessory organs of the skin and these are seen on the distal ends of the fingers and toes. Nails are made up of sheets of hardened keratinocytes. Fingernails and toenails protect the ends of fingers and toes.

Nail Anatomy (Fig. 3.20) and Functions

The following are three main parts of a nail: Root, body, and free edge (Fig. 3.20). The nail root is the portion of the nail found under the surface of the skin. The nail body is the visible external portion of the nail. The free edge is the distal end portion of the nail that has grown beyond the end of the finger or toe.

Nails grow from the nail matrix. The nail matrix is a deep layer of epidermal tissue matrix that creates new cells and old cells are pushed out distally. The nail matrix surrounds the nail root. Keratinocytes are formed from the stem cells of the nail matrix. Keratinocytes, in turn, produce keratin protein and pack into tough layers of hardened cells. The nail root slowly grows out of the skin and forms the nail body; when it reaches the surface of the skin. A layer of epidermis and dermis under the nail body is known as the nail bed (Fig. 3.20). The colour of the nail bed is pink due to the presence of blood capillaries, that support the cells of the nail body (Fig. 3.20). A whitish crescent shape known as the lunula is present near the root. The eponychium is a layer of epithelium that overlaps and covers the edge of the nail body. The eponychium is useful to seal the edges of the nail to prevent infection of the underlying tissues.

Function of the nails is to protect the fingers and toes by increasing the sensation and precision of movements.

> **Objective:** To list and describe the sudoriferous glands and their functions.

SUDORIFEROUS GLANDS (Figs 3.21 and 3.22)

BAQ: Write a note on the sudoriferous glands.

Ans: The sudoriferous glands or sweat glands are exocrine glands found in the dermis of the skin. The sweat glands are of two main types: Eccrine sweat glands and apocrine sweat glands (Figs 3.21 and 3.22).

Eccrine sweat glands are found mostly in every region of the skin. These produce a secretion of sweat containing water and sodium chloride. Eccrine sweat is delivered through a duct to the surface of the skin. Evaporation of sweat lowers the temperature of the body.

Apocrine sweat glands are found mainly in the pubic and axillary regions of the body. The ducts of apocrine sweat glands extend into the follicles of hair. The digestion of apocrine sweat by bacteria produces specific body odour.

Mammary glands are specialised sudoriferous glands situated within the breasts of females. During

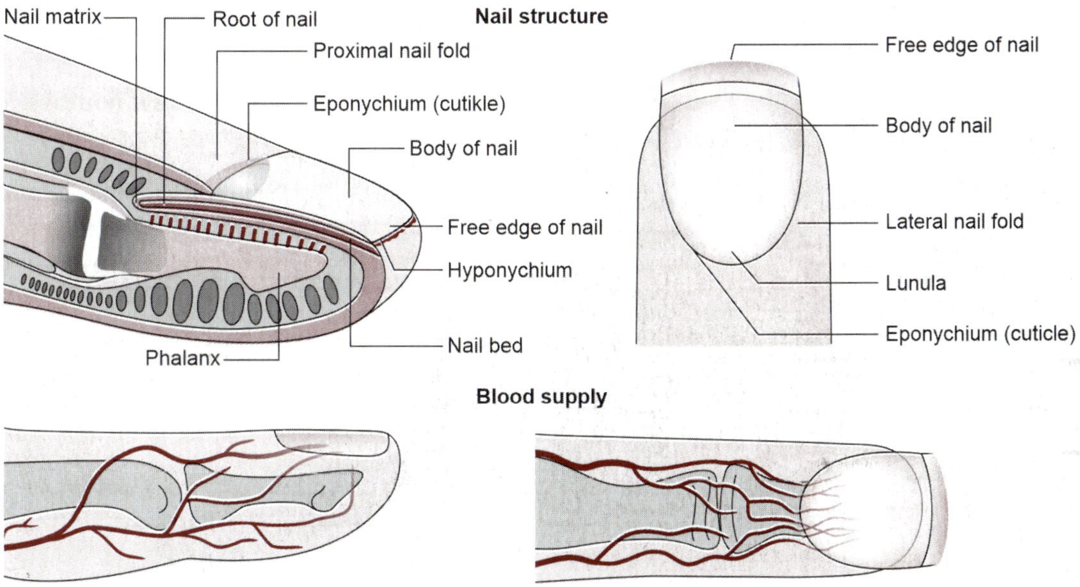

Fig. 3.20: Nail structure and blood supply

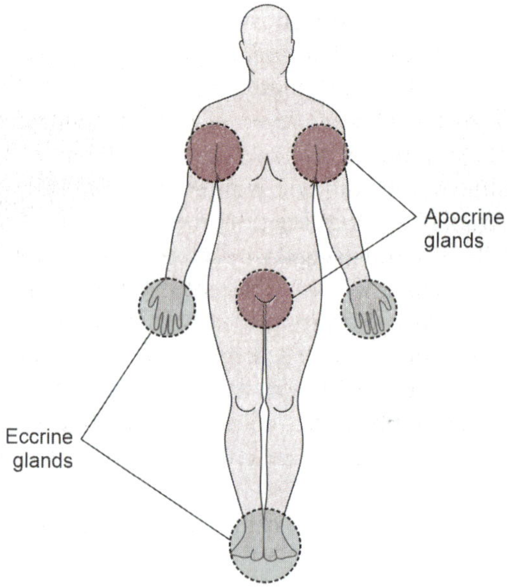

Fig. 3.21: Eccrine and apocrine gland positions

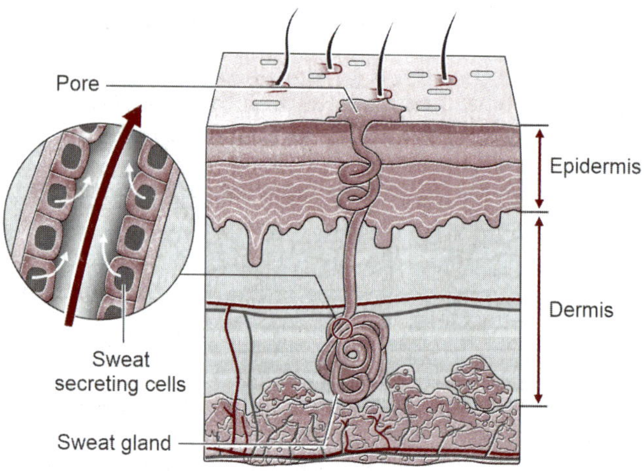

Fig. 3.22: Sudoriferous gland

the childbearing days and after the delivery, mammary glands become functional by the stimulus of pituitary and ovarian hormones and lactation takes place.

Objective: To describe the sudoriferous glands and their functions.

BAQ: Draw a labelled diagram indicating eccrine and apocrine gland positions.

Ans: Refer to Fig. 3.21.

SEBACEOUS GLANDS (Fig. 3.23)

BAQ: Write a note on the sebaceous glands.

Ans: Sebaceous glands are exocrine glands present in the dermis of the skin. These glands are present in every part of the skin except the thick skin of the palms of the hands and soles of the feet. The sebaceous glands secret sebum, an oily secretion, which is carried through ducts to hair follicles and the surface of the skin. The sebum acts as a waterproof substance and increases the elasticity of the skin. The sebum lubricates and protects the cuticles of hair.

Objective: To describe the ceruminous glands and their functions.

CERUMINOUS GLANDS (Fig. 3.24)

BAQ: Write a note on the ceruminous glands.

Ans: The ceruminous glands are typical exocrine glands present only in the dermis of the ear canals. These glands produce cerumen, a waxy secretion. The cerumen protects the ear canals and lubricates the eardrum. Foreign substances such as dust and airborne

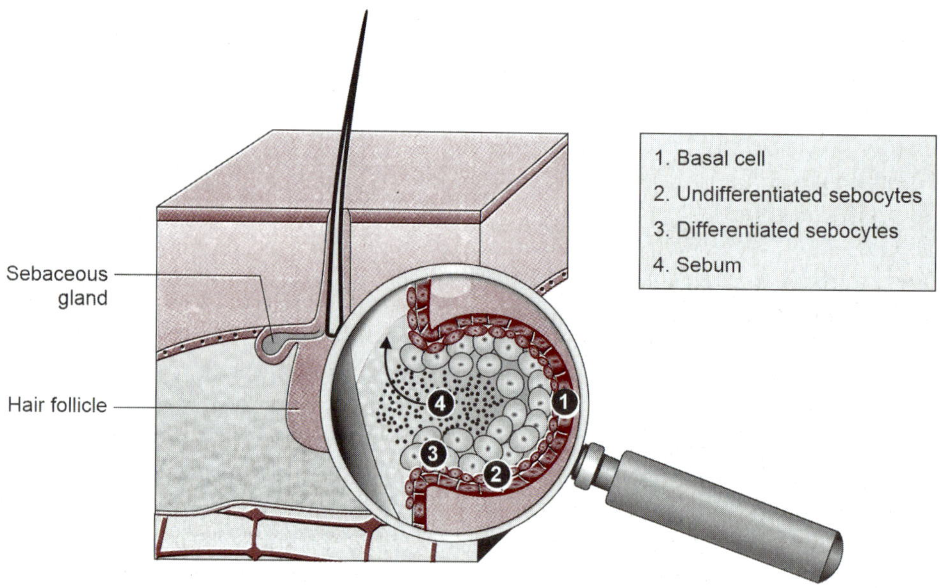

Fig. 3.23: Sebaceous gland

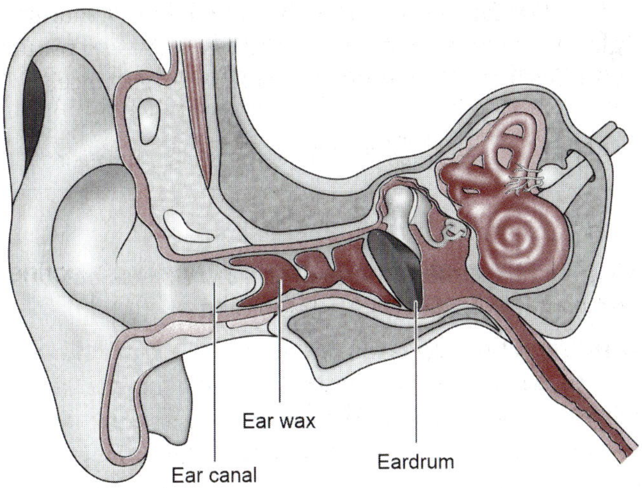

Fig. 3.24: Ceruminous glands in the ear

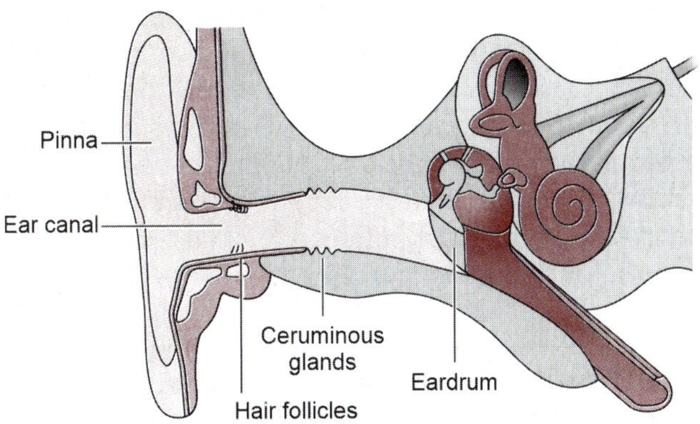

Fig. 3.25: Formation of wax in the ear

pathogens are prevented from entering the ear canal by the cerumen. The cerumen is formed continuously and accumulates as a waxy substance (Fig. 3.25). It falls out of the ear or it is manually removed.

Objective: To describe the physiology of the integumentary system.

PHYSIOLOGY OF THE INTEGUMENTARY SYSTEM

Physical Protection by Keratinization (Fig. 3.26)

BAQ: Write the significance of keratinization.

Ans: The keratinization (cornification) process is a normal accumulation of keratin within keratinocytes. The stem cells multiply and push older keratinocytes towards the surface of the skin (Fig. 3.26). When keratinocytes reach the stratum spinosum, they accumulate a significant amount of keratin and become hard, flat, and relatively more water-resistant. At this stage, since the cells do not get nutrients, the cells go through the process of apoptosis. Apoptosis is programmed cell death and the result is a tough, keratin-filled shell, which remains behind. Dead keratinocytes are tightly packed and they form a keratin barrier to protect the underlying tissues. Through this process, the skin epidermis gets an outermost layer of dead keratin, which gives protection from mechanical impacts, pressure, variations in temperature, chemicals, radiation and microbial infections.

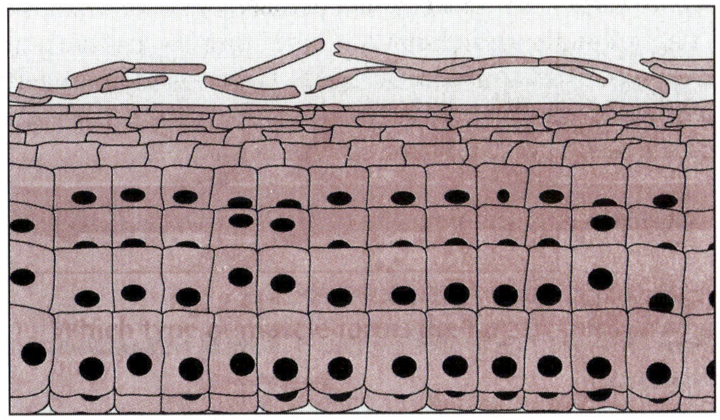
Fig. 3.26: Skin keratinization

Objective: To describe the homeostasis by the skin.

Temperature Homeostasis by the Skin

BAQ: Describe the regulation of the body temperature by the skin.

Ans: The skin can regulate the temperature of the body according to environmental changes. When body temperature rises, the skin can reduce body temperature utilizing vasodilation and sweating. Sweat begins to evaporate, which absorbs heat and cools the surface of the body. Vasodilation leads to an increase in blood circulation to the skin. Blood transports body heat deposits it in the skin and then can radiate heat out of the body into the external environment.

When body temperature decreases, the skin can raise body temperature through vasoconstriction and the contraction of the arrector pili muscles. The arrector pili form small bumps and the hair shafts remain upright from the surface of the skin. Due to this movement; air gets trapped under the hairs to insulate the surface of the body. Due to vasoconstriction, the walls of blood vessels in the dermis contract leading to a reduction in the flow of blood to the skin and blood remains in the body circulation to maintain heat and circulation to the vital organs.

Objective: To describe the role of the skin in immunity.

Role of the Skin in Immunity

BAQ: Give an account of the role of the skin in immunity.

Ans: The skin acts as the physical barrier which prevents direct entry of pathogens into the body. Thus, the skin acts as the first line of defence of the body. Myeloid cells, lymphoid cells, Langerhans cells and dermal dendritic cells present in the skin possess the property of activating the main immune system.

Skin also contains antimicrobial peptides such as defensins and cathelicidins, which are produced by the various cells in the skin, such as dendritic cells and macrophages and these are activated by proteolytic cleavage when stimulated. Lipids such as sphingomyelin and glucosylceramides are stored in the stratum corneum of the skin and display antimicrobial activity.

Objective: To describe the role of the skin in wound healing.

Role of the Skin in Wound Healing

BAQ: Write a note on the role of the skin in wound healing.

Ans: The skin plays a very important role in wound healing. When the body suffers from trauma, hemostasis, means cessation of bleeding occurs, which is followed by the inflammatory phase, and proliferative phase. During hemostasis, tissue factors located in subendothelial spaces of the skin trigger the coagulation cascade to form a fibrin clot. During the inflammatory phase, immune cells such as neutrophils and monocytes arrive at the injury site and attack pathogens, kill them and clear out debris produced by the pathogen destruction. The proliferative phase involves the multiplication of skin cells such as keratinocytes and fibroblasts, which contribute to the formation of granulation tissue, collagen and finally new extracellular matrix forms.

In the final remodelling phase, cells that are not needed undergo apoptosis and excess structures are broken down in order to restore the original skin form. Macrophages secrete matrix metalloproteases, which remove excess collagen, and remaining immature collagen matures to finalize the extracellular matrix.

Objective: To describe the various functions of the skin.

Role of the Skin in Vitamin D Synthesis

BAQ: Write a note on the role of the skin in vitamin D synthesis.

Ans: Skin contains 7-dehydrocholesterol. When skin is exposed to the sun, due to ultraviolet sunlight exposure, 7-dehydrocholesterol is converted to vitamin D_3 (cholecalciferol) in the skin. Cholecalciferol is then hydroxylated in the liver and later in the kidneys into 1,25-dihydroxy vitamin D (calcitriol), which is metabolically active. The action of calcitriol is to increase calcium absorption in the gut, which is needed for normal bone formation and also for calcium homeostasis.

Role of the Skin-in-Skin Colour Formation

BAQ: Write a note on the role of the skin-in-skin colour formation.

Ans: Three pigments, melanin, carotene, and haemoglobin play important roles in the formation of skin colour. Melanin is a brown or black pigment produced by melanocytes, which impart colour to skin and hair. Melanin production increases when the skin is exposed to high levels of UV light, which results in tanning of the skin. Carotene in the skin imparts yellow or orange colour to the skin and it is observed in people with low levels of melanin. Haemoglobin present in red blood cells imparts a red colour to the skin and it is observed in people with a small quantity of melanin.

Role of the Skin in Cutaneous Sensation

(Figs 3.27 and 3.28)

BAQ: Write a note on the role of the Merkel cells of the skin in the cutaneous sensation.

Ans: The skin can sense the external environment by picking up signals for temperature, pain, touch, pressure, vibration, etc. The Merkel disks in the epidermis connect to nerve cells in the dermis and these detect shapes and textures of objects contacting the skin. Meissner's corpuscles (tactile corpuscles) are found in the upper dermis and project into the epidermis. They respond to fine touch and pressure. Lamellar corpuscles found deep in the dermis sense pressure and vibration of the skin. There are many free nerve endings present throughout the dermis. Free nerve endings are sensitive to temperature changes and pain. The density of the sensory receptors in the skin varies throughout the body. Hence, in some regions of the body skin is more sensitive to pain, touch and temperature than other regions.

Role of the Skin in Excretion of Waste Products

BAQ: Write a note on the role of the eccine sudoriferous glands of the skin in the excretion of waste products of the body.

Ans: Eccrine sudoriferous glands of the skin excrete waste products out of the body. The sweat produced by eccrine sudoriferous glands normally contains electrolytes and trace elements. The main electrolytes excreted in sweat are sodium and chloride, however, potassium, calcium, and magnesium ions may also be excreted in very small amounts. When these electrolytes reach high levels in the blood, their excretion through sweat also increases. In addition to electrolytes, small amounts of metabolic waste products such as urea, uric acid, lactic acid and ammonia also may be excreted through sweat. Eccrine sudoriferous glands also excrete alcohol from the body of alcoholic persons.

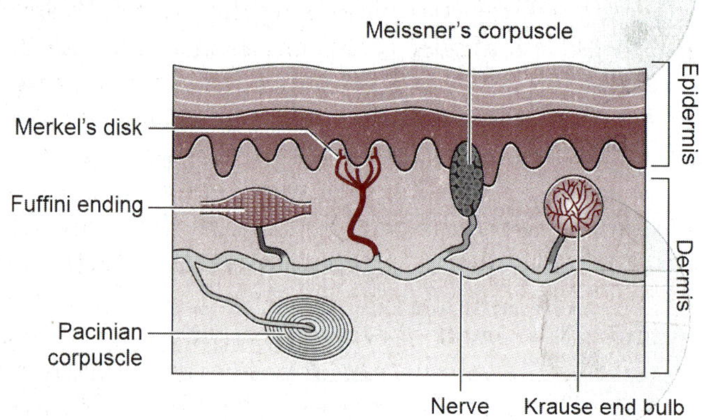

Fig. 3.27: Markel disc and Meissner's corpuscle

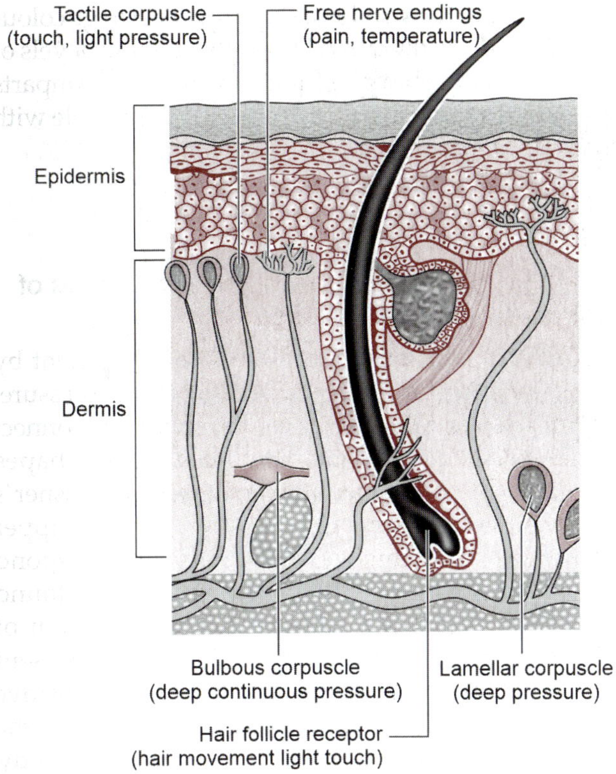

Fig. 3.28: Lamellar corpuscle and tactile corpuscle

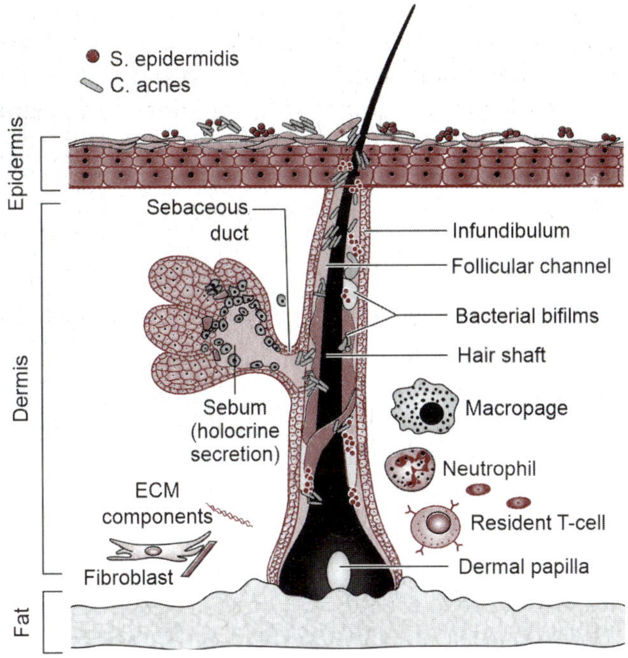

Fig. 3.29: Skin acne infections

Objective: To discuss pathophysiology related to skin disorders.

PATHOPHYSIOLOGY

Introduction

The integumentary system is directly exposed to external threats such as extreme temperatures, physical trauma, radiation and microorganisms. Hence, it is susceptible to infections, wounds, burns, etc. Skin pathologic conditions are often directly visible and the specific appearance of skin also reflects internal pathological conditions (Figs 3.15 and 3.17). Following are some common clinical conditions related to the integumentary system:

Skin Acne

BAQ: Briefly explain the pathophysiology behind the formation of acne.

Ans: Inflammation of the pilosebaceous unit is caused by the overproduction of keratin within hair follicles, increased sebum production, and *Cutibacterium acnes* infection leading to inflammation and formation of acne. Acne appears in varying forms of morphologies, such as comedones (blackheads) (Fig. 3.31), pustules, nodules, and papules with different sizes and appearances (Fig. 3.29).

For their primary sources of energy and nutrients, acnes bacteria (*Cutibacterium acnes*) use sebum, cellular debris and metabolic byproducts from the surrounding skin tissue. With elevated production of sebum by hyperactive sebaceous glands, *Cutibacterium acnes* bacteria grow and multiply (Fig. 3.30).

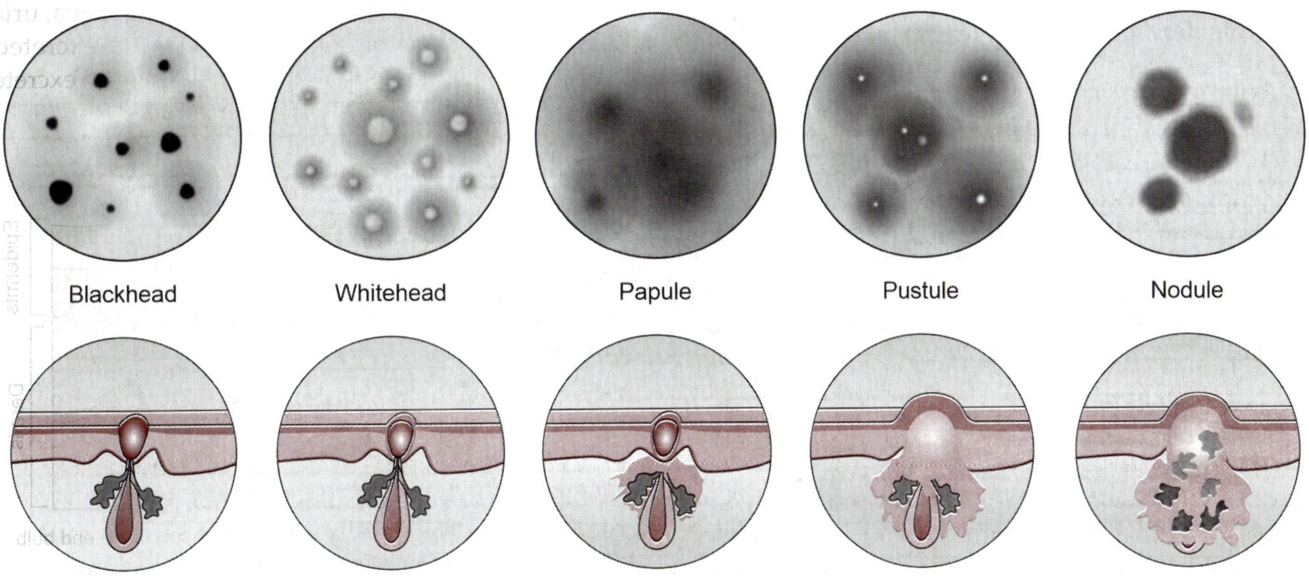

Fig. 3.30: Various types of acne

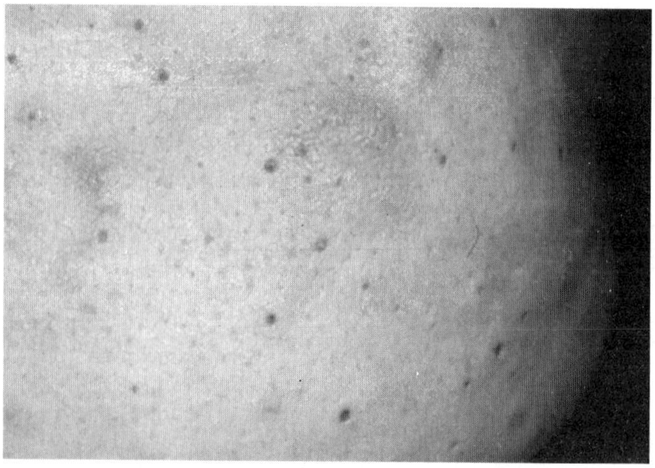

Fig. 3.31: Comedones (blackheads) on the skin

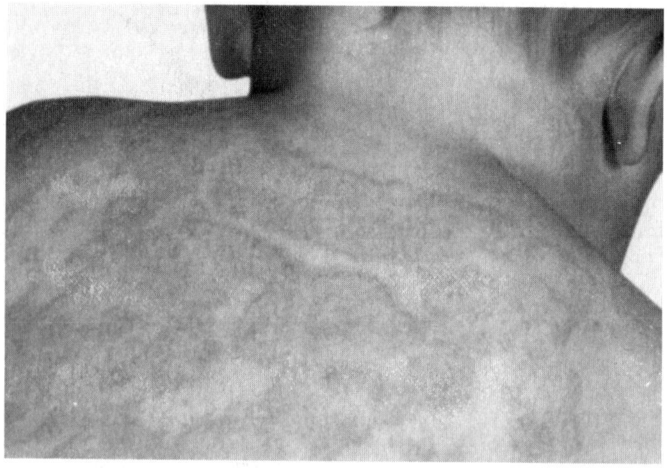

Fig. 3.33: Atopic dermatitis

Unhealthy food, skin trauma, hormonal changes and stress lead to the development of acne. In women, hormonal acne is characterized by flares involving the jawline. These get flared during menstrual cycles. Increased androgen production in circulation also contributes to acne. In this clinical condition, sebaceous glands produce sebum in response to androgens, which is required for the growth of *C. acnes* and leads to an increase in inflammatory reactions.

Atopic Dermatitis (Eczema) (Figs 3.32 and 3.33)

BAQ: Explain briefly the pathophysiology leading to eczema.

Ans: Eczema is a chronic condition that affects both children and adults. Defects in epidermal junctions reduce innate immunity in the skin, and genetics contribute to the development of this clinical condition. Filaggrin is a protein located within the stratum corneum. It links keratin intermediate filaments and creates an impenetrable outer layer. Filaggrin protein defect leads to a defective barrier function due to which increased water loss from the skin leads to characteristic symptoms of atopic dermatitis (Fig. 3.32).

Atopic dermatitis occurs mainly inside the elbows, behind the knees and in front of the neck (Fig 3.33). Atopic dermatitis is a type of eczema that leads to red and itchy skin. It is common in children, however, it can occur at any age. Atopic dermatitis is a chronic skin disorder and tends to appear periodically.

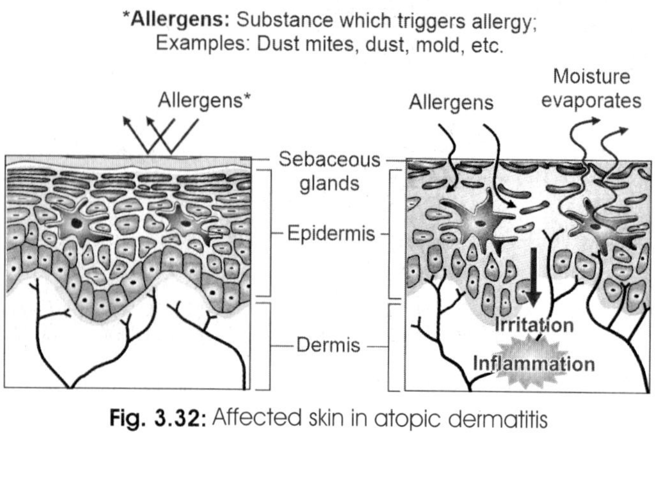

Fig. 3.32: Affected skin in atopic dermatitis

A main characteristic feature of atopic dermatitis is itching and harsh environmental factors and pollutants often trigger atopic dermatitis.

> *Note:* Eczema refers to a group of skin conditions that lead to inflamed skin. There are many types of eczema, however, atopic dermatitis is the most common type.

Psoriasis (Fig. 3.35)

BAQ: Explain briefly the pathophysiology leading to psoriasis.

Ans: The pathophysiology of psoriasis involves the hyperproliferation of keratinocytes within the epidermis and defects in the immune system. Psoriasis is an immune system disorder and infections, stress and cold conditions may trigger it. The most common symptom is a rash on the skin, but sometimes the rash involves the nails and the joints.

Psoriasis is mainly characterised by well-demarcated, erythematous plaques with overlying silvery scales. Chronic plaque psoriasis is the most common subtype of psoriasis in which edematous plaques are seen with overlying silvery scales. Lesions of 50% of patients show pruritic scales. The lesions are typically located on extensor surfaces and tend to have a symmetric distribution.

Cellulitis (Fig. 3.36)

BAQ: Briefly explain the pathophysiology leading to cellulitis.

Ans: Cellulitis is a common painful bacterial skin infection. It results from *Streptococcus pyogenes* and *Staphylococcus aureus* infection of deep dermis and subcutaneous fat. The affected skin appears swollen and red. Cellulitis usually affects the skin on the lower legs, but it can occur in other areas including the face and arms (Fig. 3.36).

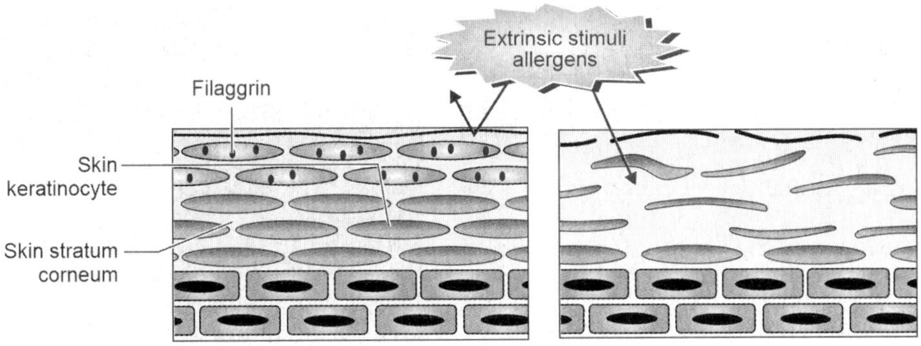

Fig. 3.34: Skin condition when Filaggrin protein is defective

Skin Cancer (Fig. 3.37)

BAQ: Briefly explain the pathophysiology leading to skin cancer.

Ans: Ultraviolet radiation is the most significant risk factor for skin cancer. UV light causes mutations in specific tumour suppressor genes and proto-oncogenes, that regulate cell growth and differentiation. Basal cell carcinoma is the most common skin cancer and it arises from the basal layer of the epidermis.

Squamous cell carcinoma is a malignant tumour that originates from epidermal keratinocytes. It is commonly observed in body parts exposed to the sun. The appearance of squamous cell carcinoma is generally present as erythematous papules, nodules or plaques that may become hyperkeratotic and may become ulcerative later on.

Melanoma is a serious type of skin cancer. It develops in melanocyte cells that produce melanin. Melanoma has the potential to metastasize quickly. It is divided into four

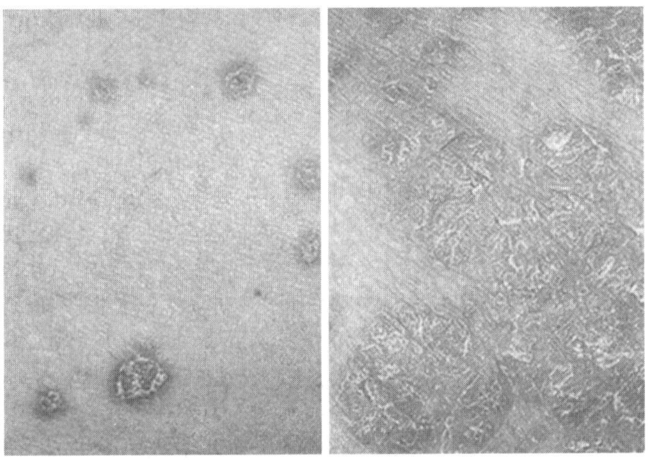

Fig. 3.35: Psoriasis

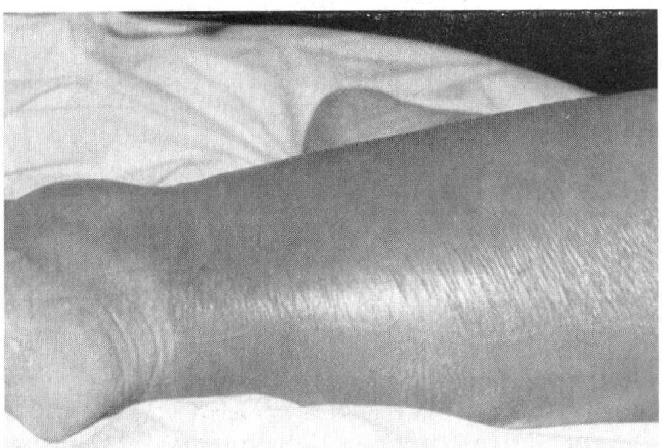

Fig. 3.36: Cellulitis

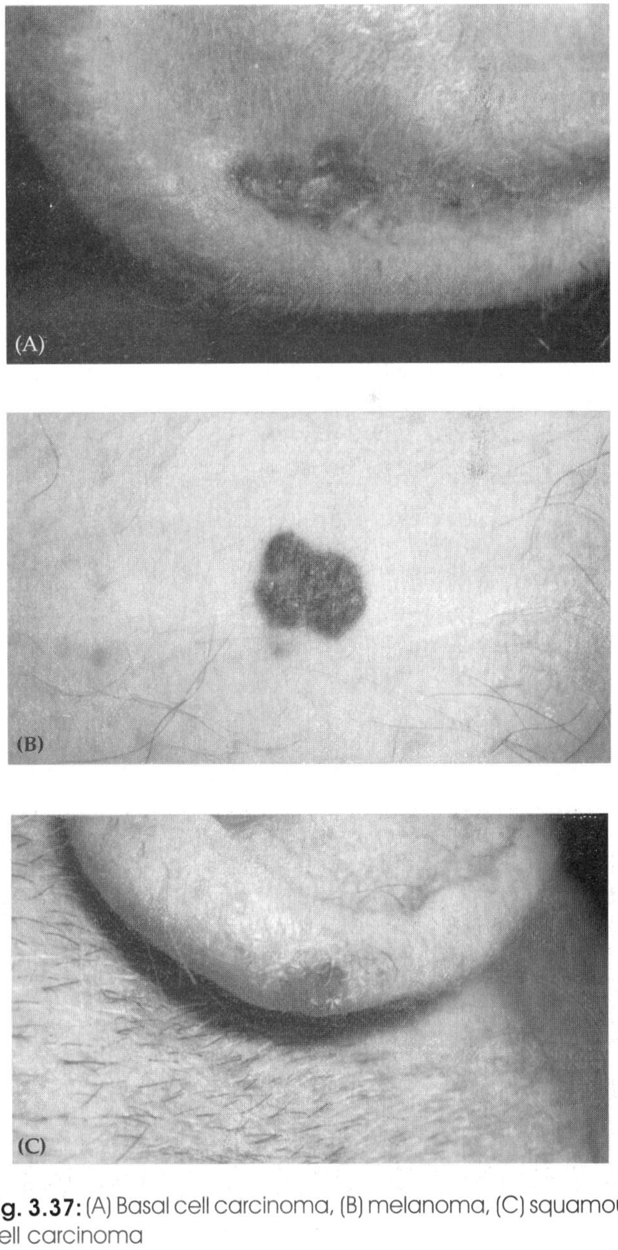

Fig. 3.37: (A) Basal cell carcinoma, (B) melanoma, (C) squamous cell carcinoma

subtypes, superficial spreading, lentigo maligna form, nodular form, and acral lentiginous form.

Objective: To describe the pathophysiology of burns.

Pathophysiology of Burns

LAQ: Briefly explain the pathophysiology caused by burns.

Ans: Burns are tissue damage that results from heat, corrosive chemicals, radiation, or electrical contact and can be minor medical problems or life-threatening emergencies. Burns are treated as emergencies since severe burns can lead to dehydration, sepsis, and death.

Burn severity can be determined by grading the depth of the burn and the area of skin involvement. Burn depth can be classified as superficial thickness, partial thickness, full thickness and fourth-degree type.

First-degree (superficial thickness) burn: It involves only the epidermal layer with no blisters. Lesions are red, dry, pale and painful. Injuries generally heal without scarring (Fig. 3.38A).

Second-degree (partial-thickness) burn: It involves the epidermis and dermis partially. Superficial partial-thickness lesions form painful blisters. This type of burns damages glandular tissue and hair follicles. Partial thickness burn damage can cause hypertrophic scarring and functional impairment and healing takes longer time (up to 4 to 8 weeks) (Fig. 3.38B).

Third-degree (full-thickness) burn involves all the layers of the dermis and often subcutaneous tissue and healing may take more than 8 weeks.

Fourth-degree burns are the most severe burns that extend beyond the skin into soft tissue and also involve underlying structures. Fourth-degree burns affect all the layers of the skin, muscles, tendons and related bones and are very serious and painful. These types of burns require surgery or grafting most of the time to close the wounds. may require a very long period for complete recovery.

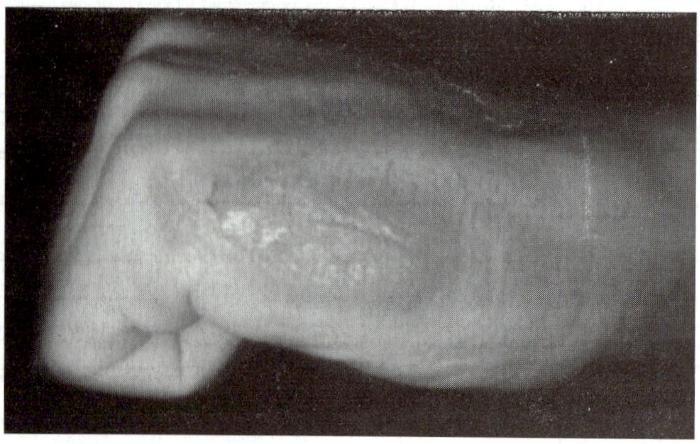

Fig. 3.38A: First-degree (Superficial thickness) burn

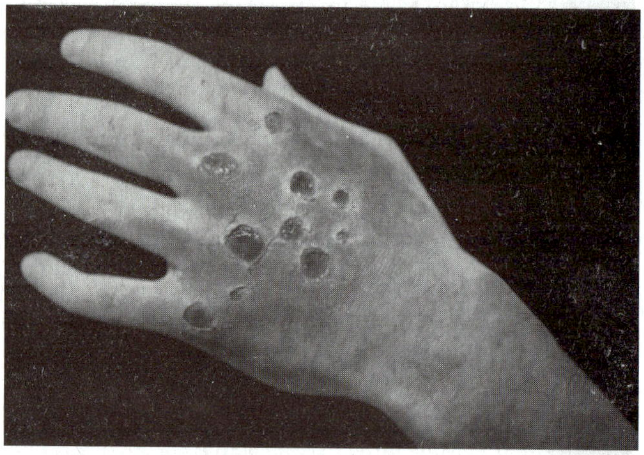

Fig. 3.38B: Second-degree (partial thickness) burn

Objective: To describe the various hair disorders.

HAIR DISORDERS

BAQ: Briefly explain the pathophysiology leading to alopecia areata.

Alopecia Areata (Fig. 3.39)

Ans: Alopecia areata is an autoimmune condition and it occurs when the immune system of the body attacks its hair follicles leading to hair loss (Fig. 3.39). The hair loss appears in patches. Hair loss can occur all over the body. The hair may regrow on its own. However, persons with alopecia areata may experience many recurrences of hair loss during their lives.

Folliculitis

BAQ: Briefly explain the pathophysiology leading to folliculitis.

Ans: Folliculitis (Fig. 3.40) is an inflammation of the hair follicle. Clinically, folliculitis appears with follicular pustules and erythematous papules. Bacterial, viral, parasitic or fungal infections may lead to folliculitis. *Staphylococcus aureus* infection of hair follicles is the most common causative bacterial infection and pruritus over hair-bearing areas is seen with occasional appearance of painful pustules and papules.

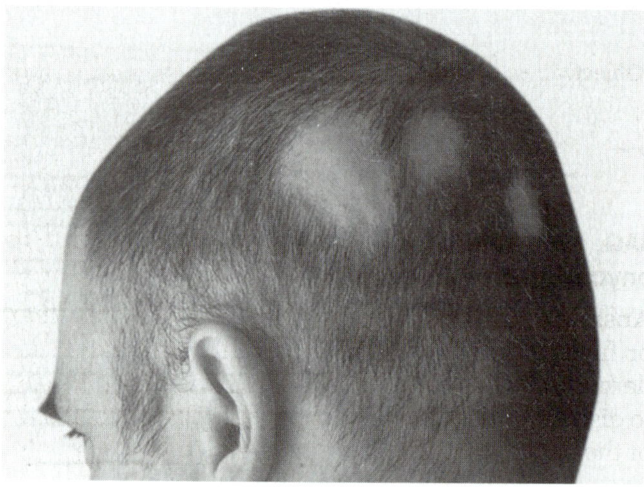

Fig. 3.39: Alopecia areata

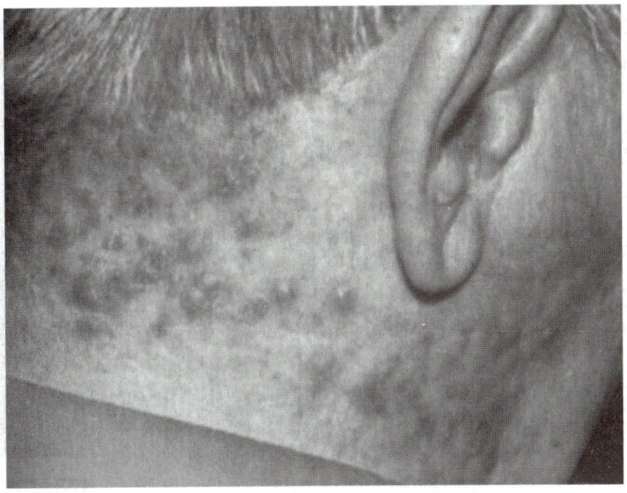

Fig. 3.40: Folliculitis

Male Pattern Balding (Fig. 3.41)

BAQ: Write a note on the male pattern of balding.

Ans: The male pattern baldness (androgenic alopecia) is the most common type of hair loss in men. This clinical condition has a genetic predisposition with a family history of baldness. Male pattern baldness is associated with androgens. Each hair on the head has a growth cycle. With male pattern baldness, this growth cycle becomes weak and the hair follicles shrink. This leads to shorter and finer strands of hair. Eventually, the growth cycle for each hair ends early and no new hair growth appears.

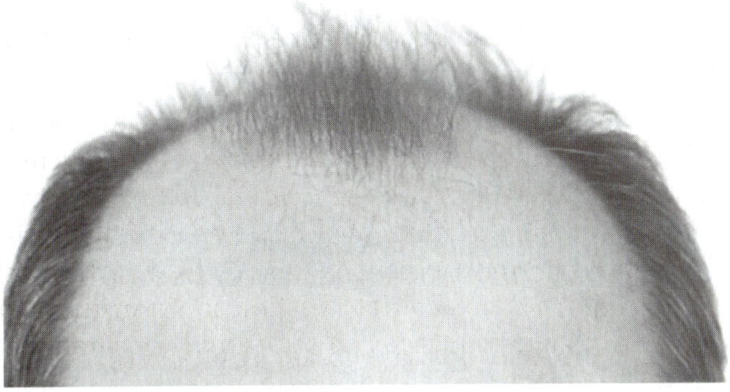

Fig. 3.41: Male pattern balding

Objective: To describe the various nail disorders.

NAIL DISORDERS

Onychomycosis

BAQ: Briefly explain the pathophysiology leading to onychomycosis.

Ans: Onychomycosis is a fungal infection of the toenails or fingernails. It can result from dermatophytes, non-dermatophyte moulds and yeasts. Onychomycosis leads to discolouration, thickening, and splitting or destruction of the nail plate (Fig. 3.42).

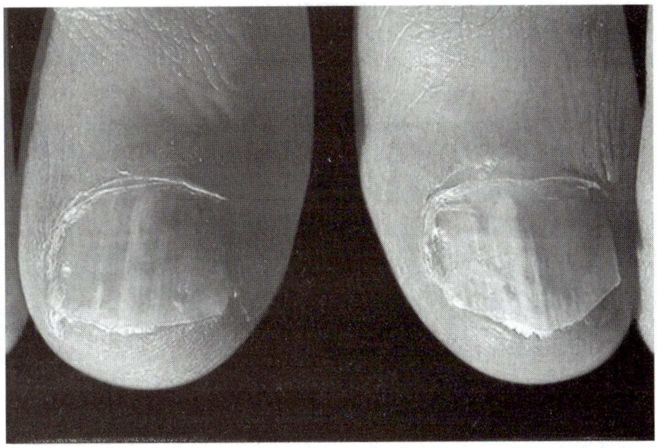

Fig. 3.42: Onychomycosis

Nail Pitting (Fig. 3.43)

SAQ: What is nail pitting?

Ans: Nail pitting occurs in conditions such as eczema, psoriasis, and alopecia areata. It is due to focal abnormal keratinization of the nail matrix. In this clinical condition, irregular, deep pits are seen within the nail plate as it grows beyond the cuticle.

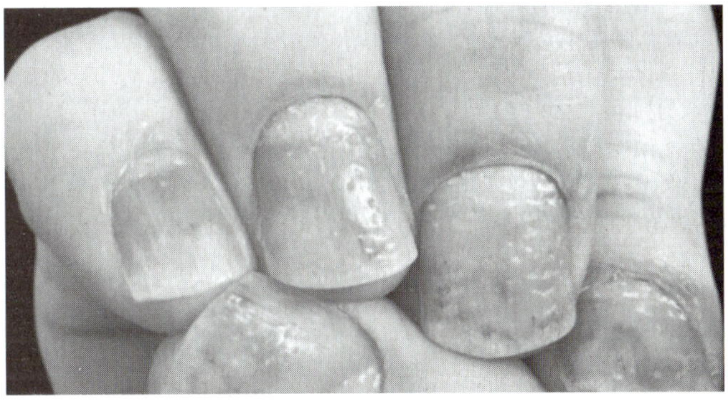

Fig. 3.43: Nail pitting

Koilonychia (Fig. 3.44)

SAQ: Describe briefly the clinical condition, koilonychia.

Ans: Koilonychia (spoon nails) are soft nails that look like spoons. Spoon nails may be a sign of iron deficiency anaemia, hemochromatosis or due to idiopathic (unknown cause) reasons.

Nail Clubbing (Fig. 3.45)

SAQ: What is nail clubbing?

Ans: Nail clubbing is characterized by increased thickening and nail plate curvature. It is caused by platelet precursors that fail the fragmentation process. These platelet precursors get trapped in the distal digit vasculature, release platelet-derived growth factor and vascular endothelial growth factor leading to nail clubbing.

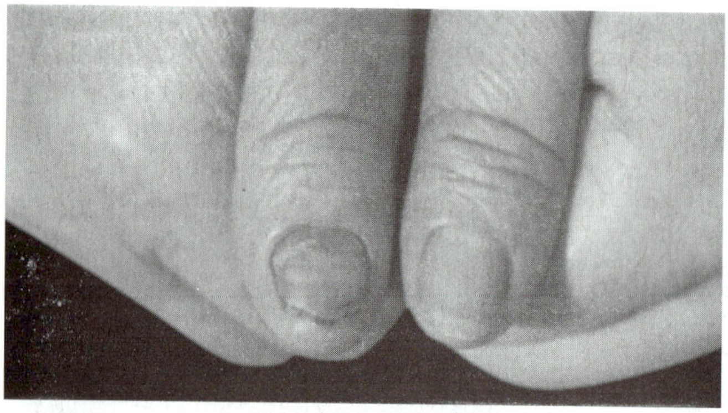

Fig. 3.44: Koilonychia

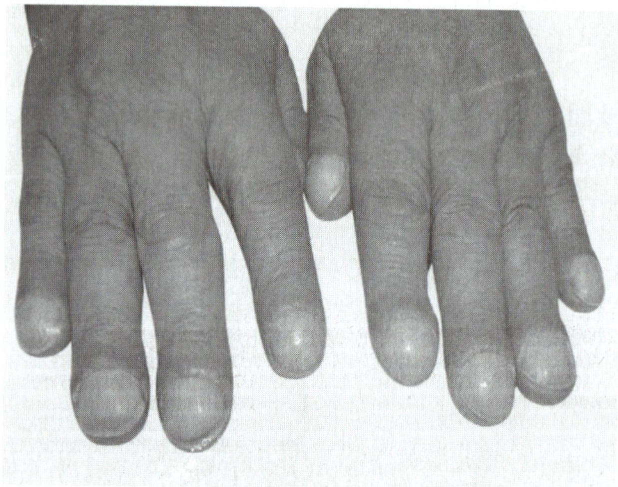

Fig. 3.45: Nail clubbing

Objective: To describe various disorders of the skin glands.

DISORDERS OF SKIN GLANDS

Seborrheic Dermatitis

BAQ: Briefly explain the pathophysiology leading to seborrheic dermatitis.

Ans: Seborrheic dermatitis is a skin disease that causes dandruff (Fig. 3.46). It also causes an itchy rash with flaky scales. Seborrheic dermatitis is also called seborrhea, seborrheic eczema, and seborrheic psoriasis. It usually appears on the scalp, however, it can be seen on any part of the body skin. The following factors may lead to seborrheic dermatitis: Genetic factors, stress, fungal infection, cold and dry weather, an immune system response and certain medicines.

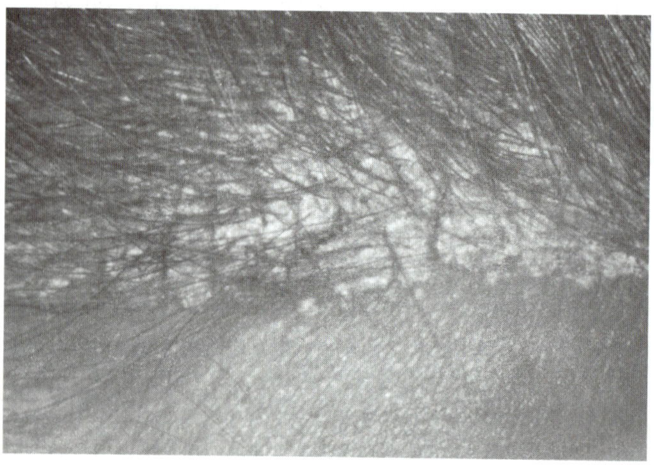

Fig. 3.46: Seborrheic dermatitis

Hyperhidrosis (Fig. 3.47)

SAQ: What is hyperhidrosis?

Ans: Hyperhidrosis is abnormally excessive sweating. It may not be related to exercise or heat. Hyperhidrosis may be an abnormal central response to normal emotional stress, which leads to increased sympathetic signalling to endocrine glands through cholinergic autonomic neurons. This causes excessive sweating beyond the physiological need for temperature regulation.

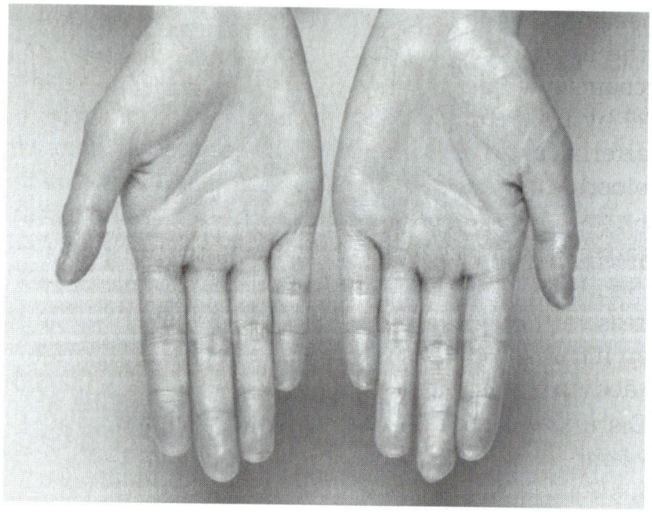

Fig. 3.47: Hyperhidrosis

Objective: To describe the role of the skin in the regulation of body temperature.

REGULATION OF BODY TEMPERATURE

LAQ: Write a note on the regulation of body temperature.

Ans: The normal average body temperature of a healthy individual is 37°± 0.5°C (98.6° ± 0.9°F). This temperature range is required for the enzyme-catalysed normal performance of the metabolic reactions of the body. Body temperature rises slightly during exercises, in the evening, and in women just after ovulation. Thermoregulation is the maintenance of normal body temperature by balancing heat loss with heat generation. The lowest body temperature is observed by 4 am, and the highest body temperature is observed by 6 pm.

The body temperature rises when the metabolic rate increases. Heat is produced mainly by the following various activities:

1. Chemical reactions involved in digestion and peristalsis actions of the gastrointestinal tract.
2. Skeletal muscular activities.
3. Metabolic activities of the liver.

Most of the heat generated by the body is lost through the skin, which can be regulated. Heat is also lost in expired air, urine and faeces, which cannot be controlled.

The endocrine gland hypothalamus (situated deep in the brain); is responsible for the temperature regulation of the body. It uses the thermoregulatory centre present inside the gland. The temperature sensors present in the thermoregulatory centre receive temperature-related information through nerve cells called thermoreceptors. The body has central and peripheral thermoreceptors. The central thermoreceptors are found in the viscera, spinal cord, and hypothalamus and sense the core temperature. The peripheral thermoreceptors are located in the skin and these sense surface temperatures. The variations in the body temperature are responsible for activating these thermoreceptors in the hypothalamus. When body temperature decreases, the thermoreceptors in the hypothalamus then activate heat regulation mechanisms to control body temperature at a normal level by the following mechanisms: (1) Constriction of arterioles in the dermis, which leads to a decrease of blood flow to the skin and (2) shivering of skeletal muscles. Once normal temperature is restored, the negative feedback to the hypothalamus is stopped.

Similarly, when body temperature rises, heat loss is increased by dilation of arterioles in the dermis, leading to an increase in blood flow to the skin and increasing the activities of sweat glands.

Disruption in the thermoregulation can lead to very low temperature (hypothermia) or very high temperature (hyperthermia) of the body. Extreme variations in the body temperature can lead to organ failure, coma, and death ultimately.

Fever

BAQ: Write a note on fever.

Ans: Fever is a body temperature that is higher than the normal average temperature, which is 98.6°F (37°C). The following various factors can lead to fever: Infection, inflammation, medicines, autoimmune reactions, or malignancy. Mainly, pyrogens such as interleukins (cytokines: Specific proteins) released by white blood cells, in response to microbial infections are responsible for fever. The interleukins trigger the thermoregulatory centre of the hypothalamus, which leads to an increase in the temperature of the body. Shivering (chills) and vasoconstriction are the body response actions that respond to the fever. The thermoregulatory system in the hypothalamus then tries to reset the body temperature by heat-loss reactions such as vasodilation, flushed pink skin and profuse sweating (rigours).

Effects of Hot Climatic Conditions on the Body

BAQ: What are the effects of hot climatic conditions on the body?

Ans: As the environmental temperature increases, the body tends to warm up. The body's internal "thermostat" (hypothalamic control) maintains a constant inner body temperature by pumping more blood to the skin and by increasing sweat production. Evaporation of sweat on the surface of the skin lowers the temperature of the body to some extent. The body increases the rate of heat loss to balance the heat burden created by the environment. In a very hot environment, the rate of "heat gain" exceeds the rate of "heat loss" and the body temperature begins to rise. A rise in the body temperature results in heat illnesses. "Heat stress" is a net heat burden on the body from the combination of the body heat generated while working, and due to environmental factors such as air temperature, humidity, air movement, radiation from the sun or hot surfaces and sources and clothing requirements.

SAQ: What is a heat stroke?

Ans: A heat stroke is due to environmental exposure to heat, resulting in an abnormally high body temperature. In severe cases, temperatures can exceed 40°C (104°F).

SAQ: What is heat syncope?

Ans: Heat syncope is heat-induced giddiness and fainting induced by temporarily insufficient flow of blood to the brain while a person is standing. It is caused by the loss of body fluids through sweating, and by lowered blood pressure due to the pooling of blood in the legs. Recovery is rapid after rest in a cool area and intake of water-containing electrolytes.

BAQ: Write a note on hyperthermia.

Ans: Hyperthermia is defined as a temperature greater than 37.5–38.3°C (100–101°F). Hyperthermia is an elevated body temperature due to failed thermoregulation. Hyperthermia occurs when the body produces or absorbs more heat than it can dissipate. When the elevated body temperatures are sufficiently high, hyperthermia is a medical emergency and requires immediate treatment to prevent disability or death.

The most common causes of hyperthermia are heat stroke and adverse reactions to drugs. Heat stroke is an acute condition of hyperthermia that is caused by prolonged exposure to excessive heat or heat and humidity. Malignant hyperthermia is a rare complication of some types of general anaesthesia.

Hot, dry skin is a typical sign of hyperthermia. The skin may become red and hot as blood vessels dilate in an attempt to increase heat dissipation, sometimes leading to swollen lips. An inability to cool the body through perspiration causes the skin to feel dry. The dehydration associated with heat stroke can produce nausea, vomiting, headaches, and low blood pressure. This can lead to fainting or dizziness, especially if the person stands suddenly.

When the body temperature reaches about 40°C, or if the affected person is unconscious or showing signs of confusion, hyperthermia is considered a medical emergency that requires treatment in a proper medical facility. In a hospital, more aggressive cooling measures are available, including intravenous hydration, gastric lavage with iced saline, and hemodialysis to cool the blood.

Non-exertional heat stroke is predominant in the young and the elderly. It can be precipitated by medications that reduce vasodilation, sweating, and other heat-loss mechanisms, such as anticholinergic drugs, antihistamines, and diuretics. In this situation, the body's tolerance for excessive environmental temperatures can be too limited to cope with the heat, even while resting.

Effects of Cold Climatic Conditions

LAQ: Write a note on the effects of cold climatic conditions on the body.

Ans: When exposed to extremely cold environmental conditions, internal thermostatic mechanisms are unable to replenish the heat that is being lost and a drop in the core temperature occurs. As the body temperature decreases, characteristic symptoms occur such as shivering and mental confusion due to hypothermia.

Hypothermia is defined as any body temperature below 35.0°C (95.0°F). Hypothermia is a condition in which core temperature drops below the required normal average temperature for normal metabolism and body functions which is normally at 35°C (95°F). Body temperature is usually maintained near a constant level of 36.5–37.5°C (98–100°F) through biological homeostasis or thermoregulation.

In very cold conditions, symptoms of mild hypothermia are shivering, hypertension, tachycardia, tachypnea, and vasoconstriction (due to sympathetic nervous system excitation). These are all physiological responses to preserve heat. Cold diuresis, mental confusion, as well as hepatic dysfunction may also be present. Glucose consumption by cells and insulin secretion both decrease and tissue sensitivity to insulin may be decreased.

In moderate hypothermia, the following symptoms are observed: Low body temperature, violent shivering, slow and laboured movements, and mild confusion, although the victim may appear alert. Surface blood vessels of the affected person contract further as the body focuses its remaining resources on keeping the vital organs warm. The victim becomes pale and the lips, ears, fingers and toes of the affected person may become blue.

In severe hypothermia, as the temperature decreases, physiological systems are affected leading to a decrease in heart rate, respiratory rate, and blood pressure. In the case of the affected person, difficulty in speaking, sluggish thinking, and amnesia are observed with the inability to use hands and stumbling. Below 30°C (86°F), the skin of the affected person becomes blue and puffy with difficulty in walking due to disturbed muscle coordination and also exhibits incoherent and irrational behaviour. Pulse and respiration rates decrease significantly, with ventricular tachycardia and atrial fibrillation. If not treated in time, the major organs of the affected person fail leading to clinical death.

Objective: To describe the healing of wounds.

WOUND HEALING

LAQ: Write a note on wound healing.

Ans: Wound healing, takes place through four precisely and highly programmed phases: Hemostasis, inflammation, proliferation, and remodelling. For successful wound healing, all four phases must occur in the proper sequence and in the normal time phase. The wound healing can be primary or secondary. In primary healing minimum destruction of tissue takes place as seen in surgical incisions. In secondary healing large amount of tissue destruction takes place.

Primary Wound Healing (Fig. 3.48)

The primary wound-healing process takes place in the following phases:

1. **Hemostasis:** By (A) vascular constriction and (B) by platelet aggregation and fibrin formation.
2. **Inflammation:** The cut surfaces become inflamed, blood clots and tissue debris fill the gaps, neutrophils accumulate there, monocytes differentiate into macrophages, phagocytes remove clots and tissue debris, and fibroblasts secrete collagen fibres, that bind broken tissue margins.
3. **Proliferation:** Epithelial cells grow till full tissue recovery is restored. The clot above the tissue becomes a dry crust and separates subsequently. Development of granulation tissue takes place with new buds, phagocytes, fibroblasts and angiogenesis. Microorganisms are removed by phagocytosis and clot formation due to collagen fibres.
4. **Maturation:** Granulation tissue is removed by fibrous scar tissue. Collagen fibers rearrange and the strength of formed tissue increases. The scar tissue changes to a less vascular type and full recovery takes place in a few weeks.

Secondary Wound Healing

The stages of secondary healing are the same as those for primary wound healing. The only difference is, in this case, a few more months are required for full recovery of the wound, which also depends on certain factors such as the nature of the wound, appropriate care of the patient, nutrition, medication, and the control of other accompanying conditions (if present), such as diabetes mellitus, hypertension, etc.

Fibrosis (Fibrotic Scarring)

BAQ: What is fibrosis?

Ans: Fibrosis (fibrotic scarring) means the formation of fibrous tissue, which cannot function like normal

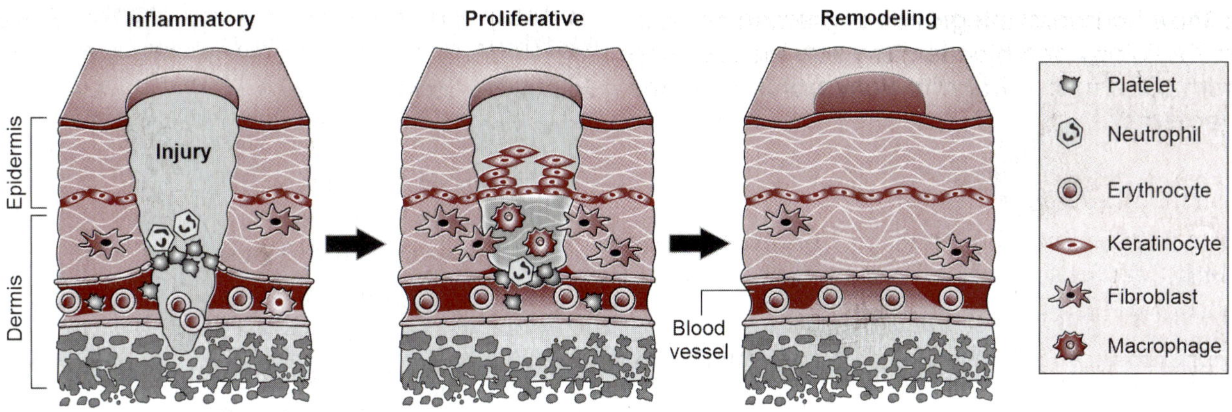

Fig. 3.48: Stages of wound healing

tissue. It may form during the secondary wound healing. The main reasons for the formation of fibrous tissue are extensive trauma, long-term ischemia and chronic inflammation. Excessive accumulation of collagen is produced by fibroblasts, leading to the formation of a permanent fibrotic scar. In the process of fibrosis, normal parenchymal tissue is replaced by connective tissue leading to permanent formation of scar tissue. The deposition of connective tissue interferes with the normal structure and function of the underlying normal tissue and organ.

Pus Formation

BAQ: Write a note on pus formation.

Ans: Pus is green, white-yellow, or yellow-coloured exudate formed at the site of inflammation caused by bacterial or fungal infection. An accumulation of pus inside a tissue space is known as an abscess. A visible collection of pus within or beneath the epidermis is known as a pimple or a pustule. Pus consists of mainly dead neutrophils and other white blood cells in a protein-rich fluid produced due to the immune response of the body.

Objective: To describe the effects of ageing on the skin.

Effects of Ageing on the Skin

BAQ: Write a note on the effects of ageing on the skin.

Ans: Changes in the skin start taking place mainly after the first three decades of life. The following changes occur in the skin due to ageing:

1. The activity of the basal layer of the skin decreases.
2. Thinning of the dermis and epidermis takes place.
3. Decrease in the dermis, elastic fibres and collagen fibres lead to the formation of wrinkling and sagging of the skin.
4. Decrease in the underlying fat layer takes
5. The skin loses some of its elasticity.
6. The skin becomes drier due to the impaired barrier function and decreased production of essential oils such as sebum.
7. The number of nerve endings in the skin decreases, leading to a decrease in the sensation of the skin.
8. The number of sweat glands and blood vessels decreases; leading to the reduction of the ability of the skin to respond to heat exposure.
9. Decrease in the synthesis of vitamin D; leading to increased risk of osteoporosis.
10. Decrease in the number of melanocytes, which decreases protection against ultraviolet radiation.
11. A decrease in the activity of sweat glands, that increases the risk of heat stroke and hyperthermia.
12. Decrease in the active hair follicles leading to the loss of hair on the skin of the head.

All of these changes make the skin more susceptible to damage and slower response to heal skin damage.

Objective: To understand and explain the central theme of competency-based medical and paramedical education (CBME): Horizontal and vertical integration of subjects.

BAQ: Show horizontal integration of physiology and biochemistry with the following anatomical change: Red, tender, inflamed and painful skin of a leg (cellulitis).

Ans:

Horizontal Integration with Physiology

Affected blood circulation in the leg.

Horizontal Integration with Biochemistry

Circulation of inflammatory factors such as prostaglandins, leukotrienes, C-reactive protein, etc., which are responsible for the inflammation of the leg.

BAQ: Show vertical integration of microbiology and pharmacology with the following anatomical change: Red, tender, inflamed and painful skin of a leg (cellulitis).

Ans:

Horizontal Integration with Microbiology

Diagnosis of microbial infection, which is responsible for cellulitis.

Horizontal Integration with Pharmacology

Selection of appropriate antibiotics to cure infection that leads to cellulitis.

BAQ: Show horizontal integration of premedical subjects: Physiology and biochemistry with the following anatomical change: Dry and itchy patches on the skin (eczema).

Ans:

Horizontal Integration with Physiology

Defects in epidermal junctions and reduced innate immunity reactions.

Horizontal Integration with Biochemistry

Defective production of the protein filaggrin, that usually keeps the skin hydrated.

BAQ: Show vertical integration of the paramedical subject: Pharmacology, with the following anatomical change: Dry and itchy patches on the skin (eczema).

Ans:

Vertical Integration with Pharmacology

Selection of an appropriate drug to manage normal skin conditions.

BAQ: Show horizontal integration of premedical subjects: Physiology, and biochemistry, with the following anatomical change: Well-demarcated, erythematous plaques with overlying silvery scales (psoriasis).

Ans:

Horizontal Integration with Physiology

Hyperproliferation of keratinocytes within the epidermis and defects in immune system functions.

Horizontal Integration with Biochemistry

Defects in normal immunological reactions and rapid epidermal turnover lead to an increase in serum uric acid.

BAQ: Show vertical integration of the paramedical subject: Pharmacology, with the following anatomical change: Well-demarcated, erythematous plaques with overlying silvery scales (psoriasis).

Ans:

Vertical Integration with Pharmacology

Selection of an appropriate drug to manage normal skin conditions.

BIBLIOGRAPHY

1. Godkar PB, Godkar DP. Medical Biochemistry. 1st ed. New Delhi, India: CBS Publishers; 2023.
2. Godkar PB, Godkar DP. Textbook of Medical Laboratory Technology. 4th ed. Mumbai, India: Bhalani Publishing House; 2024.
3. Gray H, Standring S, eds. Anatomy of the Human Body. 42nd ed. Elsevier; 2020.
4. Grant AW, Waugh A, Wilson KJW. Ross & Wilson Anatomy and Physiology in Health and Illness. 13th ed. 2018.
5. Schaum's Outline of Theory and Problems of Human Anatomy and Physiology. 2nd ed. New Delhi, India: Tata McGraw-Hill Publishing Company Limited; 1997.

MULTIPLE CHOICE QUESTIONS (MCQs)

Select the correct option.

1. This is not the function of the skin:

(A) Vitamin A synthesis
(B) Vitamin D synthesis
(C) Regulation of body temperature
(D) Pathogen entry prevention

2. The function of melanin in the skin is to:

(A) Prevention of infection
(B) Protection against UV light
(C) Regulation of body temperature
(D) Both (A) and (B)

3. Body fluid loss through the skin is prevented by:

(A) Stratum basale
(B) Carotene
(C) Keratinised dead squamous cells
(D) Melanocytes

4. The system that is the largest in the human body is:

(A) Respiratory system (B) Integumentary system
(C) Digestive system (D) Excretory system

5. This structure is a vascular stratified squamous epithelium and oxygen diffuses from capillaries in the dermis:

(A) Epidermis (B) Dermis
(C) Hypodermis (D) Mesoderm

6. This is the clear layer that is found only in thick skin and covers granulosum.

(A) Stratum granulosum (B) Stratum lucidum
(C) Stratum corneum (D) Stratum spinosum

7. The stratum corneum is this type of layer:

(A) Clear layer (B) Horny layer
(C) Grainy layer (D) Spiny layer

8. This layer of dermis consists of areolar tissue and contains small capillaries and sensory neurons:

(A) Reticular layer (B) Papillary layer
(C) Epidermis layer (D) Subcutaneous layer

9. This layer of dermis consists of collagen and elastic fibres:

(A) Grainy layer (B) Papillary layer
(C) Reticular layer (D) Spiny layer

10. This is the structure of the nails and pale crescent at the base of the nail:

(A) Lunula (B) Eponychium
(C) Nail fold (D) Cuticle

11. Human skin originates from:

(A) Mesoderm
(B) Ectoderm
(C) Mesoderm and ectoderm
(D) Ectoderm and endoderm

12. The outermost layer of skin is:

(A) Stratum granulosum (B) Stratum spinosum
(C) Stratum lucidum (D) Stratum corneum

13. Eleiden protein is found in:

(A) Stratum corneum (B) Stratum lucidum
(C) Stratum spinosum (D) Stratum granulosum

14. The deepest layer of the epidermis is:

(A) Stratum corneum (B) Stratum granulosum
(C) Stratum spinosum (D) Stratum basale

15. The following are skin derivatives:

(A) Nails (B) Sebaceous glands
(C) Sweat glands (D) All of the above

16. The sebaceous gland is an example of:

(A) Holocrine glands (B) Apocrine glands
(C) Mesocrine glands (D) Apocrine glands

17. The barrier layer of the skin is called:

(A) Stratum spinosum (B) Stratum lucidum
(C) Stratum corneum (D) Stratum granulosum

18. The melanin pigment present in the hair is found in:

(A) Cuticle (B) Medulla
(C) Cortex (D) All of the above

19. The function of the fat layer found below the skin is:

(A) To provide shape to the body
(B) Storing fat
(C) Temperature resistant
(D) All of the above

20. The epidermis has how many sub-layers?

(A) Six
(B) Three
(C) Five
(D) Four

ANSWERS

1. A 2. B 3. C 4. B 5. A 6. B 7. B
8. B 9. C 10. A 11. C 12. D 13. B 14. D
15. D 16. A 17. B 18. C 19. D 20. C

MATCH THE COLUMNS

I	II
1. Melanin	A. Regulation of body temperature
2. Sweat glands	B. Secretory epithelial cells
3. Hair colour	C. Collagen fibres
4. Sebaceous glands	D. Moist skin
5. Vitamin D	E. Tyrosine
6. Fibroblasts	F. Sunlight
7. Pus formation	G. Striated keratinised epithelial cells
8. Sebum	H. Connective tissue
9. Epidermis	I. Bacterial or fungal infection
10. Dermis	J. Melanin

ANSWERS

1. E 2. A 3. J 4. B 5. F 6. C 7. I
8. D 9. G 10. H

CHAPTER

4

Skeletal System

SAQ: Short answer question: Marks: 2
BAQ: Brief answer question: Marks: 4 or 5
LAQ: Long answer question: Marks: 9 or 10

MCQs: Multiple choice questions: Marks: 0.5 each
Match the columns: Marks: 0.5 each
Draw a labelled diagram: Marks: 5

INTRODUCTION

The human skeleton (Fig. 4.1) is the internal bony framework of the human body. This framework consists of many individual bones, cartilages, and bands of fibrous connective tissue, the ligaments and the tendons. The following are the major functions of the skeletal system: Providing support to the body, body part movement facilitation, internal organ protection, blood cell formation and storage of minerals and fat.

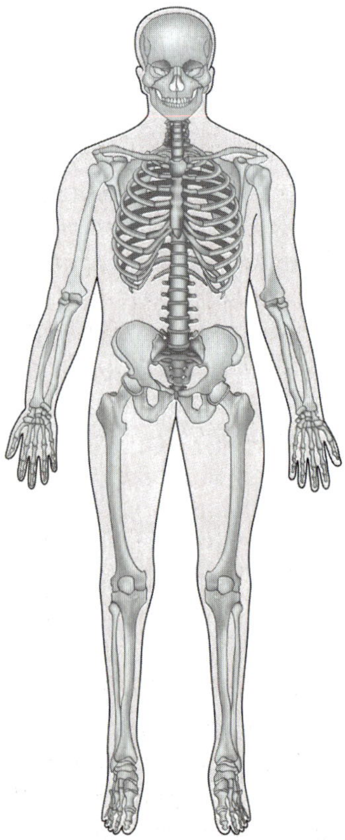

Fig. 4.1: Skeletal system

The skeletal system in an adult body is made up of an average of 206 individual bones. These bones are arranged into two major divisions: The axial skeleton and the appendicular skeleton.

Objective: To describe the functions of the skeletal system.

FUNCTIONS OF BONES

BAQ: What are the various functions of bones?

Ans: Bones:

1. Provide shape and support to the body.
2. Protect internal organs such as lungs, liver, brain, heart, etc.
3. Anchor muscles, which are necessary for the movement of the body parts.
4. Act as storage material for minerals such as calcium and inorganic phosphorus.
5. Contain red bone marrow, responsible for the production of red blood cells.

Objective: To describe the microscopic structure of bone.

MICROSCOPIC STRUCTURE OF BONE (Figs 4.2 and 4.3)

LAQ: Write a note on the microscopic structure of bone.

Ans: The skeleton makes up about 30–40% of the body mass of an adult. The skeleton is made up of a non-living bone matrix and a large number of small bone cells. About 50% of the bone mass of the bone matrix is water and the remaining 50% of bone mass is made up of collagen protein, calcium carbonate and calcium phosphate crystals.

The bone cells are responsible for the growth and development of bones. Bone cells are also responsible for the repair of bones following an injury and daily wear and tear. Bone cells also facilitate the release of their stored minerals, when the body needs these minerals.

CROSS SECTION OF BONE (Figs 4.2 and 4.3)

The bone is covered in periosteum, which is a thin layer of dense irregular connective tissue. The periosteum contains many strong fibres of collagen protein that are used to firmly anchor tendons and muscles to the bone, which facilitates movement. The periosteum contains stem cells and osteoblast cells. These cells are involved in the growth and repair of the outside of the bone due to injury and stress. Blood vessels are present in the periosteum. Blood nutrient circulation provides energy to the cells on the surface of the bone. Blood vessels penetrate the bone to supply nutrients to the cells inside of the bone. The periosteum also contains nervous tissue and many nerve endings, which make bone sensitive to pain.

Inside the periosteum, compact hard bone is present. Compact bone is made of a hard matrix of mineral salts, and it becomes stronger with the presence of tough collagen fibres. Many osteocytes live in small spaces in the matrix and these can maintain the strength and integrity of the compact hard bone.

Spongy bone is a region of bone where the bone tissue grows in thin columns called trabeculae with spaces in which bone marrow is present. The trabeculae resist outside stresses. Long bones have a porous spongy type of bone on their ends and have a hollow medullary cavity in the middle of the diaphysis. The medullary cavity contains red bone marrow during childhood. Red bone marrow turns into yellow bone marrow after puberty.

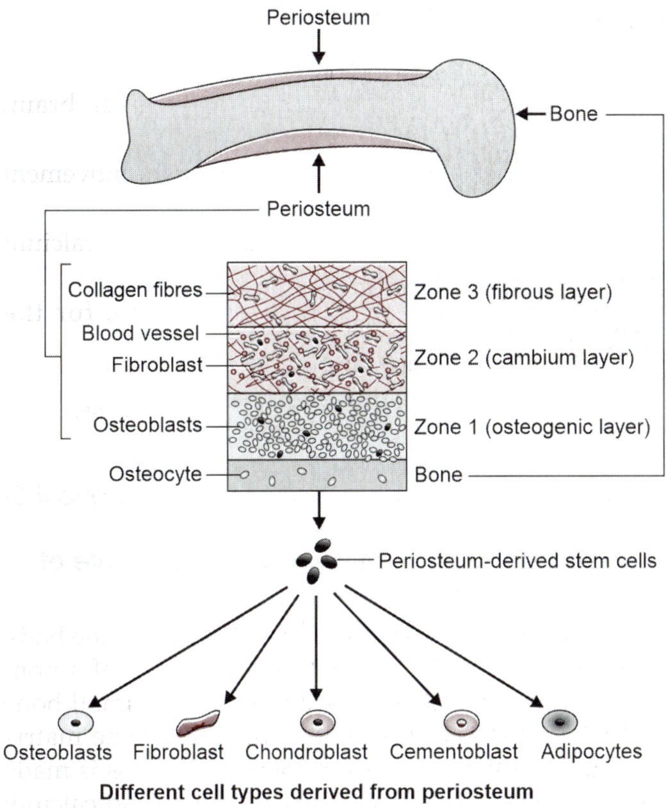

Fig. 4.2: Bone—cross section

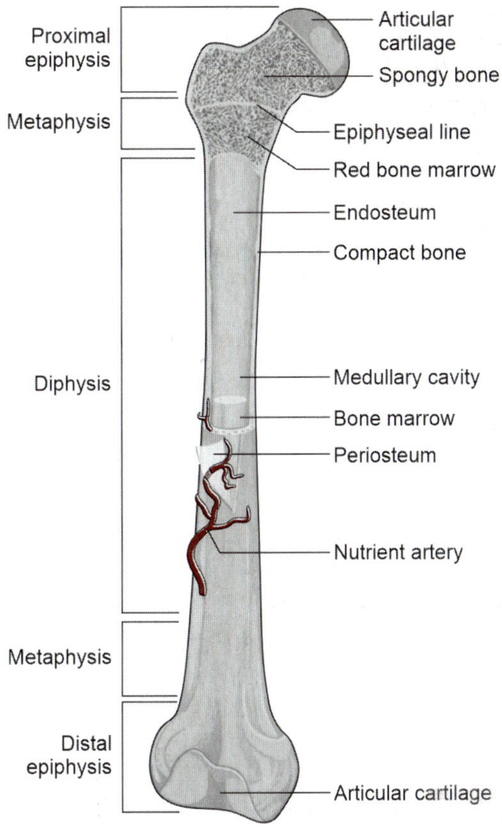

Fig. 4.3: Bone structure and parts

BAQ: Draw a labelled diagram of bone structure and parts.

Ans: Refer to Fig. 4.3.

Haversian Canals

SAQ: What are the Haversian canals?

Ans: The Haversian canals are a series of tubes around narrow channels formed by plates of tissues (lamellae). The canals and the surrounding lamellae are called the Haversian system. The Haversian canals are present surrounding blood vessels and nerve fibers throughout the long bones and these communicate with the bone cells. A Haversian canal generally contains nerve fibres and one or two blood capillaries.

Objectives:
- To describe the surface features of the bones.
- To describe the parts of bones.

PARTS OF BONES (Fig. 4.3)

BAQ: Describe the parts of a bone.

Ans: Each end bone is called an epiphysis. The middle bone is called a diaphysis. The epiphyses and diaphysis grow towards one another and eventually fuse into one bone. The region of growth and fusion between the epiphysis and diaphysis is called the metaphysis.

Table 4.1: Surface features, definition and examples of the bone		
Surface feature	***Definition***	***Examples***
Openings and depressions		
Sinus	Cavity (hollow space)	Frontal sinus of the frontal bone
Fovea	Small depression	Femur bone's fovea capitis femoris
Fossa	Shallow depression	Temporal bone's mandibular fossa
Fissure	Narrow slit-like opening	Sphenoid bone's superior orbital fissure
Meatus (canal)	Tubelike passageway	Temporal bone's external acoustic meatus)
Foramen	Round opening through a bone	Occipital bone's foramen magnum
Alveolus	Deep socket (pit)	Maxillary alveoli of teeth
Articulating surface		
Facet	Shallow or flattened articulating surface	Costal facet of a thoracic vertebra
Head	Prominent articulating end	Femur head
Condyle	Rounded articulating surface	Condyle of the occipital bone
Non-articulating projections		
Epicondyle	Projection above a condyle	Femur epicondyle
Crest	A long narrow projection	Iliac crest of the os coxae
Process	Extension of bone	Temporal bone's mastoid process
Tuberosity	Large rough process	Radial tuberosity of radius
Tubercle	Small rounded process	Humerus greater tubercle
Spine	Slender and sharp process	Spine of the scapula

The articular cartilage covers the epiphysis of long bones in the knee (Fig. 4.4). It acts as a shock absorber and gliding surface between the bones to facilitate movement at the joint.

BAQ: Draw a labelled diagram of articular cartilage.

Ans:: Refer to Fig. 4.4.

BAQ: What is the periosteum of bone and its function?

Ans: The periosteum is a thin layer of connective tissue that covers the outer surface of all the bones except at joints. It consists of an outer fibrous layer, an inner cambium layer and an osteogenic layer (Fig. 4.4). The fibrous layer is made up of dense irregular connective tissue, containing fibroblasts, while the cambium layer is highly cellular containing progenitor cells that develop into osteoblasts. These osteoblasts are responsible for increasing the width of a long bone and the overall size of the other bone types. After a bone fracture, the progenitor cells develop into osteoblasts and chondroblasts, which are essential for the healing process. The outer fibrous layer and the inner cambium layer can be differentiated under electron micrography. The periosteum contains sensory neurons and blood vessels and connects back to the circulatory system which supplies oxygen-rich blood to bones.

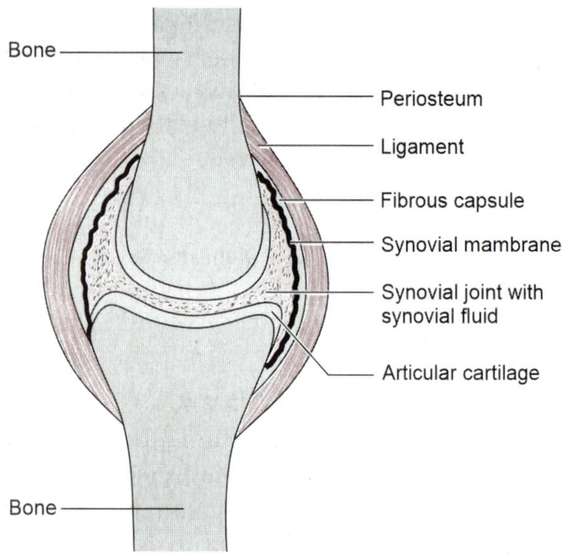

Fig. 4.4: Articular cartilage

BAQ: What are the osteogenic cells of the bone?

Ans: The osteogenic cells are stem cells. These are located in the surface lining of bones and the bone marrow. The osteogenic cells are undifferentiated bone cells and in response to specific stimuli such as bone damage or bone injury; these cells can give rise to osteoblasts that are responsible for the formation of bone structure. Osteoblasts can form osteocytes that can maintain the bone structure by regulating the mineral concentration of the matrix. Osteoclasts act to dissolve bone according to the biochemical changes taking place in the body and also to break down old or damaged bone cells. These three cells of bone maintain normal bone structures continuously through the processes called remodelling of bones that involve various steps such as bone formation, mineralization, and bone resorption.

BAQ: Write a note on the blood and nerve supply of bones.

Ans: A typical long bone has the following main sources:

1. The nutrient artery
2. The metaphyseal arteries
3. The epiphyseal arteries, and
4. The periosteal arteries.

Blood supply to the marrow is mainly provided by the nutrient arteries. These arteries extend along the longitudinal axis of the bone and provide radial branches throughout the marrow.

The metaphyseal arteries supply blood to the metaphysis, which is the most vascular region of the bone.

The epiphyseal arteries, enter the epiphyses and form branches of small vessels that supply blood to the red bone marrow and spongy bone.

The periosteal arteries seen in the proximity of the periosteum supply blood to the outer part of the compact bone.

Nervous System in Bones

The bone has a rich nerve supply of sensory nerves, which are abundant in the periosteum of the bone. The nerves detect tension or damage to the bone and relay the pain signals to the brain.

Objective: To distinguish between short bones, long bones, flat bones, and irregular bones and provide an example of each.

TYPES OF BONES

LAQ: Describe various types of bones with examples.

Ans: All of the bones of the body can be divided into five types: Long, short, flat, irregular, and sesamoid (Fig. 4.5).

Long Bones (Fig. 4.5)

Long bones are major bones of the limbs. Examples of long bones are femur, tibia, fibula, metatarsals, and phalanges.

Long bones in adults are responsible for height. Long bone contains a hollow medullary cavity in the centre in which bone marrow is stored.

Short Bones (Fig. 4.5)

Short bones: Examples of short bones are the carpal bones of the wrist and the tarsal bones of the foot.

Flat Bones (Fig. 4.5)

Flat bones vary greatly in size and shape but have the common feature of being very thin in one direction and do not have a medullary cavity. Examples of flat bones are frontal, parietal, and occipital bones of the cranium, rib and hip bones.

Irregular Bones (Fig. 4.5)

Irregular bones examples are the vertebrae, sacrum, coccyx of the spine, the sphenoid, ethmoid, and zygomatic bones of the skull.

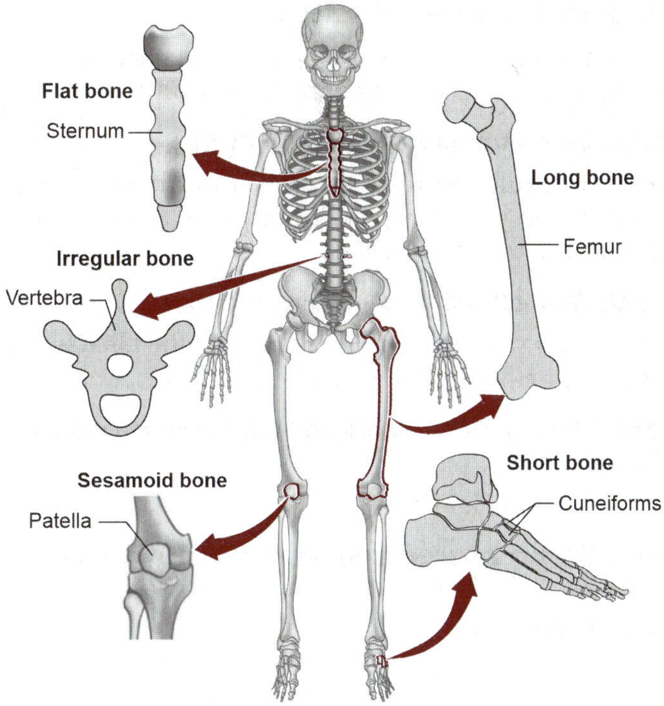

Fig. 4.5: Various types of bones

Sesamoid Bones (Figs 4.6A and B)

The sesamoid bones are formed after birth inside of tendons, which run across the joints. The sesamoid bones grow to protect the tendons from stresses and strains at the joint and give a mechanical advantage to muscles pulling on the tendon. Examples of sesamoid bones are the patella and the pisiform bone of the carpals.

SAQ: Give examples of long bones.

Ans: Examples of long bones are, the femur, tibia, fibula, metatarsals, and phalanges.

SAQ: Give examples of short bones.

Ans: Examples of short bones are the carpal bones of the wrist and the tarsal bones of the foot.

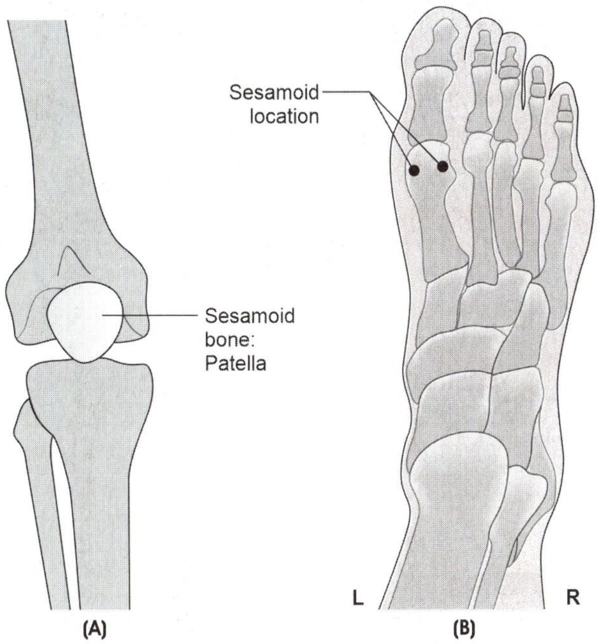

Figs 4.6A and B: Sesamoid bone

SAQ: Give examples of flat bones.

Ans: Examples of flat bones are frontal, parietal, and occipital bones of the cranium, rib and hip bones.

SAQ: Give examples of irregular bones.

Ans: Irregular bones examples are, the vertebrae, sacrum, coccyx of the spine, the sphenoid, ethmoid, and zygomatic bones of the skull.

SAQ: Give examples of sesamoid bones.

Ans: Examples of sesamoid bones are, the patella and the pisiform bone of the carpals.

BAQ: Draw a labelled diagram of the short and long bones

Ans: Refer to Fig. 4.5.

BAQ: Draw a labelled diagram of the flat and irregular bones.

Ans: Refer to Fig. 4.5.

Objective: To distinguish the difference between axial and appendicular skeletal systems.

AXIAL SKELETON (Figs 4.7 and 4.8)

SAQ: What are the main parts of the axial skeleton?

Ans: The axial skeleton runs along the body's midline axis and is made up of 80 bones in the following regions: skull, auditory ossicles, hyoid, ribs, sternum and vertebral column (Fig. 4.8).

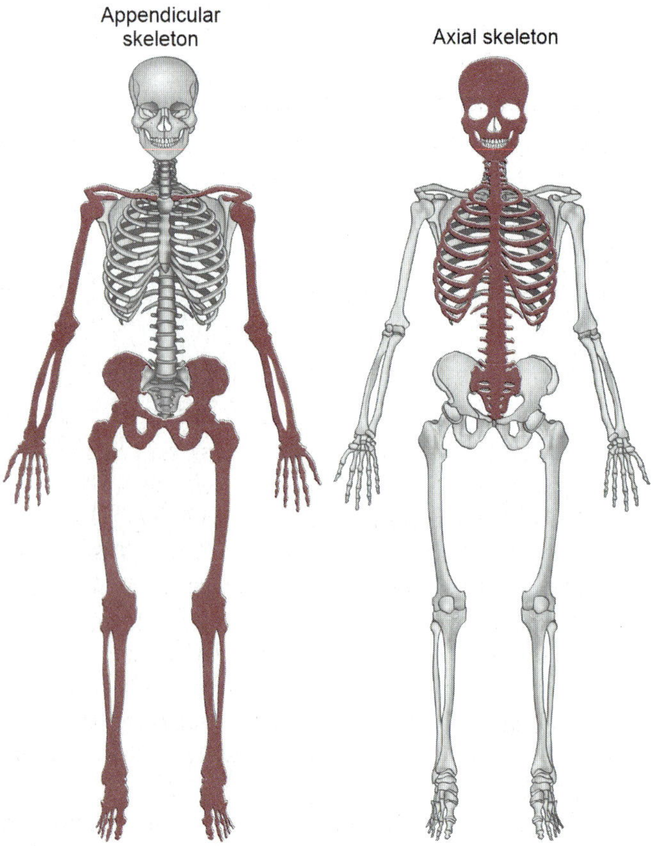

Fig. 4.7: Appendicular skeleton and axial skeleton

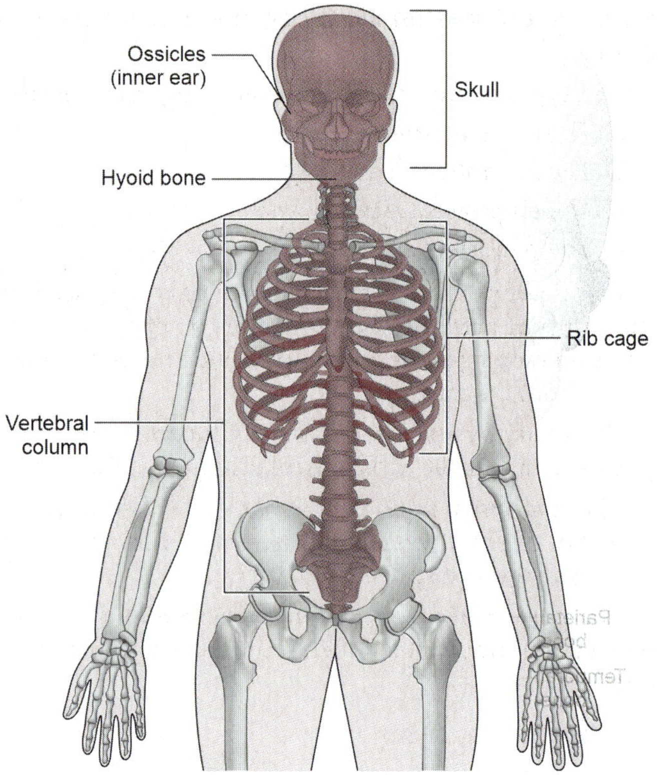

Fig. 4.8: Axial skeleton

Objective: To list the skull bones and describe the anatomical features of the skull.

Skull (Figs 4.9–4.11)

LAQ: Write a note on the bones of a skull.

Ans: The skull is composed of 22 bones that are fused except the mandible bone. Mandible is the largest bone and only movable part in the human skull and it holds the lower teeth in place. Mandible bone forms the lower jawline and assists in mastication (Fig. 4.9).

Twenty-one fused bones of the skull are different in children to allow the skull and the brain to grow. These bones fuse later on in adults to give added strength and protection.

The bones of the superior portion of the skull are known as the cranial bones and these protect the brain from damage (Fig. 4.10). The cranial main bones are the frontal bone (1), parietal bones (2), occipital bone (1), Temporal bones (2), sphenoid bone (1), and ethmoid bone (1).

The bones of the anterior portion and inferior portion of the skull are known as facial bones and support the nose, eyes and mouth (Fig. 4.11).

BAQ: Draw a labelled diagram of cranial bones.

Ans: Refer to Fig. 4.10.

SAQ: What are the various functions of the bones of the skull?

Ans: The main function of the skull is to give protection to the brain and orbits of the eyes. The skull provides an anchor for the muscular and tendinous attachments of the muscles of the face and the scalp.

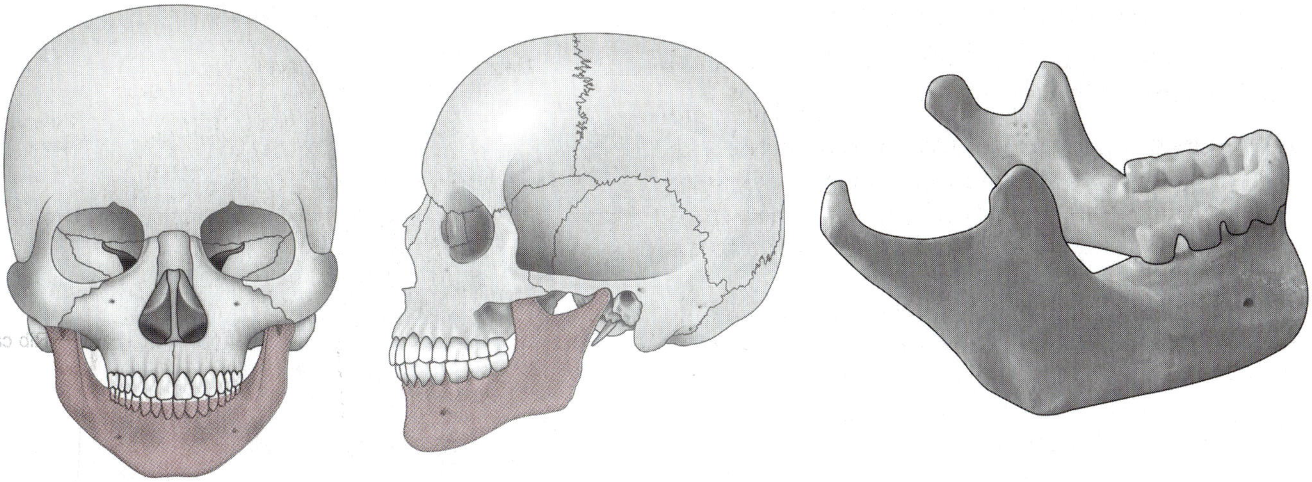

Fig. 4.9: Mandible bone

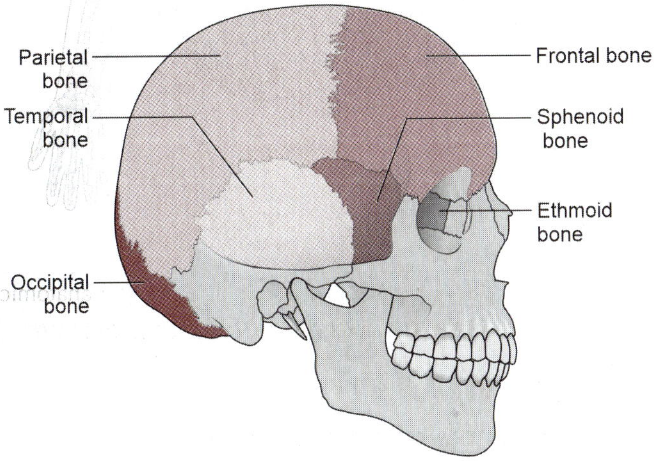

Fig. 4.10: Cranial bones

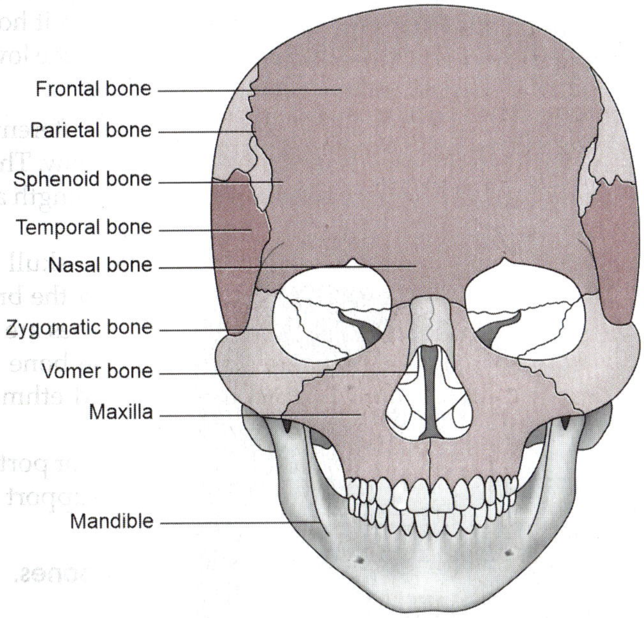

Fig. 4.11: Facial and cranial bones

SAQ: What are sutures? Describe the locations of the principal sutures of the skull.

Ans: The sutures of the skull (Fig. 4.12) are fibrous joints that connect the skull bones. These sutures appear as intricate thin lines between the bones.

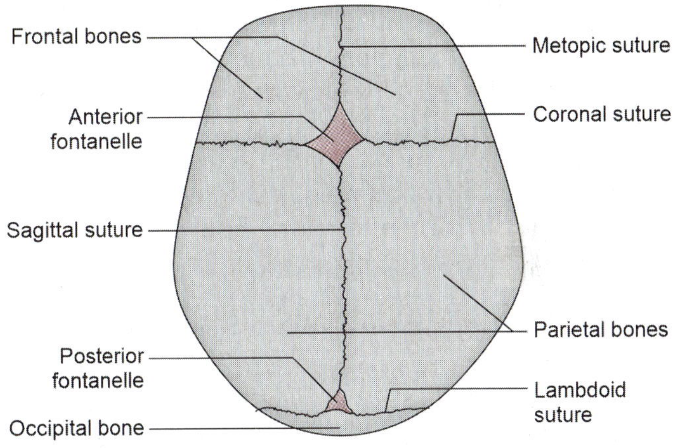

Fig. 4.12: Cranial sutures

- The frontal bone is joined to the two parietal bones at the coronal suture.
- The parietal bones meet at the sagittal suture.
- The occipital bone meets the parietal bone at the lambdoid suture.
- The parietal bone joins the temporal bone at the squamous suture.

Objective: To describe the anatomical features of the facial bones.

Facial Bones (Fig. 4.11)

The main facial bones are the maxilla (1), nasal (2), zygomatic (3), vomer (1), palatine (2), and mandible (1). The facial bones protect the brain and the organs responsible for sight, smell, and taste. The facial bones are made up of soft tissues and structures that help in various processes such as eating, breathing, talking and facial expressions.

Maxillae are a pair of bones that form the main portion of the face. The maxillae hold the tooth roots, form most parts of the nasal apertures and floor and are the major part of the hard palate, and the parts of the orbits (Fig. 4.11).

The nasal bones are symmetrical oblong two bones. These have two surfaces and four borders. Nasal bones are present in the junction of the midface. These bones anchor the upper lateral nasal cartilages inferiorly and form the bridge of the nose superiorly (Fig. 4.11).

The zygomatic bones are two in number. These are diamond-shaped and irregularly shaped bones. The zygomatic bones form the prominence of the cheeks, one part of the lateral wall, the orbit floor, and some part of the temporal fossa and infratemporal fossa and protrude laterally (Fig. 4.11).

The vomer is situated in the median plane. It is a thin and moderately quadrilateral in shape. It forms the hind and lower parts of the nasal septum. The vomer has two surfaces and four borders. The vomer joins with the left and right maxillary bones, the ethmoid, sphenoid, and the left and right palatine bones (Figs 4.11 and 4.13).

The palatine bones are two irregular bones. These are L-shaped bones; that form a part of the nasal cavity and palate. The palatine bones are situated between the maxilla bone and the sphenoid bone (Figs 4.10 and 4.11).

The mandible is the largest and strongest bone of the face. It is located inferiorly in the facial skeleton. It is the only movable part of the skull. The mandible forms the lower jaw and holds the lower teeth. It joins on either side with the temporal bone and forms the temporomandibular joint (Fig. 4.11).

Objective: To describe the anatomical features of sinuses.

Sinuses

A sinus is a cavity or sac in any tissue or organ. The paranasal sinuses are the cavities in the cranial bones near the nose and these are connected to the nose. The paranasal sinuses are extensions of the nasal cavity. These are air-filled and are present in the frontal, maxillary, ethmoid and sphenoid bones. These sinuses are lined with ciliated mucus membranes.

Objective: To describe the anatomical features of the hyoid bone and the auditory ossicles.

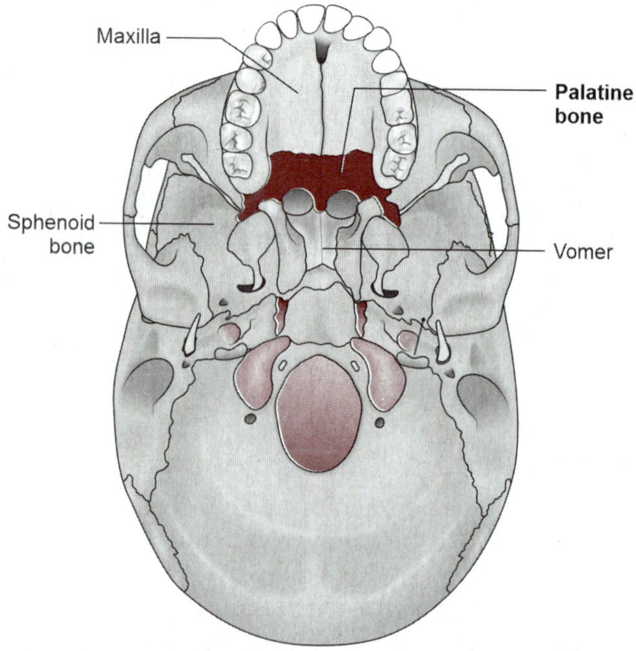

Fig. 4.13: Palatine bones

HYOID BONE AND AUDITORY OSSICLES

(Figs 4.14–4.16)

BAQ: Draw a labelled diagram of paranasal sinuses.

Ans: Refer to Fig. 4.14.

BAQ: Write a note on the hyoid bone.

Ans: The hyoid is a U-shaped small bone seen just below the mandible bone. It is the only bone in the body that does not form a joint with any other bone. A hyoid is a floating bone (Fig. 4.15).

Function: The function of the hyoid bone is to help in holding the trachea open and it forms a bony connection for the tongue muscles.

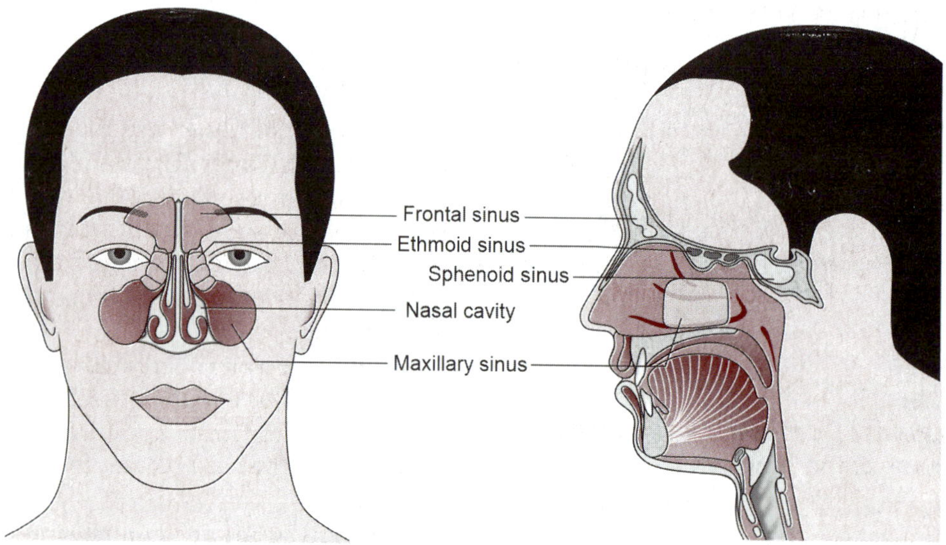

Fig. 4.14: Paranasal sinuses

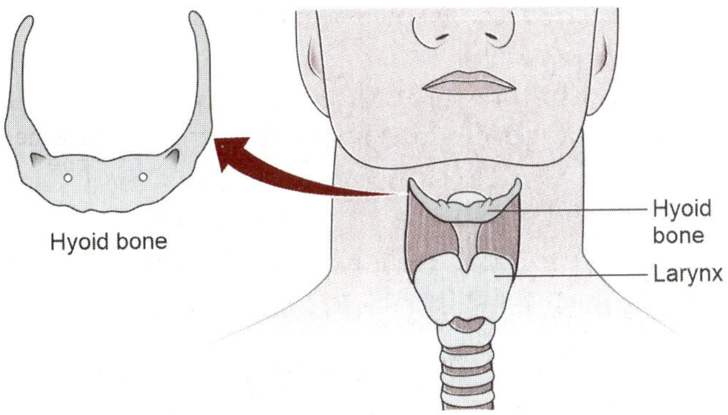

Fig. 4.15: Hyoid bone

Auditory Ossicles (Fig. 4.16)

BAQ: Write a note on the auditory ossicles.

Ans: The auditory ossicles are the malleus, the incus, and the stapes bone and these are the smallest bones in the body. These are collectively known as the auditory bone and are found in a small cavity inside the temporal bone. ***Function:*** These bones serve to transmit and amplify sound from the eardrum to the inner ear.

BAQ: Draw a labelled diagram of auditory ossicles.

Ans: Refer to Fig. 4.16.

> **Objectives:**
> - To list the bones of the vertebral column.
> - To describe the anatomical features of the vertebral column bones.
> - To describe the functions of the vertebral column.

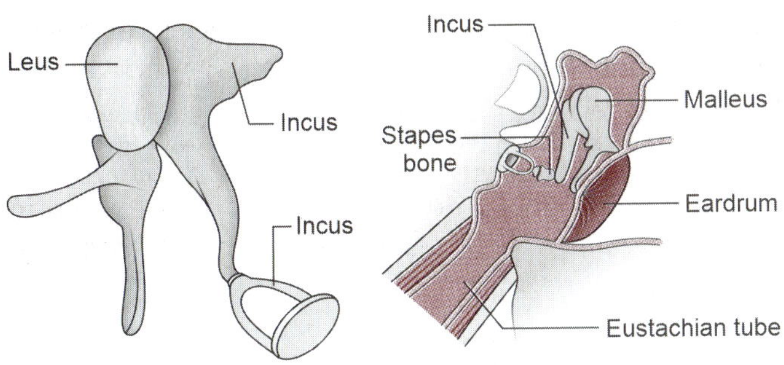

Fig. 4.16: Auditory ossicles: The malleus, incus and stapes bones in the ear

Vertebral Column (Spine or Backbone)

SAQ: Briefly describe the vertebral column.

Ans: The vertebral column (spine or backbone) indicates the defining characteristic of the vertebrate endoskeleton and it is the prominent part of the axial skeleton. The vertebral column contains a series of segmented irregular bones called vertebrae, which are separated by specific discs (Figs 4.17 and 4.18). In the dorsal portion of the vertebral column, the spinal canal (a cavity) is present.

BAQ: Enumerate the functions of the spinal cord.

Ans: Functions of spinal cord:

1. Helps to maintain the balance of the body
2. Supports the head
3. Protests the spinal cord
4. Absorbs shocks while walking
5. Serves as an attachment point to the ribs pelvic girdle, and muscle of the upper limb and back
6. Enables the following movements of the body: Forward, backwards, sideways and rotation.

VERTEBRAE (Fig. 4.17)

LAQ: Write a note on the vertebrae.

Ans: The vertebrae are the bones of the spinal column. These are 33 individuals, with interlocking bones. Each vertebra has three main functional components:

1. The vertebral body is meant for load-bearing,
2. The vertebral arch which protects the spinal cord, and
3. Transverse processes meant for ligament attachment.

Twenty-six vertebrae form the vertebral column of the human body (Figs 4.17A and B). They are named by the region of the spinal cord as follows:

Cervical (neck) region: It is made up of 7 vertebrae
Thoracic (chest) region: It is made up of 12 vertebrae
Lumbar (lower back) region: It is made up of 5 vertebrae
Sacrum region: It is made up of 1 vertebra
Coccyx (tailbone) region: It is made up of 1 vertebra.

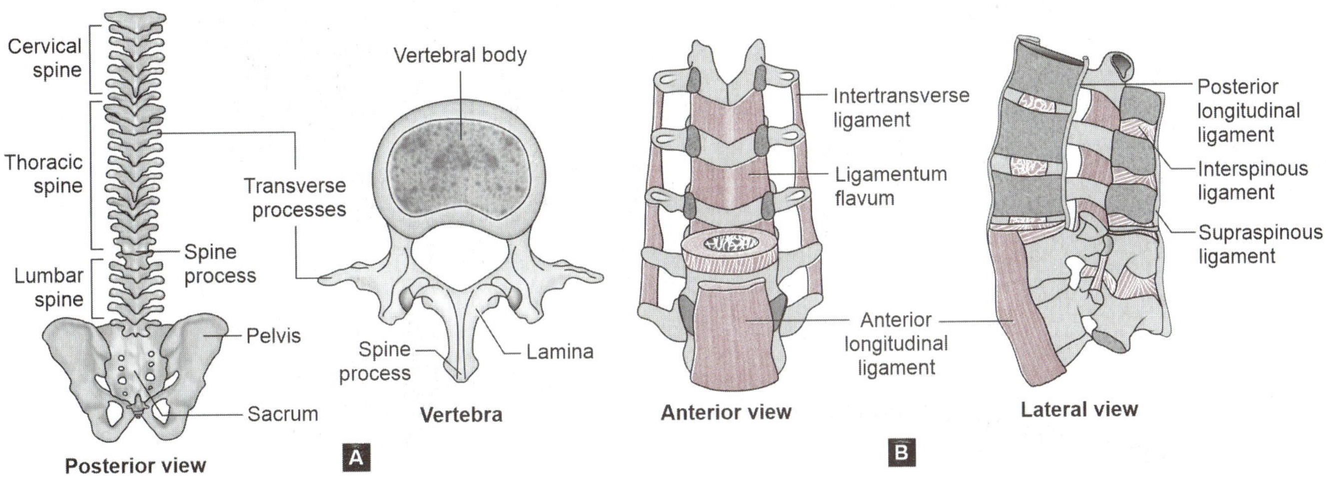

Figs 4.17A and B: (A) Vertebrae and (B) the connected ligaments

Each vertebra is named for the first letter of its region and its position along the superior-inferior axis, except the singular sacrum and coccyx bones. For example, the most superior thoracic vertebra is called T1 and the most inferior thoracic vertebra is called T12 (Fig. 4.17).

BAQ: Write a note on the specific features of the vertebrae.

Ans: The vertebrae are different in features. However, the following types have specific features (Fig 4.18):

Cervical vertebrae: These have transverse foramina for the passage of vessels to the brain.

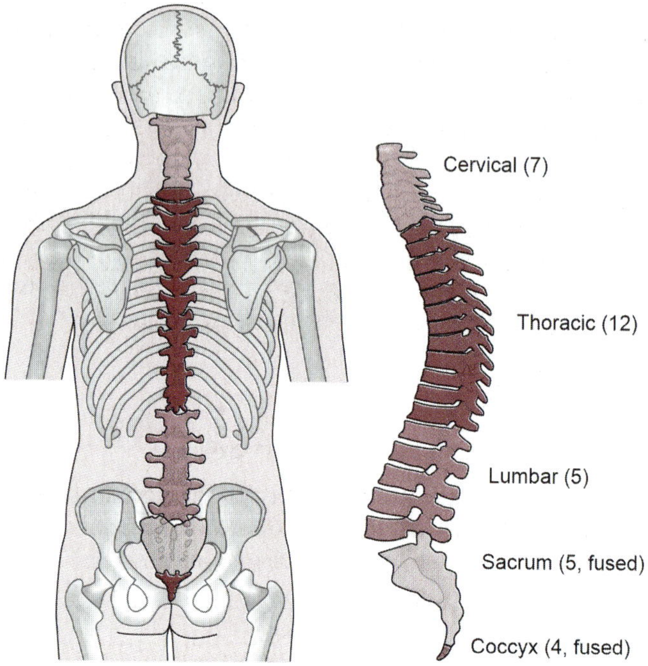

Fig. 4.18: Regions of the spinal cord

Thoracic vertebrae: These have facets for the articulation with the heads of the rib.

Large lumbar vertebrae: These have prominent processes for muscle attachment

Sacrum: It is made up of four to five fused sacral vertebrae and it connects to the pelvic girdle

Triangular coccyx: It is made up of four to five coccygeal vertebrae which are fused.

> **Objective:** To describe the anatomical features and functions of the vertebra.

BAQ: Describe a lumbar vertebra.

Ans: Each vertebra has a vertebral body. The body has a large anterior middle portion (centrum) and a posterior vertebral arch (neural arch). The body is made up of cancellous bone (spongy bone), which is covered by a thin coating of cortical bone (compact bone). The vertebral arch is formed by pedicles and laminae.

The vertebral parts, the vertebral arch and processes have moderately thick coverings of cortical bone. The upper and lower surfaces of the body of the vertebra are flattened and rough, which gives attachment to the intervertebral discs. The upper and lower surfaces are the vertebral endplates. These connect with the intervertebral discs and form the joint. The function of the endplates is to adjust the adjacent discs, to facilitate the spread of the applied loads, evenly. Endplates also provide anchorage to the collagen fibers of the disc. Endplates also serve as a semi-permeable interface for the exchange of solutes through water (Figs 4.20A and B).

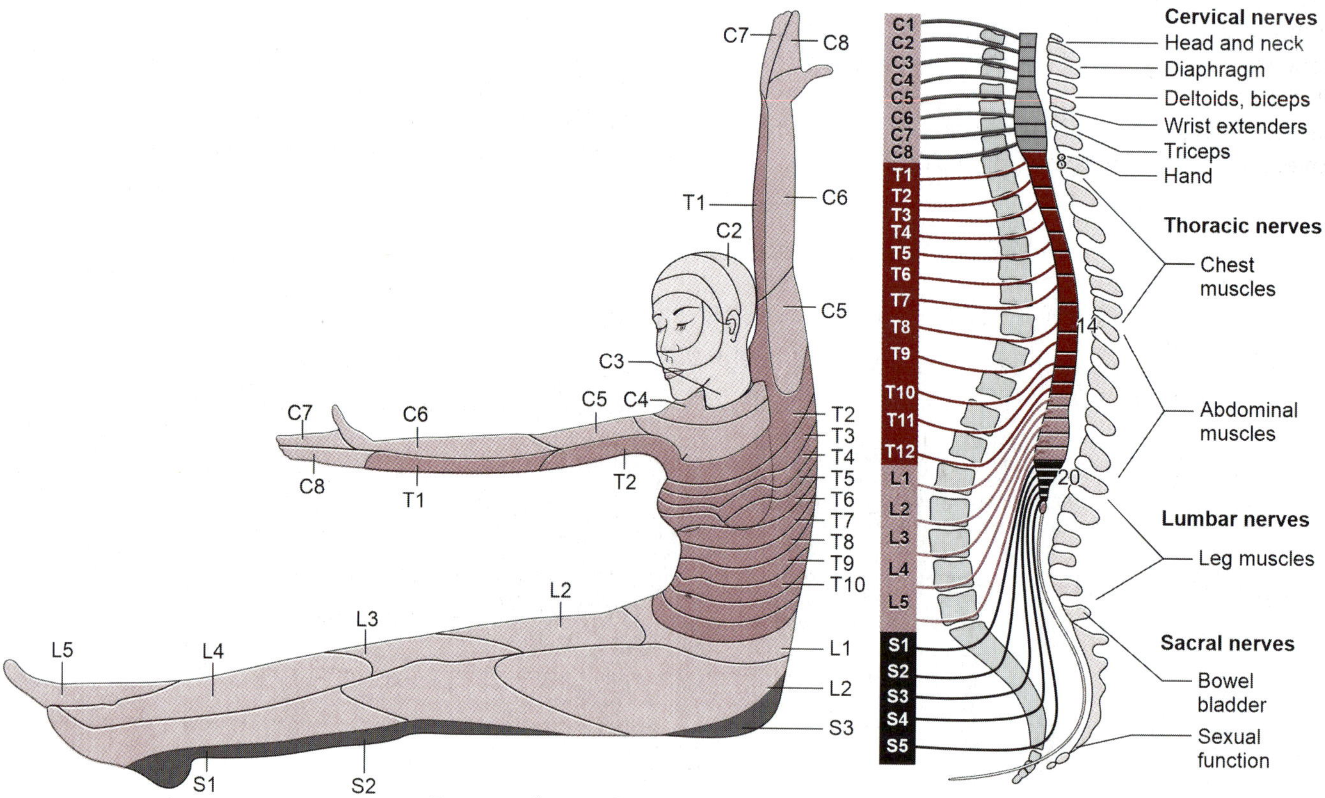

Fig. 4.19: Innervation of the vertebral bones

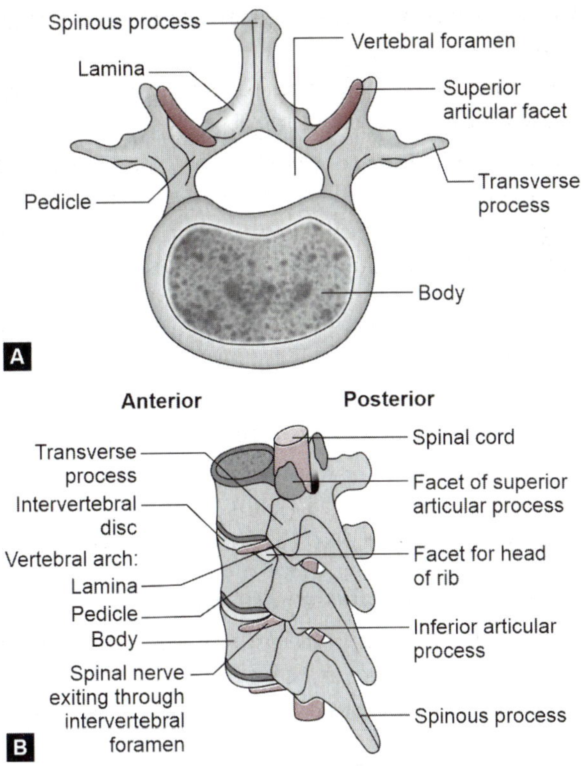

Figs 4.20A and B: The lumbar vertebra

BAQ: Draw a labelled diagram of the lumbar vertebra.

Ans: Refer to Fig. 4.20A.

Anatomy of a Vertebra

BAQ: Write a note on the anatomy of a vertebra.

Ans: Each vertebra has a vertebral body. The body has a large anterior middle portion and a posterior vertebral arch (neural arch). The body is made up of cancellous bone (spongy bone), which is covered by a thin coating of cortical bone (compact bone). The vertebral parts, vertebral arch and processes have moderately thick coverings of cortical bone (Fig. 4.20B).

The vertebral arch is formed by the pedicles and the laminae. Two pedicles extend from the sides of the vertebral body to connect the body to the arch. The pedicles are short thick processes. These extend posteriorly (one from each side), from the junctions of the posteriolateral surfaces of the centrum, on its upper surface. From each pedicle, a lamina (a broad plate), projects backwards to join and complete the vertebral arch, which forms the posterior border of the vertebral foramen leading to the completion of the triangle of the vertebral foramen.

The upper surfaces of the laminae are attached to the ligamenta flava (Fig. 4.17). These ligaments connect the laminae of the adjacent vertebra along the length of the spine from the second cervical vertebral level. Shallow depressions (vertebral notches) are present above and below the pedicles. When the vertebrae join, the notches align with those on adjacent vertebrae and form the openings of the intervertebral foramina. This facilitates the entry and exit of the spinal nerves from each vertebra (Fig. 4.20B), together with associated blood vessels. The connected vertebrae provide a strong support like a pillar to the body.

Objectives:
- To list the bones of the rib.
- To describe the anatomical features of ribs and sternum and their functions.

RIBS AND STERNUM (Fig. 4.21)

LAQ. Write a note on the rib cage (thoracic cage), the ribs and the sternum.

Ans: The rib cage (thoracic cage) is a bony and cartilaginous structure. It surrounds the thoracic cavity. The rib cage is comprised of the ribs, vertebral column and the sternum. It supports the pectoral girdle and forms a core portion of the human skeleton (Fig. 4.21).

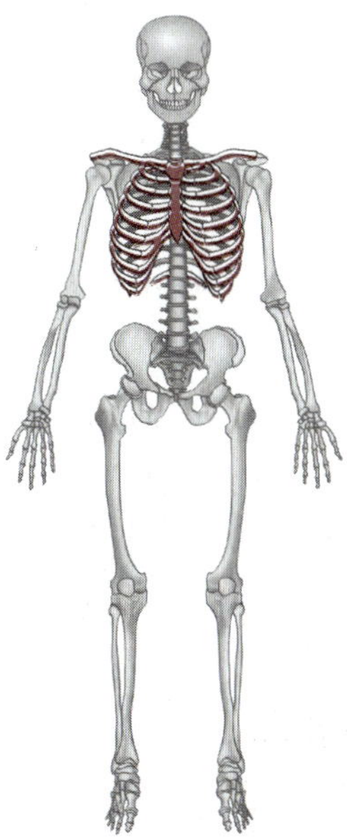

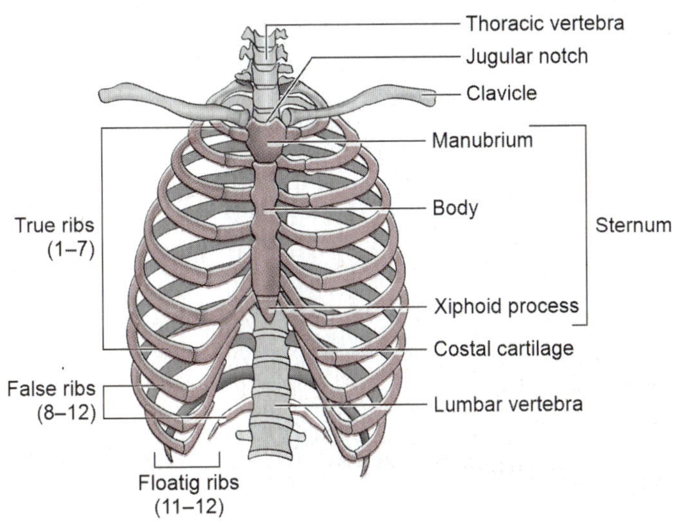

Fig. 4.21: Ribs, thoracic cage (rib cage) and the sternum

There are 12 pairs of ribs. These 12 pairs of bones are connected to the sternum bone. The 12 pairs of ribs together with the sternum form the ribcage. The sternum (breastbone) is a thin, knife-shaped bone located along the midline of the front side of the thoracic region of the skeleton. The sternum is connected to the ribs by the costal cartilage, which are thin bands of cartilage. The ribs are attached posteriorly to the 12 thoracic vertebrae. In females, the volume of the rib cage is about 10% smaller than that in males having the same height. The main function of the thoracic cage is to protect the heart and the lungs (Fig. 4.22).

The first seven ribs are known as "true ribs", since these connect the thoracic vertebrae directly to the sternum through costal cartilage. Ribs 8, 9, and 10 are known as the false ribs, since, all these ribs do not connect to the sternum directly; but connect to the sternum through cartilage that is connected to the cartilage of the seventh rib. Ribs 11 and 12 are false floating ribs since these do not have any cartilage attachment to the sternum.

BAQ: Explain the terms, "the true ribs" and "the false ribs".

Ans: The first seven ribs are known as "true ribs" since these connect the thoracic vertebrae directly to the sternum through costal cartilage. Ribs 8, 9, and 10 are known as "the false ribs' since all these ribs do not connect to the sternum directly but connect to the sternum through cartilage that is connected to the cartilage of the seventh rib. Ribs 11 and 12 are false floating ribs, since, these do not have any cartilage attachment to the sternum.

SAQ: Enumerate three classes of ribs.

Ans:

1. True ribs
2. False ribs
3. Floating ribs.

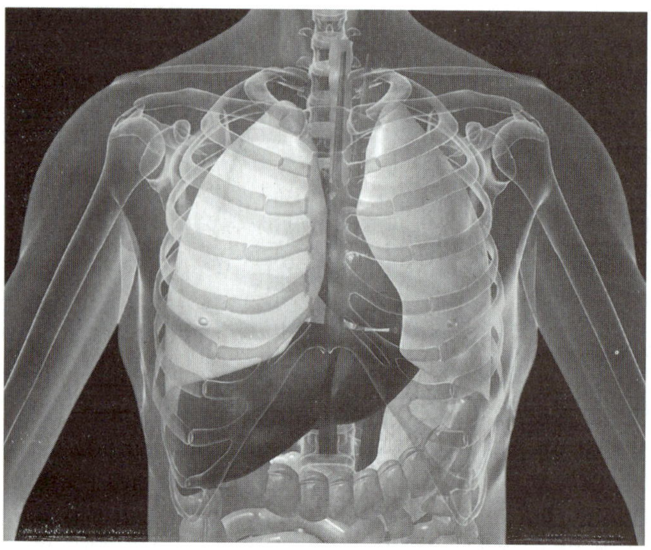

Fig. 4.22: Thoracic cage protecting the heart and lungs

BAQ: Enumerate functions of the rib cage.

Ans: Functions of rib cage:

1. **Protection:** It encloses and protects the lungs and heart. It protects parts of the nervous, immune, and digestive systems.
2. **Respiration:** The ribs and rib muscles contract and expand with normal breathing.
3. **Support:** Provides support to the pectoral girdle and the upper extremities of the skeleton.

Objectives:
- To list the bones of the appendicular skeleton.
- To describe the anatomical features and functions of the appendicular skeleton.

APPENDICULAR SKELETON (Fig. 4.23)

SAQ: What is the appendicular skeleton?

Ans: The appendicular skeleton is made up of 126 bones in the following regions: Upper limbs, lower limbs, pelvic girdle and pectoral (shoulder) girdle.

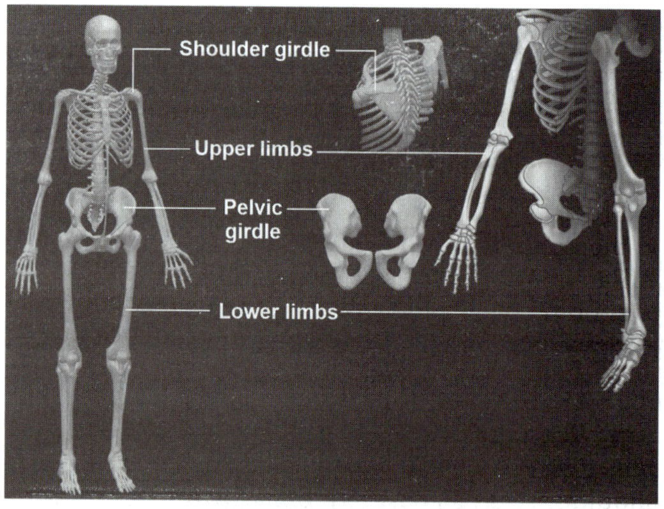

Fig. 4.23: Appendicular skeleton

BAQ: Draw a labelled diagram of the appendicular skeleton.

Ans: Refer to Fig. 4.23.

PECTORAL GIRDLE AND UPPER LIMB BONES (Fig. 4.24)

SAQ: Write a note on the pectoral girdle.

Ans: The pectoral girdle is the bony structure present on either side of the body. It is connected to the upper limb (arm) bones. Upper limb bones are connected to the axial skeleton and consist of the left and right clavicles and left and right scapulae. The pectoral girdles on either side of the body are not connected.

Functions of the Pectoral Girdle

SAQ. What are the functions of the pectoral girdle?

Ans: The functions of the pectoral girdle are as follows:

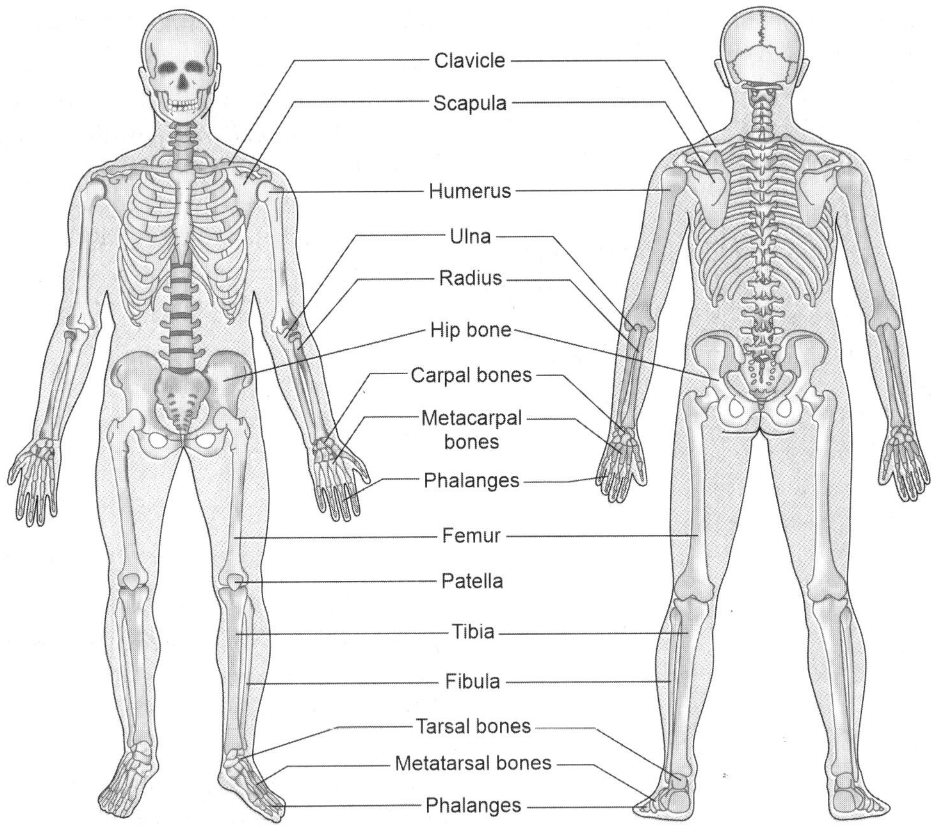

Fig. 4.24: Various bones of the appendicular skeleton

Functions of Pectoral Girdles

1. Provide structural support to the shoulder region on the left and right side of the body.
2. Facilitate a large range of motion necessary for shoulder and arm movement with the help of the connected muscles.

SAQ: Describe the humerus bone.

Ans: Bone of the upper arm is called the humerus (Fig. 4.24). It forms the ball and socket joint of the shoulder with the scapula bone; which leads to the formation of the elbow joint with the lower arm bones.

SAQ: What are the functions of the humerus bone?

Ans: Functions of humerus bone are:

1. It helps the arm to move, flex and rotate.
2. It holds about 13 muscles in place.
3. It stabilizes the elbow and hand.

SAQ: Describe the forearm bones.

Ans: The forearm bones are radius and ulna. The ulna is towards the right side of the forearm. The ulna bone forms a hinge joint with the humerus at the elbow. Due to the radius bone, the forearm and hand can turn over at the wrist joint.

SAQ: What are the functions of the forearm bones?

Ans: Functions of forearm bones are:

1. The radius and ulna together serve as the primary support structure of the forearm by joining with the humerus and carpal bones.
2. The radius and ulna also serve as origins and insertions for muscles responsible for flexion and extension of the forearm, wrist, and fingers.

SAQ: Describe the wrist joint and the carpal bones.

Ans: The lower arm bones form the wrist joint with the carpal bones. The wrist joint (the radiocarpal joint) is a condyloid synovial joint of the distal upper limb that connects and serves as a transition point between the forearm and the hand.

Carpals are a group of eight small bones that give additional flexibility to the wrist. The carpals are connected to the five metacarpals that form the bones of the hand (Fig. 4.24). Metacarpals are connected to each of the fingers. Each finger contains three bones known as phalanges, except the thumb, which contains two phalanges.

SAQ: What are the functions of the wrist joint (radio-carpal joint) and the carpal bones?

Ans: The wrist joint is condyloid. It is a modified ball and socket joint, hence, facilitates various movements such as extension (increase in the angle at the joint), flexion (clinching fist), adduction (a movement towards the midline), and abduction, movements (a movement away from the midline).

BAQ: Draw a labelled diagram of the carpal bones.

Ans: Refer to Fig. 4.25.

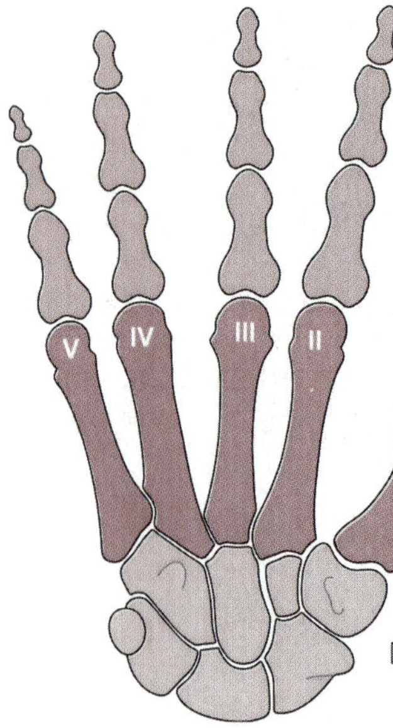

Fig. 4.25: Carpal bones

PELVIC GIRDLE AND LOWER LIMB BONES (Fig. 4.26)

Objective: To describe the anatomical features and functions of the pelvic girdle.

SAQ: Describe the pelvic girdle.

Ans: The pelvic girdle is a part of the appendicular skeleton. It connects the lower limbs to the axial skeleton (Figs 4.26 and 4.27). The pelvic girdle is formed by the connection of the right and left hip bone and it connects the lower leg (limb) bones to the axial skeleton.

The pelvic girdle is formed by a single hip bone. The hip bone attaches the lower limb to the axial skeleton through its articulation with the sacrum. The right and left hip bones, the sacrum and the coccyx, together form the pelvis.

Pelvis

SAQ: Describe the pelvis.

Ans: The pelvis consists of two hipbones, connected in front at the pubic symphysis and behind by the sacrum. Each hip bone is made up of three bones: The blade-shaped ilium (upper side), the ischium (behind and

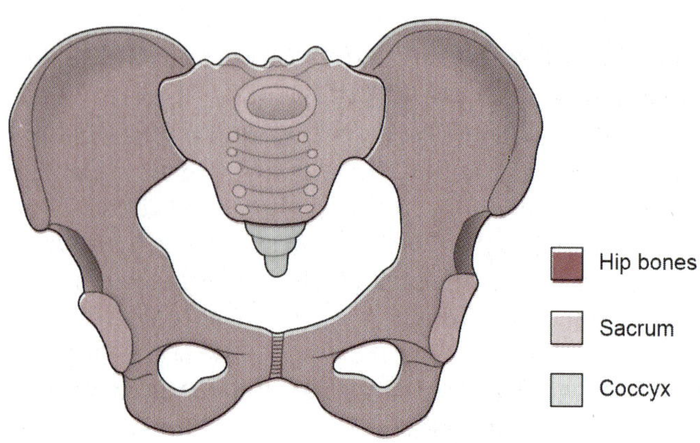

Fig. 4.26: Pelvic girdle

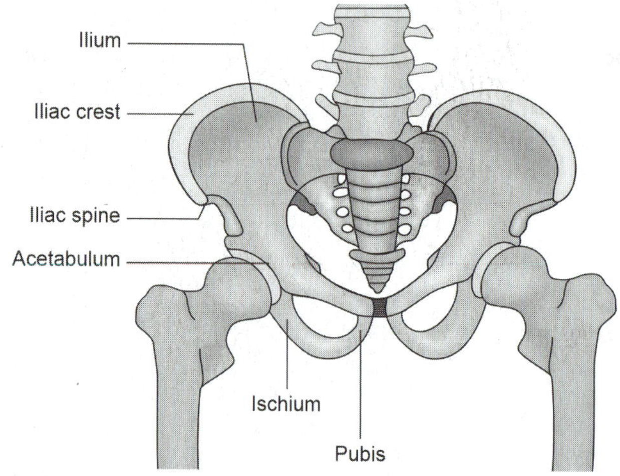

Fig. 4.27: Pelvic girdle bones

below), on which the weight rests in the sitting position; and the pubis (in front).

SAQ: What are the functions of the pelvic girdle?

Ans: The various functions of the pelvic girdle (Fig. 4.26) are as follows:

1. To transfer the weight of the upper body to the lower limbs while standing and sitting.
2. To provide attachment points for muscles that help with posture and locomotion.
3 To provide support and protection for the abdominopelvic structures.

SAQ: What are the general functions of the pelvis?

Ans: The various functions of the pelvis are as follows:

1. To help in walking, running and sitting positions.
2. To protect bladder, rectum and reproductive systems.
3. To help to transfer the weight of the body on the legs.

SAQ: What are the specific functions of the female pelvis?

Ans: The specific functions of the female pelvis are as follows:

1. To provide adaptation to childbearing.
2. To provide support to the gravid uterus.
3. To provide a passageway for the fetus to exit during the delivery.

SAQ: What is the difference between a false pelvis and a true pelvis?

Ans: The false pelvis is related to the abdominal cavity anteriorly and superiorly. It contains the major part of the small intestine, parts of the colon, and the common iliac vessels. The true pelvis contains some parts of the rectum, the small intestine, the urinary bladder, and the reproductive organs.

SAQ: What are the main differences between male and female pelvis?

Ans: The differences between male and female pelvis are as follows (Fig. 4.28):

1. Female pelvis is larger and wider than the male pelvis.
2. Female pelvis has a rounder pelvic inlet.

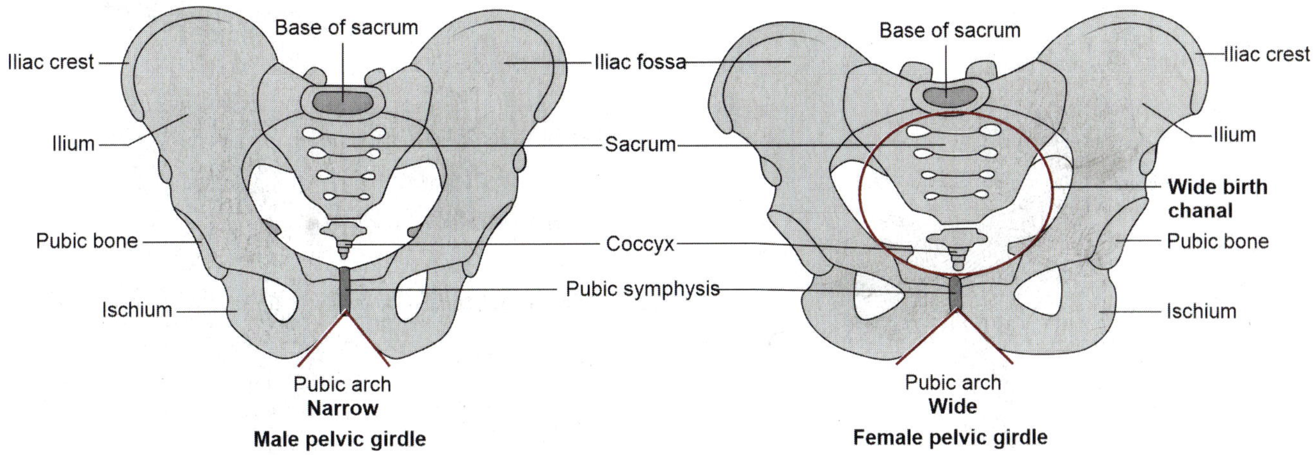

Fig. 4.28: Difference between male and female pelvic girdles

3. Male iliac crests are higher than females.
4. Male false pelvis looks taller and narrower.
5. Male sacrum is straight, longer, and narrow and has a prominent sacral compared to the female sacrum.

Objective: To describe the anatomical features of the hip bone.

SAQ: Write a note on the hip bone (os coxae, Fig. 4.29)

Ans: The hip bone (os coxae) is an irregularly shaped, bilateral compound structured bone of the bony pelvis. It is also known as the coxal bone, pelvic bone or innominate bone. The hip bone is formed of the following three smaller bones: The ilium, the pubis and the ischium.

BAQ: Draw a labelled diagram of the hip bone.

Ans: Refer to Fig. 4.29.

Objective: To describe the anatomical features of the leg bones.

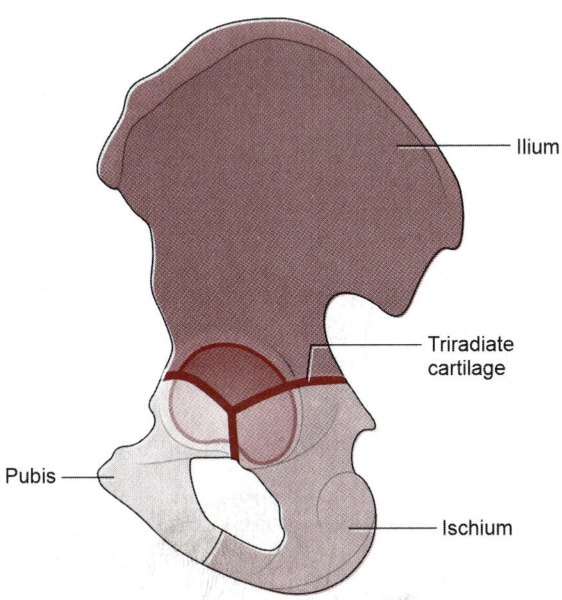

Fig. 4.29: The hip bone

Thigh Bone (Fig. 4.30)

SAQ: Write a note on the thigh bone.

Ans: The thigh bone is the femur and it is the largest bone in the body (femoral region). The femur has the ball and socket hip joint with the hip bone and it forms the knee joint with the tibia and patella (Fig. 4.30). The patella bone (knee cap) bone is not present at birth, however, it forms in early childhood. The patella supports the knee for walking and crawling.

Lower Leg Bones (Fig. 4.30)

SAQ: Write a note on the lower leg bones.

Ans: The lower leg bones are tibia and fibula. The tibia is larger than the fibula and it bears most of the body's weight. The fibula is a muscle attachment point and it is useful for maintaining balance. The tibia and fibula form the ankle joint with the talus bone, which is one of the seven tarsal bones in the foot (Figs 4.30 and 4.31).

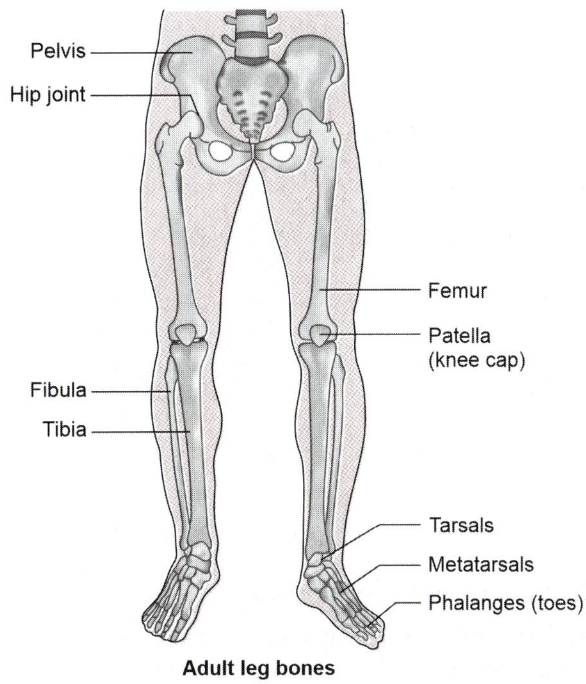

Fig. 4.30: Pelvic girdle and the lower limbs

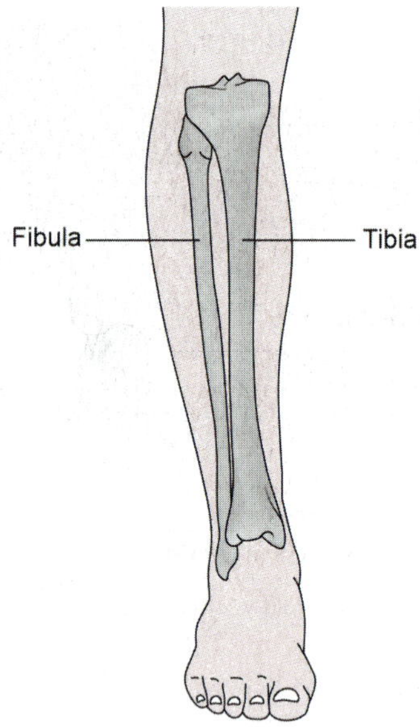

Fig. 4.31: Tibia and the fibula bones

BAQ: Draw a labelled diagram of the pelvic girdle and the lower limbs.

Ans: Refer to Fig. 4.30.

Fibula Bone

SAQ. Write a note on the fibula bone.

Ans: Fibula is a long bone in the lower leg. It is positioned on the lateral side of the tibia. It is a smaller and thinner bone compared to the tibia. The head of the tibia joins (articulates) with the lateral condyle of the tibia bone and forms the proximal tibiofibular joint. The lower end of the fibula joins with the tibia to form the lateral malleolus (Fig. 4.32), which stabilises the ankle joint.

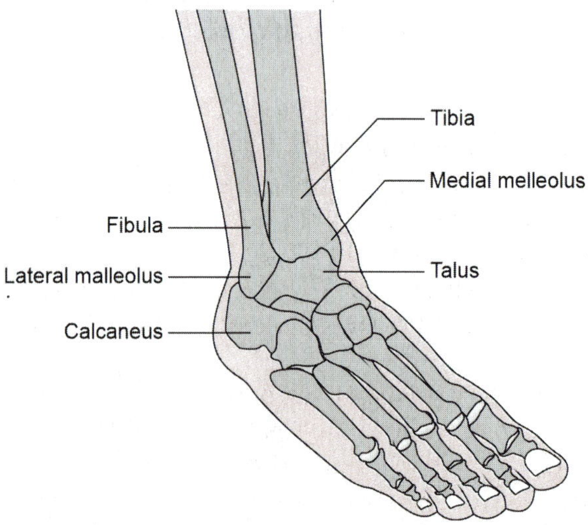

Fig. 4.32: Ankle joint: Lateral malleolus and medial malleolus

PATELLA (KNEE CAP) (Fig. 4.33)

SAQ: Write a note on the patella.

Ans: The patella (knee cap) is the largest sesamoid bone located at the front of the knee joint. It is present within the patellofemoral groove of the femur. The patella

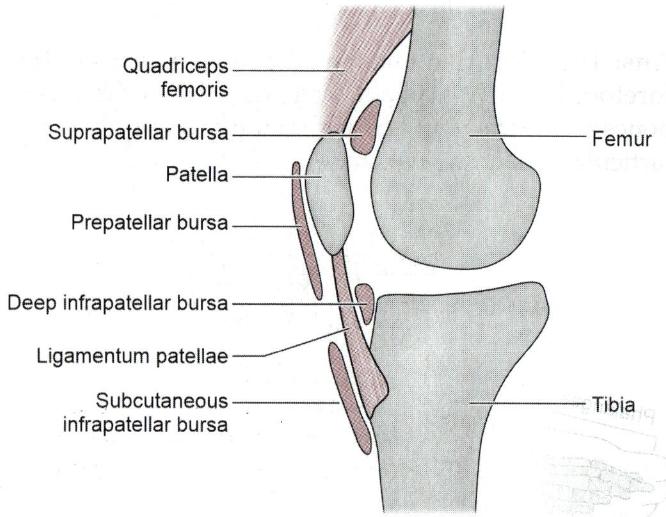

Fig. 4.33: Patella (knee cap)

helps the quadriceps muscle to move the leg. It also protects the knee joint and supports important muscles, ligaments and tendons.

Tarsals (Fig. 4.34)

SAQ: Write a note on the tarsals.

Ans: The tarsals form the posterior end of the foot and heels. These are a group of seven small bones that form joints with the five long metatarsals of the foot. Each of the metatarsals forms a joint with one of the set of phalanges in the toes (Fig. 4.34). Each toe contains three phalanges, except the big toe. The big toe contains only two phalanges.

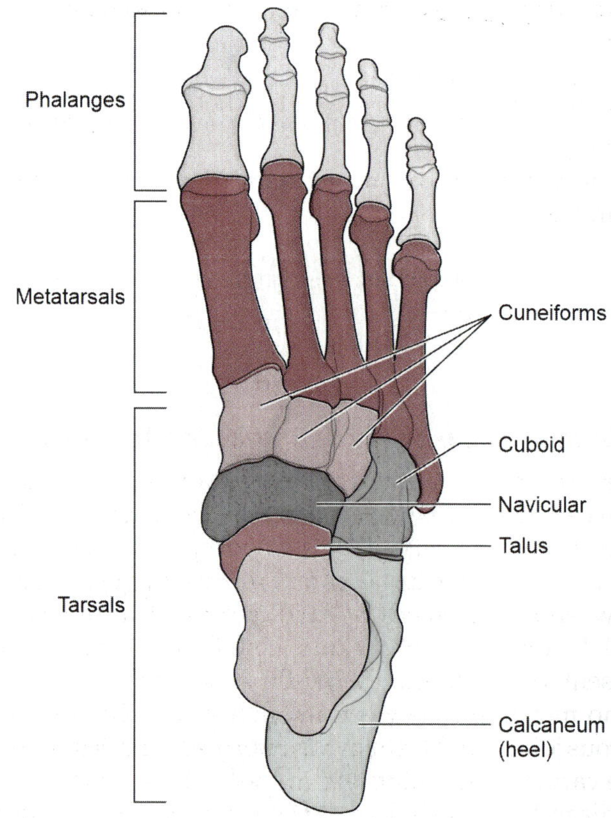

Fig. 4.34: Tarsals

Metatarsals and the Toe Bone (Fig. 4.35)

Ans: There are five metatarsal bones, which are the forefoot bones. They join (articulate) with the tarsal bones at the proximal end and their distal end, they join (articulate) with the phalanges.

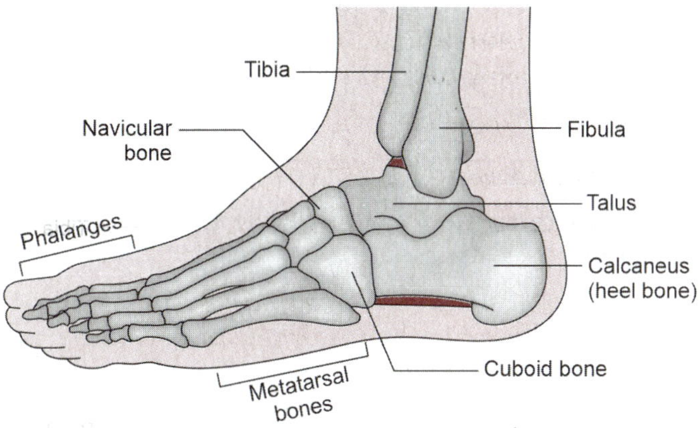

Fig. 4.35: Articulations of the metatarsals

SAQ: What is the important function of the tarsal bones?

Ans: The tarsals are in combination with the metatarsal bones. These bones together form a longitudinal (running lengthwise) arch in the foot, which is adapted for carrying and transferring weight while walking (on two legs). Thus, tarsal bones facilitate, weight-bearing and walking.

SAQ: Enumerate the functions of the metatarsal bones.

Ans: Functions of metatarsal bones:

1. These are an important component of the arches of the foot.
2. As the part of arches of the foot, these help in the walking balance, force absorption and support to the body.
3. These are insertion sites for many muscles of the lower limb and foot.

> **Objective:** To describe and discuss the articulations in the skeleton.

ARTICULATIONS

SAQ: Write a note on the articulations in the skeleton.

Ans: An articulation is a joint. It is a point of contact between bones, between a bone and cartilage. It is also a joint between a bone and a tooth. Synovial joints (Fig. 4.36) are the most common small gaps present between bones. Synovial fluid is present in the gaps, which lubricates the joints. The fibrous joints are present where bones are tightly joined and offer little to no movement between the bones. The Gomphosis fibrous joints hold teeth in their bony sockets (Fig. 4.37). The cartilaginous joints are formed where bone meets cartilage. Due to gel-like consistency, these joints provide a small amount of flexibility in the joint.

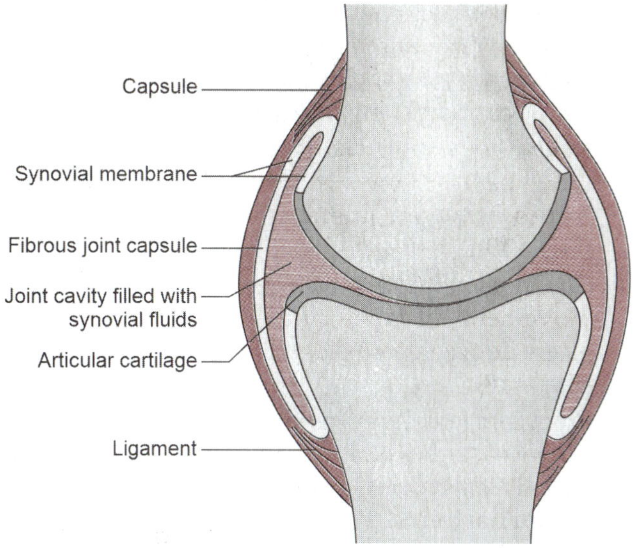

Fig, 4.36: Synovial joint

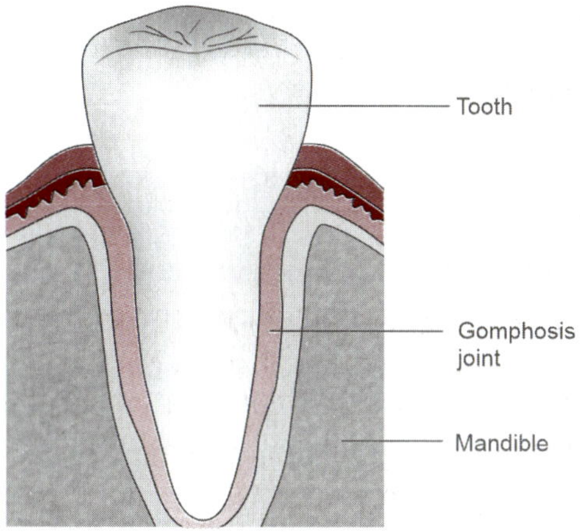

Fig. 4.37: Gomphosis fibrous joint

The joints can be classified into the following types according to the range of their movements:

1. Fixed joints
2. Slightly movable cartilaginous joints and
3. Freely movable synovial joints.

1. **Fixed joints:** In this type of joint, there is a fibrous tissue between the ends of the bones and there is no movement between the bones.

   Examples: The joints between teeth and mandible (Fig. 4.37) and the joints between bones of the skull (Fig. 4.9).
2. **Slightly movable cartilaginous joints:** In this type of joint, there is a pad of cartilage between the joints, which allows slight movement of the bones.

   Examples: Joints between the bones of vertebrae.
3. **Synovial joints (freely movable joints):** These types of joints allow free movement of the bones. The following are the various examples of synovial joints (Fig. 4.36):
   a. *Ball and socket joint:* In this type of joint, a globular head of one of the bones fits into the socket of another bone. *Examples:* Shoulder joint (between scapular and humerus) and hip joint (between hip bone and femur) (Fig. 4.29).

b. *Hinge joint:* These joints allow the movement of bones in only one direction. *Examples:* Knee joint (between femur and tibia, fibula) and elbow joint (between radius, ulna and humerus).

c. *Double hinge joint:* These types of joints allow the movement of bones in two directions. *Example:* Joints between metacarpals and phalanges (Fig. 4.19).

d. *Gliding joints (plane joint):* These types of joints allow movements of bones in all directions. *Examples:* Joints between carpels and joints between tarsals (Fig. 4.18).

e. Pivot joint (axial joint): In this type of joint, one bone turns on another bone and movement is around the axis. *Example:* Joints between femur and tibia and radioulnar joints.

f. *Saddle joint:* In this type of joint, one bone is movable on another bone in many directions. *Example:* Thumb joints.

Objectives: To describe the physiology of the skeletal system.

SKELETAL SYSTEM PHYSIOLOGY

Support and Protection

LAQ: What are the various functions of the skeletal system?

Ans:

1. **Primary function:** The primary function of the skeletal system is to support and protect various organs of the body and anchor the skeletal muscles. The bones of the axial skeleton protect the internal organs such as the heart and the brain. The appendicular skeleton bones provide flexibility and support at the joints and anchor the muscles, which are responsible for moving the limbs.
2. **Movement:** The bones of the skeletal system are attachment points for the skeletal muscles of the body. The joints act as central points for the movement of the bones.
3. **Hematopoiesis:** In adults, active bone marrow is found inside various bones such as the skull, the shoulder bone, the spine, the breast bone, rib bones, and the hip. The bone marrow in the spine and the hip has the richest source of bone marrow cells. The bone marrow produces bone marrow stem cells, which are responsible for the production and development of various blood cells, such as red blood cells, white blood cells and platelets. The process of the bone marrow that creates various blood cells is called hematopoiesis.
4. **Storage:** The skeletal system stores many different types of essential minerals mainly, calcium, inorganic phosphorus, magnesium, potassium, fluoride and protein to facilitate the growth and repair of the body. Osteocalcin hormone is secreted by the osteoblasts, which plays an important role in the calcium deposition of bone.

The yellow bone marrow contains specific stem cells; which produce cartilage, fat and bone matter. The yellow bone marrow also facilitates the storage of fats in adipocyte cells. The red bone marrow stores iron in the form of ferritin, which is useful for the mobilization of iron and mainly used to synthesize haemoglobin in red blood cells.

Growth and Development of Bones

LAQ: Write a note on the growth and development of a bone.

Ans: At birth, the skeleton of a newborn has about 300 bones. These bones grow together and fuse into about 206 bones in adults.

The skeleton begins to form early during fetal development; which is made of hyaline cartilage and dense irregular fibrous connective tissue. These tissues act as a soft, growing framework for the adult bony skeleton. As development progresses, blood vessels grow inside the soft fetal skeleton and stem cells and nutrients facilitate bone growth.

Influence of Hormones on Bone Growth

Calcium and inorganic phosphorus play a very important role in the growth of bone. The calcium and phosphorus metabolism are controlled by the following hormones:

1. **Parathyroid hormone:** It is secreted by the parathyroid gland. The actions of the parathyroid hormone are as follows:
   a. It activates osteoclasts and osteocytes to promote dissolution of the matrix, breakdown of bone salts, and liberation of calcium and phosphate.
   b. It facilitates increases in phosphate excretion by diminishing the tubular reabsorption of phosphorus and increasing the reabsorption of calcium.
2. **Calcitonin:** It is secreted by C cells of the thyroid gland. It is a calcium- and phosphate-lowering hormone. Calcitonin inhibits osteoclast function and decreases renal resorption of calcium and inorganic phosphorus.
3. **Other hormones:** Thyroxin stimulates osteoclast activity. Estrogen and androgens influence bone metabolism by promoting the production of bone matrix. Glucocorticoids, by their action on protein catabolism, affect the production of bone matrix.

Role of Vitamin D in the Growth of a Bone

Vitamin D (calciferol) promotes the absorption of both calcium and phosphorus in the small intestine. It also acts directly on the bone to promote normal growth, development, and utilization of calcium.

Objective: To describe skeletal homeostasis.

SKELETAL HOMEOSTASIS

LAQ: Write a note on the skeletal homeostasis.

Ans: Skeletal homeostasis means the maintenance of a balance of calcium and inorganic phosphorus metabolism to maintain normal bone health and bone mass of the skeleton. Skeletal homeostasis is dependent on the specific balance between bone formation and bone resorption. The osteoblasts are located along the bone-forming surface. These are responsible for laying down the osteoid seam (unmineralized matrix), which is calcified after about 10 days. Osteoclasts form multinucleated giant cells in the lacunar (empty) spaces and are responsible for bone resorption.

Eighty per cent of the skeletal mass is made up of cortical bone, which is a compact structure of dense bone. About 20% of trabecular bone consists of a delicate interlacing of dense bone with bone marrow. Although cortical bone makes up the majority of the skeletal mass, its surface area and the resorptive surface are much less than that of the trabecular bone.

The major protein component of bone is collagen. About 10% of the organic bone matrix consists of non-collagen components. These include osteocalcin, osteonectin (glycoprotein), osteopontin (one type of matrix protein), acid mucopolysaccharides, and lipids. The inorganic components of bone are primarily composed of calcium and phosphate in the form of hydroxyapatite crystals.

Bone remodelling is a continuous process consisting of bone formation, mineralization, and bone resorption. Insulin, insulin-like growth factors I and II, androgens, estrogens, growth hormone, and thyroid hormone increase the rate of bone formation. Calcitonin, increased phosphates, and diphosphonates inhibit bone resorption. Parathyroid hormone increases osteoclastic activity and subsequent bone resorption and releases calcium into the circulation. Vitamin D facilitates intestinal absorption of calcium and inorganic phosphorus and increases renal reabsorption of calcium, leading to an increase in blood calcium. Glucocorticoids decrease the rate of bone formation and increase the rate of bone resorption, which leads to a net loss of bone.

Objective: To discuss the bone fractures and healing of bone fractures.

BONE FRACTURES

SAQ: Describe types of bone fractures.

Ans: The following are the different types of bone fractures:

1. Simple type
2. Compound type and
3. Pathological type.

Simple bone fractures: In this type of fracture, the bones do not cut through the skin.

Compound bone fractures: In this type of fracture, the bones cut through the skin.

Pathological bone fracture: In this type of fracture, the bones are damaged by specific clinical conditions. For example, bacterial or viral infection of bones.

HEALING OF BONE FRACTURE

LAQ: Write a note on the healing of bone fractures.

Ans: The healing of a bone is a complicated regenerative process in which the damaged bone attains normal cellular composition and normal state. The healing of a fractured bone consists of the following four steps:

1. Hematoma formation
2. Granulation tissue formation
3. Bony callus formation and
4. Bone remodelling (Fig. 4.38).

Hematoma Formation

The blood vessels of the bone and the periosteum are damaged during the fracture. A hematoma forms at the fracture site, which contains hematopoietic cells. The

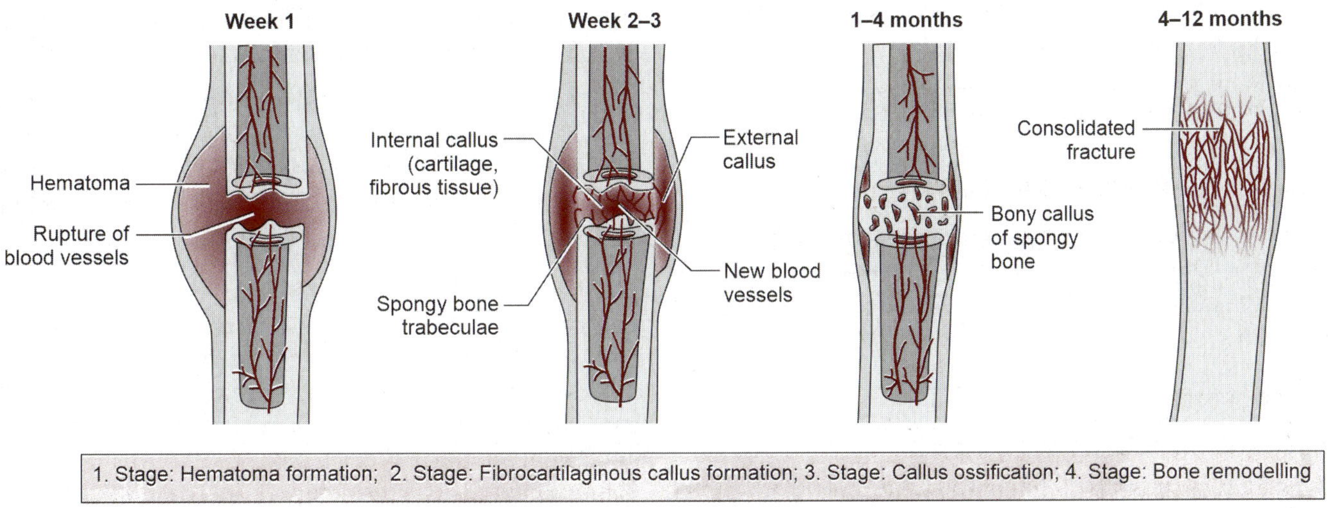

Fig. 4.38: The stages of healing of bone fracture

hematoma in clot formation becomes the temporary frame for subsequent healing. Macrophages phagocytes the dead bone cells and matrix. Fibroblasts migrate to form collagen fibres. Osteoblasts are responsible for joining bone ends. New blood capillaries begin to grow to restore blood supply in the process of bone damage repairs. Platelets also contribute to the bone repair mechanism by secreting specific helpful proteins (cytokines).

Granulation Tissue Formation

Granular tissue formation takes place within two to three weeks of the bone damage. This provides provisional stability to the damaged bone. The osteoblasts begin to calcify the bone. With the deposition of the callus as a spongy bone, the fractured splints get sealed.

Bone Remodelling

It is a continuous process for several months. With the continued actions of osteoblasts and osteoclasts, the hard callus undergoes repeated bone-remodelling processes and the centre of the callus is finally replaced by a compact bone. The remodelling of the blood vessel networks also occurs along with remodelling changes. Finally, the regeneration of the normal bone structure is completed.

Objectives: To define and describe endochondral ossification and related functions.

BAQ: Define and describe endochondral ossification and related functions.

Ans: Endochondral ossification is the bone tissue formation during fetal development of the skeletal system. Endochondral ossification processes initiate from a precursor mesenchymal tissue, which turns into an intermediate cartilage stage, ultimately substituted by a bone. Endochondral ossification is responsible for the development of most long and short bones, the bones of the skull, the part of the clavicle bone, the bones of the axial skeleton and the appendicular skeleton. The endochondral ossification also plays a very important role in the healing of fractures.

Objectives: To describe the main diseases related to bones.

MAIN DISEASES RELATED TO BONES

Several disorders affect the skeletal system The two most common disorders of the skeletal system are osteoporosis and osteoarthritis. Bone fractures and cancer are other prominent disorders of the skeletal system.

Osteoporosis

BAQ: Write a note on osteoporosis.

Ans: Osteoporosis is a systemic skeletal disorder caused by low bone mass and micro-architectural deterioration of the bone tissue. Osteoporosis leads to bone fragility and an increase in the risk of a fracture. It is a common reason for bone fractures in the elderly. Bones that are commonly affected include the bones of the forearm, the hip and the vertebrae in the spine. A person suffering from osteoporosis may have chronic pain and decreased ability to carry out normal activities.

Low levels of estrogen hormone in the case of females, after menopause may lead to osteoporosis. Other factors responsible for osteoporosis are hyperthyroidism, anorexia, alcoholism, kidney disease, and surgical removal of the ovaries.

Osteoarthritis

BAQ: Write a note on osteoarthritis.

Ans: Osteoarthritis is a degenerative bone joint disease. The common symptoms of osteoarthritis are joint stiffness and pain and the symptoms progress slowly. Other symptoms of osteoarthritis may include decreased mobility, joint swelling and weakness of the arms and legs.

Various reasons that lead to osteoarthritis are congenital factors that lead to weakness of arms and legs, mechanical injury to bone joints, loss of strength in the muscles that support a joint impairment of peripheral nerves, etc.

Rheumatoid Arthritis (RA)

BAQ: Write a note on rheumatoid arthritis (RA).

Ans: Rheumatoid arthritis (RA) is an autoimmune and inflammatory disease. The immune system of a patient's body produces specific proteins (RA factors) that attack healthy cells in the body joints causing inflammation in the affected parts of the body joint. RA factors mainly attack the joints of the hands, wrists, and knees. The lining of the joint becomes inflamed and causes damage to the joint tissue, which may lead to chronic pain, bone deformity and loss of balance while walking. RA may also affect other tissues in the body.

SAQ: What is the main difference between osteoarthritis and rheumatoid arthritis?

Ans: Osteoarthritis is caused by the mechanical wear and tear on joints and rheumatoid arthritis (RA) is an autoimmune disease. In RA immune system of a patient's body attacks tissues of the joints of the body.

Paget's Disease

This chronic skeletal disorder affects 3 to 4% of both men and women over the age of 50 years. The cause of this disease may be genetic or acquired. In Paget's disease, increased bone resorptive activity and an increased number of abnormally enlarged osteoclasts are observed. These osteoclasts have greatly increased number of nuclei coupled with the ability of rapid osteoblast-mediated bone formation. This results in architecturally inferior bone formation. The abnormal bone and its increased tendency to fracture can cause compression of neural structure. Laboratory tests related to bone profile tests and mainly increased values of serum alkaline phosphatase indicate an increase in bone turnover and markers of bone formation and bone resorption. Paget's disease treatment is usually focused on the management of the related clinical conditions.

> **Objective:** To understand and explain the central theme of competency-based medical and paramedical education (CBME): Horizontal and vertical integration of subjects.

BAQ: Show horizontal integration of physiology, and biochemistry with the following anatomical change: Weak and brittle bones (rickets).

Ans:

Horizontal Integration with Physiology

The ossification process of the bone is affected.

Horizontal Integration with Biochemistry

The general biochemical change observed in rickets is very low levels of serum calcium, and inorganic phosphorus due to vitamin D deficiency.

Horizontal Integration with Nutrition

The diet given to the patient should contain a good percentage of protein and vitamin D necessary for the normal ossification of the bones.

BAQ: Show vertical integration of pharmacology, and preventive medicine with the following anatomical change: Weak and brittle bones (Rickets).

Ans:

Vertical Integration with Pharmacology

Use of appropriate medication to treat rickets.

Horizontal Integration with Preventive Medicine.

Use of preventive measures (foods containing adequate vitamin D, and calcium) to prevent rickets in children.

BAQ: Show horizontal integration of premedical subjects: Physiology and biochemistry with the following anatomical change: Swelling of the bone joints (rheumatoid arthritis).

Ans:

Horizontal Integration with Physiology

The flexor and extensor muscle activities of the bone are affected.

Horizontal Integration with Biochemistry

Production of antibodies that attack the cells in the bone joints.

BAQ: Show vertical integration of the paramedical subject, pharmacology with the following anatomical change: Swelling of bone joints (rheumatoid arthritis).

Ans:

Vertical Integration with Pharmacology

Use of appropriate medicines (immunosuppressive) to treat (rheumatoid arthritis).

BIBLIOGRAPHY

1. Medical Biochemistry, 1st Edition (2023). Godkar PB, Godkar DP, CBS Publishers, New Delhi, India.
2. Textbook of Medical Laboratory Technology, 4th Edition, (2024). Godkar PB, Godkar DP, Bhalani Publishing House, Mumbai, India.
3. Anatomy of the Human Body. 42nd Edition. Henry Gray, Editor-in-chief: Susan Standring, Elsevier (2020).
4. Ross and Wilson Anatomy and Physiology in Health and Illness, 13th Edition, by Allison Wynn Grant, Anne Waugh, and Kathleen J.W. Wilson (2018).
5. Schaum's outline of theory and problems of Human Anatomy and Physiology, 2nd Edition (1997), Tata MaGraw-Hill Publishing Company Limited, New Delhi, India.

MULTIPLE CHOICE QUESTIONS (MCQs)

Select the correct option.

1. The skeletal system in an adult body is made up of:

(A) Average 200 bones (B) Average 306 bones
(C) Average 236 bones (D) Average 206 bones

2. A shallow and flattened articulate bone surface of a bone is called:

(A) A fossa (B) A facet
(C) A fovea (D) A tubercle

3. This is not a part of the axial skeleton:

(A) Sacrum (B) Sphenoid bone
(C) Clavicle (D) Hyoid bone

4. This is the only bone in the body that does not form a joint with any other bone:

(A) Sacrum (B) Sphenoid bone
(C) Clavicle (D) Hyoid bone

5. The number of bones the skull is composed of is:

(A) 11 (B) 33
(C) 22 (D) 13

6. The auditory ossicles do not contain the following bone:

(A) Malleus (B) Sacrum
(C) Incus (D) Stapes bone

7. The optic foramen is present in:

(A) The occipital bone (B) The sphenoid bone
(C) The palatine bone (D) The ethmoid bone

8. Tendons and ligaments are:

(A) Muscular tissue (B) Connective tissue
(C) Skeletal tissue (D) Fibrous connective tissue

9. Skeletal muscle bundles are held together by a common connective tissue layer known as:

(A) Fascia (B) Perimysium
(C) Aponeurosis (D) Endomysium

10. The composition of the bone marrow is made of:

(A) Adipose tissue
(B) Adipose, areolar tissue and blood
(C) Adipose and areolar tissue
(D) Adipose tissue and fibroblasts

11. The formation of erythrocytes in foetus takes place in:

(A) Red bone marrow (B) Sarcoplasm
(C) Liver and spleen (D) Blood

12. Nasal septum damage recovery requires healing of this cartilage:

(A) Elastic cartilage (B) Fibrous cartilage
(C) Calcified cartilage (D) Hyaline cartilage

13. The membrane that surrounds the bone is known as as:

(A) Pericardium (B) Periosteum
(C) Perichondrium (D) Endosteum

14. The mammalian pinna is supported by:

(A) Elastic cartilage
(B) Hyaline cartilage
(C) White fibrous connective tissue
(D) Calcified cartilage

15. Hyaline cartilage does not have:

(A) Blood capillaries (B) Cells
(C) Lacunae (D) Fibres

16. Major inorganic component(s) of vertebrate bone is/are:

(A) Potassium hydroxide (B) Calcium phosphate
(C) Calcium carbonate (D) None of the above

17. Haversian canals occur in:

(A) Humerus (B) Scapula
(C) Pubis (D) Clavicle

18. A shallow articulating surface of a bone is known as a:

(A) Fovea (B) Facet
(C) Tubercle (D) Fossa

19. This is an example of a gliding joint:

(A) The radiocarpal joint (B) The intervertebral joint
(C) The phalangeal joint (D) The intercarpal joint

20. This is not a part of the os coxae:

(A) Ischium (B) Pubis
(C) Capitulum (D) Obturator foramen

21. This bone does not contain a paranasal sinus:

(A) Vomer bone (B) Ethmoid bone
(C) Maxila bone (D) Sphenoid bone

22. The characteristic feature of the false pelvis is:

(A) Found in male and female
(B) Found only in male
(C) Broader in male compared to female
(D) Narrower in male compared to female

23. This type of bone lacks a styloid process:

(A) Radius (B) Ulna
(C) Sphenoid bone (D) Temporal bone

24. Rheumatoid arthritis (RA) is related to:

(A) An autoimmune type of disease
(B) A viral disease
(C) Inflammatory type of disease
(D) Both (A) and (C)

25. These hormones decrease the rate of bone formation:

(A) Insulin
(B) Parathyroid hormones
(C) Androgens
(D) Thyroid hormone

ANSWERS

1. D 2. A 3. C 4. D 5. C 6. B 7. B
8. D 9. A 10. B 11. C 12. D 13. B 14. A
15. D 16. B 17. A 18. B 19. D 20. C 21. A
22. D 23. C 24. D 25. B

MATCH THE COLUMNS

I	II
1. Process	A. Narrow ridgelike projection
2. Tubercle	B. Shallow depression
3. Crest	C. Narrow slit-like opening
4. Fossa	D. Rounded opening through a bone
5. Sulcus	E. Anybody extension
6. Fissure	F. Small rounded process
7. Foramen	G. Small pit
8. Sinus	H. Deep pit
9. Fovea	I. Cavity
10. Alveolus	J. Grove that contains tendon, nerve or a vessel

ANSWERS

1. E 2. F 3. A 4. B 5. J 6. C 7. D
8. I 9. G 10. H

CHAPTER

5

Muscular System

SAQ: Short answer question: Marks: 2
BAQ: Brief answer question: Marks: 4 or 5
LAQ: Long answer question: Marks: 9 or 10
MCQs: Multiple choice questions: Marks: 0.5 each
Match the columns: Marks: 0.5 each
Draw a labelled diagram: Marks: 5

Objective: To describe the types and process of basic formation of the muscular system.

INTRODUCTION

The muscular system (Fig. 5.1) consists of the skeletal, smooth and cardiac muscles. It is responsible for the movement of the body. The muscular system is controlled through the nervous system. However, some muscles can be completely autonomous. About 700 muscles are attached to the bones of the skeletal system and these make up approximately 50% body weight of an individual. Each of these muscles is a discrete organ made up of skeletal muscle tissue, blood vessels, tendons, and nerves. Muscle tissue is also present inside the organs such as the heart, digestive organs, and blood vessels. In these organs, muscles serve to move various substances throughout the body.

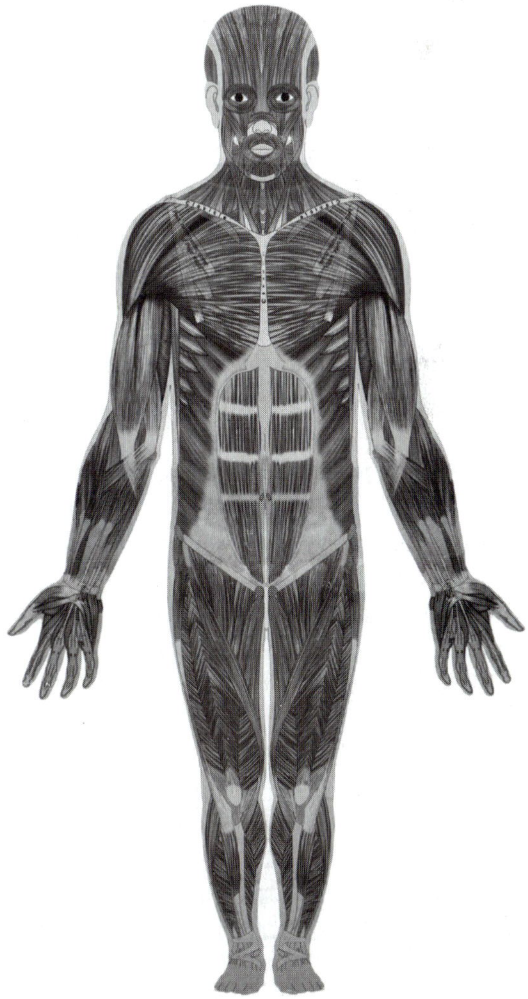

Fig. 5.1: Muscular system

MUSCLE TYPES

SAQ: How many muscle types are present in a body?

Ans: There are three types of muscle tissues: The visceral muscle, the cardiac muscle, and the skeletal muscle.

SAQ: Which type of muscle forms the largest portion of a body?

Ans: The skeletal muscle forms the largest portion of a body. It constitutes about 40% of the body's weight. About 3% of cardiac muscles and smooth muscles are present in an average size of a normal body.

BAQ: How does muscle tissue form in the body?

Ans: The muscle tissue of the body forms from the embryonic mesoderm. The skeletal muscles, except those of the limbs and head, develop from mesodermal somites (Fig. 5.2) which are segmental axial structures of the vertebrate embryos. The somites give rise to the vertebral column, ribs, skeletal muscles, and subcutaneous tissues. The skeletal muscle in the head and limbs develops from the general mesoderm.

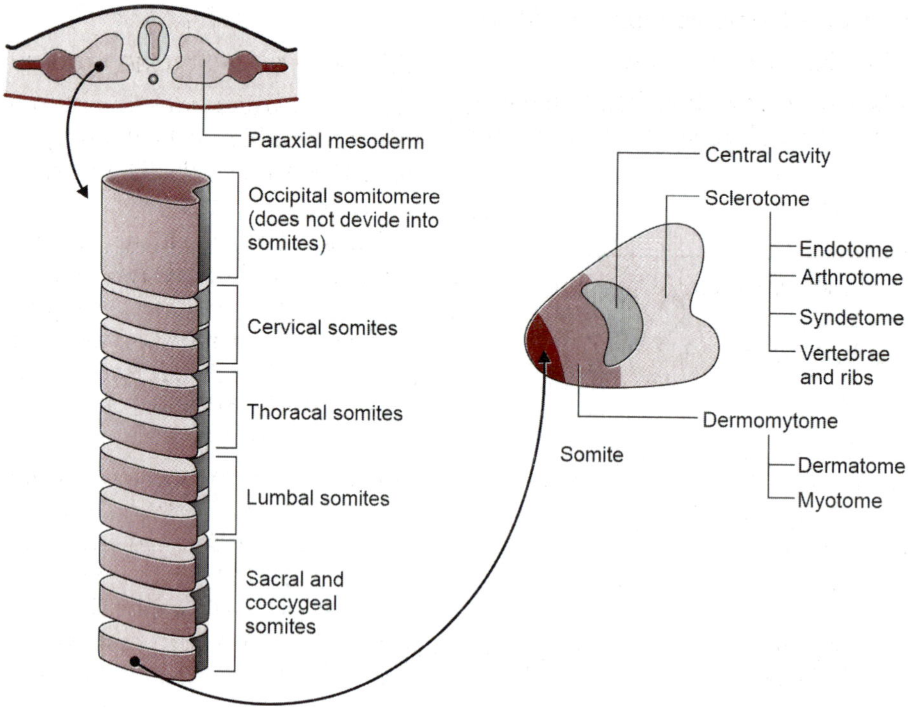

Fig. 5.2: Somites

The muscle tissue cells have the special ability to shorten or contract to facilitate movement of the body parts.

Objective: To enumerate and discuss the functions of the muscular system.

FUNCTIONS OF THE MUSCLES

BAQ: Enumerate the various functions of the muscles.

Ans: The following are the various functions of the muscles:

1. **Mobility:** Muscles facilitate; large and coordinated motions such as walking, running, climbing, and swimming, etc. and smaller movements, such as facial expressions, speaking, writing, etc.
2. **Stability:** Muscle tendons are useful for the stability of the body and the body parts.
3. **Posture:** Skeletal muscles help to attain a proper position (posture) for sitting or standing postures.
4. **Blood circulation:** The muscles of the heart facilitate the pumping of blood throughout the body. Smooth muscle in the arteries and veins plays a very important role in the circulation of blood around the body. These muscles also play an important role in the maintenance of normal blood circulation and blood pressure.
5. **Respiration:** The muscles of the diaphragm play a very important role in the breathing process.
6. **Digestion:** Smooth muscles of the gastrointestinal tract control the movement of the digestion process, the movement and passage of the digested and non-digested food.
7. **Urination:** The urinary system is comprised of both smooth and skeletal muscles. With the help of nerves, they can hold and release urine from the bladder.
8. **Vision:** The skeletal muscles around the eye control the eye movements.
9. **Organ protection:** Muscles in the torso protect the internal organs from all sides of the body with the help of the bones of the spine and ribs. Muscles are also able to protect the organs and bones by absorbing shock and reducing friction in the various types of joints.
10. **Temperature regulation:** Maintenance of normal body temperature is an important function of the muscular system.
11. **Childbirth:** The movements of the smooth muscles in the uterus that push the baby through the vagina.

Objectives:
- To describe the nomenclature related to the muscular system.
- To describe functions of specific types of muscles.
- To describe the actions of different types of muscles.

MUSCLE NAMES

BAQ: Write a note on "muscle names".

Ans: Muscle names are derived from the following various factors: Location, orientation, shape, relative position and functions. The following are the various examples:

Location: Brachii (upper arm muscle). Intercostal (between the ribs). Pectoralis (of chest region).

Orientation

- Transverse (across).
- Rectus (straplike)

Shape: Biceps (two heads). Rhomboides (rhomboid-like)

Relative position: Medialis, external, lateralis

Function: Pronator (assists in pronation (bends inwards), flexor (flexes (bends) a joint, abductor (control position in the frontal plane).

MUSCLE ACTIONS

The following terms are related to the specific muscle actions:

Table 5.1: Muscle actions, definitions, examples

Action	*Definition*	*Examples*
Abduction	An appendage moves away from the middle	Deltoid
Adduction	An appendage moves towards the middle	Adductor longus
Depression	Lowers a body part	Depressor labii inferioris
Elevation	Raises a body part	Levator scapulae
Eversion	Turns a part (the sole outwards	Peroneus tertius
Extension	Increases a joint angle	Triceps brachii
Inversion	Turns the sole inwards	Tibialis anterior
Flexion	Decreases a joint angle	Biceps brachii
Rotation	Turns a bone around its longitudinal axis	Sternocleidomastoid

Objective: To discuss the various types of muscles and their functions.

Visceral Muscle

SAQ: Write a note on the visceral muscle.

Ans: The visceral muscles are found inside the blood vessels, stomach and intestines. It has a very smooth and uniform appearance. Hence, these muscles are also called smooth muscles. The visceral muscle tissue is weak compared to other muscle tissues. The visceral muscles are involuntary. These muscles function and contract without conscious control and are controlled by the autonomic nervous system. The main function of the visceral muscle is in the contraction of related organs to move substances through the organ.

BAQ: Draw a labelled diagram of the visceral muscle.

Ans: Refer to the Fig. 5.2A.

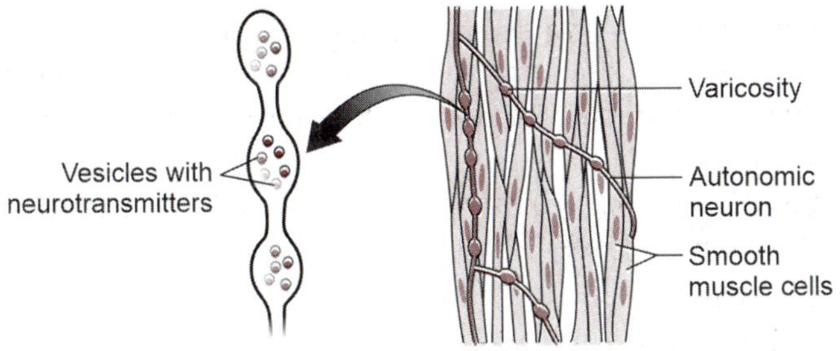

Fig. 5.2A: Visceral muscle

Cardiac Muscle (Fig. 5.3)

BAQ: Write a note on the cardiac muscle.

Ans: The cardiac muscle is found only in the heart. It is responsible for facilitating pumping of the blood throughout the body. The cardiac muscle tissue is an involuntary muscle.

The cells of the cardiac muscle tissue are striated (having thin, long, lines, marks, or strips of colour, Fig. 5.3). They appear to have light and dark stripes when observed under a light microscope. The arrangement of protein fibres inside the cells of the cardiac muscle is responsible for the striated appearance. The cardiac muscle is very strong.

The cells of the cardiac muscle are branched X or Y-shaped cells. These cells are tightly connected by special junctions called intercalated disks (Fig. 5.3). The intercalated disks interlock and create a strong bond between the cells. The branched structure and intercalated disks are responsible for making strong muscle cells; which resist high blood pressures and also sustain the strain of pumping blood throughout a lifetime. The specific features of the cardiac muscle are also responsible for spreading electrochemical signals quickly from cell to cell and the heart then beats as a unit.

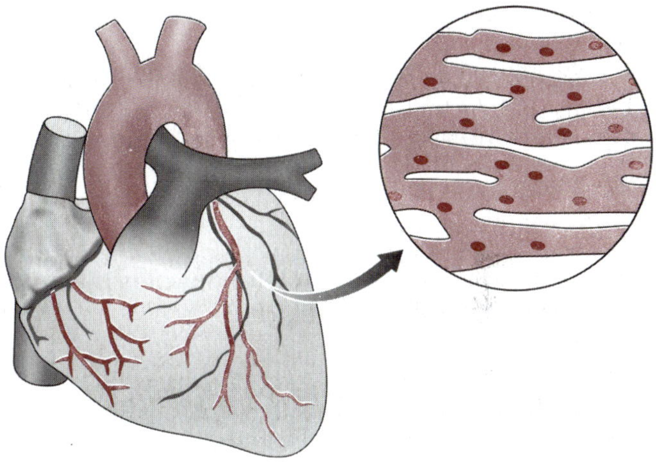

Fig. 5.3: Cardiac muscles

BAQ: Draw a labelled diagram of the cardiac muscle.

Ans: Refer to the Fig. 5.3.

Skeletal Muscle (Fig. 5.4)

SAQ: Write a note on the skeletal muscle.

Ans: The skeletal muscle is voluntary muscle tissue in the body. The voluntary muscles are under conscious control. They are attached to the bones. The voluntary muscles are responsible for the movement of the body parts. Every physical action of a person like speaking, walking, or writing is possible due to skeletal muscles.

The skeletal muscle is strong, since, the muscle cells contain strong straight, and long multinucleated fibers (Fig. 5.4). The skeletal muscles always connect to the skeleton in at least one place.

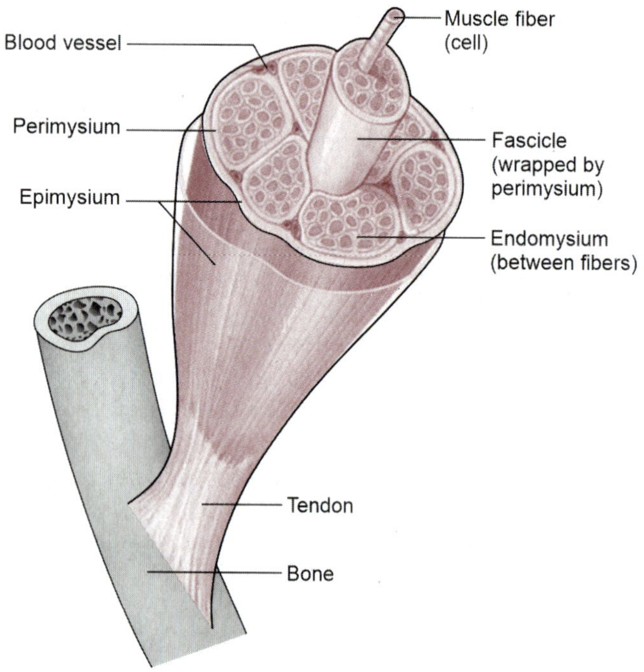

Fig. 5.4: Skeletal muscle

BAQ: Draw a labelled diagram of the skeletal muscle.

Ans: Refer to the Fig. 5.4.

NAMES OF SKELETAL MUSCLES (Fig. 5.5)

Skeletal muscles are named based on their location, shape, size, direction, function, origin, number of origins, and insertion. The following are some examples:

Skeletal Muscles Named Based on the Location (Anatomical Region)

SAQ: Write two names of skeletal muscles based on the location (anatomical region).

Ans: The rectus abdominis and transversus abdominis are found in the abdominal region (Fig. 5.5). The tibialis anterior, are named after the part of the bone (the anterior portion of the tibia), where they are attached (Fig. 5.6).

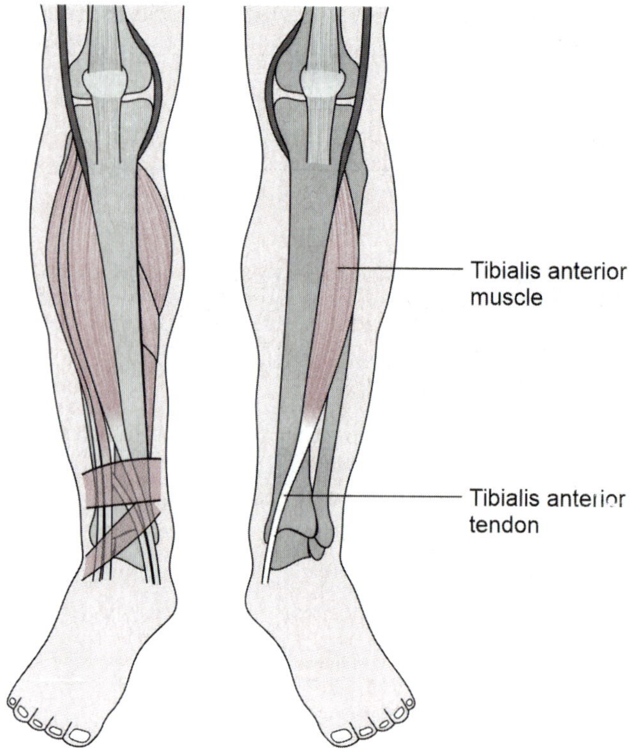

Fig. 5.6: Tibialis anterior muscle

Skeletal Muscles Name Based on Origins

SAQ: Write two names of skeletal muscles based on origins.

Ans: Some muscles connect to more than one bone or more than one place on a bone. They have more than one origin. A muscle with two origins is called a biceps (Fig. 5.7). A muscle with three origins is a triceps muscle and a muscle with four origins is a quadriceps muscle (Fig. 5.8).

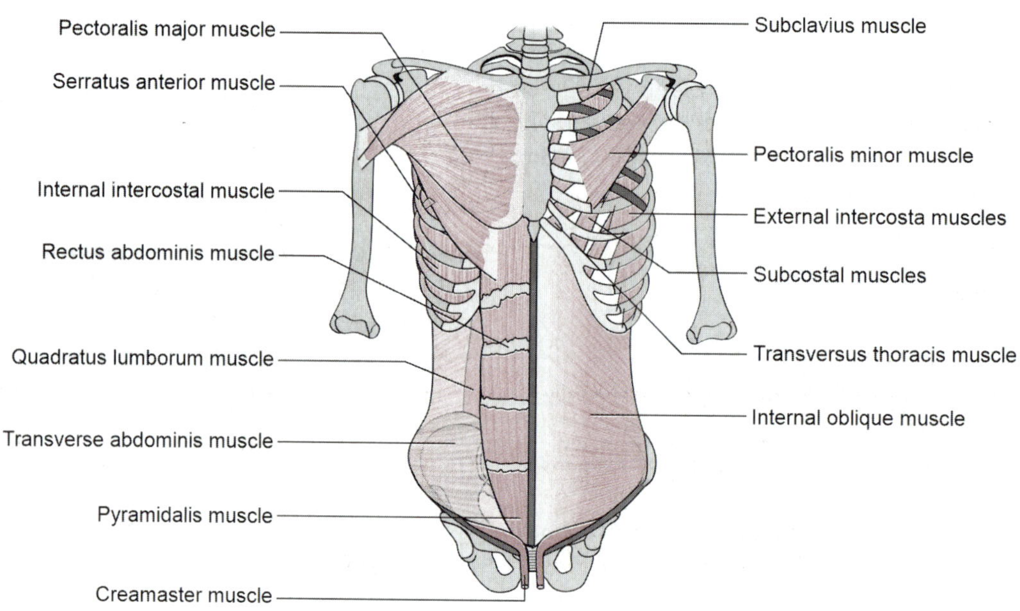

Fig. 5.5: Abdominal skeletal muscles

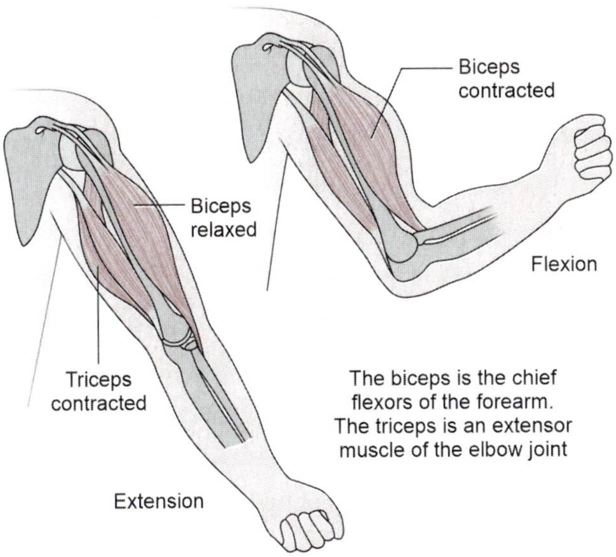

Fig. 5.7: Biceps and triceps

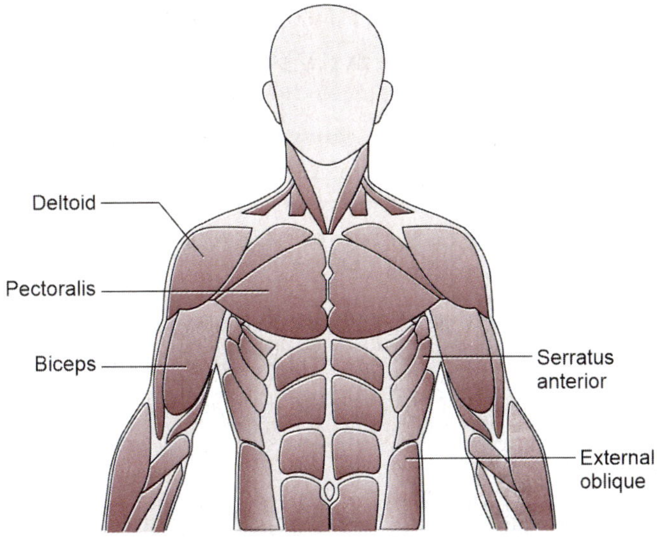

Fig. 5.9: Deltoid and serratus muscles

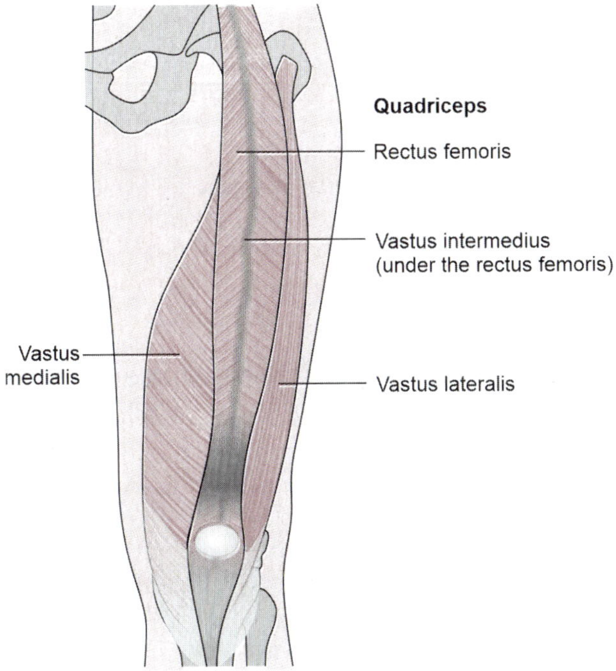

Fig. 5.8: Quadriceps

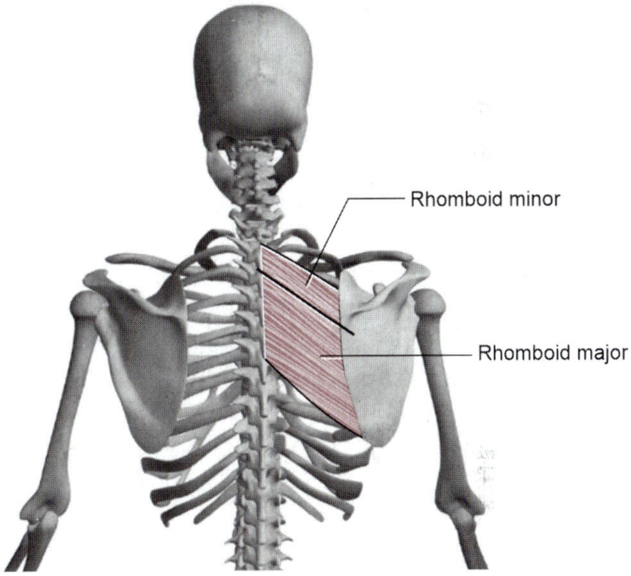

Fig. 5.10: Rhomboid muscles

Skeletal Muscles Names Based on Shape

SAQ: Write two names of skeletal muscles based on shape.

Ans: The deltoids have a delta or triangular shape. The serratus muscles have a serrated or saw-like shape (Fig. 5.9). The rhomboid major has a rhombus or diamond shape (Fig. 5.10).

Skeletal Muscles Names Based on Size

SAQ: Write three names of skeletal muscles based on size.

Ans: The size of the muscle is useful to distinguish between two muscles found in the same region. The gluteal region contains the following three muscles differentiated by size: (1) The gluteus maximus (large), (2) the gluteus medius (medium) and (3) the gluteus minimus (smallest) (Fig. 5.11).

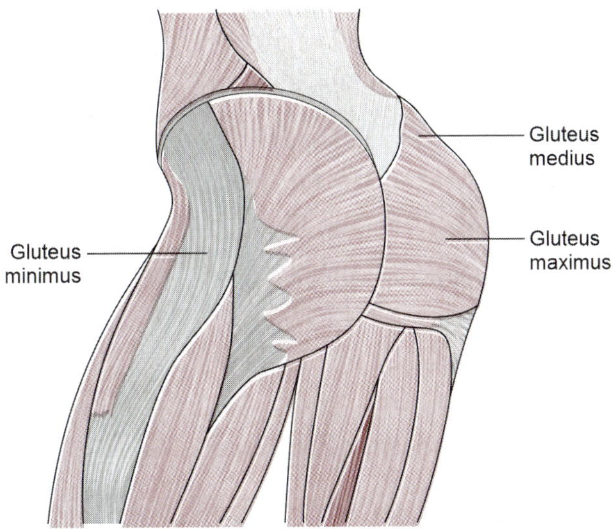

Fig. 5.11: Gluteus muscles

Skeletal Muscles Names Based on Direction

SAQ: Write three names of skeletal muscles based on the directions.

Ans: Rectus abdominis is the muscle whose fibres run straight up and down (Fig. 5.12). Transverse abdominis are the muscles running transversely (left to right) (Fig. 5.12), and the muscles running at an angle are the external obliques (Fig. 5.12).

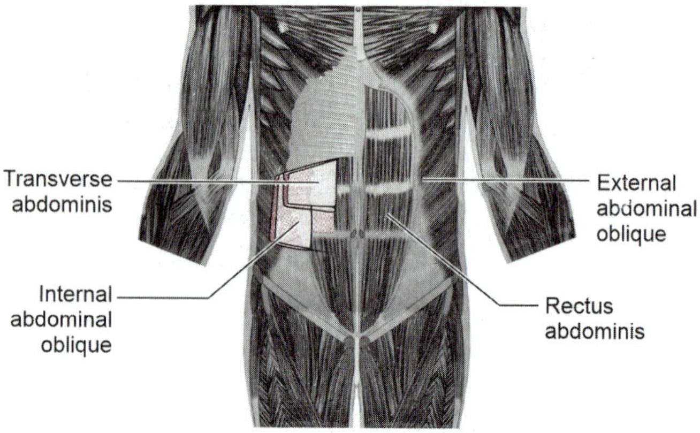

Fig. 5.12: Rectus abdominis and transverse abdominis

Skeletal Muscles Names Based on Functions

SAQ: Write three names of skeletal muscles based on functions.

Ans: The flexor group of the forearm muscles flexes the wrist and the fingers (Fig. 5.13). The supinator is a muscle that turns (supinates) the wrist by rolling it over to the facepalm in an upward direction (Fig. 5.14). The role of adductor muscles in the leg is to pull together (adduct) the legs (Fig. 5.15).

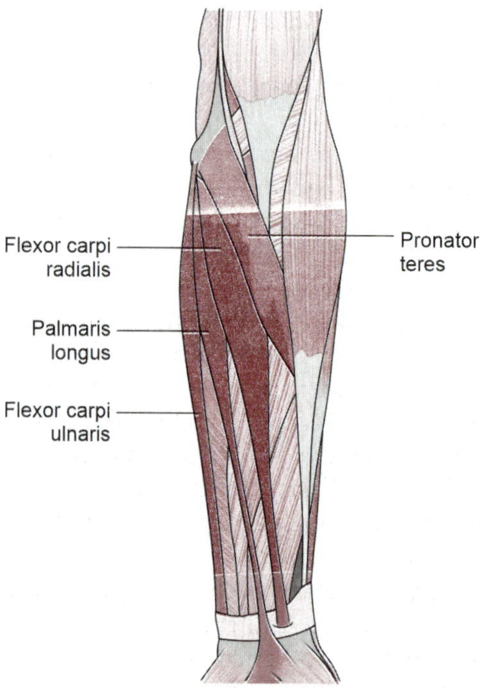

Fig. 5.13: Flexor muscles

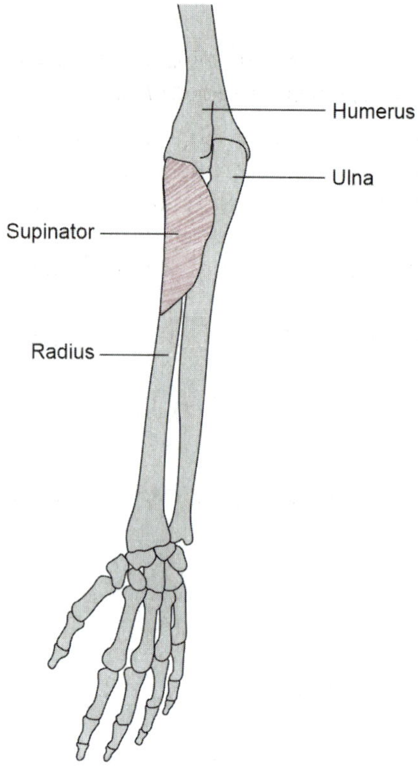

Fig. 5.14: Supinator muscle

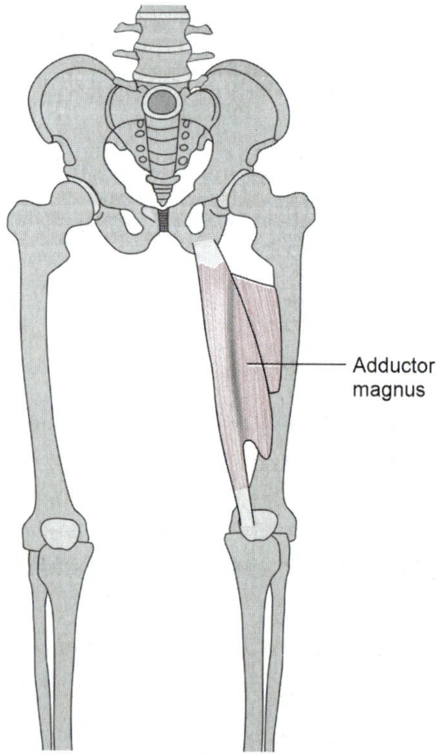

Fig. 5.15: Adductor muscle

BAQ: Draw a neat and labelled diagram of the following muscles: The flexor, the supinator and the adductor.

Ans: Refer to Figs 5.13–5.15.

Objective: To discuss the group actions of the skeletal muscles.

GROUP ACTIONS IN SKELETAL MUSCLE

SAQ: What are agonist and antagonist skeletal muscles and their related functions?

Ans: The skeletal muscles work in groups to produce precise movements. The muscle that produces any specific movement of the body is known as an agonist muscle (Fig. 5.16). The agonist muscle always pairs with an antagonist muscle that produces the opposite effect on the same bones. For example, the biceps brachii muscle flexes the arm at the elbow. The triceps is the antagonist muscle, which extends the arm at the elbow. When the agonist muscle contracts, the antagonist muscle relaxes and vice versa (Fig. 5.16).

BAQ: Draw a labelled diagram of agonist and antagonist muscles.

Ans: Refer to Fig. 5.16.

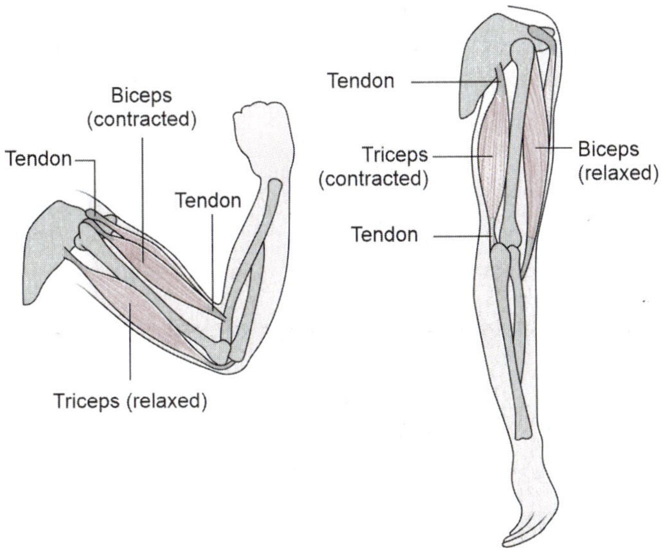

Fig. 5.16: Agonist and antagonist muscles

SAQ: What are synergist muscles?

Ans: The synergist muscles work to support the movements of the agonist. Synergists act to stabilize a movement and reduce extraneous movements. Synergists are usually found in regions near the agonist and often connect to the same bones (Fig. 5.17).

LAQ: Write a note on the fixator muscles.

Ans: The fixator muscle acts as a stabilizer and helps the agonist work effectively as one part of the body during the movement of another part. When heavy material is lifted with the arms, fixators in the trunk region hold the body upright in an immobile condition to maintain the balance of the body while lifting the weight (Fig. 5.18). The following are the examples of fixator muscles:

(1) The levator scapulae muscle, (2) the rhomboid muscles and (3) the trapezius muscle.

1. **The levator scapulae muscle (Fig. 5.17):** The levator scapulae muscle is a synergist with the upper trapezius

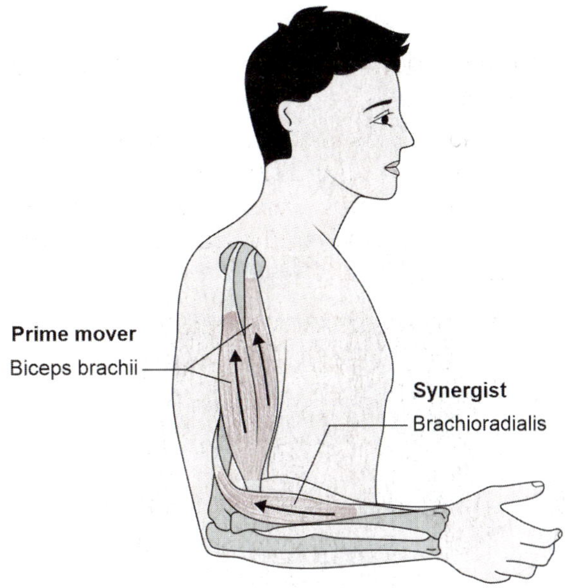

Fig. 5.17: Synergistic muscle

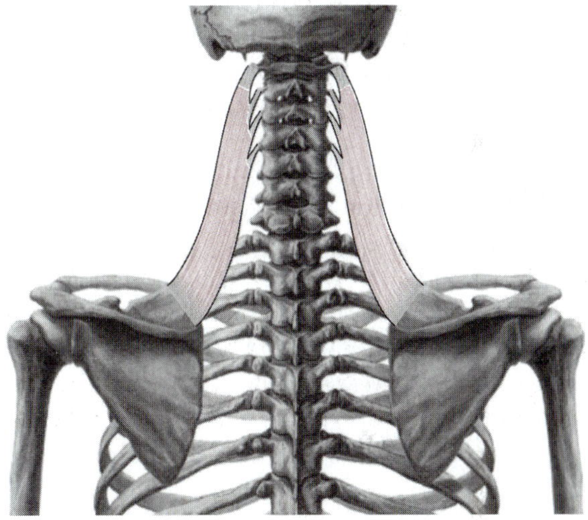

Fig. 5.18: Levator scapulae muscle

muscle for scapular elevation and adduction, however, it is an antagonist for scapular rotation.

Synergistic action: With the fixed spine, the concentric contraction of the levator scapulae muscle causes adduction, elevation and downward rotation of the scapulae.

2. **Rhomboid muscles (Fig. 5.19):** The rhomboids are two types of muscles: (1) Rhomboid major and (2) rhomboid minor. The two rhomboids are arranged deep into the trapezius to form parallel bands. These parallel bands pass inferolaterally (below and at one side) from the vertebrae to the medial border of the scapula. The rhomboid major is a thin and flat muscle. It is two times wider than the thicker rhomboid minor which is placed superior to it.

Synergistic action: The rhomboid major muscle helps to hold the scapula and the upper limb onto the ribcage. Other muscles such as serratus anterior and pectoralis minor, which are both rhomboids, also act to retract the scapula, by pulling it towards the vertebral column.

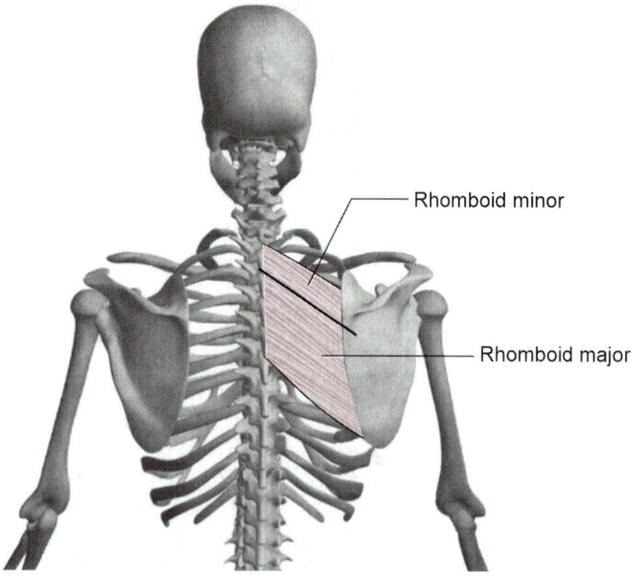

Fig. 5.19: Rhomboids muscles (major and minor)

3. **Trapezius muscle** (Fig. 5.20): The trapezius muscle is a large superficial muscle of the back. It extends from the external protuberance of the occipital bone to the lower thoracic vertebrae and laterally to the spine of the scapula.
   Synergistic action: The upper trapezius (Fig. 5.21) acts synergistically with the sternocleidomastoid muscle in some head and neck movements.

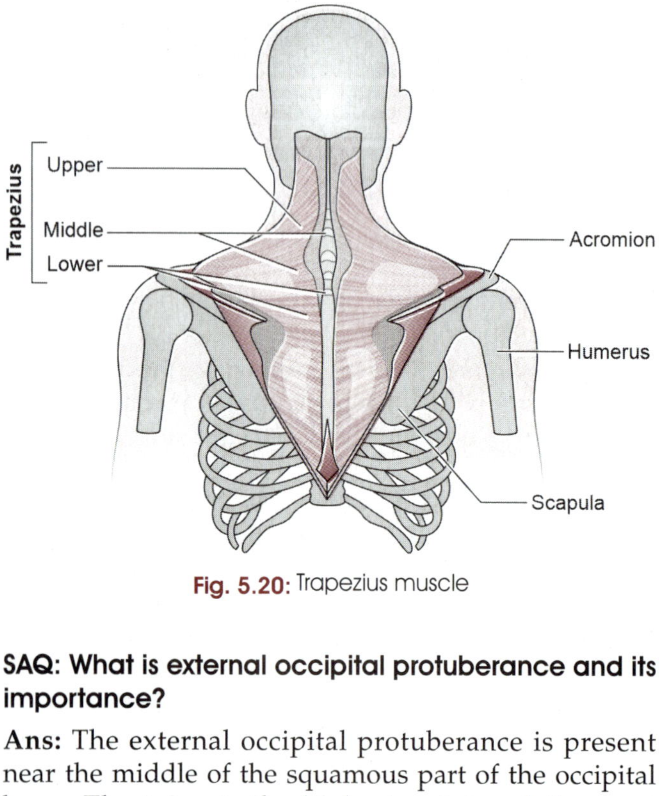

Fig. 5.20: Trapezius muscle

SAQ: What is external occipital protuberance and its importance?

Ans: The external occipital protuberance is present near the middle of the squamous part of the occipital bone. The inion is the highest point and the most prominent projection of the protuberance, located at the posteroinferior (rear lower) part of the human skull. The nuchal ligament and trapezius muscle attach to it. The inion is used as a prominent point in the electroencephalography (EEG) recording.

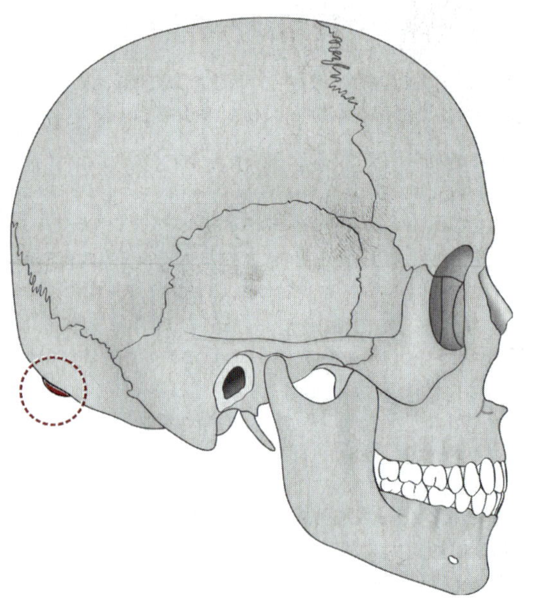

Fig. 5.21: External protuberance of the occipital bone

BAQ: Draw neat and labelled diagrams of the following muscles: The rhomboids and the trapezius.

Ans: Refer to Fig. 5.19–5.20.

Objective: To describe the gross anatomy of a skeletal muscle.

GROSS ANATOMY OF A SKELETAL MUSCLE

BAQ: Write a note on the gross anatomy of a skeletal muscle.

Ans: A skeletal muscle contains multiple bundles (fascicles) of muscle fibres. Each fibre and each muscle is surrounded by a connective tissue layer (fascia) (Fig. 5.22). The sarcomere units are the basic functional, contractile units of the muscle fiber. Muscle fibres are formed from the myoblasts in a process known as myogenesis and form long multinucleated cells. In these cells, the nuclei (myonuclei) are located along the inside of the cell membrane. The muscle fibres contain multiple mitochondria to meet energy requirements, for the various activities of the skeletal muscle.

The muscle fibres are composed of myofibrils. The myofibrils are composed of actin and myosin protein filaments (myofilaments). These filaments are repeated in sarcomere units, which are the basic functional, contractile units of the muscle fiber. The sarcomeres are necessary for muscle contraction (Fig. 5.22). Muscles get energy mainly from the oxidation of carbohydrates and fats. Adenosine triphosphate (ATP) molecules produced in the oxidation of carbohydrates and fats are used to power the movement of the myosin head.

Organization of Sarcomere (Fig. 5.22)

BAQ: Write a note on the organization of a sarcomere.

Ans: The organization of a sarcomere is a very important feature of the sliding filament model. Each sarcomere is composed of hundreds of myofilaments. Thick and

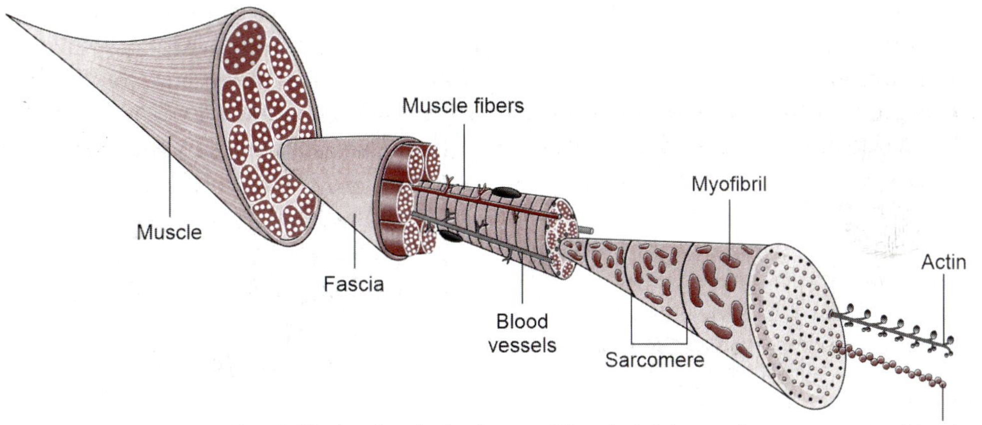

Fig. 5.22: Anatomic features of the skeletal muscle

thin filaments are the two kinds of myofilaments. Thick myofilaments are composed of several hundred molecules of a fibrous protein known as Myosin (Fig. 5.23). Thin myofilaments are composed of two helically interwound, linear polymers of actin, which is a globular protein (Fig. 5.24). Thin and thick filaments also contain accessory proteins. Each sarcomere consists of a central A-band (thick filaments) and two halves of the I-band (thin filaments) (Fig. 5.25). The I-band from two adjacent sarcomeres meets at the Z-line. The central portion of the A-band is the M-line, which does not contain actin.

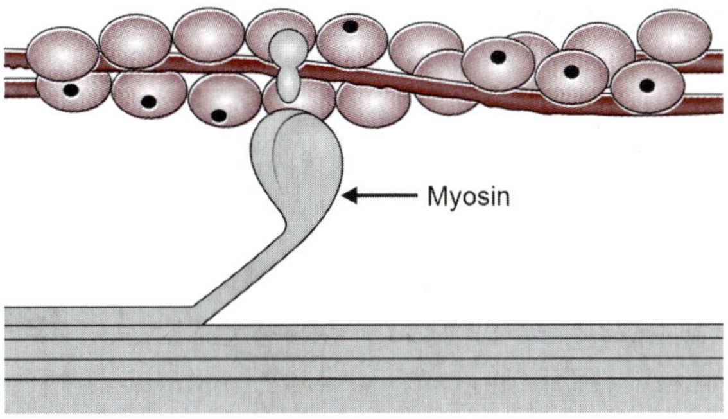

Fig. 5.23: Myosin

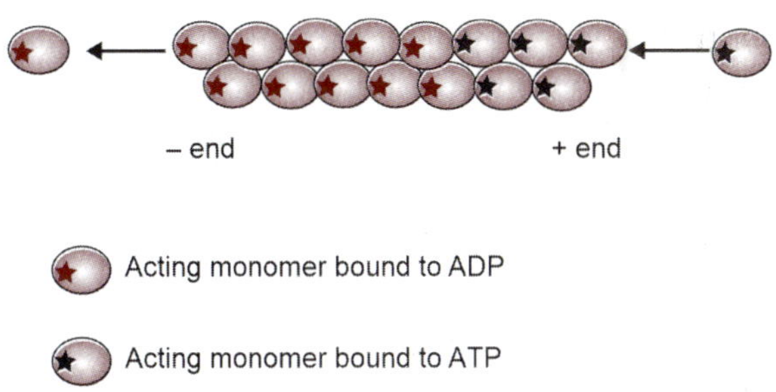

Fig. 5.24: Actin filament assembly

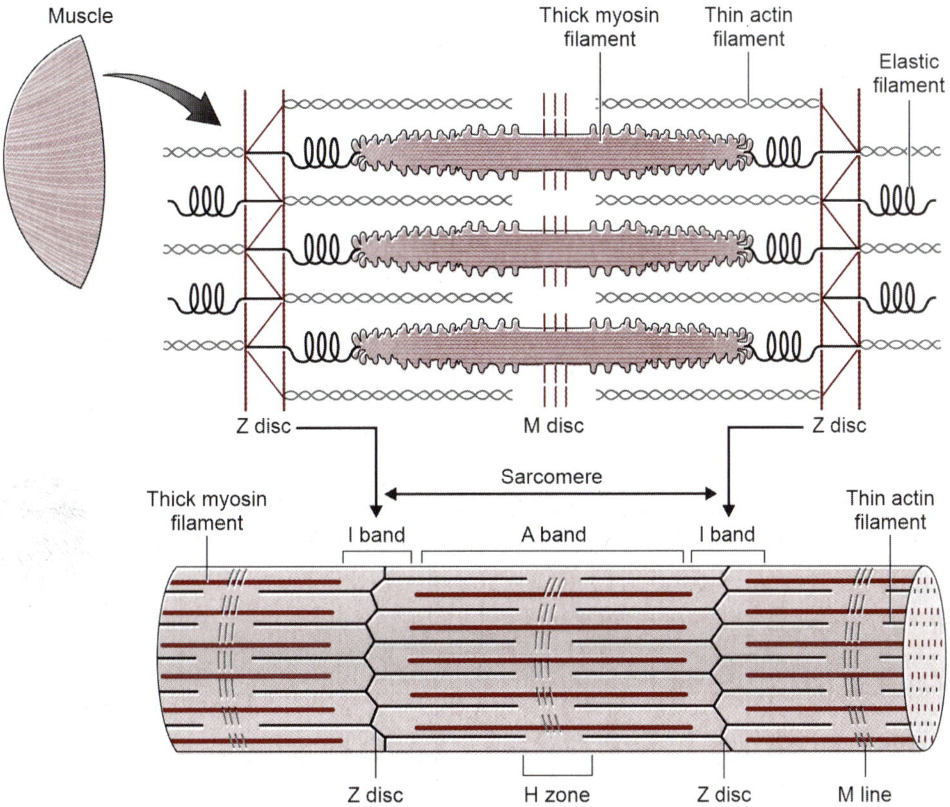

Fig. 5.25: Organization of a sarcomere

Proteins of the Z line act as embedding matrix and anchor for one end of the thin filaments, which extend toward the centre of sarcomeres on either side of the Z-line. The Z-line proteins often appear continuous across the width of a muscle fibre and keep the myofibrils within a myofiber. The distal end of each thin filament is free in the sarcoplasm and is capped with a protein known as β-actinin. The M-line is centrally located in sarcomeres. Like Z-line protein, the M-line protein aggregate acts as an embedding matrix. Thick filaments extend from their point of attachment on both sides of the M-line toward the two Z-lines that define a sarcomere.

Description of Sarcomere (Fig. 5.25)

BAQ: Define and describe a sarcomere of a microfibril.

Ans: A sarcomere is defined as the segment between two neighbouring Z-lines (or Z-discs, or Z bodies) in a microfibril. In electron micrographs of cross-striated muscle, the Z-line appears as a series of dark lines. The description of a sarcomere is as follows:

- Surrounding the Z-line is the region of the I-band.
- Following the I-band is the A-band.
- Within the A-band is a paler region called the H-band.
- Inside the H-zone is a thin M-line formed of cross-connecting elements of the cytoskeleton.

Objective: To locate and describe the types and actions of the muscles of the axial skeleton.

IMPORTANT SKELETAL MUSCLES

Muscles of the Face

LAQ: Write a note on the muscles of the face.

Ans: The human face contains about 30 muscles. The facial muscles are striated. These muscles connect the skin of the face to the bone of the skull to perform important functions such as mastication and expression of emotions. The following are the positions of various important facial muscles (Fig. 5.26):

- Buccolabial muscles in and around the mouth
- Nasal muscles around the nose.
- Epicranial muscles on the forehead, skull and neck.
- Auricular muscles around the ears.
- Orbital muscles surrounding the eyes.

The following are the facial muscles involved in chewing (Figs 5.26 and 5.27):

- A buccinator is a thin muscle in the cheek that holds each cheek toward the teeth.
- A masseter is a muscle that runs from each cheek to each side of the jaw and helps the jaw to close.
- The medial pterygoid is a thick muscle that helps the jaw to close.
- The temporalis is a fan-shaped muscle that helps the jaw close.

The following are the muscles that facilitate facial expressions: (Fig. 5.26):

1. Corrugator supercilii, which is near the eyebrow that enables frowning.
2. Depressor anguli oris, which is on each side of the chin and along with other muscles help in the expression of frown.
3. Depressor labii inferioris is a muscle in the chin that helps to control movement in the lip.
4. Levator labii superioris alaeque nasi, which helps to open the nostrils and lift the upper lip.
5. Mentalis, a pair of muscles toward the centre of the chin that help to control the lower lip.
6. Nasalis muscle allows to flare the nostrils.

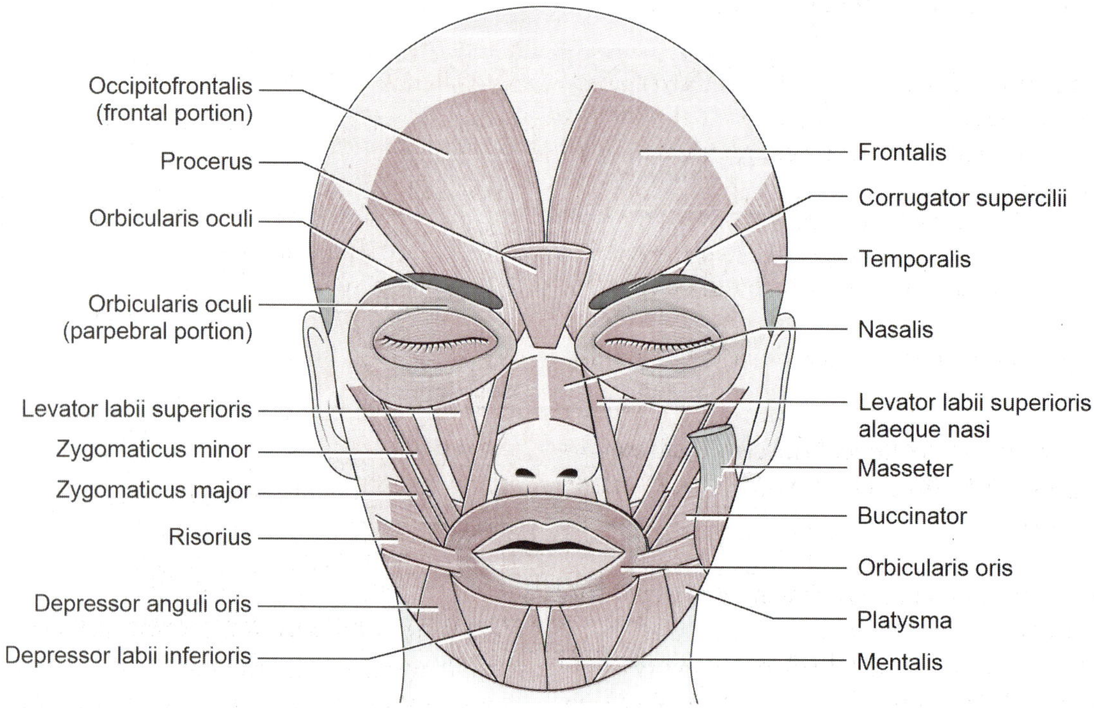

Fig. 5.26: Muscles of the face

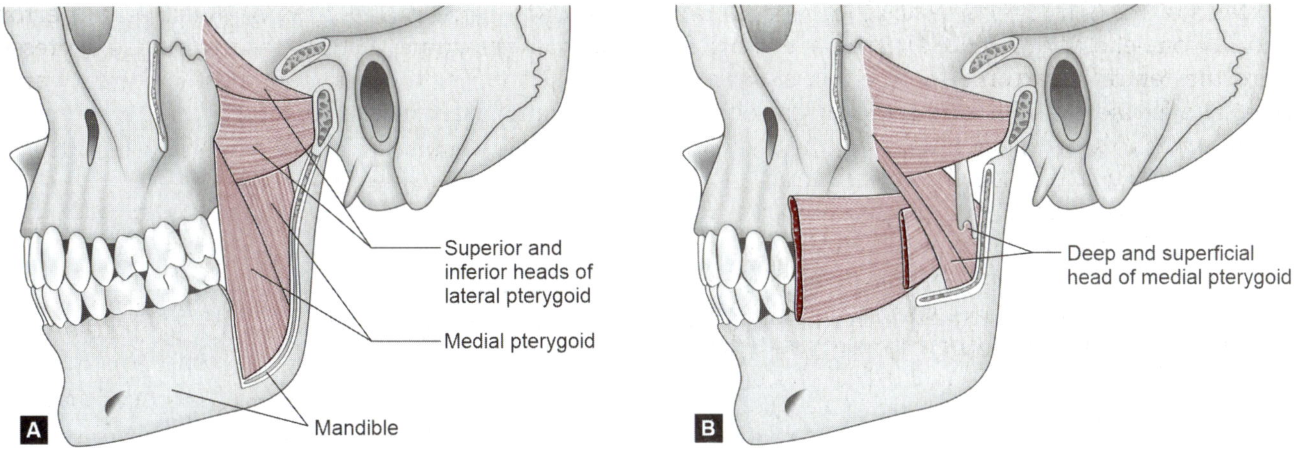

Fig. 5.27: (A) Lateral pterygoid muscle; (B) medial pterygoid muscle

7. Occipitofrontalis is a muscle that extends from the eyebrows to the top of the skull and can raise eyebrows and create wrinkles on the forehead.
8. Orbicularis oculi is useful to close the eyelids.
9. Orbicularis oris, form a circle of muscles around the mouth that closes or purses the lips.
10. Procerus is a muscle between the eyebrows that can pull eyebrows downward and help to flare nostrils.
11. Risorius is located on each side of the mouth and helps in smiling.
12. Zygomaticus major and minor muscles facilitate smile.

Other functions of the muscles of the face include the protection of the eyes, churning food and drink in the mouth, talking, singing, and whistling.

BAQ: Write names of the facial muscles that help for the following functions: (1) To hold cheeks near the teeth, (2) to open the jaw, (3) to close the jaw.

Ans:

1. The buccinator is a thin muscle in the cheek that holds each cheek toward the teeth.
2. The lateral pterygoid is a fan-shaped muscle that helps the jaw to open.
3. The masseter is a muscle that runs from each cheek to each side of the jaw and helps the jaw to close. The medial pterygoid is a thick muscle that helps the jaw to close.

   Temporalis is a fan-shaped muscle that helps the jaw to close.

BAQ: Write names of the facial muscles that enable the following expressions: (1) Frowning, and (2) movements of the lip.

Ans:

1. The corrugator supercilii, which is near the eyebrow enables frowning.

   The depressor anguli oris, which is on each side of the chin and along with other muscles helps in the expression of a frown.
2. The depressor labii inferioris is a muscle in the chin that helps to control movement in the lip. The levator labii superioris alaeque nasi, can open the nostrils and lift the upper lip. The mentalis is a pair of muscles toward the centre of the chin that helps to control the lower lip.

BAQ: Write names of the facial muscles that enable the following expressions: (1) Flaring of nostrils, (2) wrinkle creations, (3) closing of eyelids, (4) smiling.

Ans:

1. The nasalis muscle allows flaring of the nostrils.
2. The occipitofrontalis is a muscle that extends from the eyebrows to the top of the skull and can raise eyebrows and create wrinkles on the forehead.
3. The orbicularis oculi is useful to close the eyelids.
4. The risorius is located on each side of the mouth and helps in smiling. Zygomaticus major and minor muscles also help to smile.

Table 5.2: Insertion, origin and action of important muscles of facial expression

Facial muscle	*Insertion*	*Origin*	*Action*
Occipitalis	Posterior end of galea aponeurotica	Occipital bone and mastoid process	Scalp move backwards
Orbicularis	Eyelid tissue	Front surface of the eye socket	Closing of eye
Oculi Orbicularis Oris	Lip mucosa	Lip tissue	Lip closing
Lavator labbi superioris	Orbicularis oris	Zygomatic process of maxilla	Lip elevation

Muscles of the Neck (Fig. 5.28)

BAQ: Write a note on the muscles of the neck.

Ans: The muscles of the neck are responsible for the movement of the head in various directions. These are closely related to various important structures that pass

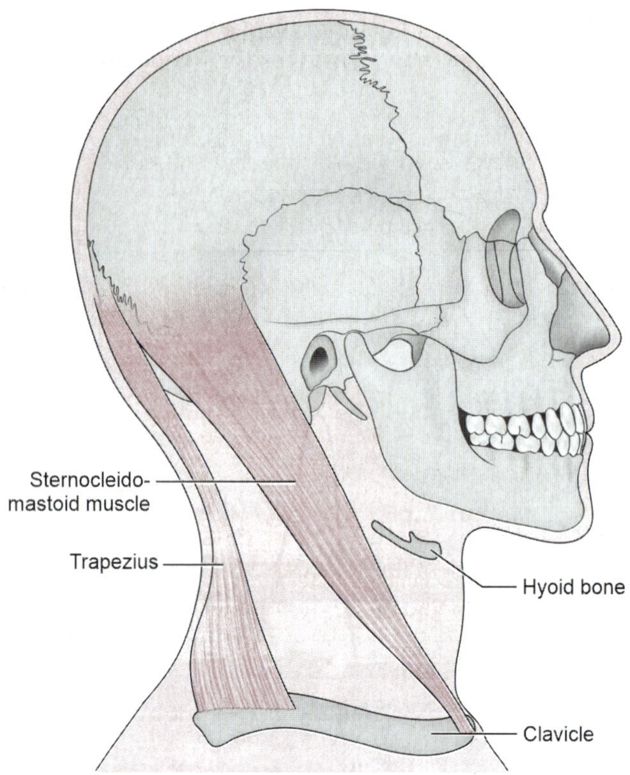

Fig. 5.28: Sternocleidomastoid muscle of neck

between the thorax and the head such as important nerves, major blood vessels, and the various important parts of the respiratory and gastrointestinal systems.

Based on their position in the neck; muscles are comprised of the following main groups: (1) Anterior group, (2) lateral group and (3) posterior groups. The musculature of the neck is further divided into more specific groups based on a number of determinants; including the depth, precise location and function. The following two large muscles play important functions: (A) The sternocleidomastoid and (B) the trapezious.

A. Sternocleidomastoid Muscle (SCM)

The sternocleidomastoid muscle is one of the largest and superficially palpable muscles that act on the neck (Fig. 5.28). The SCM has dual innervation and it performs the following various functions:

1. It draws the mastoid process (projection) of the temporal bone (Fig. 5.29) down toward the same side.
2. It helps in turning the head from side to side. It also acts as an accessory muscle in respiration. When this muscle on one side contracts, it draws the head near the shoulder. When they contract together (from both sides), the muscles of the two sides bend (flex) the neck.

B. Trapezius Muscle: Ref. page 101, Fig. 5.30.

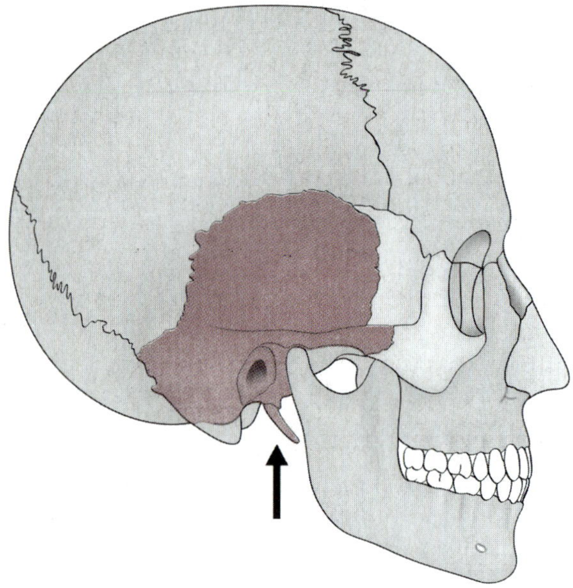

Fig. 5.29: Process of the temporal bone

BAQ: Write a note on the sternocleidomastoid muscles (SCM), with respect to: (1) Origin, (2) insertion, (3) nerve supply and action.

Ans:

1. The sternocleidomastoid muscle originates from the manubrium of the sternum and the clavicle.
2. **Insertion:** It passes across the side of the neck and inserts at the mastoid process of the temporal bone of the skull.
3. **Nerve supply:** The sternocleidomastoid muscle has a nerve supply from the accessory nerve.
4. **Action:** It helps in turning the head from side to side.

MUSCLES OF THE BACK

Trapezius Muscle (Fig. 5.30)

BAQ: Write a note on the trapezius muscle.

Ans: The trapezius muscle is a large superficial back muscle. It extends from the external protuberance of the occipital bone to the lower thoracic vertebrae. Laterally, the trapezius extends to the spine of the scapula. The trapezius has upper, middle and lower fibres. The

Table 5.3: Muscle that act on forearm

Muscle	*Insertion*	*Origin*	*Nerve supply*	*Action*
Biceps brachii	Radial tuberosity	Above glenoid fossa of scapula	The musculocutaneous nerve	Supinates forearm, flexes elbow joint
Brachioradialis	Onto the ulnar tuberosity	Distal anterior humerus	The musculocutaneous nerve	Elbow joint flexing
Brachialis	Coronoid process of ulna	Anterior part of humerus	The musculocutaneous nerve	Elbow joint flexing
Triceps brachii	The olecranon of the ulna glenoid fossa	Tuberosity below	The radial nerve	Elbow joint extension

trapezius has the following three functional parts: (1) An upper (descending) part that supports the weight of the arm; (2) a middle region, which retracts the scapula and (3) a lower (ascending) part that medially rotates and depresses the scapula.

The trapezius performs the following various actions:

1. To stabilize and move the scapula.
2. The upper fibers are able to elevate and upwardly rotate the scapula and extend the neck.
3. The middle fibers medially retract the scapula.
4. The lower fibers depress and help the upper fibers to rotate the scapula in upward direction.

The various functions performed by the trapezius muscle are as follows:

1. Pulls the head backwards.
2. Squares the shoulders
3. Controls the movements of scapula

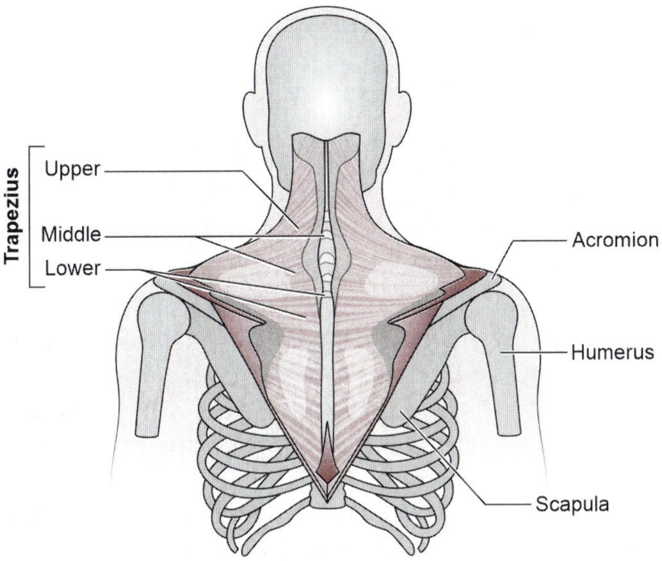

Fig. 5.30: Trapezius muscle

BAQ: Write a note on the trapezius muscle with respect to: (1) Origin, (2) insertion, (3) nerve supply and (4) action.

Ans:

1. **Origin:** The trapezius has multiple origin points. It originates on the occipital bone, the ligamentum nuchae, and the spinous processes of T01–T12.
2. **Insertion:** The trapezius has many insertion points. Mainly it inserts on the lateral third of the clavicle, the acromion and scapular spine of the scapula.
3. **Nerve supply:** The cranial nerve XI innervates the motor function of the trapezius.
4. **Action:** The trapezius stabilizes and moves the scapula.

Muscles of the Trunk (Figs 5.31 and 5.32)

The space between the ribs is called the intercostal space. There are 11 intercostal spaces, which comprise intercostal muscles and membranes and neurovascular structures. The muscles of the trunk are useful to move the vertebral column, and form the thoracic and abdominal walls, and also cover the pelvic outlet.

Erector Spinae Group of Muscles (Fig. 5.31)

The erector spinae group of muscles on each side of the vertebral column is a large muscle mass in the trunk that extends from the sacrum to the skull.

BAQ: Write a note on the erector spinae group muscles of the trunk.

Ans: The erector spinae muscles comprise the intermediate layer of the deep (intrinsic) muscles of the back. They extend on either side of the vertebral column, between the base of the cranium superiorly and pelvis inferiorly. The erector spinae are divided into three groups, from medial to lateral: (1) Spinalis muscles, (2) longissimus muscles, and (3) iliocostalis muscles (Fig. 5.31).

Function: The erector spinae group muscles are primarily responsible for extending the vertebral column to maintain erect posture.

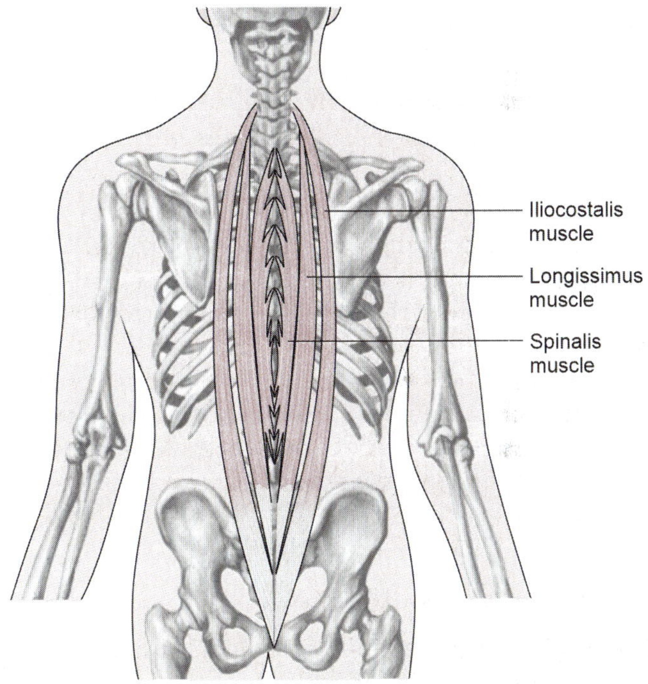

Fig. 5.31: Erector spinae muscles

Intercostal Muscles

BAQ: Write a note on the Intercostal muscles.

Ans: Eleven pairs of the intercostal muscles are situated in between the ribs that create and move the chest wall. The muscles are made up of the following three layers: External intercostal muscles (The most superficial layer), internal intercostal muscles, and the innermost intercostal muscles.

Functions: Air is expelled out, when the internal intercostal muscles contract and compress the thoracic cavity, during exhalation process. Similarly, the external intercostal muscles contract and draw the ribs up and out. During this process, space is created in the thoracic cavity for inhalation and expansion of the lungs.

Table 5.4: Muscle that move the thigh at the hip joint

Muscle	*Insertion*	*Origin*	*Nerve supply*	*Action*
Psoas major	Lesser trochanter of femur	The deeper segment originates from the first four lumbar vertebrae, the superficial segment originates along the lateral surface of the distal thoracis vertebrae	the anterior rami of L1-L4, small branches of the femoral nerve	Flexes and rotates thigh at the hip joint
Iliacus	Lesser trochanter of femur	Iliac fossa	Branches of the femoral nerve (L2, L3)	Flexes and rotates thigh at hip joint
Gluteus maximum	The iliotibial tract and gluteal tuberosity of the femur	Gluteal surface of ilium, sacrum, coccyx	Inferior gluteal nerve (root L5, S1 and S2)	Extends and rotates thigh laterally at hip jpint
Gluteus medius	Greater trochanter of femur	Ilium (lateral surface)	Superior gluteal nerve	Abducts and rotates thigh medially at hip jpint
Gluteus minimum	Greater trochanter of femur	Ilium (lower lateral surface)	Superior gluteal nerve	Abducts and rotates thigh medially at hip joint

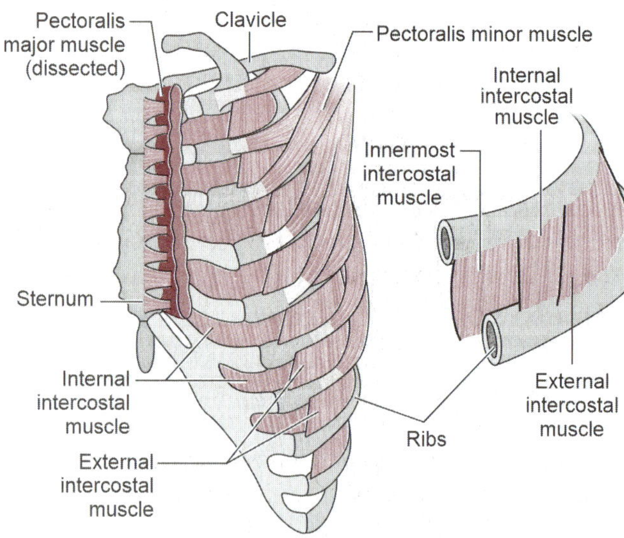

Fig. 5.32: Intercostal muscles.

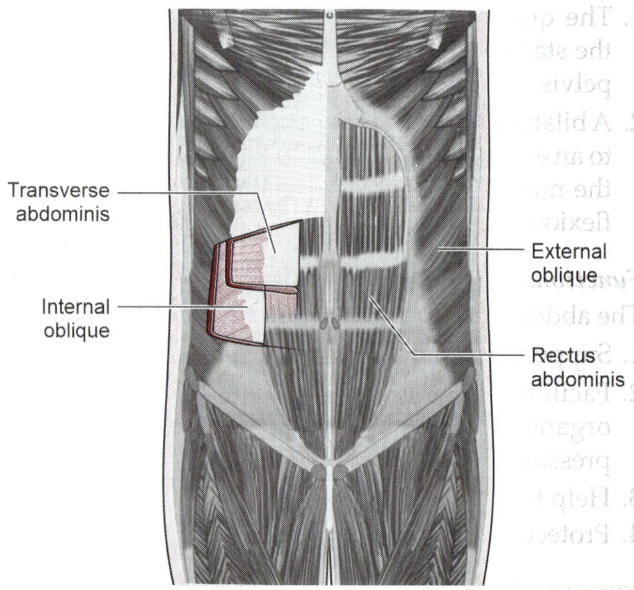

Fig. 5.33A: Main abdominal muscles

Abdominal Muscles (Fig. 5.33)

LAQ: Write a note on the abdominal muscles.

Ans: The abdomen, unlike the thorax and pelvis, does not have bony protection. The abdominal wall consists entirely of five muscle pairs. These are arranged in layers. The pelvic outlet is formed by two muscular sheets and their associated fascia. From the surface inwards, the main abdominal muscles are as follows: (1) Rectus abdominis, (2) external oblique, (3) internal oblique, (4) transversus abdominis, and (5) quadratus lumborum.

1. **Rectus abdominis (six pack muscle) (Fig. 5.33A):** The rectus abdominis is a superficial, very long and flat muscle. It extends along the whole length of the front of the abdomen. It supports the abdominal wall while straining in forced expiration or passing hard stool.
2. **External oblique muscle (Fig. 5.33A):** The external oblique muscle is the outermost abdominal muscle (Fig. 5.31). It occupies a large part of the trunk area and situated at both the sides of the abdomen. External

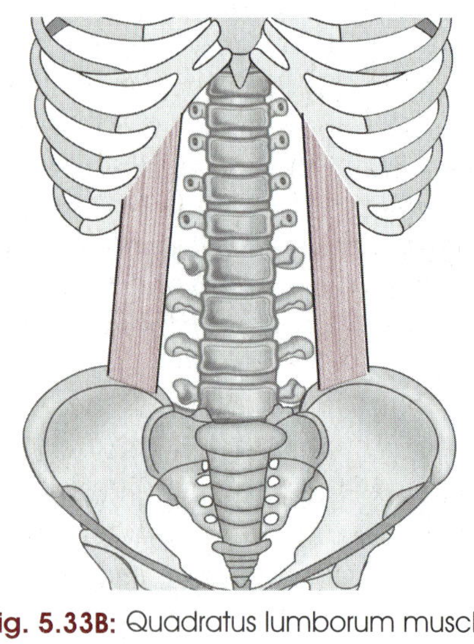

Fig. 5.33B: Quadratus lumborum muscle

oblique muscle extends from the lower half of the ribs around and down to the pelvis.

3. **Internal oblique muscle (Fig. 5.33A):** Internal abdominal oblique is a broad and thin muscle. It is placed on the lateral side of the abdomen. Internal oblique muscle forms one of the layers of the lateral abdominal wall along with the transverse abdominis on the inner side and external oblique on the outer side.
4. **Transversus abdominis (Fig. 5.33A):** The transversus abdominis muscle is the deepest abdominal muscles. It extends between the ribs and the pelvis and wraps around the trunk from front to back.
5. **Quadratus lumborum muscle (QL) (Fig. 5.33B):** The quadratus lumborum muscle is quadrilateral (four-sided) and the deepest back muscle. It is a paired muscle of the left and right posterior abdominal wall.

Functions

1. The quadratus lumborum play important role in the stabilization and movement of the spine and the pelvis.
2. A bilateral contraction of quadratus lumborum leads to an extension of the lumbar vertebral column. When the muscle is activated on one side it causes lateral flexion (the trunk is bent towards that one side).

Functions of the Abdominal Muscles

The abdominal muscles:

1. Support the trunk.
2. Facilitate movements of internal organs and hold organs in place by regulating internal abdominal pressure.
3. Help to make body stable and balanced.
4. Protect of the spine.

Table 5.5: Insertion, origin and action of important muscles of the abdominal wall

Abdominal muscle	*Insertion*	*Origin*	*Action*
Rectus abdominis	Xiphoid process of the sternum costal cartilage of ribs 5–7	Crest of the pubis bone	Flexes vertebral column
Transverse abdominis	Xiphoid process, linea alba pubic crest	Lnguinal ligament, lumbar fascia costal cartilages of last six ribs	Abdomen compression
External abdominal oblique	Iliac crest, linea alba	lateral surface of ribs lower ribs	Abdomen compression lateral rotation
Internal abdominal oblique	Linea alba, last four ribs	Iliac crest, inguinal ligament, lumbar facia	Abdominal compression lateral rotation

Muscles of the Back

BAQ: Write a note on the muscles of the back.

Ans: The muscles of the back can be divided into three distinct groups (1) The superficial group, (2) the intermediate group and (3) the deep group.

1. **The superficial group (the appendicular group):** The superficial group is composed of trapezius, latissimus dorsi, rhomboid major, rhomboid minor and levator scapulae. The superficial group is mainly associated with movement of the appendicular skeleton.
2. **Intermediate group (respiratory group):** The intermediate group is composed of serratus posterior superior muscle and serratus posterior inferior muscle. These muscles play important role in the respiration process.
3. **Deep group (intrinsic group) muscles:** The deep group muscles can be further subdivided into the four groups: Spinotransversales, Erector spinae, Transversospinales and Segmental muscles.

The following six pairs are the main muscles of the back: Trapezius, latissimus dorsi, teres major, psoas, quadratus lumborum and sacrospinalis.

Trapezius (Fig. 5.30, page 101)

BAQ: Write a note on the latissimus dorsi muscle.

Ans: The latissimus dorsi muscle (Fig. 5.34) is a broad and flat muscle. It occupies most of the lower posterior thorax.

Functions

1. The main function of the latissimus dorsi muscle is to move the upper extremity.
2. The latissimus dorsi muscle also plays an important role as an accessory muscle of respiration.

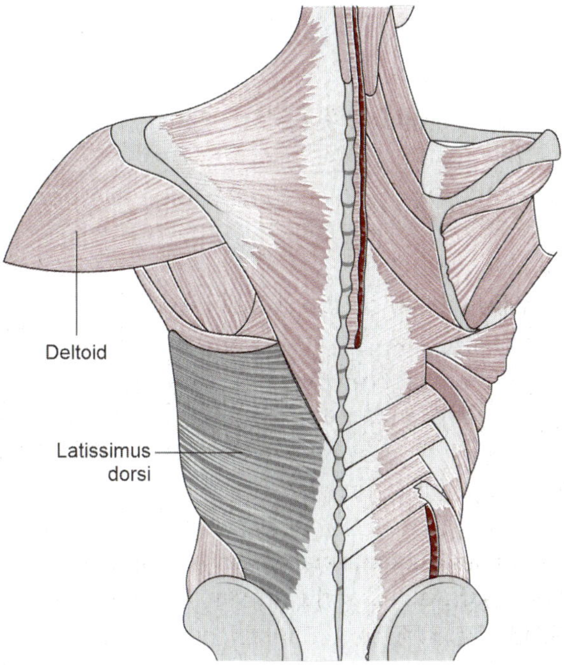

Fig. 5.34: Latissimus dorsi muscle

BAQ: Write a note on the latissimus dorsi muscle with respect to: (1) Origin, (2) insertion, (3) nerve supply and (4) action.

Ans:

1. **Origin:** Spines of lumbar, sacral and lower part of the vertebral column.
2. **Insertion:** Humerus intertubercular groove.
3. **Nerve supply:** The thoracodorsal nerve.
4. **Action:** Extends, adducts and rotates humerus.

> **Objective:** To locate and describe the types and actions of the muscles of the appendicular skeleton.

BAQ: Write a note on the teres major muscle.

Ans: The teres major muscle (Fig. 5.35): The teres major is a rectangular thick and flat muscle.

1. **Origin:** It extends from the inferior posterior scapula to the intertubercular groove of the humerus.
2. **Insertion:** Intertubercular groove of humerus.
3. **Nerve supply:** The teres major is innervated by the lower subscapular nerve.

Function: It plays important role synergistically with the latissimus dorsi to extend, adduct, and internally rotate the humerus.

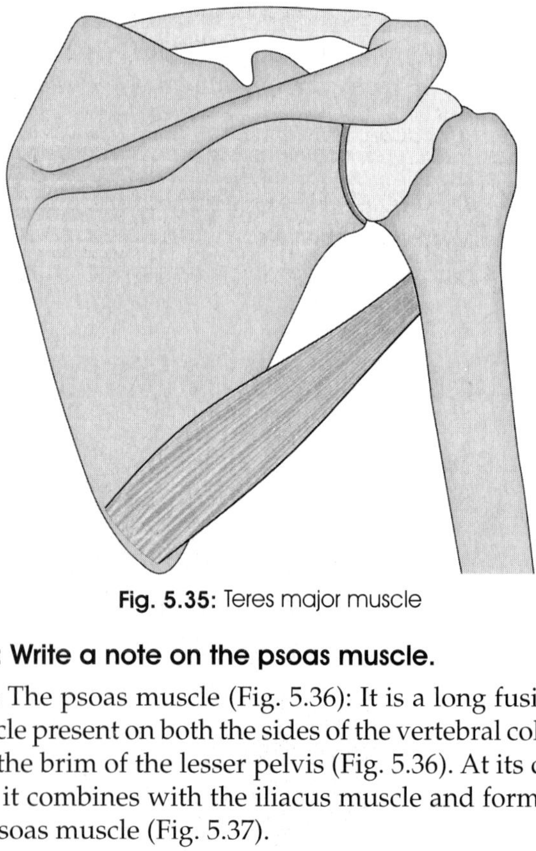

Fig. 5.35: Teres major muscle

BAQ: Write a note on the psoas muscle.

Ans: The psoas muscle (Fig. 5.36): It is a long fusiform muscle present on both the sides of the vertebral column and the brim of the lesser pelvis (Fig. 5.36). At its distal end, it combines with the iliacus muscle and forms the iliopsoas muscle (Fig. 5.37).

Functions

1. Flexion and lateral rotation of the thigh at the hip.
2. It flexes the trunk at the hip and also flexes the trunk laterally.

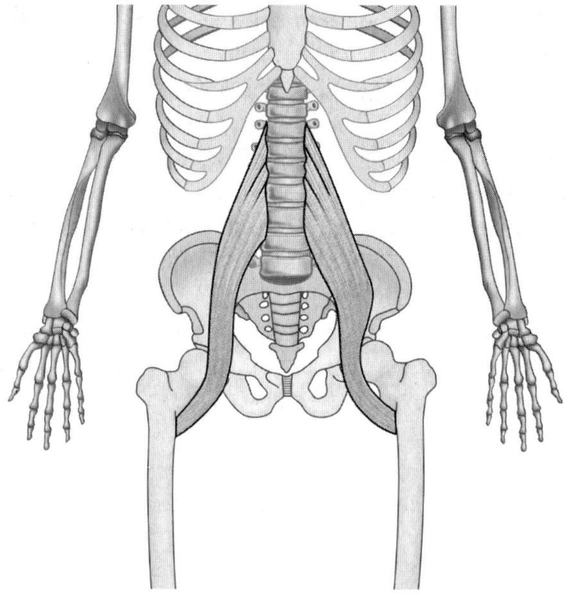

Fig. 5.36: Psoas muscle

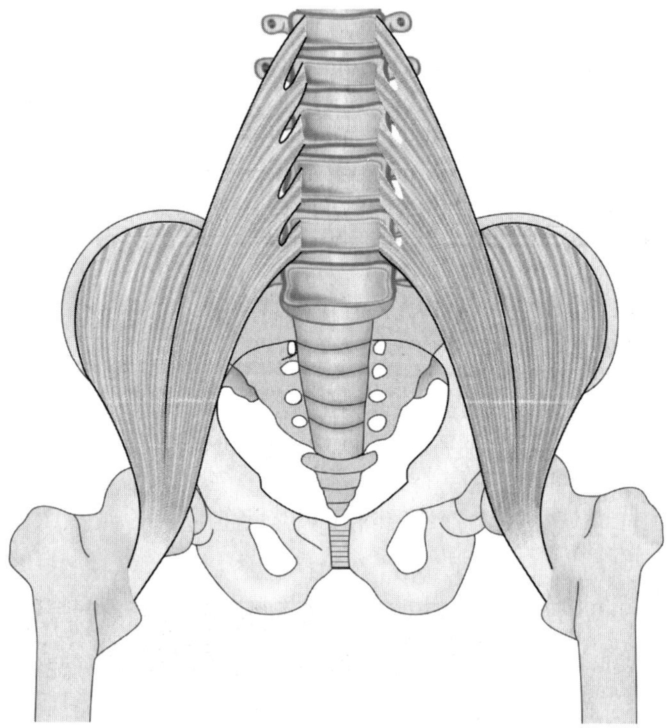

Fig. 5.37: Iliopsoas muscle

BAQ: Draw a neat and labelled diagrams of the following muscles: The psoa, The iliopsoas and the erector spinae muscle.

Ans: Refer to Figs 5.36–5.38.

BAQ: Write a note on the psoas muscle with respect to: (1) Origin, (2) insertion, (3) nerve supply and (4) action.

Ans:

1. **Origin:** The deeper segment of the muscle originates from the first four lumbar vertebrae. The superficial segment of the psoas muscle originates along the

lateral surface of the distal thoracic vertebrae and the adjacent intervertebral discs.

2. **Insertion:** The psoas muscle inserts into the lesser trochanter of the femur.
3. **Nerve supply:** The psoas major muscle is innervated through the anterior rami of L1–L4, and small branches from the femoral nerve.
4. **Action:** Flexion and lateral rotation of the thigh at the hip. It flexes the trunk at the hip and also flexes the trunk laterally.

BAQ: Write a note on the quadratus lumborum muscle with respect to: (1) Origin, (2) insertion, (3) nerve supply and (4) action.

Ans: Quadratus lumborum muscle (Fig. 5.33):

1. **Origin:** Iliac crest and lower part (lower three) of lumber vertebrae
2. **Insertion:** Twelfth rib and upper part of lumber vertebrae
3. **Nerve supply:** The twelfth thoracic nerve and the spinal rami of the lumbar spinal nerves.
4. **Action:** Stabilization and movement of the spine and the pelvis.

BAQ: Write a note on the erector spinae muscle (sacrospinalis muscle).

Ans: The erector spinae (sacrospinalis muscle) (Fig. 5.38) is a group of muscles and tendons which run on the left and the right side of the spine from the sacral region and hips to the base of the skull.

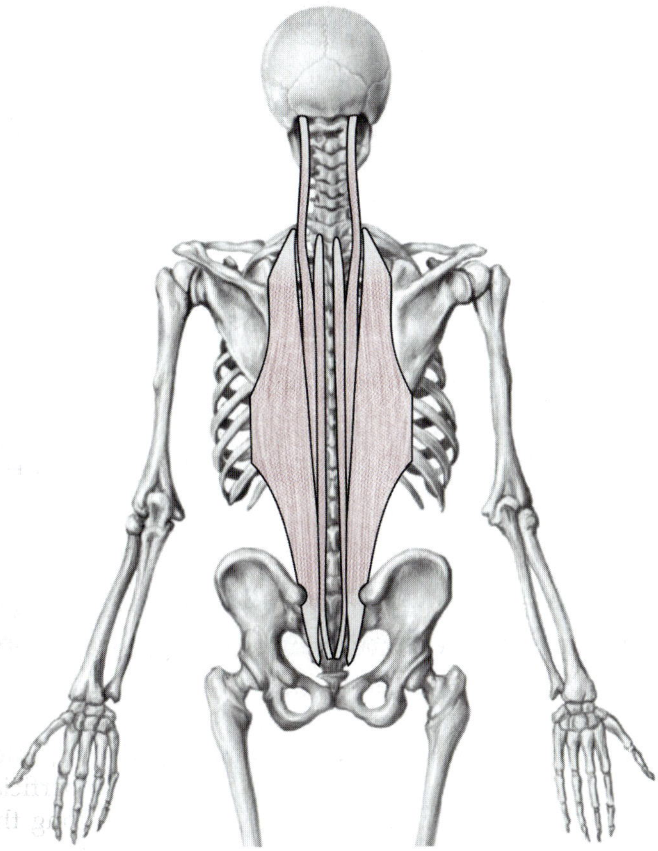

Fig. 5.38: Erector spinae muscle (sacrospinalis muscle)

Functions

1. To extend and laterally flex the spine.
2. To facilitate movements like backbends.

BAQ: Write a note on the erector spinae muscle (the sacrospinalis muscle) with respect to: (1) Origin, (2) insertion, (3) nerve supply and (4) action.

Ans:

1. **Origin:** The lumbar and lower thoracic regions of the body.
2. **Insertion:** On to the upper thoracic and cervical regions of the body.
3. **Nerve supply:** By the dorsal rami of the first cervical nerve (C1).
4. **Action:** Extends and laterally flexes the spine and facilitate the movements like backbends.

Muscles of the Pelvic Floor

SAQ: Write a note on the muscles of the pelvic floor.

Ans: The levator ani (Fig. 5.39) forms the bulk of the pelvic floor muscles. It consists of the following three muscle components: (1) pubococcygeus, (2) puborectalis and (3) iliococcygeus.

Pelvic floor muscles perform the following two important functions: (1) To provide support to the abdominal viscera and (2) to facilitate continence mechanism to the anal, urethral, and vaginal orifices (in females).

Levator Ani (Fig. 5.39)

BAQ: Write a note on the levator ani muscle.

Ans: The levator ani is a complex funnel-shaped muscle (Fig. 5.39). It is composed of the following three parts: Puborectalis, pubococcygeus, and the iliococcygeus muscles. The levator ani is located on both sides of the lower pelvis.

Functions

1. It provides support and raise the pelvic visceral structures.
2. It helps in appropriate urination, defecation, and sexual functions.

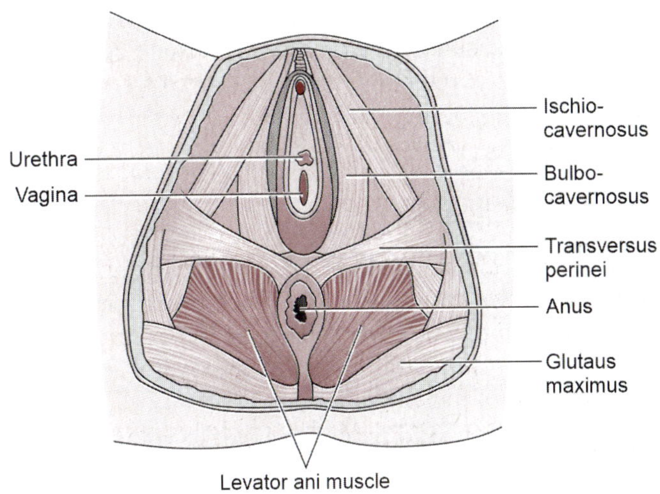

Fig. 5.39: Levator ani muscle

BAQ: Write a note on the levator ani muscle (the sacrospinalis muscle) with respect to: (1) Origin, (2) insertion, (3) nerve supply and (4) action.

Ans:

1. **Origin:** From the pubic bone (the part of the muscle).
2. **Insertion:** Into the intersphincteric groove.
3. **Nerve supply:** Sacral efferent and pudendal nerves (2, 3)
4. **Functions:** It provides support and helps in appropriate urination, defecation, and sexual functions.

Coccygeus Muscle (Fig. 5.40)

BAQ: Write a note on the coccygeus (ischiococcygeus) muscle.

Ans: The coccygeus (ischiococcygeus) muscle is a triangular-shaped muscle located posterior to the levator ani muscles in the pelvic floor. The pelvic diaphragm is formed by the combination of coccygeus muscle with the levator ani muscle.

Functions: The coccygeus (ischiococcygeus) muscle forms part of the pelvic diaphragm, and assists the levator ani muscle to support the pelvic viscera.

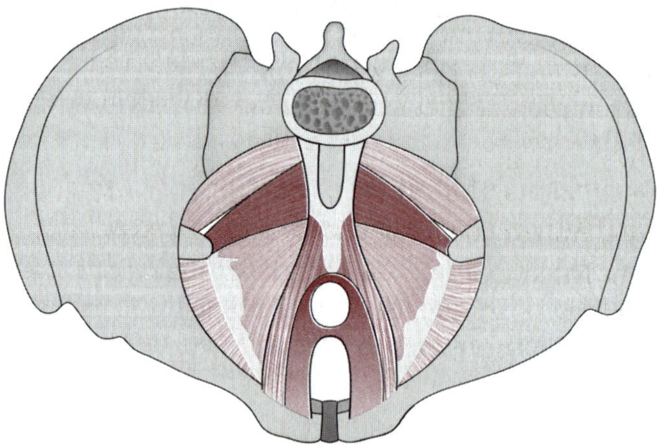

Fig. 5.40: Coccygeus muscle

MUSCLES OF THE SHOULDER AND THE UPPER LIMB

The shoulder and upper limb muscles are specialized to perform various functions of the hands. The upper limb is comprised of many muscles which act on the various joints of the hand, arm, and shoulder, maintain tone, provide stability and also facilitate smooth fluid movements.

Pectoralis Major (Fig. 5.41)

BAQ: Write a note on the pectoralis major.

Ans: The pectoralis major is a thick, fan-shaped, the largest and superior most muscle of the anterior chest wall. It lies underneath the breast tissue and forms the anterior wall of the axilla.

Function: Flexion, adduction, and medial rotation of the humerus.

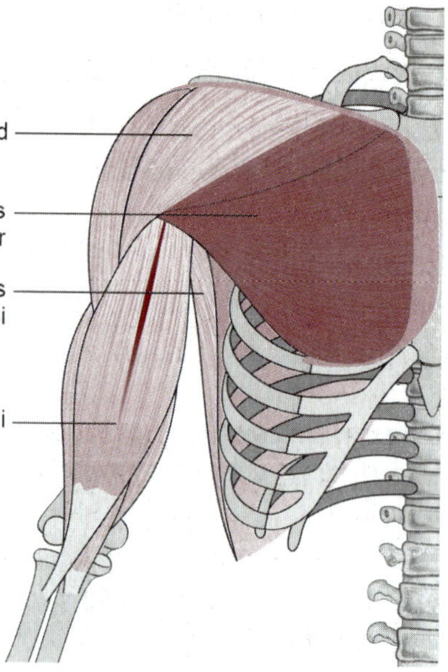

Fig. 5.41: Important upper limb muscles

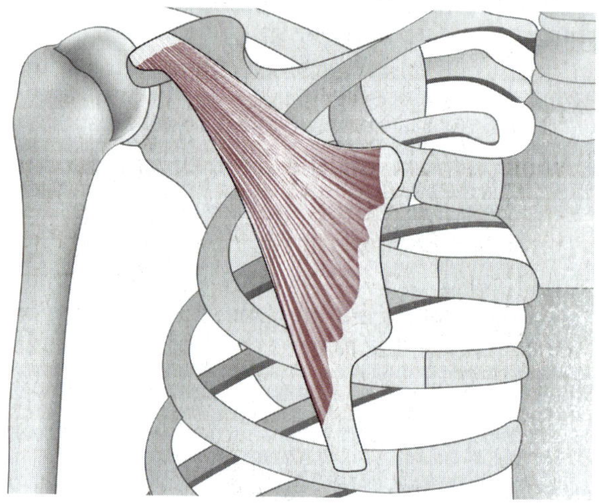

Fig. 5.42: Pectoralis minor muscle

BAQ: Write a note on the pectoralis major muscle with respect to: (1) Origin, (2) insertion, (3) nerve supply and (4) action.

Ans:

1. **Origin:** From the 3rd–5th ribs.
2. **Insertion:** Into the coracoid process of the scapula.
3. **Nerve supply:** The lateral pectoral nerve and the medial pectoral nerve.
4. **Action:** Flexes, adducts, and rotates humerus.

Pectoralis Minor Muscle (Fig. 5.42)

BAQ: Write a note on the pectoralis minor.

Ans: The pectoralis minor muscle is a thin triangular muscle. It is situated at the upper part of the chest, beneath the pectoralis major in the human body.

Function: Extension of the scapula and depression of the shoulder.

Deltoid Muscle (Fig. 5.43)

BAQ. Write a note on the deltoid muscle.

Ans: The deltoid muscle is a tringle-shaped muscle that covers the shoulder (Fig. 5.43).

Functions

1. **Anterior part:** Flexion and medial rotation of arm
2. **Middle part:** Abduction of arm
3. **Posterior part:** Extension and lateral rotation of arm.

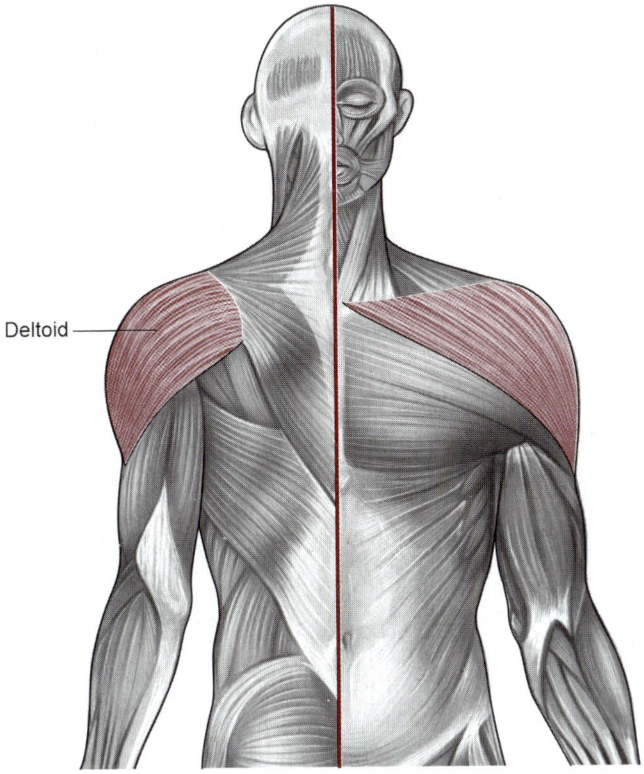

Fig. 5.43: Deltoid muscle

BAQ: Write a note on the deltoid muscle with respect to: (1) Origin, (2) insertion, (3) nerve supply and (4) action.

Ans:

1. **Origin:** Clavicle and spine of scapula.
2. **Insertion:** Deltoid tuberosity of humerus.
3. **Nerve supply:** The lateral pectoral nerve and the medial pectoral nerve.
4. **Action:** It abducts arm and flexes humerus.

Biceps Brachii (Fig. 5.44)

BAQ: Write a note on the biceps brachii.

Ans: The biceps brachii (BB, the biceps), is a thick and large muscle on the ventral portion of the upper arm. BB is composed of a short head and a long head.

Functions

1. Supination of forearm
2. Major flexion of forearm and
3. It resists dislocation of the shoulder.

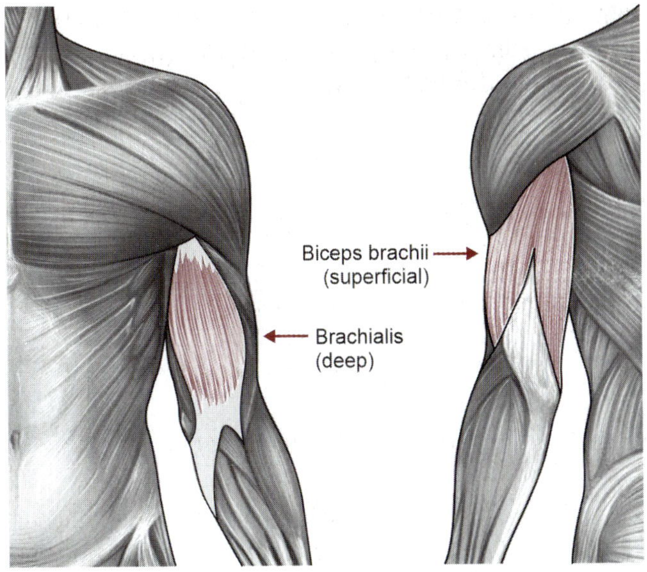

Fig. 5.44: Biceps brachii muscle and the brachialis muscle

Brachialis Muscle (Fig. 5.44)

BAQ: Write a note on the brachialis muscle.

Ans: The brachialis is one of the largest elbow flexor. It originates from the distal anterior humerus and inserts onto the ulnar tuberosity.

Function: Flexion of the forearm.

Triceps Brachii Muscle (Fig. 5.45)

BAQ. Write a note on the triceps brachii muscle.

Ans: The triceps brachii is a large and thick muscle. It is present on the dorsal part of the upper arm.

Functions

1. Major extensor of forearm and
2. Resists dislocation of the shoulder.

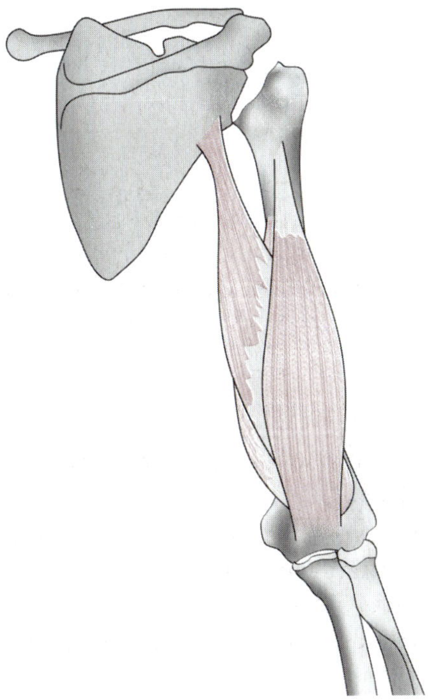

Fig. 5.45: Triceps brachii muscle

Flexor Carpi Radialis (Fig. 5.46)

SAQ: Write a note on the flexor carpi radialis muscle.

Ans: The flexor carpi radialis muscle is a superficial, long, and relatively thin muscle present on the anterior part of the forearm.

Function: Flexion and adduction at the wrist.

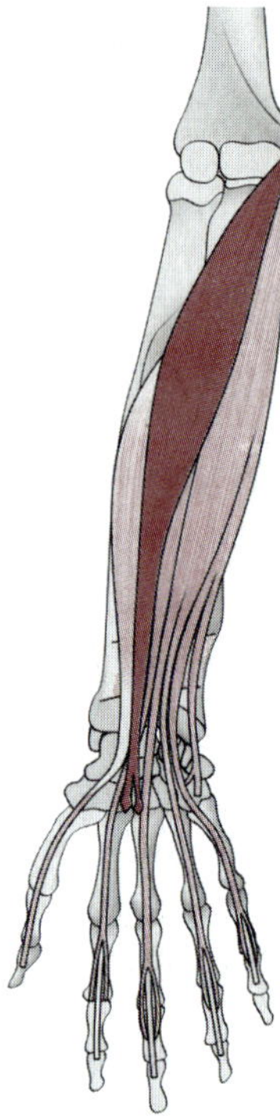

Fig. 5.46: Flexor carpi radialis

Palmaris Longus Muscle (Fig. 5.47)

SAQ: Write a note on the palmaris longus muscle.

Ans: The palmaris longus is a slender, elongated and spindle shaped muscle. It is present on the medial side of the flexor carpi radialis.

Function: Flexion at the wrist, and tensing of the palmaris aponeurosis.

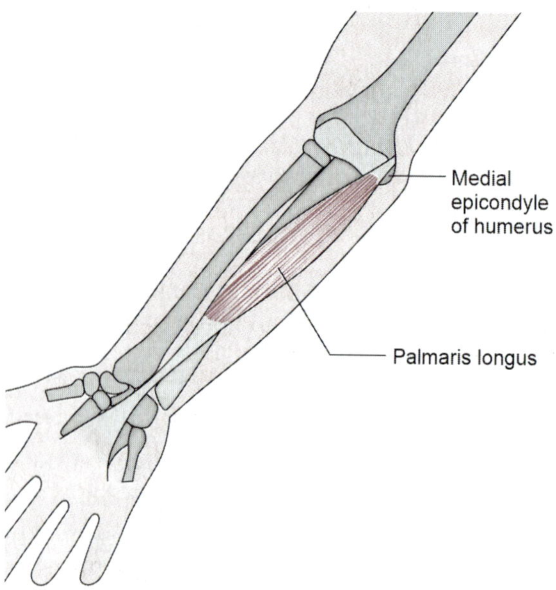

Fig. 5.47: Palmaris longus

Teres Minor Muscle (Fig. 5.48)

SAQ: Write a note on the teres minor muscle.

Ans: The teres minor is a narrow muscle. It is present below the infraspinatus, and above the teres major and the triceps brachii, and deeper to deltoid muscle. It is one of the four muscles of the rotator cuff.

Function: Lateral rotation of arm.

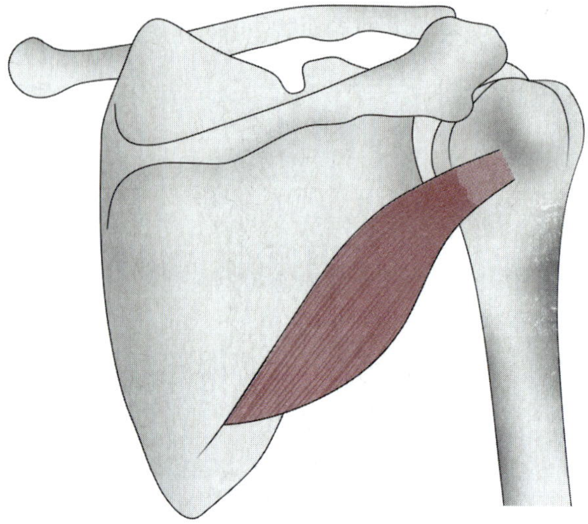

Fig. 5.48: Teres minor

Pronator Teres Muscle (Fig. 5.49)

SAQ. Write a note on the pronator teres muscle.

Ans: The pronator teres muscle is a long and round muscle. It is present on the anterior part of the forearm. The pronator muscle has two different points of origin: 1. The humeral head and 2. the ulnar head.

Function: Pronation of radio-ulnar joint.

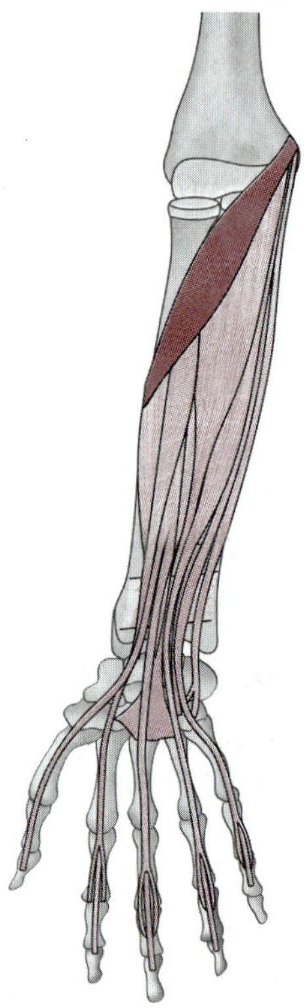

Fig. 5.49: Pronator teres muscle

Flexor Carpi Ulnaris (FCU) (Fig. 5.50)

SAQ: Write a note on the flexor carpi ulnaris (FCU).

Ans: The flexor carpi ulnaris (FCU) is a fusiform (elongated and tapering at both the end) muscle. It is located in the anterior compartment of the forearm.

Function: Flexion and adduction at the wrist.

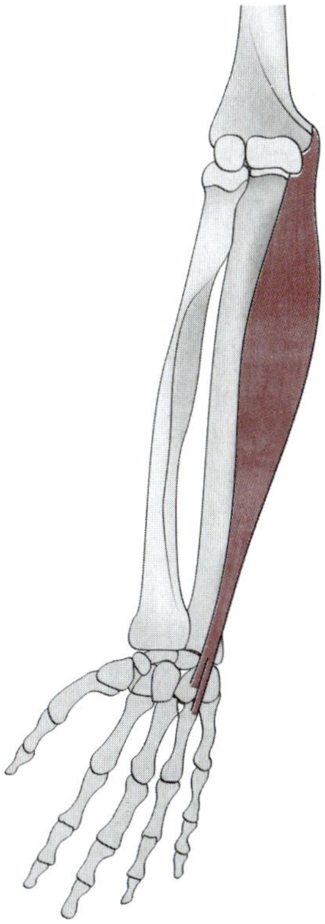

Fig. 5.50: Flexor carpi ulnaris

BAQ: Draw a neat and labelled diagram of the following muscles: The flexor carpi radialis, the triceps brachii and the flexor carpi ulnaris.

Ans: Refer to Figs 5.46, 5.45 and 5.50.

BAQ: Write a note on the flexor carpi ulnaris muscle with respect to: (1) Origin, (2) insertion, (3) nerve supply and (4) action.

Ans:

1. **Origin:** Medial epicondyle of humerus.
2. **Insertion:** Carpel and metacarpel bones.
3. **Nerve supply:** The ulnar nerve.
4. **Action:** Flexes and adducts wrist.

Brachioradialis Muscle (Fig. 5.51)

SAQ: Write a note on the brachioradialis muscle.

Ans: The brachioradialis is a superficial forearm muscle. It is located in the lateral forearm.

Functions

1 The brachioradialis primarily flexes the forearm at the elbow.
2. It supinates or pronates depending on the rotation of the forearm.

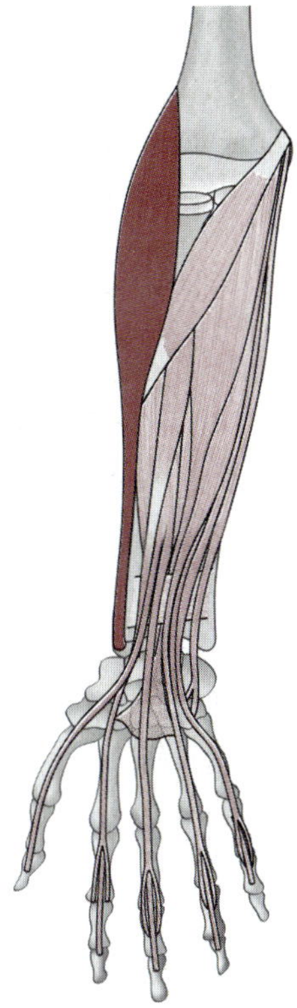

Fig. 5.51: Brachioradialis muscle

BAQ: Write a note on the brachioradialis muscle with respect to: (1) Origin, (2) insertion, (3) nerve supply and (4) action.

Ans:

1. **Origin:** Lateral supracondylar ridge of the humerus.
2. **Insertion:** Proximal to styloid process of the radius.
3. **Nerve supply:** Radial nerve.
4. **Action:** Flexes the forearm at the elbow.

Extensor Carpi Radialis Brevis (Fig. 5.52):

SAQ: Write a note on the extensor carpi radialis brevis muscle.

Ans: The extensor carpi radialis brevis muscle is a fusiform muscle. It is found in the lateral part of the posterior forearm.

Function: Extension and abduction of the wrist.

BAQ: Write a note on the extensor carpi radialis brevis muscle with respect to: (1) Origin, (2) insertion, (3) nerve supply and (4) action.

Ans:

1. **Origin:** The fascia of the extensor digitorum communis.
2. **Insertion:** On the anterior aspect of the base of the second metacarpal.
3. **Nerve supply:** The deep branch of the radial nerve (C7, C8).
4. **Action:** Extension and abduction of the wrist.

Extensor Digitorum Muscle (Fig. 5.53)

SAQ: Write a note on the extensor digitorum muscle (extensor digitorum communis).

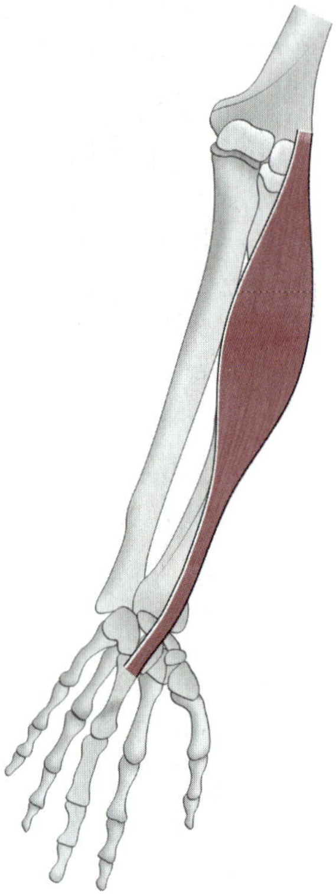

Fig. 5.52: Extensor carpi radialis brevis muscle

Ans: The extensor digitorum muscle (extensor digitorum communis) is a muscle of the posterior forearm.

Functions

1. Extension of the proximal interphalangeal joint of the second, third, fourth, and fifth finger.
2. A weaker extension action also on the metacarpophalangeal joints of the same fingers.

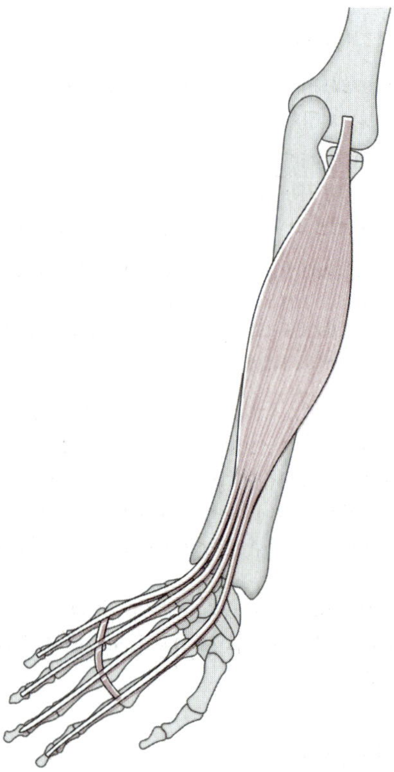

Fig. 5.53: Extensor digitorum muscle

BAQ: Write a note on the extensor digitorum muscle with respect to: (1) Origin, (2) insertion, (3) nerve supply and (4) action.

Ans:

1. **Origin:** The lateral epicondyle of the humerus.
2. **Insertion:** On the anterior part of the base of the second metacarpal.
3. **Nerve supply:** The deep branch of the radial nerve (C7, C8).
4. **Action:** Extension of the proximal interphalangeal joint of the second, third, fourth, and fifth finger.

Supinator Muscle (Fig. 5.54)

SAQ: Write a note on the supinator muscle.

Ans: The supinator is a spiral muscle. It is present in the posterior compartment of the forearm, along with brachioradialis, and the superficial and deep forearm extensors. The supinator muscle curls around the proximal part of radius and connects it with the ulna. This muscle crosses the sagittal axis of the forearm.

Function: Supination of the forearm.

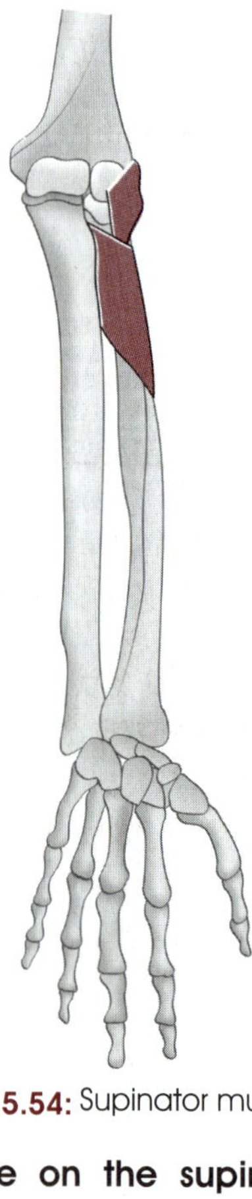

Fig. 5.54: Supinator muscle

BAQ: Write a note on the supinator muscle with respect to: (1) Origin, (2) insertion, (3) nerve supply and (4) action.

Ans:

1. **Origin:** Crest of ulna.
2. **Insertion:** Lateral surface of the radius.
3. **Nerve supply:** A branch of the radial nerve.
4. **Action:** Supinates hand.

Muscles of the Hip and Lower Limb

The hip is a ball and socket joint. It unites the femur (thigh bone) with the pelvis. The hip muscles can be divided into the following three main groups: Iliopsoas group, gluteal muscles and hip adductors. The hip joint permits movements of bones in three degrees of freedom: Abduction, adduction, flexion, extension, external rotation, internal rotation and circumduction. Flexion of the hip joint draws the thigh towards the trunk. The hip helps the lower extremity to move in three planes of motion. The hip muscles also provide shock absorption support function to the torso and upper body.

Psoas Muscle (Fig. 5.36)

SAQ: Write a note on the psoas muscle.

Ans: The psoas muscle is a long fusiform muscle present on either side of the vertebral column and the brim of the lesser pelvis. It combines with the iliacus muscle to form the iliopsoas muscle, at its distal end.

Function: The psoas muscle in combination with the iliopsoas muscle, becomes a major contributor of flexion of the hip joint.

Iliacus Muscle (Fig. 5.55)

SAQ: Write a note on the Iliacus muscle.

Ans: The iliacus muscle is a triangle-shaped muscle. It is present in the pelvic bone that flexes and rotates the thigh bone.

Function: The iliacus muscle stabilizes the pelvis and works in combination with other muscles in the hip and thigh to facilitate actions such as bending, running, walking, sitting, and to maintain correct posture.

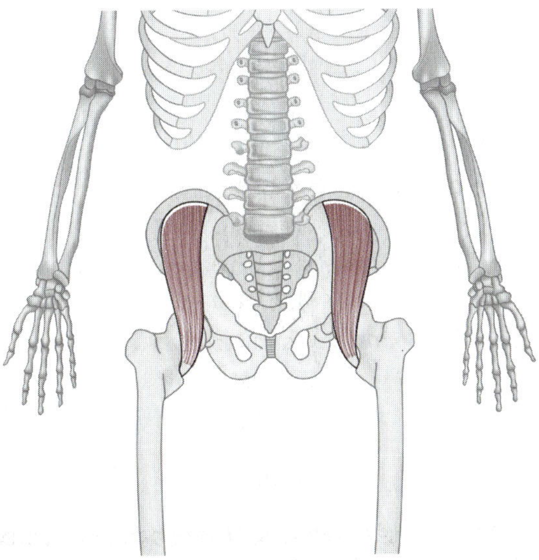

Fig. 5.55: Iliacus muscle

Quadriceps Femoris Muscles (Fig. 5.56)

SAQ: Write a note on the quadriceps femoris muscles.

Ans: The quadriceps femoris are a group of muscles at the front of the thigh.

Function: It facilitates a variety of movements such as walking, running, jumping and kicking.

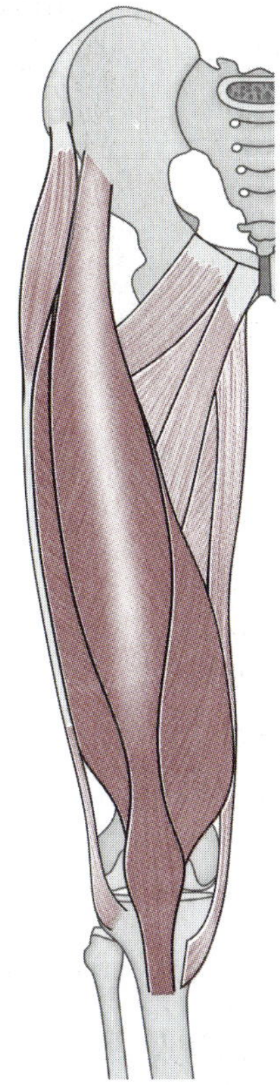

Fig. 5.56: Quadriceps femoris muscle

BAQ: Write a note on the quadriceps femoris muscle with respect to: (1) Origin, (2) insertion, (3) nerve supply and (4) action.

Ans:

1. **Origin:** Ilium, upper part of pelvis and femur.
2. **Insertion:** Tibial tuberosity.
3. **Nerve supply:** The femoral nerve.
4. **Action:** It facilitates movements such as walking, running, jumping and kicking.

Obturator Muscles (Fig. 5.57)

SAQ: Write a note on the obturator muscles.

Ans: The obturator externus and internus are bilateral-triangular shaped muscles. These originate in the pelvis and insert onto the greater trochanter of the femur.

Functions

1. The obturator muscles work together with the surrounding muscles to provide mobility to the hip.
2. The obturator externus also contributes to adduction of the flexed hip, while the obturator internus plays important role in the abduction of the flexed hip.

BAQ: Write a note on the Obturator muscle with respect to: (1) Origin, (2) insertion, (3) nerve supply and (4) action.

Ans:

1. **Origin:** The pelvis.
2. **Insertion:** The greater trochanter of the femur.

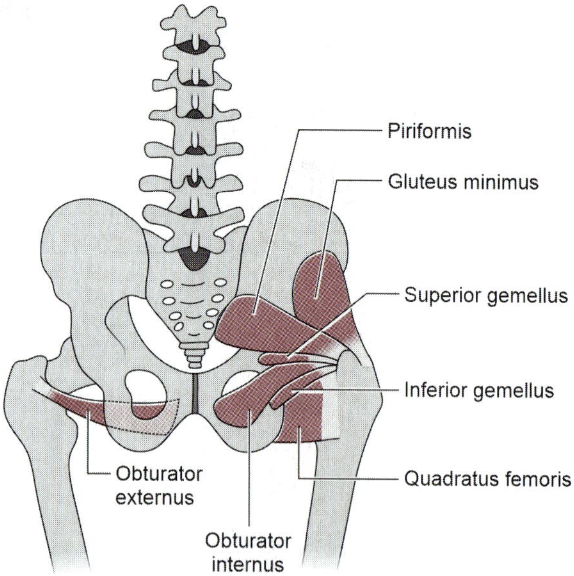

Fig. 5.57: Obturator muscles

3. **Nerve supply:** The obturator nerve from lumbar plexus.
4. **Action:** provide mobility to the hip.

Gluteal Muscles (Fig. 5.58)

SAQ: Write a note on the gluteal muscles.

Ans: The gluteal muscle muscles consists of the gluteus maximus (the most superficial and the largest in the group), gluteus medius, and gluteus minimus. These are a group of muscles that make up the area of the buttock.

Functions

1. The gluteal muscles mainly act on the hip joint to facilitate abduction and extension of the thigh.
2. These muscles also assist in the external rotation, adduction, and internal rotation of the thigh.

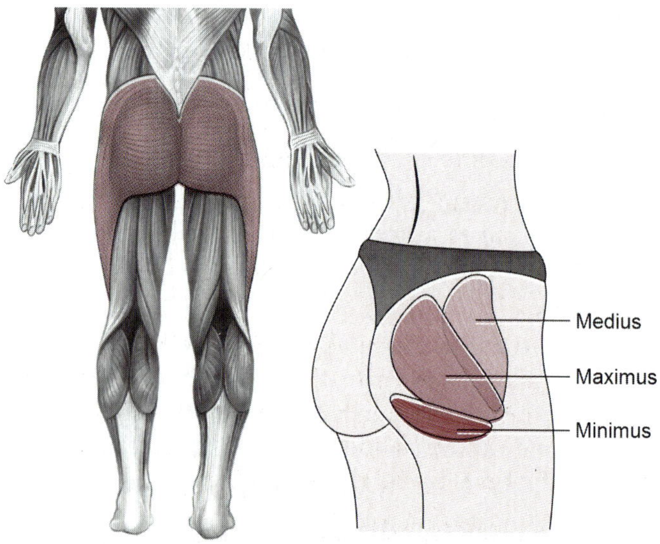

Figs 5.58A and B: Gluteal muscles

BAQ: Draw a neat and labelled diagrams of the following muscles: The Iliacus, quadriceps femoris and the gluteal.

Ans: Refer to Figs 5.45, 5.46 and 5.50.

Sartorius Muscle (Fig. 5.59)

SAQ: Write a note on the sartorius muscle.

Ans: The sartorius muscle is a thin superficial and long muscle. It is present in the anterior compartment of the thigh. It runs down the length of the thigh. It is the longest muscle in the human body.

Functions

1. At the hip it helps to flex, rotate and weakly abduct the thigh laterally.
2. At the knee, it helps to flex the leg; rotates the leg medially.
3. It plays an important part in the stabilisation of the pelvis.

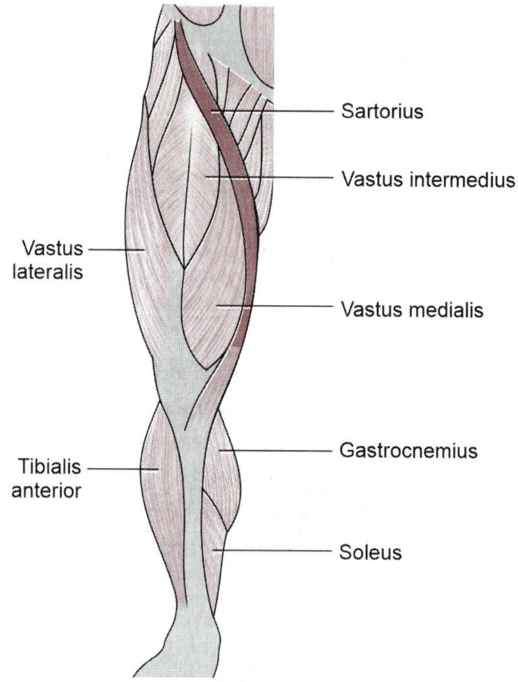

Fig. 5.59: Sartorius muscle

Hamstrings (Fig. 5.60)

SAQ: Write a note on the hamstrings.

Ans: The hamstrings are a group of three muscles in the rear of the thigh. These run from the pelvis to the lower leg bones, attaching on the sides of the bone.

Functions: The hamstring muscles help to perform the following various functions: Rotating the hip joint, bending the knee joint, and extending the hip joint.

Gastrocnemius Muscle (Fig. 5.61)

SAQ: Write a note on the gastrocnemius muscle.

Ans: The gastrocnemius muscle is the main complex muscle of the calf of the leg. It passes to the Achilles tendon from two heads, which are attached to the femur.

Functions

1. The gastrocnemius muscle flexes the knee and foot.
2. It plays important role in maintaining posture and walking.

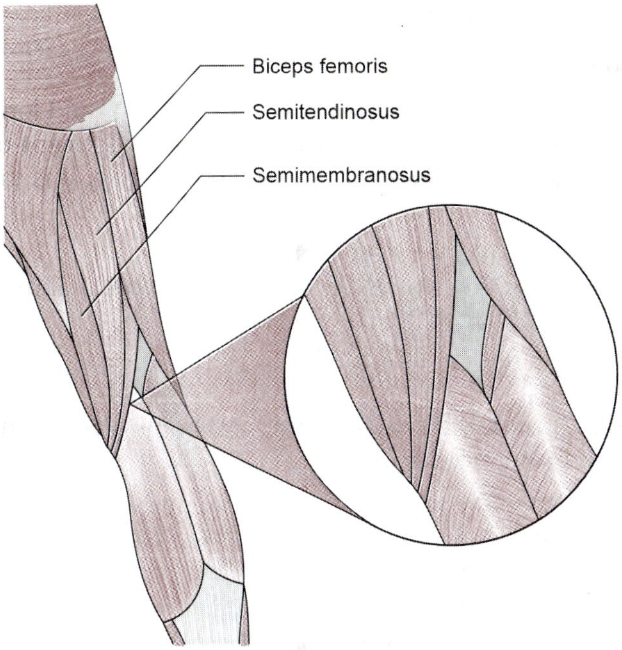

Fig. 5.60: Hamstrings

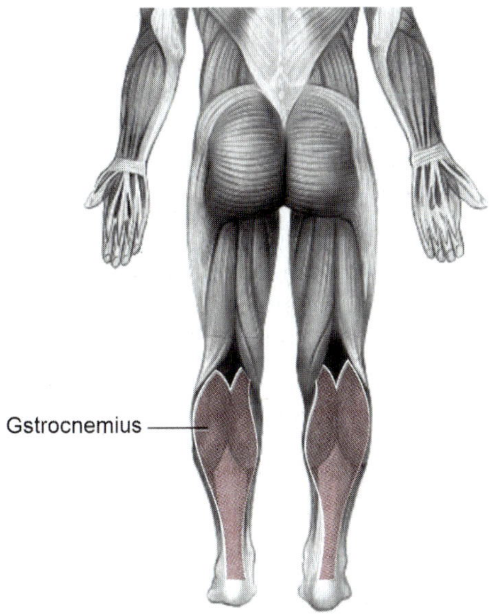

Fig. 5.61: Gastrocnemius muscle

Anterior Tibialis Muscle (Fig.5.62)

SAQ: Write a note on the tibialis anterior muscle (the tibialis anticus).

Ans: The tibialis anterior muscle (the tibialis anticus), is a thick and the largest muscle in the anterior compartment of the leg.

Functions: The anterior tibilis muscle plays an important role in the activities such as walking, kicking any object and hiking action by stabilizing the ankle joint.

Soleus Muscle (Fig. 5.63)

SAQ: Write a note on the soleus muscle.

Ans: The soleus muscle is a powerful lower limb muscle. It is situated deep to the gastrocnemius muscle. It forms the calf muscle in conjunction with gastrocnemius and plantaris muscles.

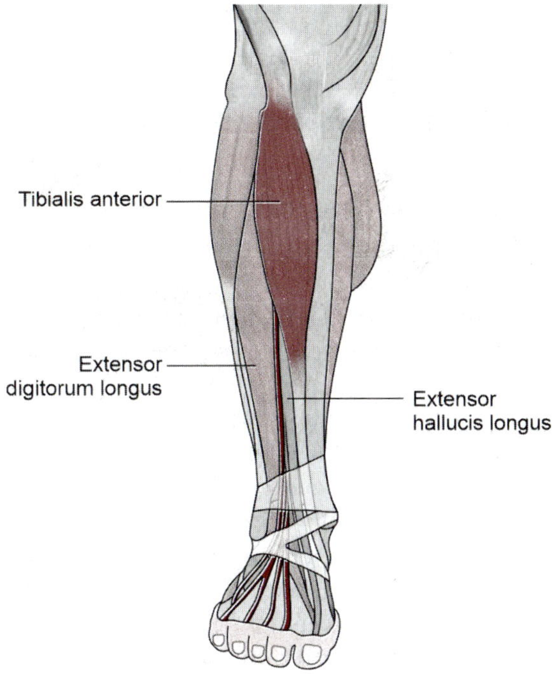

Fig. 5.62: Anterior tibialis

Functions

1. The soleus muscle, along with other calf muscles contributes in various actions such as walking, running, and dancing.
2. It also plays important role in maintaining proper posture.

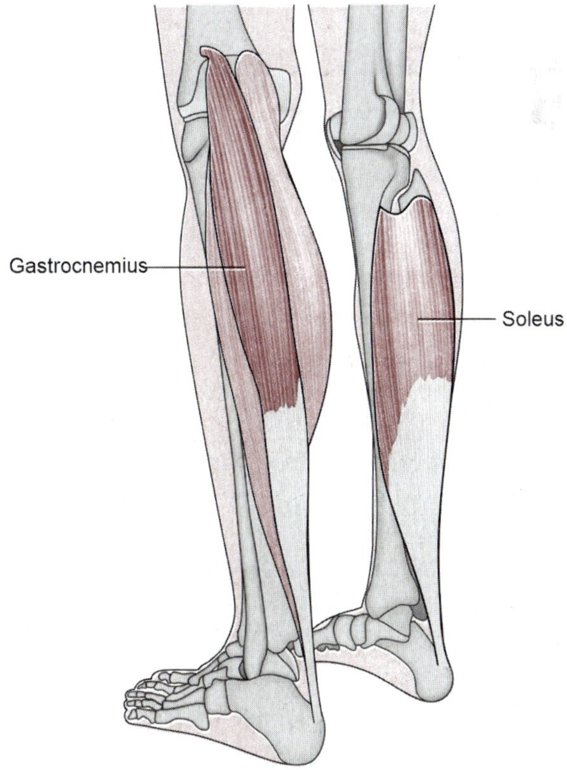

Fig. 5.63: Soleus muscle

Objective: To describe the muscle physiology.

Muscle Contraction (Figs 5.64–5.65)

LAQ: Describe the events involved in muscle contraction. Or

Describe physiology of neuromuscular junction.

Ans: The following steps are involved in the muscle contraction (Fig. 5.64):

1. The sequence of events leading to contraction is initiated somewhere in the central nervous system, either as voluntary activity from the brain or as reflex activity from the spinal cord.
2. A motor neuron in the ventral horn of the spinal cord is activated, and an action potential passes outward in a ventral root of the spinal cord.
3. The axon branches to supply a number of muscle fibers called a motor unit, and the action potential is conveyed to a motor end plate on each muscle fiber.
4. At the motor end plate, the action potential causes the release of enzyme acetylcholine into the synaptic clefts on the surface of the muscle fiber (Fig. 5.23).

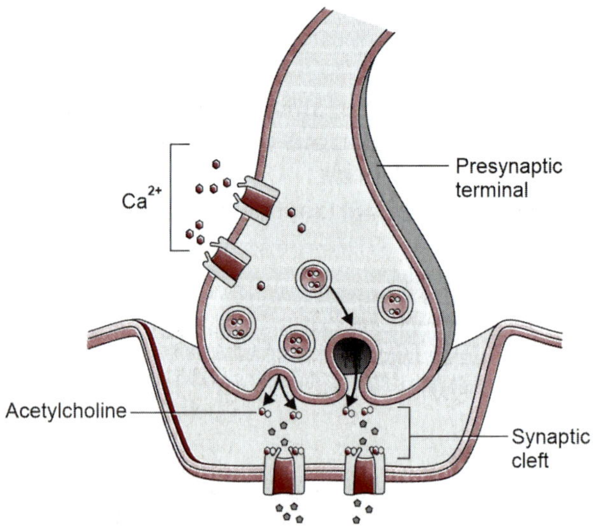

Fig. 5.64: Function of acetyl choline at neuromuscular junction

5. Acetylcholine action changes the electrical resting potential under the motor end plate and initiates an action potential which passes in both directions along the surface of the muscle fiber.
6. The action potential spreads inside the muscle fiber.
7. The action potential causes the sarcoplasmic reticulum to release Ca^{2+} ions.
8. The released calcium ions result in movement of troponin and tropomyosin on their thin filaments. This is the driving force for the muscle contraction (Fig. 5.65).

Contraction is turned off by the following sequence of events:

1. Acetylcholine at the neuromuscular junction is broken down by acetylcholinesterase, and this terminates the stream of action potentials along the muscle fiber surface.
2. The sarcoplasmic reticulum ceases to release calcium ions, and immediately starts to isolate all the calcium ions that have been released.
3. In the absence of calcium ions, a change in the configuration of troponin and tropomyosin then blocks the action of the myosin molecule heads, and contraction ceases.
4. An external stretching force, such as gravity or an antagonistic muscle, pulls the muscle back to its original length.

Smooth Muscle Contraction (Figs 5.66 and 5.67)

LAQ: Describe the events involved in the smooth muscle contraction.

Ans: Smooth muscles contain actin and tropomyosin molecules. The contraction of the smooth muscles takes place by the following events:

1. In the smooth muscle cells, a neurological impulse from the autonomic nervous system causes Ca^{2+} gates in the cell membrane to open and allow rush of calcium ions into the cells from the extracellular medium. Calcium then combines with a protein called calmodulin to form calcium–calmodulin complex.
2. The myosin light chain kinase (MLCK) gets activated, when it combines with calcium–calmodulin complex. MLCK is capable of activating myosin light chain (ML) by adding phosphate molecules to the light chain (phosphorylation).
3. The phosphorylation of light chain initiates binding of myosin head to actin molecule and contraction of smooth muscle takes place.

> *Note:* Calmodulin is a protein molecule that senses calcium levels and relays signals to various calcium-sensitive enzymes, ion channels and other proteins.

Relaxation of Smooth Muscle (Fig. 5.67)

Relaxation of smooth muscle occurs by the following events:

1. When sarcoplasmic calcium (Ca^{2+}) falls below 10^{-7} mol/L, calcium dissociates from calmodulin.
2. Calmodulin in turn dissociates from the myosin light chain kinase, which then becomes inactive.
3. Relaxation of smooth muscle occurs when myosin head detaches from the actin filament.

Contraction of the Cardiac Muscle

LAQ: Describe the events involved in the contraction of cardiac muscle.

Ans: The action potentials initiate the contraction of the heart. The contraction of the cardiac muscle is triggered in a different way than contraction of the skeletal muscle. The heart cells do not have motor nerve terminals attached to them. Heart cells communicate with each other directly by passing electrical impulse to their neighbouring cells through special channels

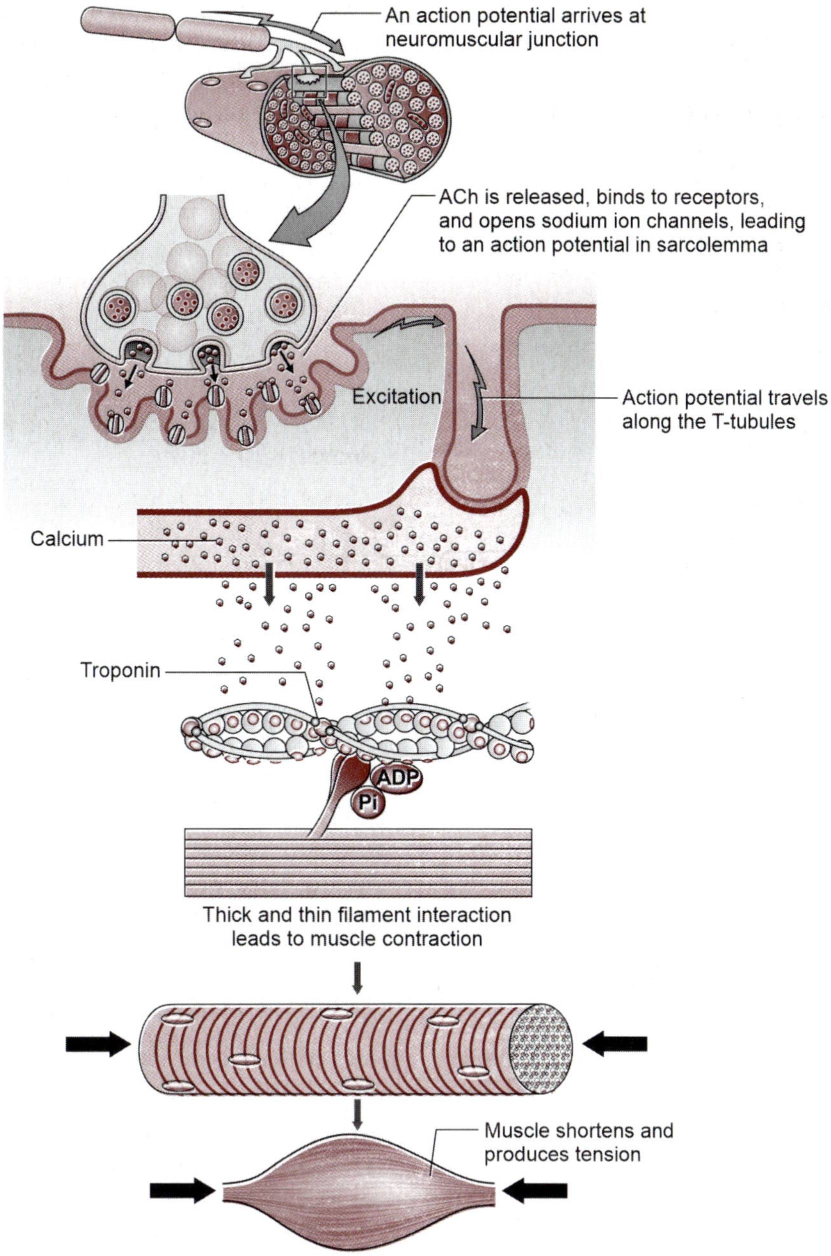

Fig. 5.65: Muscle contraction

called gap-junctions (Fig. 5.68). This enables the heart to be stimulated at only one location, with the electrical impulse passing on to the rest of the heart muscle, causing it to contract.

Inside each cardiomyocyte there are compartments filled with calcium. The action potential causes these compartments to release the calcium ions into the cell. These calcium ions allow myosin heads to bind to actin filaments and pull them by "power stroke". That is the way action potential causes the individual muscle cells to contract.

Importance of ATPs and Creatin in Muscle Physiology

Although three types of muscles (skeletal, cardiac and smooth) have significant differences, all three types of muscles use the movement of actin against myosin to create contraction.

Muscular activity accounts for much of the energy consumption of the body. All muscle cells produce adenosine triphosphate (ATP) molecules which are used to power the movement of the myosin heads. Muscles conserve energy in the form of organic compounds known as creatine phosphate. It is generated from ATPs and can regenerate ATP when needed using creatine kinase enzyme. The muscles also keep a storage form of glucose in the form of glycogen. Glycogen can be rapidly converted to glucose when energy is required for sustained and powerful contractions.

Within the voluntary skeletal muscles, the glucose molecule can be metabolized anaerobically in glycolysis which produces two ATP and two lactic acid molecules. Muscle cells also contain fat globules, which are used for energy during aerobic exercise. The aerobic energy systems take longer to produce ATP molecules, but

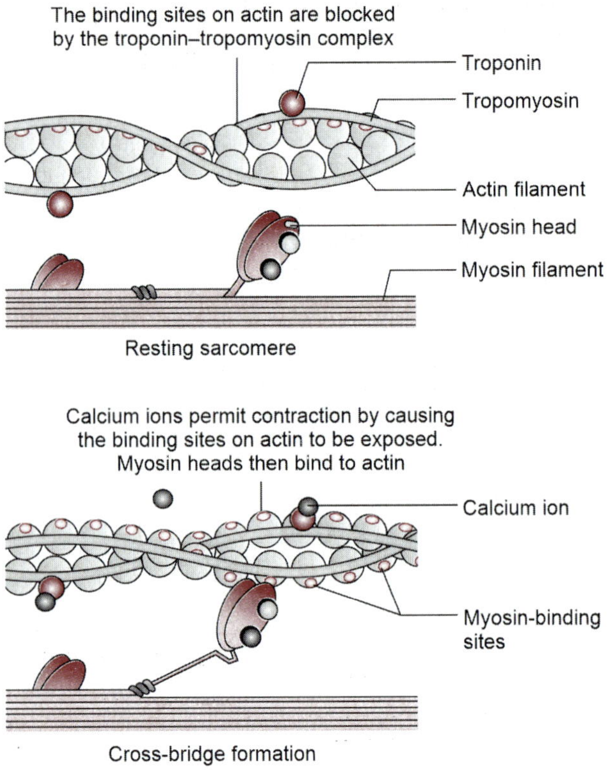

Fig. 5.66: Resting sarcomere and cross-bridge formation by calciumions

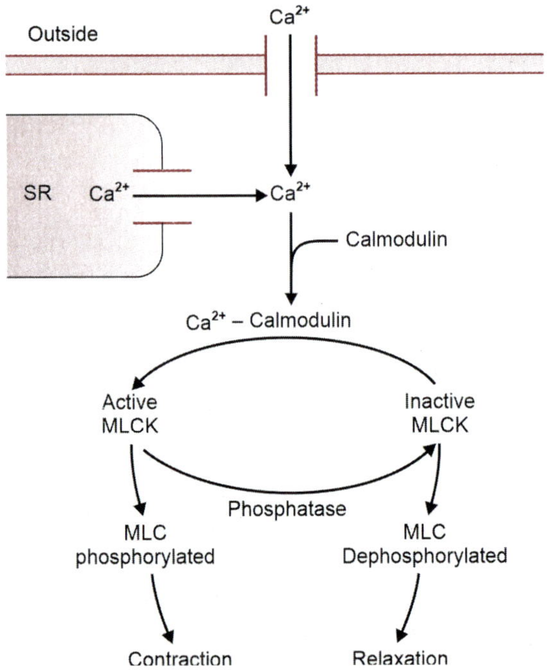

Fig. 5.67: Contraction and relaxation of smooth muscle

produces significantly more ATPs than anaerobic glycolysis. Cardiac muscle on the other hand, can readily consume any of the three macronutrients such as glucose, fat or protein aerobically and usually extracts maximum ATP molecules. The heart, liver and red blood cells also use glucose for energy formed from lactic acid molecules.

Objective: To describe the clinical conditions related to muscle diseases.

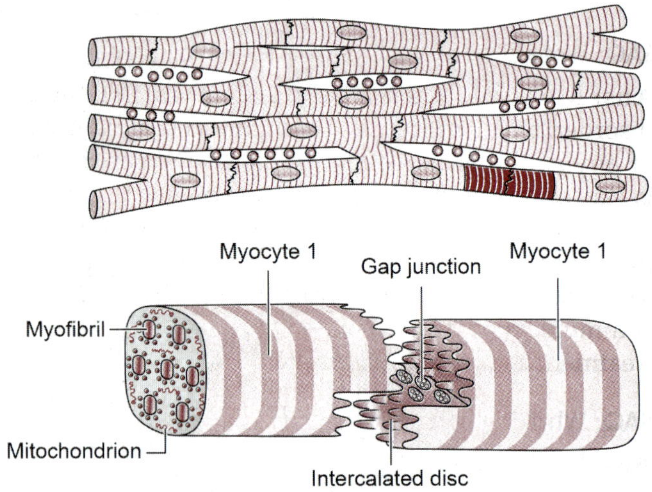

Fig. 5.68: Cardiac muscle microfibril, intercalated discs and gap junctions

IMPORTANT MUSCLE DISEASES

Introduction

Symptoms of muscle diseases may include weakness, spasticity, myoclonus and myalgia. There are many diseases and conditions which cause a decrease in muscle mass, known as muscle atrophy. Examples include cancer and AIDS, which induce a body wasting syndrome called cachexia. Other syndromes or conditions which can induce skeletal muscle atrophy are congestive heart disease and some diseases of the liver.

Multiple Sclerosis (MS)

SAQ: Write a brief note on multiple sclerosis (MS).

Ans: Multiple sclerosis is an autoimmune inflammatory disease in which the fatty myelin sheaths around the axons of the brain and spinal cord are damaged, due to the specific antibodies. This clinical condition leads to the demyelination and scarring.

Specific symptoms of MS include muscle weakness, loss of sensation, loss of coordination, vision loss, etc. The disease onset usually occurs in young adults, and it is more common in women. Presently, treatment of MS is only supportive.

Muscular Dystrophy (MD)

SAQ: Write a brief note on muscular dystrophy (MD).

Ans: Muscular dystrophies (MD) is a genetic and clinically heterogeneous group of rare neuromuscular disease that leads to progressive weakness and breakdown of skeletal muscles. MD is characterized by progressive skeletal muscle weakness, defects in muscle proteins, and the death of muscle cells and tissue. The most types of MD are multi-system disorders which affect the body systems such as the heart, the gastrointestinal and nervous systems, endocrine glands, skin, eyes and the brain. The condition may also lead to mood swings and learning difficulties. Presently, treatment of MD is only supportive.

Myasthenia Gravis

SAQ: Write a brief note on myasthenia gravis.

Ans: Myasthenia gravis (MG) is a neuromuscular disorder, characterized by weakness and rapid fatigue of any of the muscles under voluntary control. MG is caused by an abnormal immune reaction, in which specific antibodies inappropriately attack neuromuscular junctions in muscles that receive nerve impulses. MG leads to the significant decrease in the normal communication between nerves and muscles. Presently, treatment of myasthenia gravis is only supportive.

SAQ: What is sarcopenia?

Ans: During aging, there is a gradual decrease in the ability to maintain skeletal muscle function and mass, known as sarcopenia. Sarcopenia is a normal aspect of aging, and is not a disease state. Sarcopenia can be linked to injuries that occur in the case of the elderly.

Objective: To understand and explain the central theme of competency based medical and paramedical education (CBME): Horizontal and vertical integration of subjects.

BAQ: Show horizontal integration of premedical subjects, physiology, and biochemistry with the following anatomical change: Weak muscles that get rapidly fatigued (myasthenia gravis, MG).

Ans:

Horizontal Integration with Physiology

Affected normal transmission of nerve impulses, leading to the significant decrease in the normal communication between nerves and muscles.

Horizontal Integration with Biochemistry

Circulation of antibodies that attack neuromuscular junctions, leading to abnormal immunological responses.

BAQ: Show vertical integration of paramedical subject: Pharmacology with the following anatomical change: Weak muscles that get rapidly fatigued.

Ans:

Horizontal Integration with Pharmacology

Selection of appropriate drugs for the management of MG.

BIBLIOGRAPHY

1. Medical Biochemistry, 1st Edition (2023). Godkar PB, Godkar DP, CBS Publishers, New Delhi, India.
2. Text book of Medical Laboratory Technology, 4th Edition, (2024). Godkar PB, Godkar DP, Bhalani Publishing House, Mumbai, India.
3. Anatomy of the Human Body. 42nd Edition. Henry Gray, Editor-in-chief: Susan Standring, Elsevier (2020)
4. Ross and Wilson Anatomy and Physiology in Health and Illness, 13th Edition, by Allison Wynn Grant, Anne Waugh, and Kathleen J. W. Wilson (2018).
5. Schaum's outline of theory and problems of Human anatomy and Physiology, 2nd Edition (1997), Tata MaGraw-Hill Publishing Company Limited, New Delhi, India.

MULTIPLE CHOICE QUESTIONS (MCQs)

Select the correct option.

1. Which type of muscle forms the largest portion of a body?

(A) Visceral muscle (B) Cardiac muscle
(C) Skeletal muscle (D) None of these

2. The visceral muscle is found inside of:

(A) Blood vessels (B) Stomach
(C) Intestines (D) All of these

3. This is a flexor muscle of the shoulder joint:

(A) Teres major (B) Trapezius
(C) Supraspinatus (D) Pectoralis major

4. This muscle is not attached to the humerus:

(A) Teres major (B) Biceps brachii
(C) Pectoralis major (D) Brachialis

5. This is not synergist in flexing the elbow joint:

(A) Brachialis (B) Biceps brachii
(C) Brachioradialis (D) Coracobrachialis

6. The length of this part of the muscle gets reduced during the muscle contraction:

(A) Sarcomere (B) I-Band
(C) A-Band (D) H-Zone

7. This is true about muscle fibres:

(A) These are better adapted for slow sustained activities
(B) For energy, they are depended on anaerobic glycolysis
(C) For energy, they are only depended on aerobic glycolysis
(D) They do not possess mitochondria

8. This muscle planter flexes and invers the foot when it supports the arches:

(A) Tibialis posterior
(B) Flexor hallucis longus
(C) Gastrocnemius
(D) Flexor digitorum longus

9. The accumulation of this leads to muscle fatigue:

(A) Lactic acid (B) Glucose
(C) Creatine phosphate (D) Carbon dioxide

10. Duration of one muscle twitch is:

(A) 1 second (B) 0.5 seconds
(C) 10 seconds (D) 0.1 seconds

11. This is a common connective tissue layer that holds together the skeletal muscle bundles:

(A) Aponeurosis (B) Endomysium
(C) Fascia (D) Perimysium

12. This muscle causes rotation of the hand with the palm faces posteriorly:

(A) Abductors (B) Supinators
(C) Adductors (D) Flexors

13. These muscles are synergistic to the diaphragm during inspiration:

(A) The abdominal muscles
(B) The internal intercostal muscles
(C) The external intercostal muscles
(D) Both (A) and (C)

14. This is a muscle that helps in the mastication process:

(A) The temporalis (B) The mentalis
(C) The buccinator (D) The zygomaticus

15. This muscle extends and helps to rotate the thigh:

(A) The gluteus maximum (B) The gluteus minimum
(C) The gluteus medius (D) The psoas major

16. During muscle contraction calcium ions bind with:

(A) TpT (B) Tropomyosin
(C) TpC (D) TpI

17. The stimulation of muscle fibers by a motor neuron takes place at:

(A) The neuromuscular junction
(B) The myofibril
(C) The transverse tubules
(D) The sarcoplasmic reticulum

18. These face muscles enable frowning:

(A) The corrugator supercilii
(B) The depressor anguli oris
(C) The depressor labii inferioris
(D) Both (A) and (B)

19. This face muscle enables movements in the lip:

(A) The corrugator supercilii
(B) The depressor anguli oris
(C) The depressor labii inferioris
(D) The depressor labii inferioris

20. This face muscle helps to control lower lip:

(A) The corrugator supercilii
(B) The mentalis
(C) The depressor labii inferioris
(D) The depressor labii inferioris

21. This muscle is a large superficial back muscle:

(A) The depressor labii inferioris
(B) The depressor labii inferioris
(C) The trapezius
(D) The corrugator supercilii

22. This is a broad and flat muscle that occupies most of the lower posterior thorax:

(A) The depressor labii inferioris
(B) The depressor labii inferioris
(C) The trapezius
(D) The latissimus dorsi muscle

23. One of the following statements is not correct, regarding the visceral muscles:

(A) Visceral muscle is found inside of blood vessels, stomach and intestines.
(B) Visceral has a very smooth and uniform appearance.
(C) Visceral muscles are involuntary muscles.
(D) Visceral muscles are voluntary muscles.

24. All of the statements regarding the cardiac muscle and cells are correct, *except:*

(A) The cells of cardiac muscle tissue are striated.
(B) The cells of cardiac muscle appear to have light and dark stripes when observed under a light microscope.
(C) The cardiac muscle is very weak.
(D) The cardiac muscle is very strong.

25. All of the statements regarding the skeletal muscle and cells are incorrect, *except:*

(A) Skeletal muscle is voluntary muscle tissue in the body.
(B) Skeletal muscles are not attached to the bones.
(C) Skeletal muscles are not responsible for the movement of body parts.
(D) The physical actions of a person like speaking and walking, or writing do not require skeletal muscle.

ANSWERS

1. C 2. D 3. D 4. B 5. D 6. C 7. B
8. A 9. A 10. D 11. C 12. B 13. D 14. A
15. B 16. C 17. A 18. D 19. C 20. B 21. C
22. D 23. D 24. C 25. A

MATCH THE COLUMNS

I	II
1. Gracilis	A. Flexes the elbow joint
2. Trapezius	B. Adducts the hip joint
3. Psoas major	C. Flexes the joints of the vertebral column
4. Deltoid	D. Extends the joints of the vertebral column
5. Rectus abdominis	E. Extends the joints of the lumber region of the vertebral column
6. Quadratus lumborum	F. Abducts and medially rotates the hip joint
7. Gluteus medius	G. Abducts the scapula
8. Vastus lateralis	H. Flexes the hip joint and joins the vertebral column
9. Latissimus dorsi	I. Adducts the scapula
10. Brachialis	J. Extends the knee joint
	K. Adducts and extends the shoulder joint

ANSWERS

1. B 2. I 3. H 4. G 5. C 6. E 7. F
8. J 9. K 10. A

CHAPTER 6

Nervous System

SAQ: Short answer question: Marks: 2
BAQ: Brief answer question: Marks: 4 or 5
LAQ: Long answer question: Marks: 9 or 10
MCQs: Multiple choice questions: Marks: 0.5 each
Match the columns: Marks: 0.5 each
Draw a labelled diagram: Marks: 5

Objectives: To distinguish and describe central nervous system, peripheral nervous system and autonomous nervous syste.

INTRODUCTION

BAQ: Write a brief note on the nervous system.

Ans: The nervous system (Fig. 6.1) consists of the brain, spinal cord, meninges, sensory organs, and all the nerves that connect the various organs with the rest of the body (Fig. 6.3). It is mostly made up of neural tissue. The nervous system consists of two main parts:

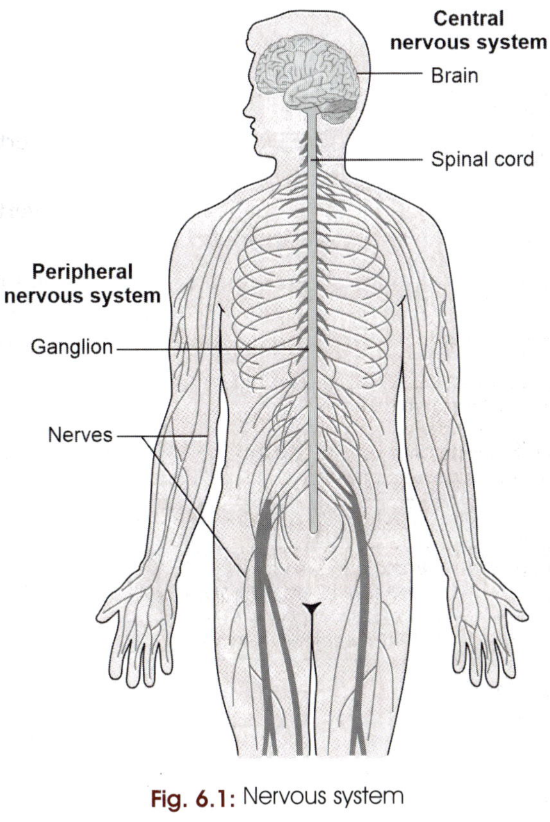

Fig. 6.1: Nervous system

1. The central nervous system (CNS) (Fig. 6.2A) and
2. The peripheral nervous system (PNS) (Fig. 6.2B). The CNS contains the brain and spinal cord. The PNS consists of nerves, which are long fibers that connect the CNS to every part of the body. The PNS also includes peripheral ganglia, sympathetic and parasympathetic ganglia, and the enteric nervous system, which controls the gastrointestinal system.

The brain makes up the largest portion of the central nervous system (CNS). The spinal cord is a bony structure that begins at the bottom of the brain stem and ends in the lower back (Fig. 6.3). The meninges are membranous connective tissues that cover the brain and spinal cord. A fold (ridge) in the cortex is termed a gyrus (plural gyri) and a groove is termed a sulcus (plural sulci).

The nervous system is the main regulatory, controlling and communicating system in the body. It plays very important role in all the mental activities such as thinking,

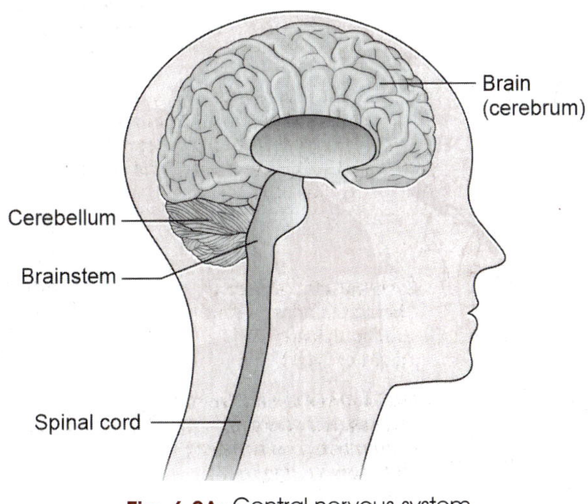

Fig. 6.2A: Central nervous system

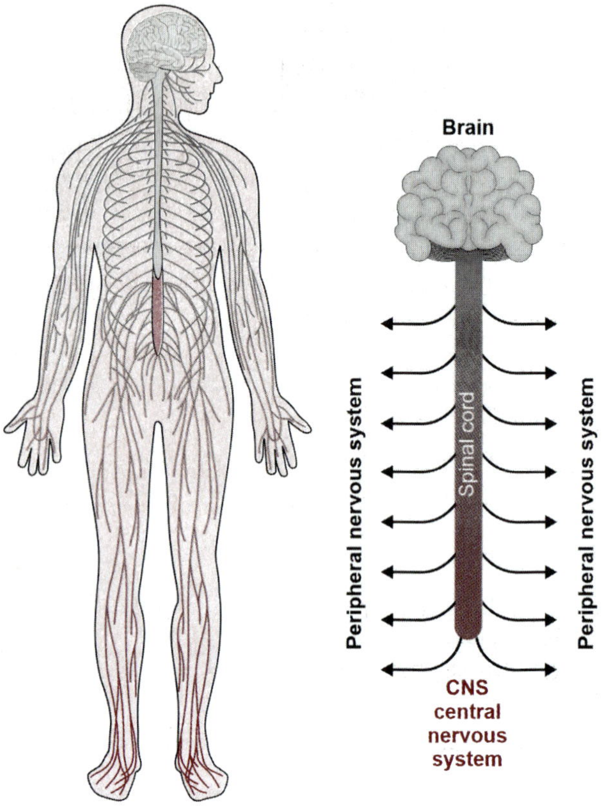

Fig. 6.2B: Peripheral nervous system

learning, and memory processes. In coordination with the endocrine system, the nervous system is responsible for the regulation and maintenance of homeostasis.

Objectives: To enumerate and discuss the functions of the nervous system.

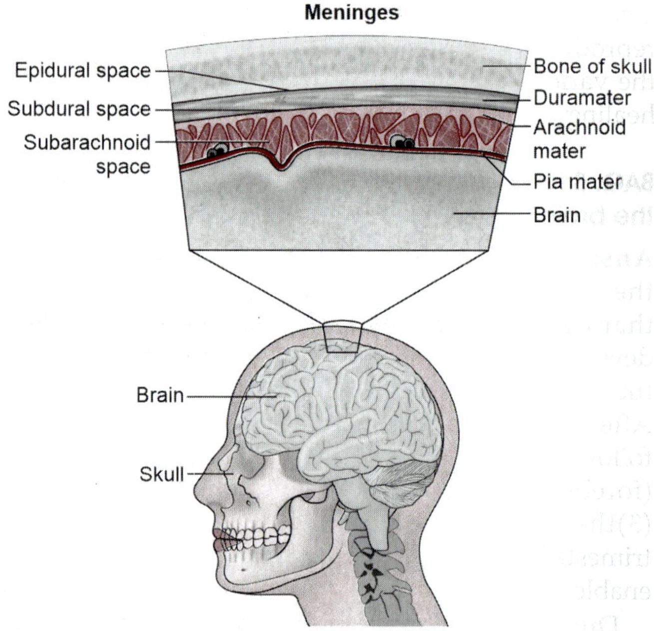

Fig. 6.3: Meninges

FUNCTIONS OF THE NERVOUS SYSTEM

SAQ: Explain and enumerate the functions of the nervous system.

Ans: The nervous system plays very important role in practically every aspect of health and well-being of the body. The nervous system controls various daily activities such as the maintenance of homeostasis, interpretation of sensory information, creation of motor responses; that involves the movements of the body parts and control of various actions such as breathing, eating, talking, learning, memorising, thinking, sleeping,

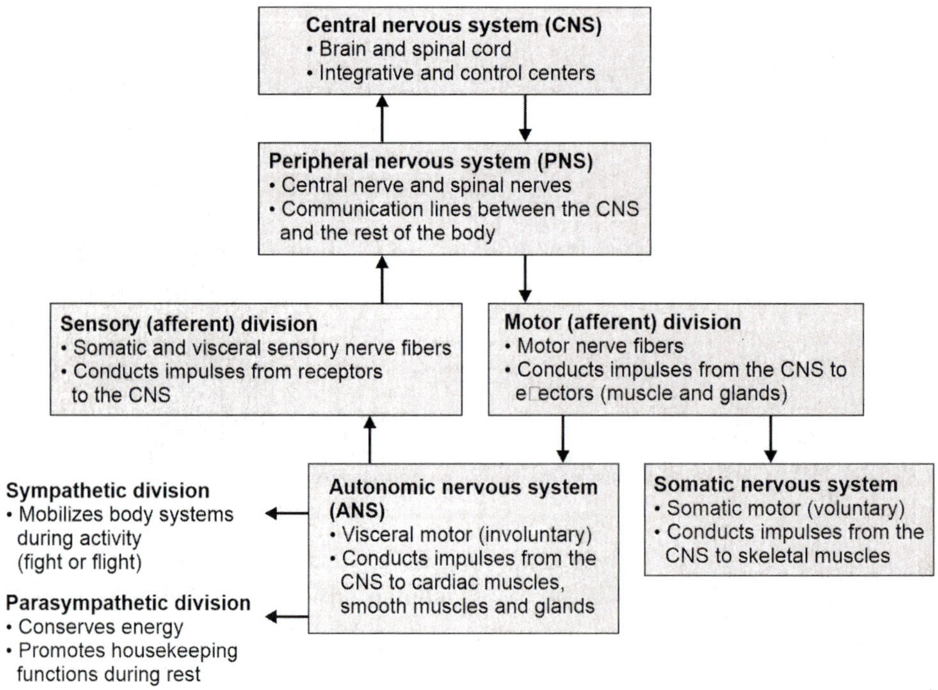

Fig. 6.4: Central nervous system and the peripheral nervous system tabular description

awaking, expressing emotions, control of digestion and reproductive activities, and it plays important role in the various processes such as the stress management, healing, rehabilitation, etc.

BAQ: Briefly describe the embryonic development of the brain.

Ans: The neural tube forms in the embryo after the conception. The neural tube is a hollow tube that contains early brain and the spine. The brain development takes place from the front end of the neural tube, with rapid cell development and differentiation. After the conception, by end of the fourth week, the following three parts develop: (1) The prosencephalon (forebrain), (2) the mesencephalon (midbrain) and (3)the rhombencephalon (hindbrain). In the first trimester of pregnancy nerve connections are built that enable the baby to move in the womb.

During the fifth week, from the forebrain, the telencephalon and the diencephalon parts develop, the midbrain does not change and from the hind brain metencephalon and myelencephalon parts form. In the second trimester, nerve connections increase and the brain tissue formation takes place.

In the third trimester, the cerebrum develops prenatally from the forebrain (prosencephalon) and the dorsal telencephalon develops into the cerebral cortex, and the ventral telencephalon, becomes the basal ganglia. The cerebral cortex begins to develop from the brain stem and prepares the baby for the development of the learning ability. The gyri (folds, ridges) and sulci start developing in the cortex. These surface convolutions appear during fetal development and continue to mature after birth through the process of gyrification.

By the time of the delivery, the baby is fairly able to hear and also able to see around. The average brain weighs about 350–400 grams at the birth. It grows to about average 800 grams during the childhood and it develops further and the average weight of an adult brain attains about 1.3 kg to 1.4 kg.

Objective: To discuss and describe the organization of the nervous system and related functions.

CENTRAL NERVOUS SYSTEM

BAQ: Briefly describe the central nervous system.

Ans: The central nervous system (CNS) is the part of the nervous system consisting primarily of the brain and spinal cord. The brain coordinates and influences the activity of all the parts of the body.

The CNS is contained within the dorsal body cavity and the brain is situated in the cranial cavity within the skull. The spinal cord is present in the spinal canal (cavity) within the vertebrae (Fig. 6.5). The inter-neuronal space within the CNS is filled with a large amount of neuroglia.

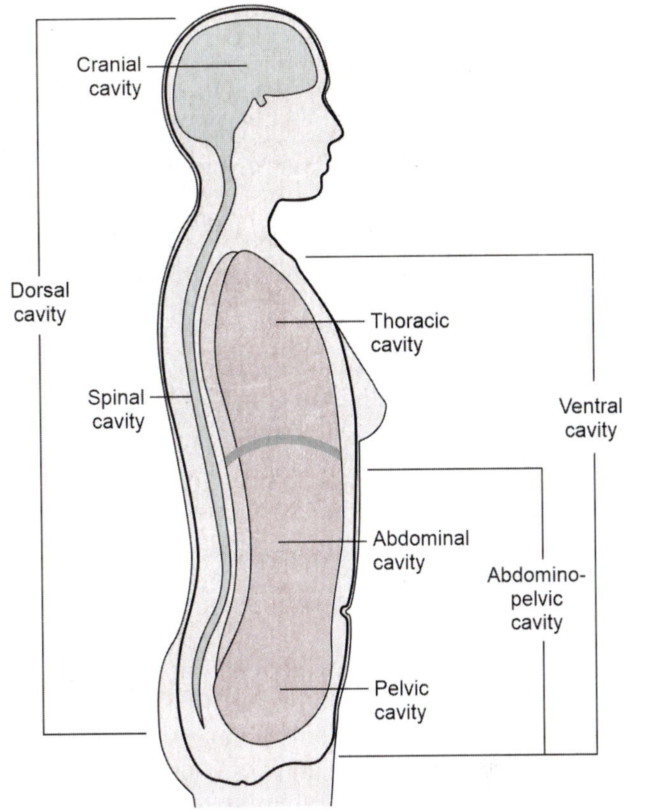

Fig. 6.5: Body cavities

BRAIN (Figs 6.5 and 6.6)

BAQ: Write a brief note on the brain.

Ans: The brain makes up the largest portion of the central nervous system (CNS). It is the major functional part of the central nervous system (CNS). The average brain weighs about 350–400 grams at the birth. It grows to about average 800 grams during the childhood. The average weight of an adult brain is about 1.3 kg to 1.4 kg.

Brain Tissue and Cells

The brain is made up of two types of cells: Neurons and neuroglia (glia). Percentage of neuron cells is about 10% in the brain and compared to the neurons, large number of glial cells are present in brain. The functions of neuron is sending and receiving nerve impulses or signals. The functions of glial cells is to provide support and nutrition, form myelin, facilitate signal transmission in the nervous system and play important role in the maintenance of homeostasis.

The brain is divided into specific parts that serve related important functions (Figs 6.6 and 6.7). The following are the main five main lobes of the brain: 1. Frontal lobe, 2. parietal lobe, 3. occipital lobe, 4. temporal lobe and 5. insular lobe.

The important parts of the brain are: The cerebrum, the cerebral cortex, the brain stem, hypothalamus, thalamus, pituitary gland, pineal gland, amygdala, and hippocampus.

The cerebrum (telencephalon) (Fig. 6.7A) is the largest part of the brain. It contains the cerebral cortex and the

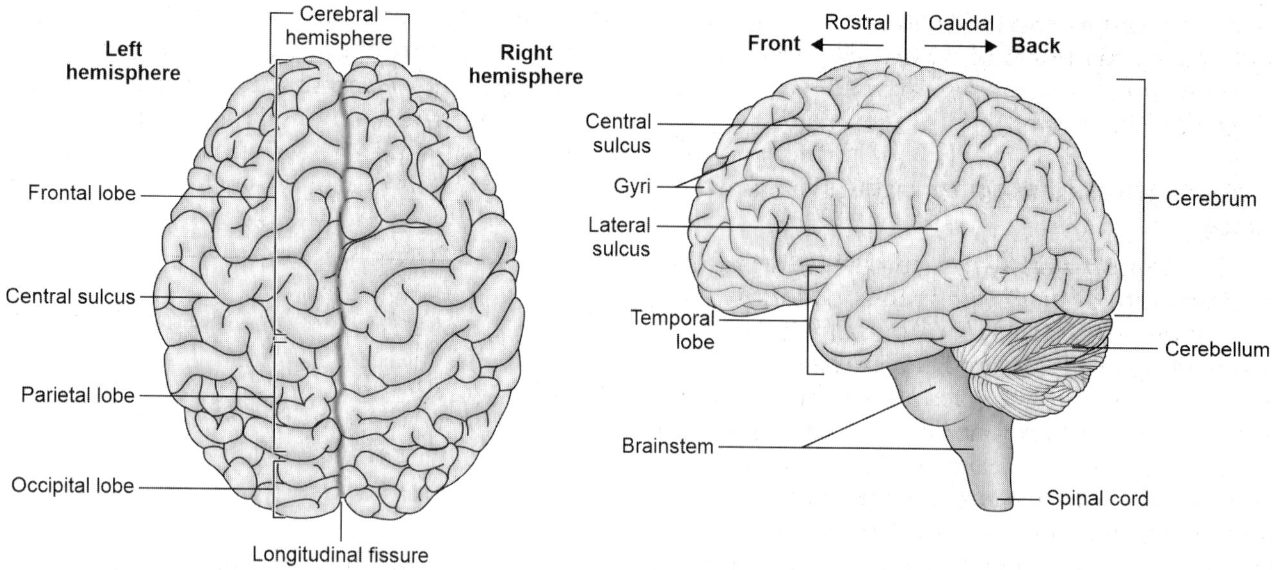

Fig. 6.6: Left and right cerebral hemispheres

other subcortical structures such as the hippocampus, basal ganglia, and olfactory bulb. The cerebrum is the uppermost region of the central nervous system. The cerebral cortex is the outer layer of neural tissue of the cerebrum Mostly, it consists of the six-layered neocortex and 10% of the allocortex. It is separated into two cortices, by the longitudinal fissure, which divides the cerebrum into the left and right cerebral hemispheres (Fig. 6.6). These two hemispheres join beneath the cortex by the corpus callosum (Fig. 6.7). The corpus callosum is the primary junctional part of the brain that contains white matter tracts, which connect the left and right cerebral hemispheres.

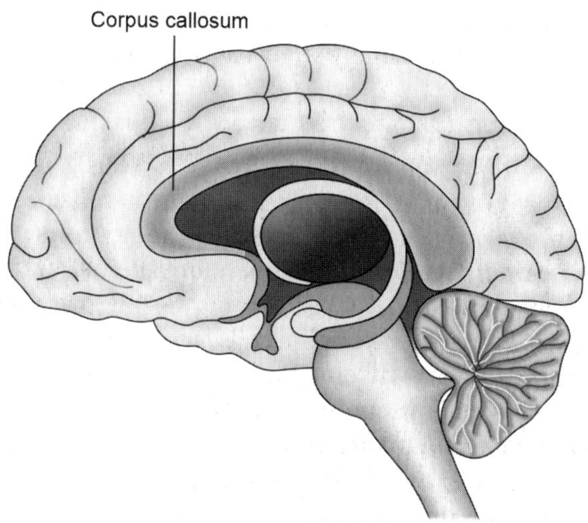

Fig. 6.7: Corpus callosum

The cerebral cortex (Fig. 6.8) contains the largest neural integration in the central nervous system. It displays the gyri and the sulci (Fig. 6.9). The cerebral cortex is buried in the sulci. The major sulci and gyri mark the divisions of the cerebrum into the lobes of the brain. The cell bodies of neurons are clumped together to form ganglia, which are sites for synapses of neurons

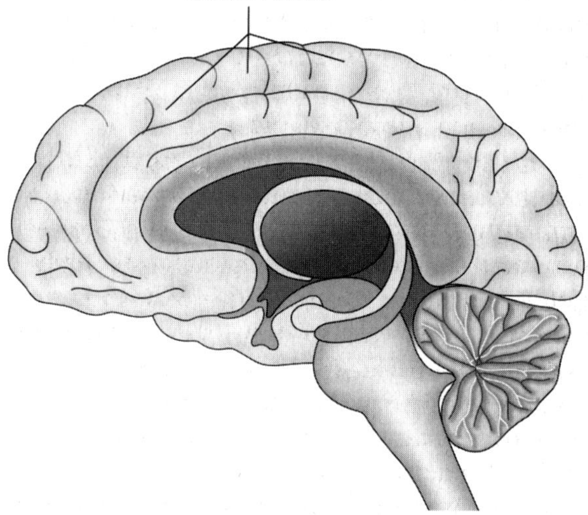

Fig. 6.8: Cerebral cortex

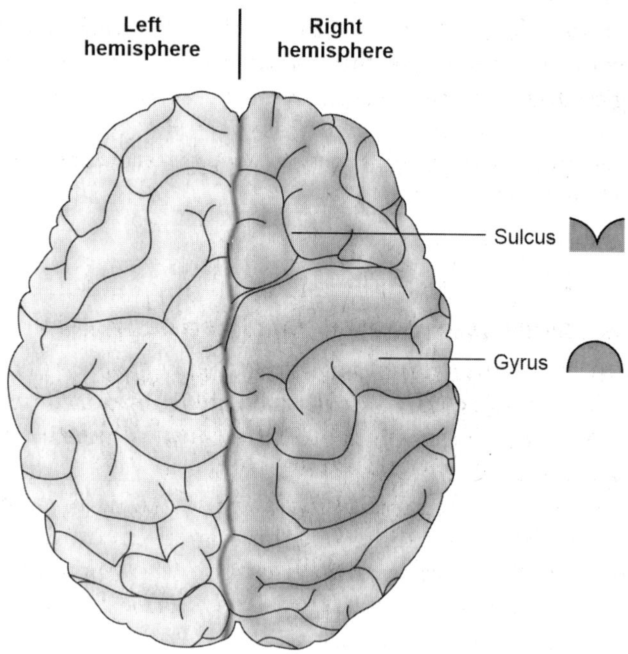

Fig. 6.9A: Sulci and gyri on the cerebral cortex

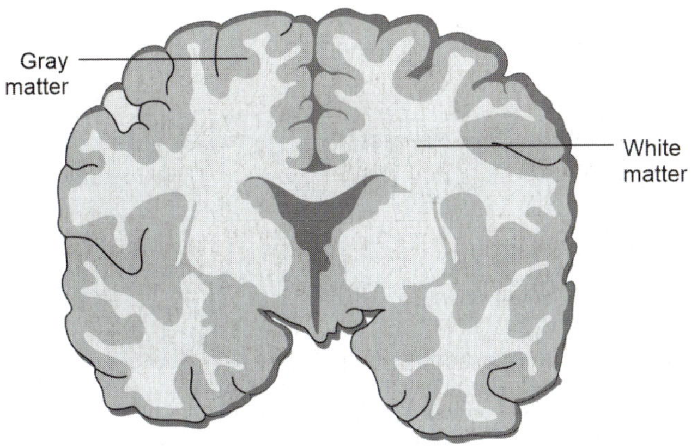

Fig. 6.9B: Gray matter and white matter of the brain

between spinal cord and the body organs. The basal ganglia (basal nuclei) are specialized paired masses of grey matter present deeply inside the white matter.

The cerebral cortex appears grey, since nerves in this area lack the myelin insulation. Due to myelin most other parts of the brain appear white (Fig. 6.9B). The surface of the brain appears wrinkled. Beneath the cerebral cortex connecting fibers between the neurons form the "white matter."

Messages in the brain travel from gyri to gyri, from one lobe to another lobe, from one side of the brain to the other side of brain and from one lobe of the brain to a structure such as thalamus (Fig. 6.11) that is found deep in the brain or from the deep structures of the brain to another part in the central nervous system. The right side of the brain controls the left side of the body and vice versa.

The brain and the spinal cord are both enclosed in the meninges (Fig. 6.2C). The meninges provide a barrier to chemicals dissolved in the blood and protect the brain from most neurotoxins present in the blood circulation. Within the meninges the brain and spinal cord are bathed in cerebral spinal fluid.

The brain serves many important functions. It receives messages through the five senses of touch, taste, sight, smell and hearing. The brain controls memory, thinking and speech procedures. It controls arm and leg movements and the functions of many organs within the body. The brain also responds to the stressful situations by regulating breathing and heart beat rates.

The signals in the brain are transported along specific pathways. Destruction of brain tissue at any point can disrupt the communication between different parts of the brain. The result is then indicated by a loss of functions such as the reading ability or the ability to follow simple spoken commands and also speech.

SAQ: What are gyri and sulci on the surface of the cerebral cortex?

Ans: A gyrus is a ridge-like elevation present on the surface of the cerebral cortex and gyri are surrounded by the depressions known as sulci (Fig. 6.9).

GANGLIA

SAQ: What are ganglia and their functions?

Ans: The cell bodies of neurons are clumped together to form ganglia, which are sites for synapses of neurons between spinal cord and the body organs. The ganglia facilitate passing of signals back and forth from spinal cord and various body organs by means of nerve impulses.

Basal Ganglia (Basal Nuclei)

SAQ: Write a note on the basal ganglia (basal nuclei).

Ans: The basal ganglia (basal nuclei) are specialized paired masses of the grey matter present deeply inside the white matter. These are made of the corpus stratum and other parts of the mesencephalon. The corpus stratum consists of the lentiform nucleus and the caudate nucleus. The lentiform nucleus consists of globus, pallidus and putamen parts.

In the case of brain injury involving basal nuclei or in neural diseases such as Parkinson's disease, variety of motor dysfunctions are observed, which lead to tremor, rigidity, and absurd movements of the body parts.

SAQ: Write a note on the meninges.

Ans: The meninges are three layers of membranes that cover the brain and the spinal cord (Fig. 6.3). The inner

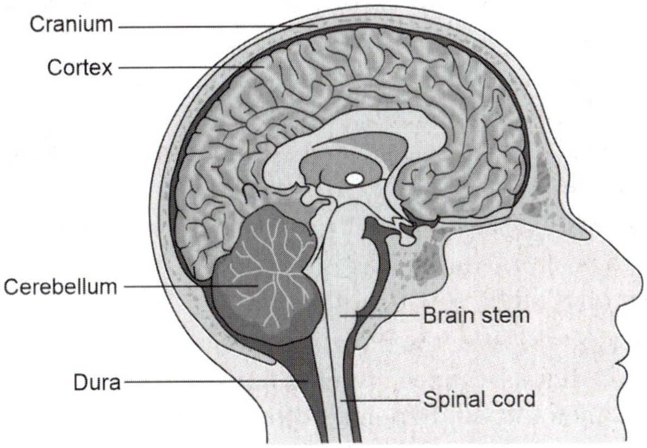

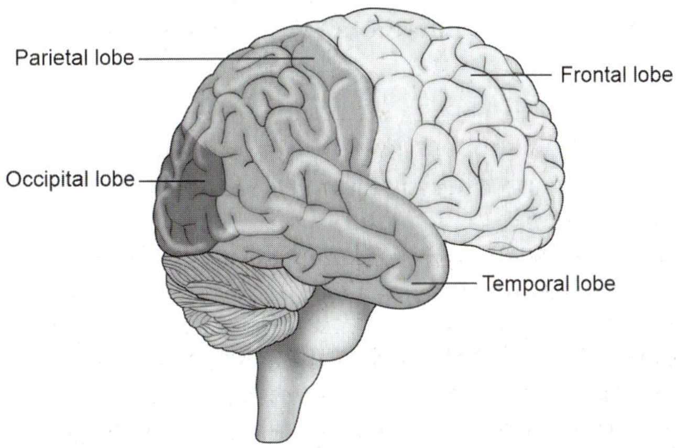

Fig. 6.10: Main lobes of the brain and other anatomical features

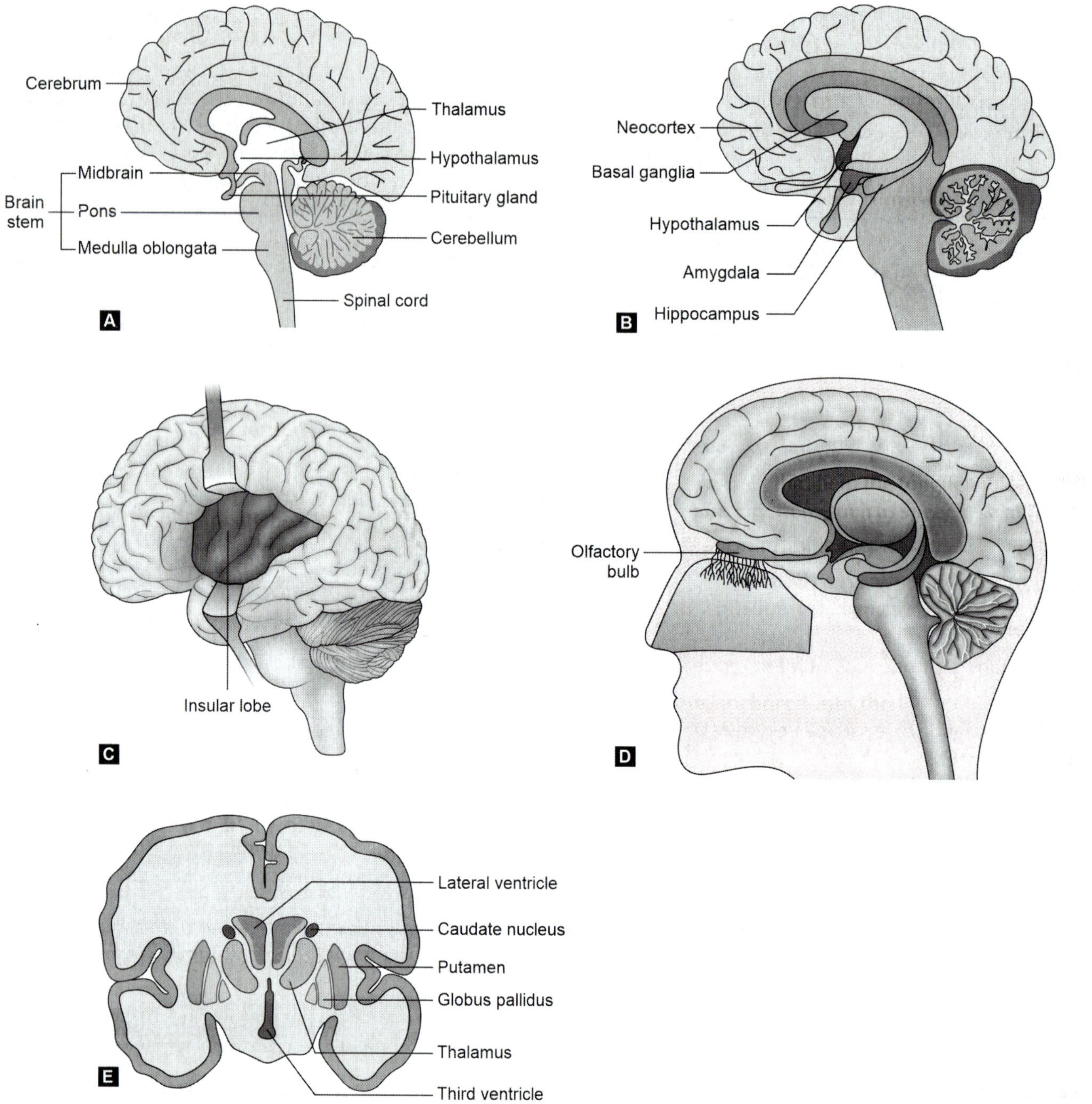

Figs 6.11A–E: Main anatomical parts and the features of the brain

layer is delicate and called the pia mater. The middle layer is the arachnoid. It is a web-like structure and filled with fluid that cushions the brain. The tough outer layer is called the dura mater.

Functions

1. Protect and support the sensitive areas of the brain.
2. Give support to nerves, blood vessels, and lymphatics in the brain
3. Give support and protection to the cerebrospinal fluid in the central nervous system.

BAQ: Write a note on the various lobes of the brain and related functions.

Ans: The brain has an organized anatomical structure. It is divided into many components that serve specific and important functions (Fig. 6.11). The following are the five main lobes of the brain and their respective functions:

1. **Frontal lobe:** This part controls the attributes, such as reasoning, planning, speech, general movements of body parts, emotions, reasoning, smell and personality.
2. **Parietal lobe:** It is vital for sensory perception and integration, including the management of taste, hearing, sight, touch, and smell.
3. **Occipital lobe:** It is the visual processing area of the brain. It is associated with the visuospatial processing, distance and depth perception, colour determination, object and face recognition, and memory formation and retaintion.

4. **Temporal lobe:** It helps to process sensory input, including pain and auditory stimuli. It also helps to understand language, retain visual memories, and to process and remember emotions.
5. **Insular lobe (insular cortex, insula):** It controls the autonomic functions by the regulation of the sympathetic and parasympathetic systems. It also plays an important role in the regulating the immune system.

BRAIN COMPONENTS AND FUNCTIONS

BAQ: What are the principal regions and the main structures of the brain and their general functions?

Ans: The following Table 6.1 indicates the principal regions, the main structures and functions of the brain:

BAQ: Draw a neat labelled diagram of functional areas of the brain.

Ans: Refer to Fig. 6.12A.

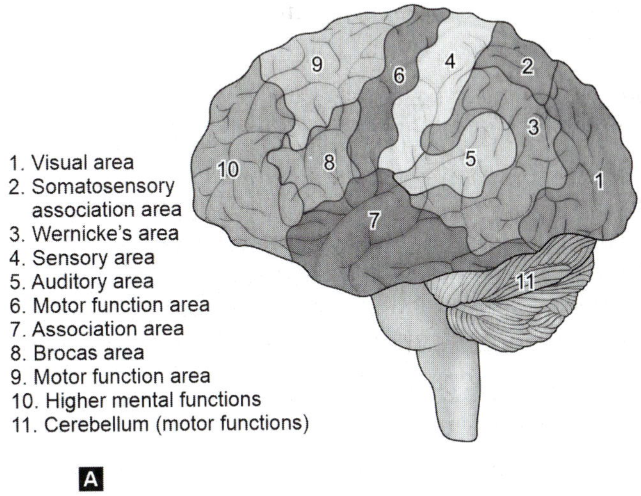

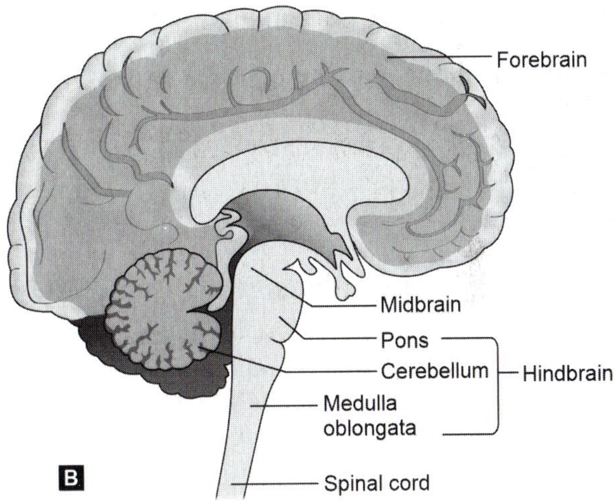

Figs 6.12A and B: (A) Functional areas of the brain; (B) hindbrain

SAQ: What is hindbrain?

Ans: The hindbrain is the lower part of the human brain. It is near the brainstem and is also known as rhombencephalon.

SAQ: How nerve types are described? What are the different types of nerves?

Ans: The nerve types can be described in the following four types on the basis of their functions: Motor nerves, sensory nerves, autonomic nerves and cranial nerves.

SAQ: What are motor nerves (motor neurons)?

Ans: The motor nerves (motor neurons) send impulses from the brain and spinal cord to all the muscles of the body. This facilitates actions such as talking, walking, running, jumping, talking, blinking of eyes, etc. Motor nerve damage can lead to muscular weakness.

SAQ: What are sensory nerves (sensory neurons)?

Ans: Sensory nerves (sensory neurons) collect information about temperature, pain, pressure, etc. from the sensors in the skin, muscles and internal organs and send it back to the spinal cord and the brain. Damage to the sensory nerves may cause numbness, pain, tingling, oversensitivity and numbness in the affected region of the body.

SAQ: What are autonomic nerves?

Ans: The autonomic nerves are part of the peripheral nervous system that regulates involuntary physiologic

Table 6.1: Regions and principal structures of the brain with their functions

Region	*Structure*	*Functions*
1. Telencephalon	Cerebrum	Control of sensory (touch, smell) and motor activities (walking, running)
2. Diencephalon	Thalamus	Impulses relay center
	Hypothalamus	Regulation of homeostasis
	Pituitary gland	Regulation of other endocrine systems in the body
3. Mesencephalon	Superior colliculus	Visual reflexes
	Inferior colliculus	Auditory reflexes
	Cerebral peduncles	Reflex coordination
4. Metencephalon	Cerebellum	Motor coordination and balance
	Pons	Contain respiratory nuclei and relay center
5. Myelencephalon	Medulla oblongata	Visceral autonomic center (heart beat, respiration, vasoconstriction), relay center)

processes such as blood pressure, respiration, digestion, heartrate, sexual arousal, etc.

SAQ: What are cranial nerves?

Ans: The cranial nerves (Fig. 6.27) are a set of twelve paired nerves at the back of the brain. The cranial nerves send electrical signals from brain to face, neck and other parts of the body. The cranial nerves are responsible for the sensations such as smell, taste, temperature, climate changes, etc. The cranial nerves are also responsible for facial expressions, eye blinks and movement of tongue.

SAQ: What is the importance of the motor function area of the brain?

Ans: The main function of the motor function area is to generate signals to direct the various movements of the body parts and the general activities of the body.

SAQ: What is the importance of the sensory area of the brain?

Ans: The sensory areas of the brain receive and process sensory information received from hearing, sight, touch, taste, smell, etc.

SAQ: What is the importance of the somatosensory area of the brain?

Ans: The primary function of the somatosensory area of the brain is to detect sensory information from the body regarding touch, pain, temperature, perception of the location, body part activities, texture, etc.

SAQ: What is the importance of the auditory area of the brain?

Ans: The auditory area of the brain is highly organized processing unit of sound in the brain that plays very important role in the various activities such as hearing, language communication and music performances.

SAQ: What is the importance of the Broca's area in the brain?

Ans: The Broca's area is a component of a complex speech network known as the motor speech area. This area interacts with the flow of sensory information from the temporal cortex by creating a process for speaking and passing it to the motor cortex, which is responsible to control the movements of the mouth. In general, the mental activity in the motor speech area creates selective stimulation of motor centers in the frontal lobe of the brain. These stimulations cause coordinated contraction of the skeletal muscles in the larynx and pharynx.

SAQ: What are aphasias clinical conditions?

Ans: Aphasias clinical conditions are speech and language disorders. Aphasias may be congenital or acquired. Congenital aphasias is due to genetic disorder. Acquired aphasias may be result of damage to the language center in the amygdala, due to trauma or infection.

SAQ: What is the importance of the Wernicke's area in the brain?

Ans: The Wernicke's area is a region of the brain that contains motor neurons, which play important role in the comprehension (understanding) of speech.

SAQ: What is the importance of the visual area of the brain?

Ans: The visual area in the brain contributes to the ability of an individual to successfully accommodate and pass through the physical space and interact with various individuals and objects around.

SAQ: What is the importance of the higher mental function area of the brain?

Ans: The higher mental function area of the brain facilitates understanding of images, speech, memory retention and use, increase in focus, logical thinking, colour differentiation, perception of the depth of the surrounding, etc.

CEREBRUM (Fig. 6.11A)

BAQ: Write a brief note on the cerebrum.

Ans: The cerebrum is the uppermost region of the central nervous system and is the largest part of the brain (Fig. 6.11A). It contains the cerebral cortex and the other subcortical structures such as the hippocampus, basal ganglia, and the olfactory bulb.

The cerebrum contains specific functional areas such as the visual, somatosensory association, sensory, auditory, motor function, higher mental function, Broca's and Wernicke's area.

Functions

The cerebrum controls the sensory actions such as touch, smell, etc. and the motor activities such as walking, jumping, running, eating, reading, observing, etc. It controls the body posture and equilibrium of the body. The higher mental function area of the cortex facilitates understanding of images, speech, memory retention and use, increase in focus, logical thinking, colour differentiation, and perception of the depth of the surrounding,

Cerebral Cortex (Fig. 6.8)

BAQ: Write a brief note on the cerebral cortex.

Ans: The cerebral cortex is the outer layer of neural tissue of the cerebrum. In consists mainly of the six-layered neocortex and 10% of the allocortex. The cerebral cortex is average 2.5 mm thick and consists of six layers of nerve cells. It contains about 21–26 billion nerve cells. It is separated into two cortices, by the longitudinal fissure, which divides the cerebrum into the left and right cerebral hemispheres. These two hemispheres join beneath the cortex by the corpus callosum. The cerebral cortex contains the largest neural integration in the central nervous system. It contains the convolutions that displays the gyri and the sulci. The convolutions significantly increase the surface area of grey matter and the nerve cell bodies. The cerebral cortex is buried in the sulci. The major sulci and gyri mark the divisions of the cerebrum into the lobes of the brain. The cerebral cortex is divided into main four lobes: Frontal, parietal, temporal and occipital, which are responsible for processing different types of information.

Functions

The cerebral cortex is responsible for specific brain functions that include motor, sensory, and higher intellectual functions. It controls the various processes that include, memory, language, thinking, reasoning, learning, decision-making, expression of emotions and intelligence, etc.

Brainstem (Fig. 6.11A)

SAQ. Write a brief note on the brainstem.

Ans: The brainstem consists of three structures, the midbrain, pons and medulla oblongata. It is the lower extension of the brain and it is located in front of the cerebellum and connected to the spinal cord.

Functions

The brainstem plays an important role in passing messages back and forth between various parts of the body and to the cerebral cortex.

Midbrain (Mesencephalon) (Fig. 6.11A)

SAQ. Write a brief note on the midbrain (mesencephalon).

Ans: The midbrain is a part of the central nervous system. It is located below the cerebral cortex and at the upper part of the brainstem (Fig. 6.11A).

The midbrain can be divided into the following three portions: Tectum (posterior), tegmentum, and cerebral peduncles (anterior). It contains the corpora quadrigemina, which are the rounded elevations on the superior portion of the midbrain. The upper two superior colliculi play important role in the visual reflexes and the two posterior inferior colliculi are responsible for the auditory reflexes.

Functions

The midbrain (mesencephalon) forms a channel for the spinal cord to transmit the sensory stimuli (any event that is received by the senses) from the head and body to the brain. The sensory stimulus can be from heat, light, sound or touch. The brain then directs the specific action to respond to the specific sensory stimulus. Thus, it is functionally associated with various actions such as, motor control, sleep, awakening, vision, hearing, temperature control and alertness.

Cerebral Peduncles

SAQ: What are cerebral peduncles?

Ans: The cerebral peduncles (Fig. 6.13B) are a large collection of fiber bundles in the ventral midbrain. The cerebral peduncles originate in the cerebral cortex. These are two stalks that attach the cerebrum to the brainstem. The cerebral peduncles are present at the front of the midbrain and arise from the ventral pons. It contains the large ascending (sensory) and descending (motor) nerve tracts and also the sensory fibers. These peduncles connect by means of nerves with the nuclei in the pons, the cerebellum and the spinal cord.

SAQ. What is the difference between nuclei and ganglia?

Ans: The difference between ganglia and nuclei is that nuclei are clusters of nerve cell bodies in the central nervous system (CNS) whereas ganglia are clusters of nerve cell bodies in the peripheral nervous system (PNS).

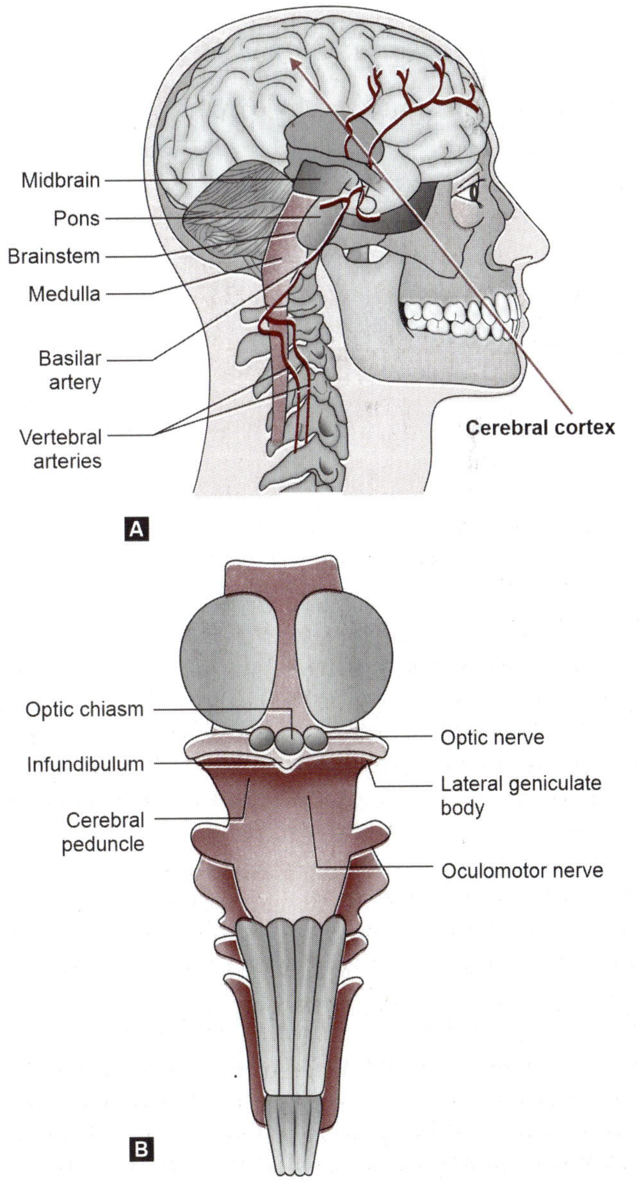

Figs 6.13A and B: (A) Midbrain and (B) cerebral peduncles the associated parts of the brain

SAQ: Briefly describe the functions of the nuclei within the midbrain.

Ans: The nuclei within the midbrain are clusters of neuron cell bodies present in the white matter. These form many networks related to cardiovascular and visceral control and movement functions. These nuclei also play important role in pain modulation in the state of consciousness and also in the waking and sleeping rhythms.

SAQ: What is the red nucleus in the midbrain?

Ans: The red nucleus is present in the grey matter; that connect the cerebral hemisphere and the cerebellum. The appearance of red nucleus is due to the presence of rich blood supply to that region (red colour of hemoglobin). It is involved in the reflexes related to the motor coordination. The substantia nigra is another dark coloured pigmented nucleus (dark colour of melanin), which is inferior to the red nucleus and involved in the inhibitory involuntary movements.

Pons (Figs 6.11A and 6.13)

SAQ. Write a brief note on the pons.

Ans: The pons is a part of the brainstem, that links the brain to the spinal cord (Fig. 6.11). In contains the apneustic center that sends signals for deep and long breaths.

Functions

The pons is involved in control of breathing, hearing, maintain balance and also plays important role in the coordination of eye, facial movements, and facial sensation.

Medulla Oblongata (Fig. 6.11)

SAQ: Write a brief note on the medulla oblongata.

Ans: The medulla oblongata is the lowest part of the brain and it is also the lowest part of the brainstem. The medulla oblongata is connected to the midbrain by the pons. It remains continuous posteriorly with the spinal cord. The medulla oblongata merges at the foramen magnum opening at the base of the skull (Fig. 6.14). It contains nuclei for cranial nerves for vital autonomic functions.

The medulla oblongata mainly consists of white matter in the form of the descending motor tracts, the ascending sensory tracts, the cardiovascular-respiratory regulation system, and origin of cranial nerves IX, X, XI, and XII. It contains the decussation area. The projection fibers from these tracts cross to other side through the pyramidal region. The grey matter of the medulla oblongata contains several nuclei for the sensory nerve signal relay to the thalamus and the motor components for the nerve signal relay from the cerebrum to the cerebellum.

Functions

The medulla oblongata plays an important role in transmitting messages between spinal cord and brain. It is essential for the regulation of cardiovascular and respiratory systems. Various processes such as breathing, heart rhythms, blood pressure and swallowing are controlled by the medulla oblongata.

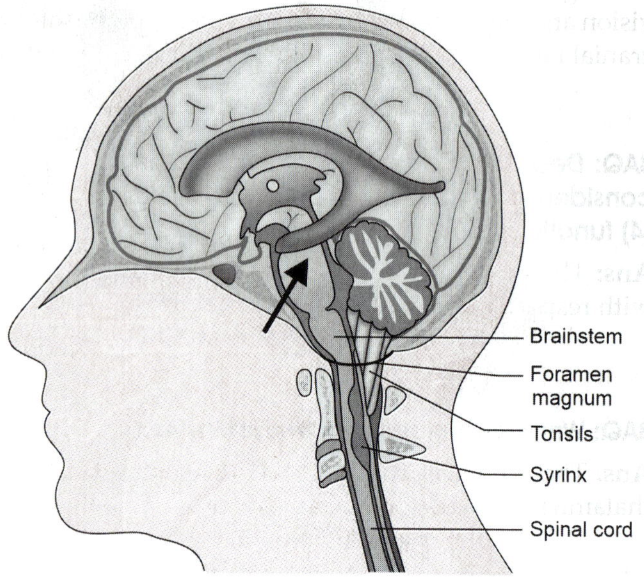

Fig. 6.14: Medulla oblongata merges at the foramen magnum opening at the base of the skull

> *Note*
> 1. Brainstem sends messages from the cortex to the spinal cord and nerves that branch from the spinal cord.
> 2. Destruction of midbrain leads to "brain death."

BAQ: What are the autonomic functions of the medulla oblongata?

Ans: The medulla oblongata contain three nuclei that function as the autonomic centers. The inhibitory fibers through the vagus nerve and accelerator fibers through the spinal nerves T1–T5 arise from the nuclei of the cardiac center. The nuclei in the medulla oblongata control the following main visceral organs:

Respiratory center: Breathing rate is controlled.

Cardiac center: Heart beat rate is controlled.

Vasomotor center: Contraction of smooth muscles in the arterioles to raise blood pressure as per the need.

SAQ: What is the reticular activating system?

Ans: In the midbrain, pons, medulla and part of the thalamus, a network of neurons is present. It is called the reticular activating system (RAS). It is involved in sleep patterns, dreaming, and controls the levels of wakefulness and flight or fight responses. Individuals are able to pay attention to the environment around and the related changes. The damage to RAS causes unconsciousness.

Cranial Nerves

LAQ: Write a brief note on the cranial nerves.

Ans: Twelve paired cranial nerves are originated in the brainstem. These nerves control the movements of the face, neck, shoulder and tongue muscles and play very important role in the eye movements, facial sensations, hearing, tasting, and swallowing. The cranial nerves for vision and smell originate in the cerebrum. Four pairs of cranial nerves originate from the pons (Fig. 6.15).

Cranial Nerves (Fig. 6.15)

BAQ: Describe cranial nerves in the tabular form by considering (1) functions, (2) types, (3) pathways and (4) functions.

Ans: The following Table 6.3 describes cranial nerves with respect to the question.

DIENCEPHALON (Fig. 6.16)

BAQ: Write a note on the diencephalon.

Ans: The two components of the diencephalon are the thalamus and the hypothalamus.

Thalamus (Fig. 6.16)

The thalamus is a small structure within the brain. It is located above the brain stem and between the cerebral cortex and the midbrain. It has large number of nerve connections to cerebral cortex and the midbrain. The primary function of the thalamus is to relay motor and sensory signals to the cerebral cortex. The thalamus relays sensory impulses from receptors in various parts of the body to the cerebral cortex. A sensory impulse travels from the body surface towards the thalamus, which is received it as a sensation. This sensation is then passed onto the cerebral cortex for interpretation as pain, touch, or temperature detection.

Hypothalamus (Fig. 6.16)

The hypothalamus is a small structure of the brain. It is located at the base of the brain and near the pituitary gland. The hypothalamus receives information from the autonomic nervous system and responds by secreting various hormones and controls functions such as eating, sleeping, sexual behaviour, regulation of blood osmotic concentration, body temperature, emotions, secretion of hormones and movement.

LIMBIC SYSTEM (Fig. 6.17)

BAQ: What is the limbic system and its functions?

Ans: The limbic system includes the hypothalamus, part of the thalamus, amygdala and hippocampus. The limbic system is mainly involved in the behavioural and emotional responses of an individual. It deals with the sexual stimulation and learning. The limbic system controls long-term memory, behaviour, motivation, long-term memory, and the sense of smell. The limbic system is linked to the endocrine and autonomic nervous systems and plays important role in the reactions of the body to the stressful conditions and environmental changes. The limbic system also controls the instincts

Table 6.3: The cranial nerve characteristic features

Cranial nerve	*Type*	*Pathway*	*Function*
Olfactory	Sensory	Olfactory epithelial to olfactory bulb	Smell
Optic	Sensory	Eye retina to thalamus	Visual fields and ability to see
Oculomotor	Motor	Mid brain to eye muscle	Eye movements; eyelid opening
Trochlear	Motor	Mid brain to superior oblique muscle Eye muscle to mid brain	Eye movements
Trigeminal	Mixed	Pons to muscles of mastication From face skin, cornea, lips, tongue, teeth	Facial sensation
Abducens	Motor	Pons to lateral rectus muscle Eye muscles to pons	Eye movements
Facial	Mixed	From pons to facial muscle And from facial muscles to pons	Movement of face, secretion of saliva, tears
Auditory/vestibular	Sensory	Ear anatomical parts to pons	Hearing; sense of balance
Glossopharyngeal	Mixed	Medulla oblongata to pharyngeal muscle and pharyngeal muscle to medulla oblongata	Taste sensation, swallowing
Vagus	Mixed	Medulla oblongata to viscera and viscera to medula oblongata	Control of neck and shoulder movements
Hypoglossal	Motor	Medulla oblongata to tongue muscle tongue muscle to medulla oblongata	Tongue movement
Accessory	Motor	Medulla oblongata to pharynx and neck muscles and from neck muscle To the medulla oblongata	Head movements and swallowing of food and other safe matter

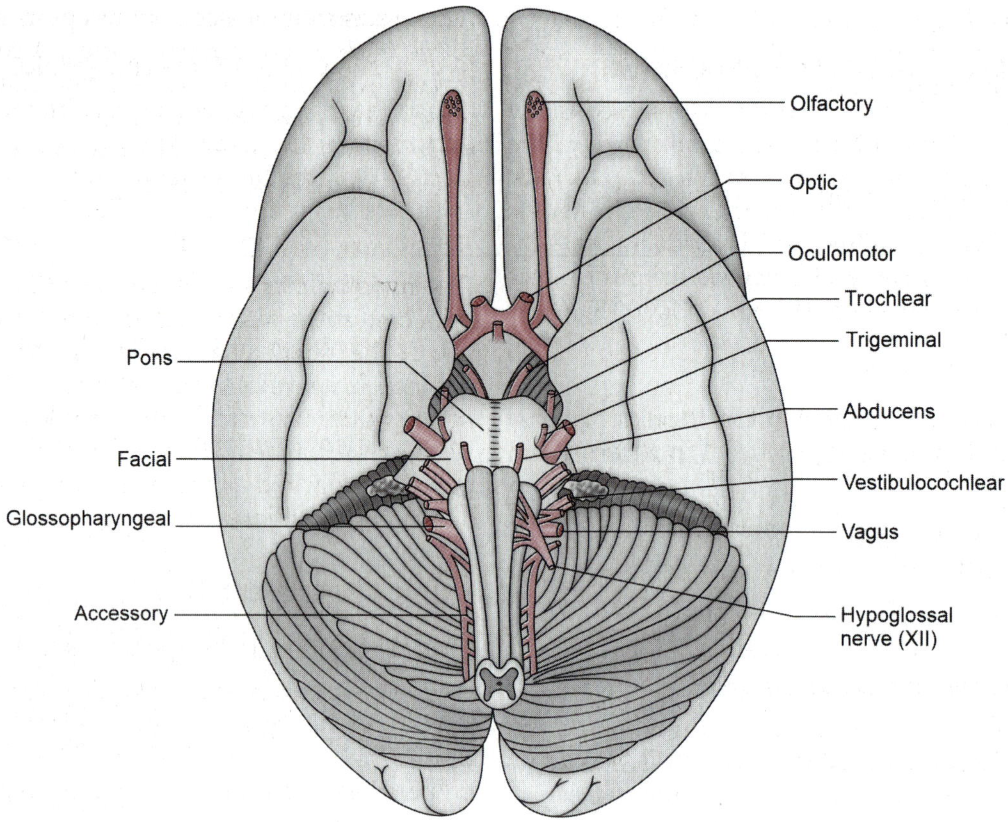

Fig. 6.15: Cranial nerves and related functions

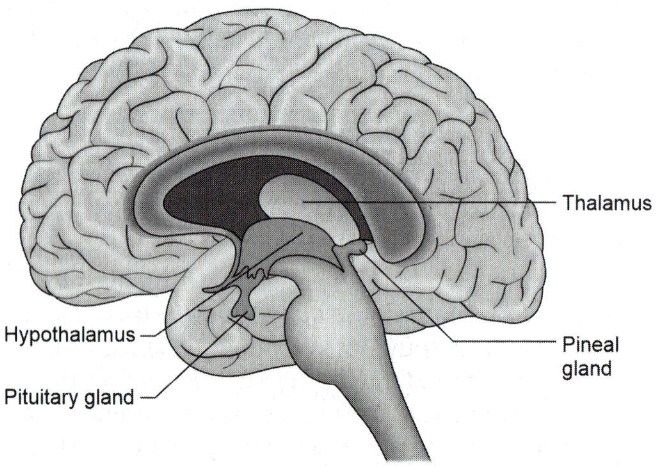

Fig. 6.16: Diencephalon

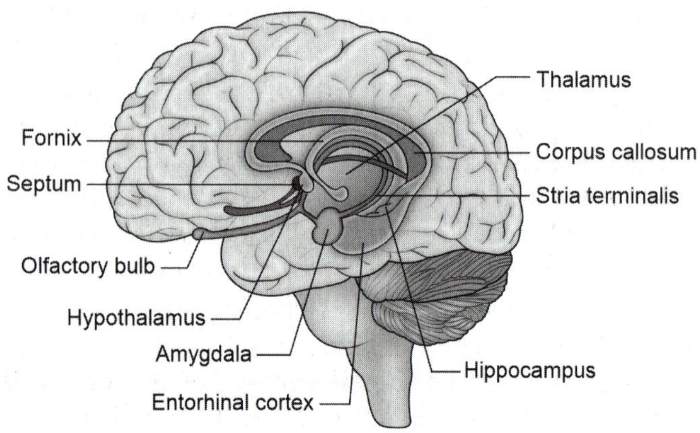

Fig. 6.17: Limbic system

of an individual for feeding, reproduction, caring for children, and response to the fight-or-flight situations.

Pineal Gland (Fig. 6.18)

BAQ: Write a note on the pineal gland.

Ans: The pineal gland is a pea-shaped small gland (5–8 mm) in the brain. It is present in the epithalamus and attached to the brain by a pineal stalk. It is involved in the production and regulation of melatonin hormone. The melatonin hormone plays an important role in the regulation of sleep patterns (circadian rhythms). The internal clock of the body is naturally aligned with the

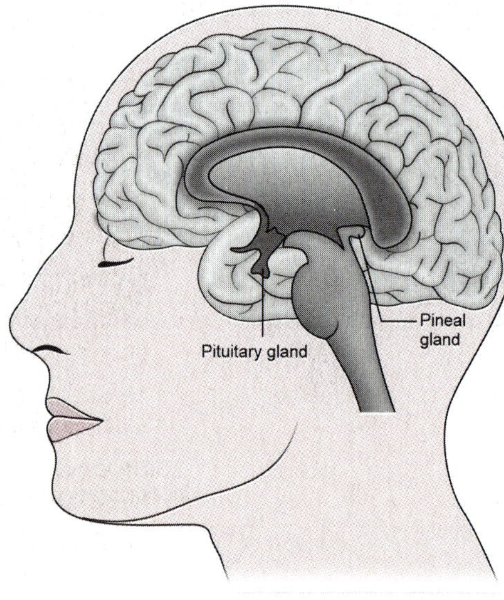

Fig. 6.18: Pineal gland and pituitary gland

cycle of day and night. The circadian rhythms influence several processes in the body that include sleepiness, alertness, body temperature and appetite.

Pituitary Gland (Fig. 6.19)

BAQ: Write a note on the pituitary gland (hypophysis).

Ans: The pituitary gland (hypophysis) is a small endocrine gland present at the base of the brain, behind the bridge of the nose and directly below the hypothalamus.

Hormones Produced by Pituitary Gland and Related Functions

The following are the major hormones produced by the pituitary gland and their related functions:

Adrenocorticotropic hormone (ACTH): It stimulates the production of cortisol (stress hormone), which maintains blood pressure and blood sugar levels.

Follicle-stimulating hormone (FSH): It stimulates the ovaries in female to produce estrogen and promotes sperm production in males.

Luteinizing hormone (LH): It stimulates testosterone production in men and ovulation in women.

Growth hormone (GH): It maintains healthy muscles and bones and manage appropriate fat distribution.

Prolactin (PRL): It controls the hormones that influence the functions of ovaries and testes, which can affect menstrual periods, sexual functions and fertility. Prolactin also stimulates breast milk production after childbirth.

Thyroid-stimulating hormone (TSH): It stimulates the thyroid gland and controls the production of thyroid hormones (T3 and T4), which regulates metabolism, energy and the nervous system.

Oxytocin: It controls breast milk flow, affects labour, behaviour and social interactions.

Antidiuretic hormone (vasopressin) (ADH): It regulates water balance and blood sodium levels.

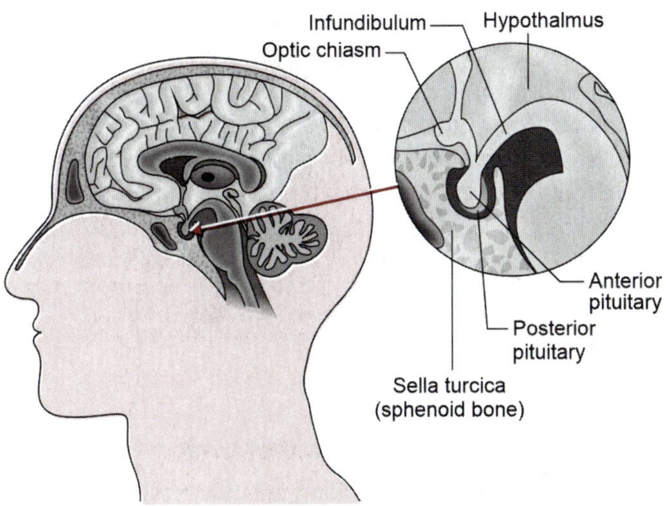

Fig. 6.19: Pituitary gland

Amygdala

SAQ: Write a note on the amygdala.

Ans: The amygdala is a small almond-shaped paired structure present in the temporal lobe of the brain. It is a part of the limbic system of the brain (Fig. 6.20). It is responsible for the "fight or flight" response. Although, it is associated with the fear and stress responses of body, it also plays important role also plays a role in the following actions: The emotions connected to memories, aggression, caretaking, handling and using unconscious memory, enabling abilities such as cycling, swimming, learning through rewards and punishment, social communication, interpretation of interactions, addiction, etc.

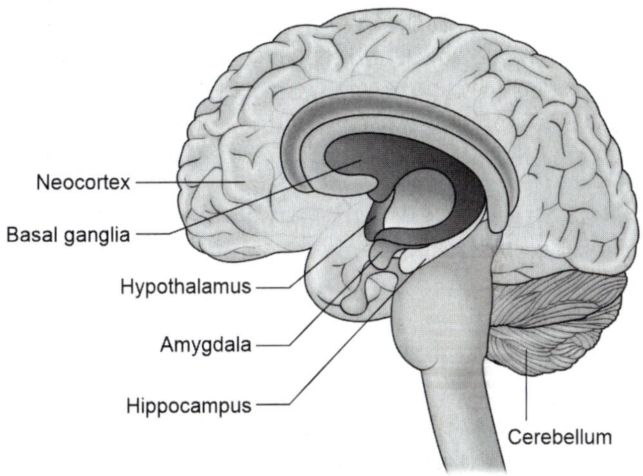

Fig. 6.20: Amygdala

CEREBELLUM

SAQ: Write a note on the cerebellum.

Ans: It is a part of the brain located below the brain and at the back of the head (Fig. 6.20). It is just above and behind the spinal cord that connects the brain. The cortical surface of cerebellum is covered with finely spaced parallel grooves. These are different from the broad irregular convolutions of the cerebral cortex. The cerebellar cortex is made up of the following types of three layers: (1) An outer synaptic layer (the molecular layer), (2) an intermediate discharge layer (the Purkinje layer), and (3) an inner receptive layer (the granular layer).

The Purkinje cells of the Purkinje layer release gamma-aminobutyric acid (GABA) neurotransmitter, which exerts inhibitory actions on specific neurons and reduces the transmission of nerve impulses. By means of this inhibitory function, the Purkinje cells are able to regulate and coordinate motor movement.

The loss of or damage to Purkinje cells can give rise to certain neurological diseases. The loss of Purkinje cells has been observed in children suffering from autism and in patients with an inherited metabolic disorder, Niemann-Pick disease type C.

The cerebellar granule cells of the granular layer play important role in coordinating the passive electric conduction, which control sleep in conjunction with GABA.

Functions: The cerebellum plays very important role in the motor movement regulation and balance control. It coordinates gait and maintains posture, controls voluntary muscle activity and muscle tone. Overall, the cerebellum controls voluntary movements such as maintaining body balance and posture, eye movements, speech, walking, and coordination. The cerebellum also plays important role in various types of motor learnings, such as swimming, bike riding, playing musical instrument, etc.

The damage to the cerebellum can lead to loss of coordination of motor movement, muscles become weak leading to unstable movements, inability to judge distance and to perform rapid alternating movements. Other symtoms observed are slurred speech and abnormal eye movements.

BAQ: Describe the communication of the cerebral hemispheres by the nerve impulses.

Ans: The cerebral hemispheres communicate with each other by the nerve impulses, that pass through the following specific three types of fiber tracts in the white matter and to the other parts of the brain: (1) Association fibers, (2) commissural fibers and (3) projection fibers.

Association fibers: These are present in the specific hemisphere and conduct nerve impulses between neurons in various lobes.

Commissural fibers: These connect the neurons and gyri of one hemisphere with another hemisphere.

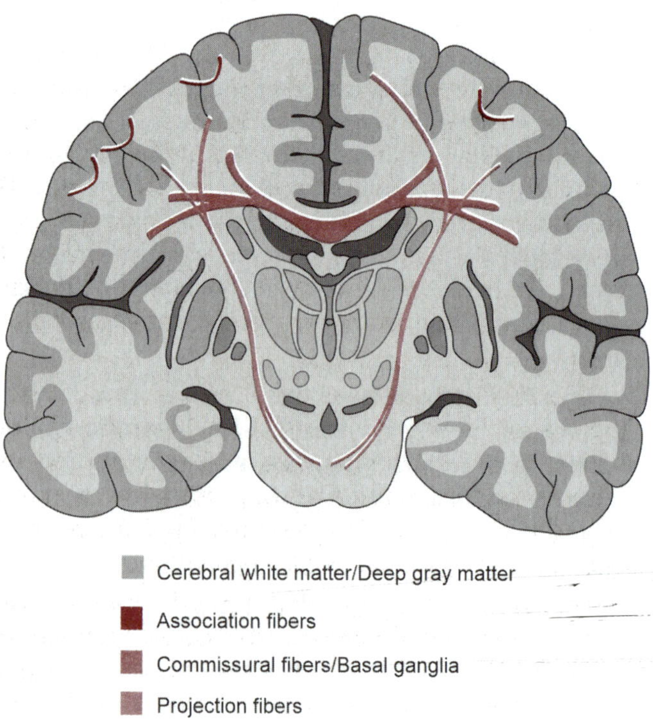

Fig. 6.21: Fiber tracts in the white matter of the brain

Projection fibers: These are of two types: Descending types and ascending types. Descending types of fibers transmit nerve impulses from the cerebrum to other parts of the brain and to the spinal cord. Ascending types of fibers transmit nerve impulses from the spinal cord and other parts of the brain to the cerebrum.

Decussation means the fibers cross from one side of the CNS to the other side.

BRAIN WAVES AS RECORDED IN AN ELECTROENCEPHALOGRAM

BAQ: Write a note on the brain waves as recorded in an electroencephalogram (EEG).

Ans: Brain waves are the collective expressions of millions of action potentials from the cerebrum neurons. During the daily personal activities, the neurons of the brain of an individual fire randomly or in a synchronized manner. The brain waves are synchronized, rhythmic electrical pulses from communicating neurons. The brain waves originate from the various cerebral lobes with different oscillating frequencies. These can be detected from the cerebral surface using an electroencephalography (EEG) equipment. The four main brain waves that are recognized by EEG are: Alpha, beta, theta, and delta waves (Fig. 6.22).

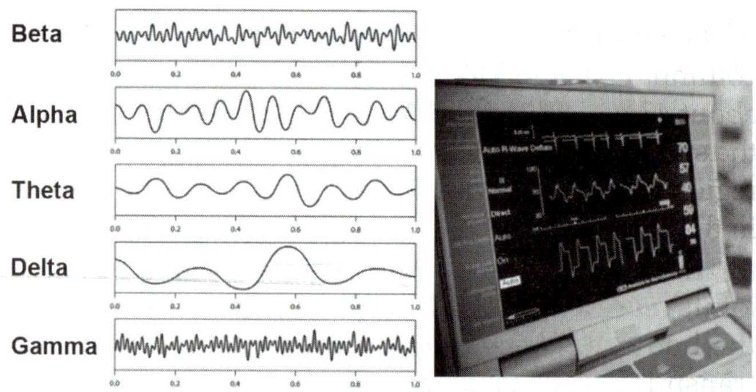

Figs 6.22A and B: (A) Brain waves; (B) ECG machine

Alpha waves (8–12 Hz) can be detected in an awake and relaxed adult. In the case of a child, the alpha waves range is 4–7 Hz. Beta waves (13–30 Hz) indicate mental and visual activity. Theta waves (4–8 Hz) are common in a newborn. However, detection of theta waves in the case of an adult indicate severe emotional stress and signs of nervous breakdown. Delta waves (1–4 Hz) are common in the case a person who is asleep. However, detection of delta waves in an awake person indicate brain damage.

> ***Note:*** It has been observed that music therapy significantly increases alpha waves and decreases beta activity in patients suffering from anxiety, depression, and schizophrenia.

Spinal Cord (Fig. 6.23)

LAQ: Write a note on the spinal cord.

Ans: The spinal cord is a long tubular structure made up of nervous tissue. It extends from the medulla oblongata

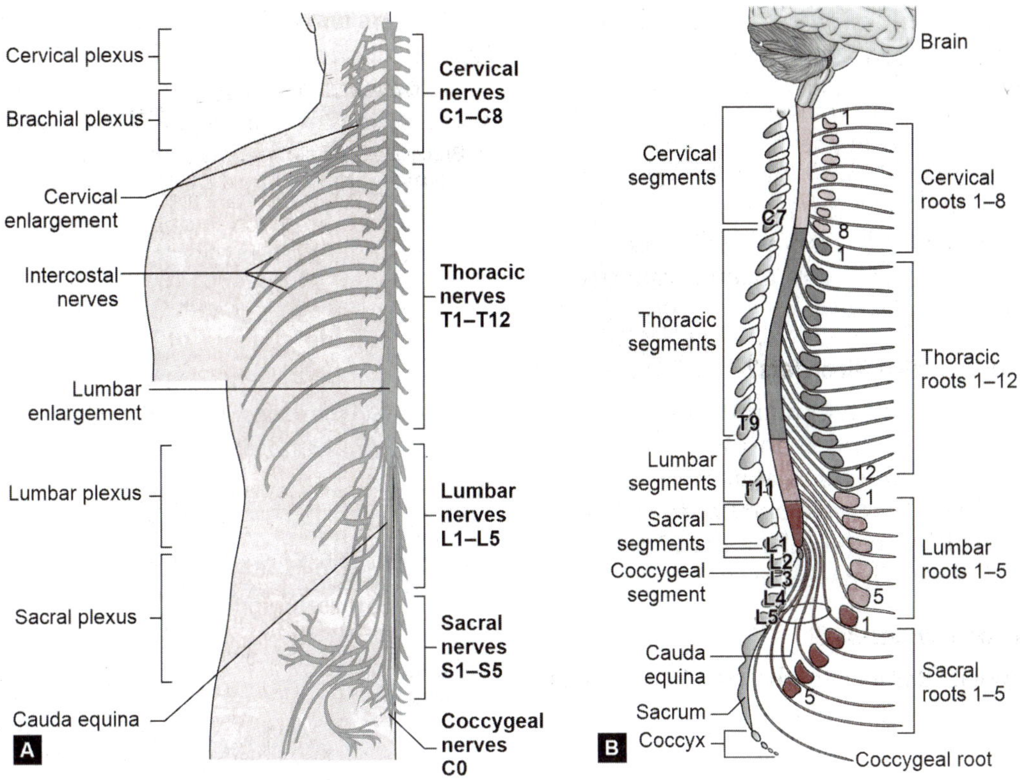

Figs 6.23A and B: Spinal cord and nerves

in the brainstem to the lumbar region of the vertebral column. It is about 45 cm (18 inch) long in men and about 43 cm (17 inch) long in women. The diameter of the spinal cord is about 13 mm (0.5 inch) in the cervical region and lumbar regions and about 6.4 mm (0.25 inch) in the thoracic area.

The spinal nerves connect the spinal cord to muscles, joints, skin, limbs and various organs and parts of the body. The spinal nerves are responsible for the transmission of efferent motor signals, and afferent motor signals. Afferent neurons bring stimuli to the brain. Efferent motor signals are motor neurons carrying neural impulses away from the central nervous system and towards muscles to cause movements of muscles, glands, and organs of the body in response to sensory input (Fig. 6.24). In the brain the signal received is integrated and processed. The brain then coordinates appropriate response through efferent signals back to the specific body parts.

The following are 31 spinal cord nerve segments in a spinal cord (Fig. 6.23B):

- Eight cervical segments forming 8 pairs of cervical nerves.
- Twelve thoracic segments forming 12 pairs of thoracic nerves.
- Five lumbar segments forming 5 pairs of lumbar nerves.
- Five sacral segments forming 5 pairs of sacral nerves.
- 1 coccygeal segment.

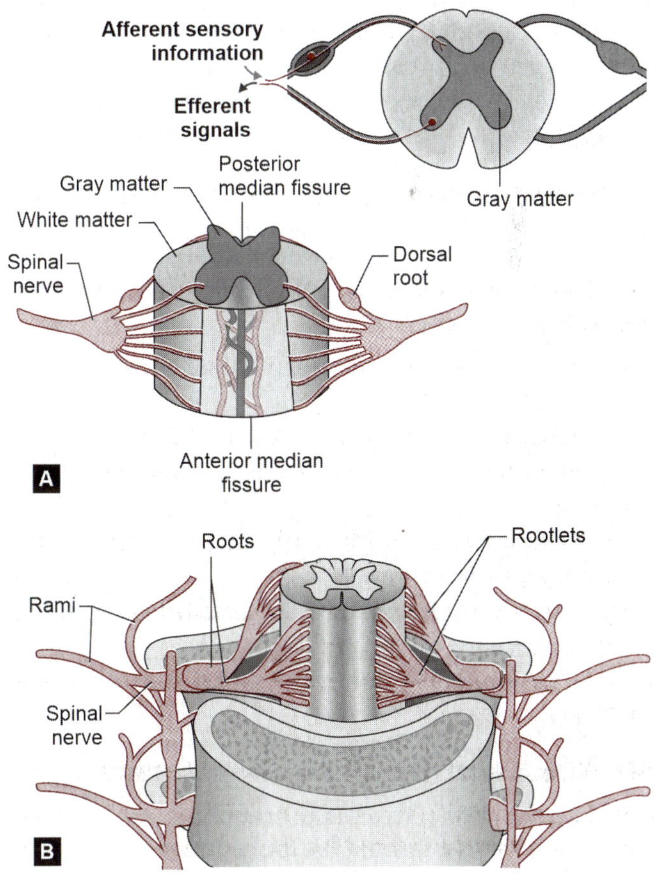

Figs 6.24A and B: (A) Spinal nerves, afferent and efferent signals; (B) spinal nerve, roots, rami and rootlets

Nerve Roots

SAQ: What is a nerve root?

Ans: A nerve root (Fig. 6.24B) is the initial part of a nerve that extends directly from the central nervous system. The following are two different kinds of nerve roots: (1) Cranial nerve roots and (2) spinal nerve roots. Cranial nerve roots extend from the nerves very close to the brain stem and spinal nerve roots extend from nerves that extend from the spinal cord.

SAQ: What are nerve root disorders?

Ans: The nerve root disorders mainly result from a herniated disk or osteoarthritis in the spine. These disorders lead to muscle weakness, abnormal sensation, and pain in the area of the related body part. The nerve root disorders are diagnosed on the basis of results of imaging tests and electrodiagnostic tests.

SAQ: What are rami of nerves?

Ans: Rami (singular: Ramus) are the branches of spinal nerves (Fig. 6.24B).

Plexuses

SAQ: What are nerve plexuses and their functions?

Ans: A nerve plexus (Figs 6.23 and 6.25) is a branching network of intersecting nerves. It is composed of afferent and efferent fibers that arise from the merging of the anterior rami of spinal nerves. The plexuses nerves contain sensory nerves and motor nerves and perform sensory and motor functions, respectively. These functions include muscle contraction, body coordination, body control, maintenance, the reactions to sensations such as pain, pressure, heat, cold, etc.

BAQ: Enumerate the main spinal plexuses and their respective connections?

Ans: The following are the main spinal plexuses and their respective connections:

1. Cervical plexus connects the head, neck and shoulders.
2. Brachial plexus connects the chest, shoulders, arms and hands.
3. Lumbar plexus connects the back, abdomen, groin, thighs, knees, and calves.
4. Sacral plexus connnects the buttocks, pelvis, buttocks, thighs, genitals, calves, and feet.
5. Coccygeal plexus connects a small part over the coccyx.

BAQ: Write a short note on the cervical plexus.

Ans: The cervical plexus is a branching network of intersecting nerves formed by the anterior rami of the first four cervical nerves. It is situated deep inside the neck opposite the cervical vertebrae 1–4 and supported by the sternocleidomastoid muscle.

Superficial branches of the cervical plexus connect side and back part of the head, front side of neck skin.

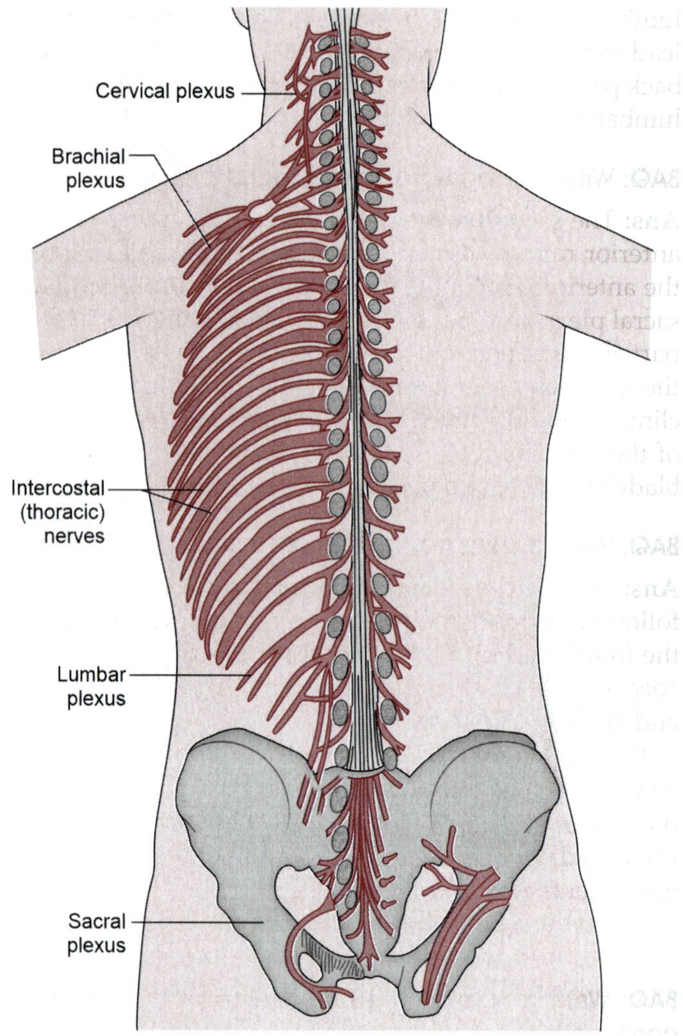

Fig. 6.25: Spinal nerve plexuses

The deep branches of the cervical plexus connect the muscles of the neck (trapezius and sternocleidomastoid). Damage to the cervical plexus due to accident or disease will lead to failure of spontaneous respiration.

BAQ: Write a short note on the brachial plexus.

Ans: The brachial plexus forms from the large part of the first thoracic nerve and lower four (C5–C8) cervical nerves. It is a network of nerves situated deep in the neck and the shoulder. The brachial plexus nerve branches connect the muscles and skin of upper limbs and part of the chest muscles. The brachial plexus facilitates movement and sensory signals from the spinal cord to the arms and hands. Brachial plexus injuries lead to pain, numbness and weakness in the arms and hands.

BAQ: Write a short note on the lumbar plexus.

Ans: The lumbar plexus is formed by the ventral primary rami of L1–L4 roots that pass through the posterior psoas muscle and anterior to the L2–L5 transverse processes. The lumbar plexus is responsible for innervating the bladder and the lower extremities. The nerves of the lumbar plexus are responsible for the functioning of the lower extremity and to maintain the ability to extend the knee, adduct the thigh, flex the hip, etc. The damage to lumbar plexus due to trauma or clinical condition may lead to numbness, feeling of tingling (paresthesia), low back pain and leg pain caused due to the damage to the lumbar nerves.

BAQ: Write a short note on the sacral plexus.

Ans: The sacral plexus is formed by combining of the anterior rami of lumbar spinal nerves L4 and L5 and the anterior rami of the sacral spinal nerves S1–S4. The sacral plexus provides motor and sensory nerves to the part of pelvis, posterior part of the thigh, lower legs, and the feet. Damage to the sacral spine due to trauma or a clinical condition may lead to loss of some movements of the legs and hips. The sacral cord injury may affect bladder control or bowel control.

BAQ: Write a short note on the coccygeal plexus.

Ans: The coccygeal plexus is formed in the pelvis by the following three nerve roots: The first coccygeal nerve, the fourth and fifth sacral nerves. The nerves from the coccygeal plexus connect the skin around the coccyx and anal area.

Damage to coccygeal plexus due to injury or a clinical condition may cause severe localized pain in the tailbone area. The pain is severe while sitting for prolonged periods of time. Similarly, straining and bowel movements are often painful.

Blood Supply of the Spinal Cord

BAQ: Write a note on the blood supply of the spinal cord.

Ans: Three arteries supply blood to the spinal cord. The three longitudinal arteries are the anterior spinal artery, and the right and left posterior spinal arteries. These travel in the subarachnoid space and send branches into the spinal cord. They form connections through the anterior and posterior segmental medullary arteries, which enter the spinal cord at various points along its length (Fig. 6.26).

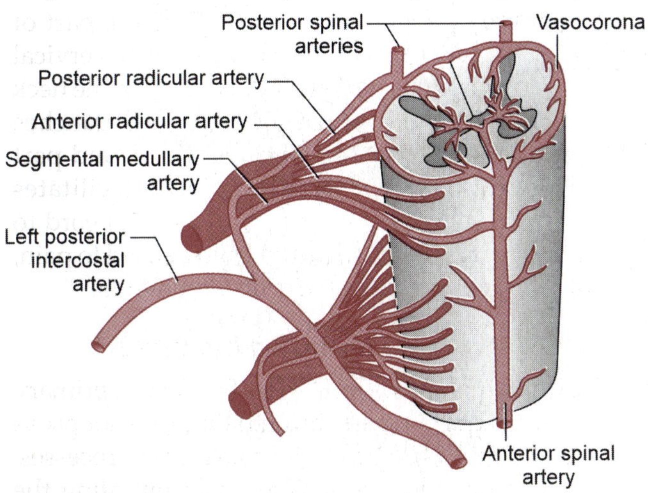

Fig. 6.26: Blood supply of the spinal cord

Objective: To discuss and describe the organization of the peripheral nervous system and related functions.

PERIPHERAL NERVOUS SYSTEM (PNS)

(Figs 6.1, 6.2 and 6.27)

BAQ: Write a brief note on the peripheral nervous system (PNS).

Ans: The peripheral nervous system (PNS) consists of the nerves and ganglia outside the brain and spinal cord. Peripheral nervous system (PNS) includes all the nerves that branch out from the CNS components, that means from brain and spinal cord and extend to all other parts of the body. PNS extends to the skin, the muscles, the glands, and the sense organs. Most of the PNS nerves are composed of mixed nerves containing motor and sensory nerves. The CNS is protected by the skull and the vertebrae of the spine, however, the nerves, and cells of the PNS are not enclosed by bones. Hence, the PNS is more susceptible to the traumatic damages.

The PNS relay information between brain and the rest of the parts of the body. For example, the sense organs are able to detect changes in the environment and relay information through the sensory nerves to the CNS. The brain then sends signals through the nerves to the muscles, resulting in the muscles to move in response.

The main functions of the PNS are the conduction of the voluntary movements. When an action is produced with the involvement of thoughts, they are called voluntary actions. The voluntary actions initiate walking, running, jumping, eating, etc. These actions are produced consciously. The PNS also regulates the unconscious body behaviours, i.e. autonomic functions such as breathing, digestion, and pumping action of the heart by beating.

The PNS is divided into the somatic nervous system and the autonomic nervous system. The somatic nervous system (SNS) and the autonomic nervous system (ANS) are both part of the peripheral nervous system. The SNS controls voluntary actions such as talking, walking, jumping, running, etc. The ANS is responsible for the control of vital functions such as breathing and heart beating. ANS is also involved in the acute stress response. In acute stress it works in association with the endocrine system to prepare the body to fight or flight.

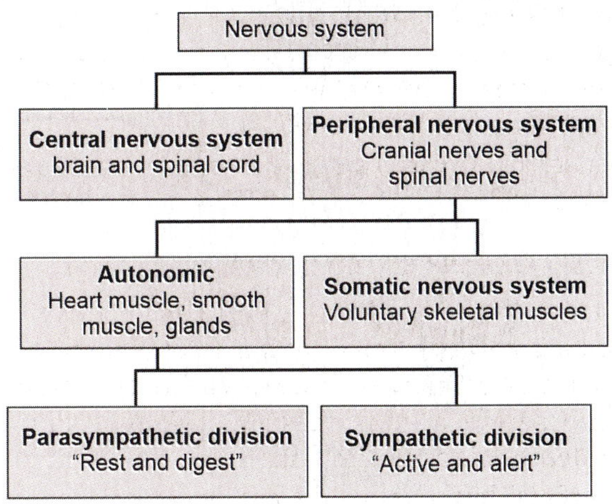

Fig. 6.27: Main divisions of the nervous system

SOMATIC NERVOUS SYSTEM (Fig. 6.27)

BAQ: Write a note on the somatic nervous system.

Ans: The somatic nervous system controls voluntary or conscious activities. It is involved in the relay of sensory and motor information to and from the CNS. The somatic nervous system is also responsible for the reflexes, which are involuntary muscle responses.

Somatic nervous system consists of motor neurons and sensory neurons. Sensory neurons are also known as afferent neurons. They send information to the CNS from the skin, muscles, glands or from the external stimuli through touch, sound, light and heat. For example, when a hot surface is touched, this information is transmitted through the sensory neurons to the brain. The brain then sends signals through motor neurons to move hand away from the hot surface by the reflux action. The motor neurons are also known as efferent neurons. They transmit signals from the CNS to the muscles to control muscle movements. Motor neurons act in response to external stimuli.

AUTONOMIC NERVOUS SYSTEM (ANS) (Fig. 6.28)

BAQ: Write a note on the autonomic nervous system (ANS).

Ans: The autonomic nervous system (ANS) consists of components within the CNS and specific nerves. The autonomic nervous system is further divided into two components: (1) Parasympathetic nervous system and (2) sympathetic nervous system.

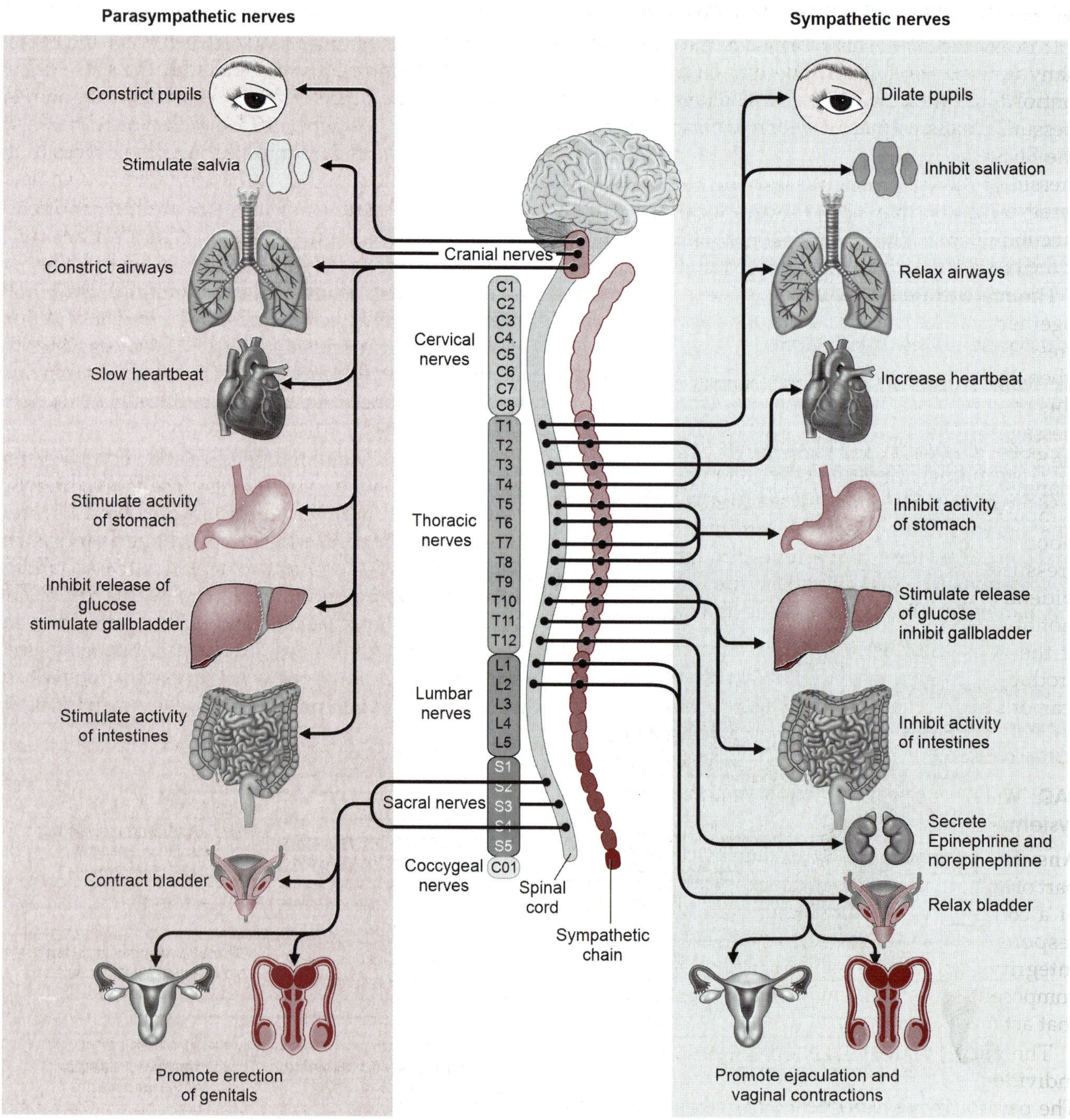

Fig. 6.28: Parasympathetic and sympathetic nerves

The autonomic nervous system is responsible for the coordinating involuntary behaviours such as breathing, beating of heart and digestion. These important functions take place without conscious thoughts and they work automatically.

SYMPATHETIC NERVOUS SYSTEM (SNS) (Fig. 6.24)

BAQ: Write a note on the sympathetic nervous system (SNS).

Ans: The sympathetic nervous system is a part of autonomic nervous system (ANS).

It is comprised of a complex network of neuronal pathways that is responsible for the maintenance of the physiologic integrity of cells, tissues and organs tissues. PNS is composed of pre-ganglionic and post-ganglionic neurons that act on effector organs.

It is an automatic nervous system as it facilitates many functions for which thinking is not required to control a specific body action such as the control of blood pressure, digestion, heart rate, sweating, urination, etc. The SNS plays very important role in responding to stressful and dangerous situations. The sympathetic and parasympathetic nervous systems have complementary functions, operating in tandem to maintain homeostasis of the body.

The actions of the sympathetic nervous system occur together with other neural or hormonal responses to stress. The sympathetic nervous system comes into play when the body needs to respond to threatening stimuli. This response is called the fight-or-flight response and messages in the form of nerve impulses travel through the SNS in a bidirectional flow. Efferent messages trigger changes in different parts of the body simultaneously. Sympathetic nervous system responds by constricting blood vessels, accelerating heart rate, raising blood pressure. These give rise to initiation of sweating, widening of the bronchial passages, decrease in the motility of large intestine, dilation of pupils, activation of the goose bumps, means a roughness of the skin produced by erection of its papillae, mainly from cold, fear, or a sudden feeling of excitement.

Parasympathetic Nervous System (PNS) (Fig. 6.24)

BAQ: Write a note on the parasympathetic nervous system.

Ans: The parasympathetic nervous system (PNS) is a part of autonomic nervous system (ANS). It is comprised of a complex network of neuronal pathways that is responsible for the maintenance of the physiologic integrity of cells, tissues and organs tissues. PNS is composed of pre-ganglionic and post-ganglionic neurons that act on effector organs.

The parasympathetic nervous system relaxes the individual once the stress related emergency has passed. The parasympathetic system aims to maintain normal bodily functions by decreasing activities related to stress. The PNS helps to reach a state of rest. The sympathetic and parasympathetic systems have complementary functions, operating in tandem to maintain homeostasis of the body.

Sensory Nerves (Afferent Nerves)

SAQ: Write a brief note on the sensory nerves (afferent nerves).

Ans: The sensory nerves (afferent nerves) carry sensory information toward the central nervous system (CNS) from different sensory receptors of sensory neurons in the peripheral nervous system present in the skin, muscles, tendons, joints, etc.

The sensory nerves of the skin: The skin is mainly innervated by the sensory nerve fibers that contain highly specialized sensory receptors. These receptors detect and respond to the physical and chemical stimuli in the environment. The skin receives stimuli from the external environment by various actions such as touch, pressure, pain, stretch, temperature changes, etc. This sensory information received through the specific stimuli are relayed to the central nervous system.

The sensory nerve fibers also innervate the internal skin structures such as the eccrine sweat glands, the apocrine sweat glands, sebaceous glands, arrector pili muscles, and arterioles. Autonomic input induces actions like thermoregulation (such as vasodilation and sweat production) and "goosebumps" (bumps at the base of the body hair) brought about by the contraction of the arrector pili muscles.

The nerves of the skin form a branching plexus in the deeper layers of the skin. In these deep layers, the sensory receptors and innervated structures such as the hair follicle and glands are found. Smaller nerve fibers extend further through the dermis to the papillary layer and form a papillary and a variety of plexus receptors are found there. Sensory receptors such as the free nerve endings terminate in the epidermis.

Functions of cevical sensory nerves:

- C2—is responsible for sensation at the back of the head.
- C3—is responsible for sensation at the scalp area and the sides of the face.
- C4—this is one of the nerves that controls the diaphragm, as well as giving motor control over some shoulder movement.

Motor Nerves (Efferent Nerves)

SAQ: Write a brief note on the motor nerves (efferent nerves)

Ans: The motor neurons (efferent neurons) are located in the motor cortex, brainstem, the spinal cord, and outside the spinal cord to control mainly muscles and glands. The following are the two types of motor neurons: (1) Upper motor neurons and (2) lower motor neurons.

Upper Motor Neurons

The upper motor neuron cell bodies are present in the primary motor area of the cerebrum. The axons of the cell bodies pass through the pons and medulla oblongata and in the spinal cord they form the lateral corticospinal tracks of the white matter (Fig. 6.29). The fibers of synapse in the upper motor neurons connect with the cell bodies of the lower motor neurons in the grey matter. The axons from the lower motor neurons carry signals from the spinal cord to the efferent neurons. The axons of the upper neurons cross each other and form a pyramid in the medulla oblongata.

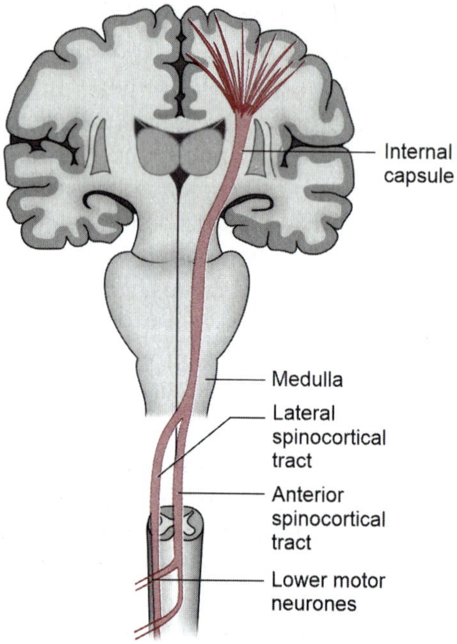

Fig. 6.29A: Lateral corticospinal tracks

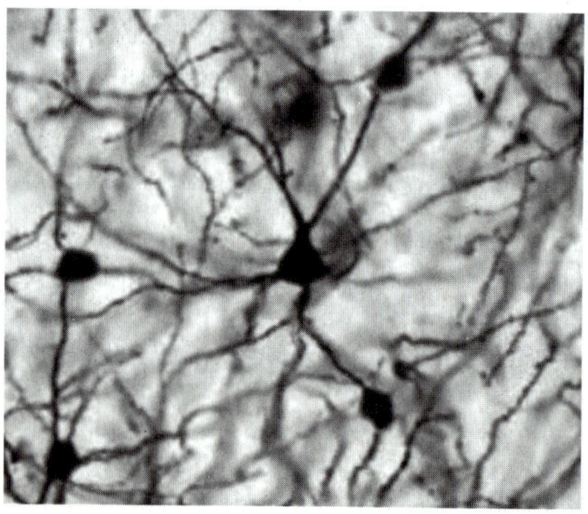

Fig. 6.29B: Pyramidal neurons of upper motor neurons

Upper Body Neuron Functions

The upper body neurons are involved in the spinal cord reflexes and stretch reflexes.

A reflex occurs through the neural pathways in the nervous system called reflex arcs.

The upper body neurons influence the muscles that help to maintain body balance and posture, muscle tension (tone) and coordinate muscle movements.

Lower Motor Neurons

The lower motor neurons represent the final common pathway for the transmission of nerve impulses to skeletal muscles. The cell bodies of lower motor neurons are controlled by the upper motor neurons that originate in the various parts of the brain and some neurons in the spinal cord, which either stimulate or inhibit the lower motor neurons.

> ***Note:*** Pyramidal neurons are the primary excitation cell types in the corticospinal tract. These are found in the various areas of the brain including the cerebral cortex, the hippocampus, and the amygdala. Pyramidal neurons in the prefrontal cortex are involved in the cognitive ability.

> **Objective:** To discuss the organization and the functions of the reflex arc.

BAQ: Write a note on the reflexes.

Ans: A reflex is an involuntary or automatic, action that a body part in response to a specific stimulus or a situation. A reflex occurs through the neural pathways in the nervous system called reflex arcs. In the neural pathways, a sudden stimulus initiates a neural signal, which is carried to a synapse. The signal is then transferred across the synapse to a motor neuron, which produces a specific response. These neural signals do not always pass to the brain. Hence, many reflexes are an automatic response to a stimulus that does not receive or need conscious thought.

The reflexes can be spinal cord reflexes, stretch body reflexes or autonomous reflexes.

The spinal cord reflexes involve sensory neurons, neurons in the spinal cord and lower body neurons. In the stretch body reflexes, the cell body of the lower motor neurons is directed simultaneously by the sensory neurons, without the involvement of the interneurons. The knee jerk is an example of stretch body reflex. To test the integrity of the reflex arc, knee jerk test is used (Fig. 6.30).

When a knee is bent and when a tendon is tapped below it, the sensory nerve endings in the tendon and in the thigh muscles get stretched. This creates a nerve impulse, that passes to the spinal cord. From the spinal cord, the nerve impulse passes to the cell body of the lower motor neuron in the anterior part of the grey matter on the same side of the body. The thigh muscles suddenly contract and the foot kicks in forward direction. This type of reflex prevents very fast joint movement and protect the muscles, ligaments and tendons from the damage, that may occur due to very fast actions.

Autonomic reflexes take place suddenly to protect a specific part of a body. For example, blinking action of eyes, in response to very bright light and also the closing of eyes to prevent entry of dust particles in a storm. Similarly, the action like taking a hand away from a very hot surface.

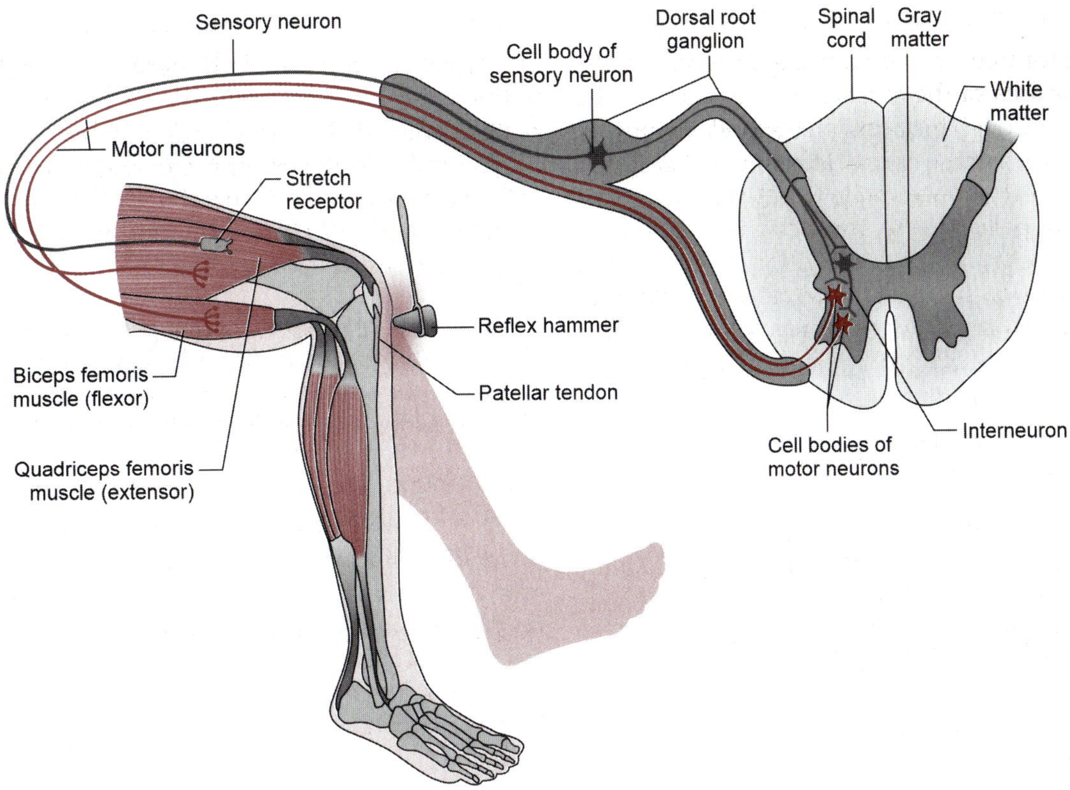

Fig. 6.30: Reflex reaction

BAQ: Write a note on a reflex arc.

Ans: A reflex arc is a neurological and sensory mechanism that controls the reflexes as an immediate response to specific particular stimuli. The reflex arcs are important mainly to maintain a balanced and stable position of the body parts. The following are the primary components of the reflex arc: (1) Receptors located within the skin, (2) the sensory neurons that receive stimulation and pass it to other nerve cells, (3) the center is an axon of an sensory neuron with associated neuron, (4) motor neuron at the synapse of the associated neuron, and (5) effectors, which are the effector muscle cells that perform the reflex action.

Example of an reflex arc: Accidently touching of a hot plate stimulates the pain receptors of the skin. The pain receptors initiate an impulse in a sensory neuron. The impulse produced travels to the spinal cord where it passes, by means of a synapse, to a relay neuron situated in the spinal cord and a person realises the damage made to the skin of the hand by the hot plate and a prompt action is taken to move the hand away from the hot plate to prevent further damage to the skin of the hand.

BAQ: What is a three-neuron arc? Give example.

Ans: Three-neuron arc is mainly consists of the following components: (1) A receptor, (2) an interneuron (or adjustor), and (3) a motor neuron unit. Three neurons together form a functional group. Sensory cells carry afferent impulses from the receptor to a central interneuron, which makes contact with a motor neuron. The motor neuron carries efferent impulses to the specific part of the body (effector), which produces the response. Most reflex arcs involve only three neurons. The following is an example of functioning a three neuron arc: A needle stick stimulates the pain receptors of the skin. The pain receptors initiate an impulse in a sensory neuron. The impulse produced travels to the spinal cord where it passes, by means of a synapse, to a relay neuron situated in the spinal cord and a person realises the damage made by a needle stick and takes a prompt action to prevent further complications.

BAQ: What is a two-neuron arc? Give example.

Ans: In a two-neuron arc, simple reflexes are automatic, prompt and short-lived and involve only a part of the body. Example of a simple reflex is the blink of an eye in response to very bright light, contraction of a muscle in response to stretching and saliva production in mouth at the sight of food. Reflexes of these types are usually involved in to maintain homeostasis.

BAQ: Write a note on somatic and autonomic reflex arcs.

Ans: The following two types of reflex arcs are observed: 1. Somatic reflex arc, that affect muscles, 2. autonomic reflex arc, that affect inner organs.

Somatic reflexes involve skeletal muscles and are voluntary, while autonomic reflexes involve smooth muscle, cardiac muscle, and glands and are involuntary. Autonomic reflexes may involve the spinal cord and some somatic reflexes may be mediated by the brain rather than the spinal cord.

BAQ. Give an example of somatic reflux.

Ans: The following is an example of pathway of nerve signals during a somatic reflux:

Stimulus → Sensory receptors → Sensory neuron → Spinal cord → Motor neuron → Muscles → Response

1. A specific stimulus activates somatic receptors in the skin, muscles or tendons.
2. Afferent nerve fibers present in these body parts carry signals from the somatic receptors to the posterior horn of the spinal cord or to the brainstem.
3. Efferent nerve fibers carry motor nerve signals from the anterior horn to the muscles
4. Innervated effector muscle by the efferent nerve fibers carries out the response.

SAQ. Enumerate the components in a reflex arc.

Ans: The following are the components of a typical reflex arc:

(1) Receptor (located within the skin), (2) sensory neuron, (3) center (in the spinal cord in the gray matter, (4) motor neuron, (5) effector (muscle or gland).

BAQ: Draw a neat labelled diagram of a reflux arc.

Ans: Refer to Fig. 6.31.

BAQ: What are monosynaptic reflexes and poly-synaptic reflexes?

Ans: The monosynaptic reflex arc takes place without the involvement of an associated neuron. Example of a monosynaptic reflex is knee-jerk reflex.

When a patellar ligament is tapped, stretching of quadriceps femoris muscle takes place, leading to nerve impulse provocation. The nerve impulses are conducted along the sensory neurons to the spinal cord. The sensory neuron synapses with a motor neuron, leading to the contraction of the quadriceps femoris muscle.

The polysynaptic reflex arc takes place with more than one associated neurons. An example of polysynaptic reflex arc is the withdrawal reflex.

When a hot article is touched, it stimulates sensory receptors of the skin. The sensory receptors initiate an impulse. The impulse produced travels to the spinal cord where it passes by means of a synapse to a relay neuron situated in the spinal cord and two or more neurons are stimulated. The stimulated neuron generates nerve impulse to a motor neuron. The motor neuron initiates a response by a withdrawal action of the hand away from the hot article.

A person realises the damage made to the skin of the hand by the hot plate and a prompt action is taken to move the hand away from the hot plate to prevent further damage to the skin of the hand.

SAQ: Name the cranial nerves that innervate the eyes for eyeball movements.

Ans: The following six extrinsic eye muscles control the movements of the eyeballs: The superior, inferior and medial recti muscles and the inferior oblique muscle are innervated by the oculomotor nerve. The lateral rectus muscle is innervated by the abducens nerve and the superior oblique muscle is innervated by the trochlear nerve.

BAQ: Which are the most important cranial nerves involved in the dental practice?

Ans: The study of paired trigeminal nerves is important for the education of the dentists. These nerves convey sensory information from the teeth, jaw, tongue, nasal area and face to the brain. These nerves also provide motor innervation for the process of mastication to the gums and teeth of the lower jaw, major part of the tongue, mouth mucosa, lower part of the face, and ear auricle. The mandibular nerve also provides motor innervation to the muscle meant for the process of mastication. The maxillary nerve provides sensory innervation to the inferior mucosa of the nasal cavity, teeth, gums, palate and part of the pharynx. The ophthalmic nerve provides sensory innervation to the upper mucosa of the nasal cavity, tear glands, and skin of the upper eyelids.

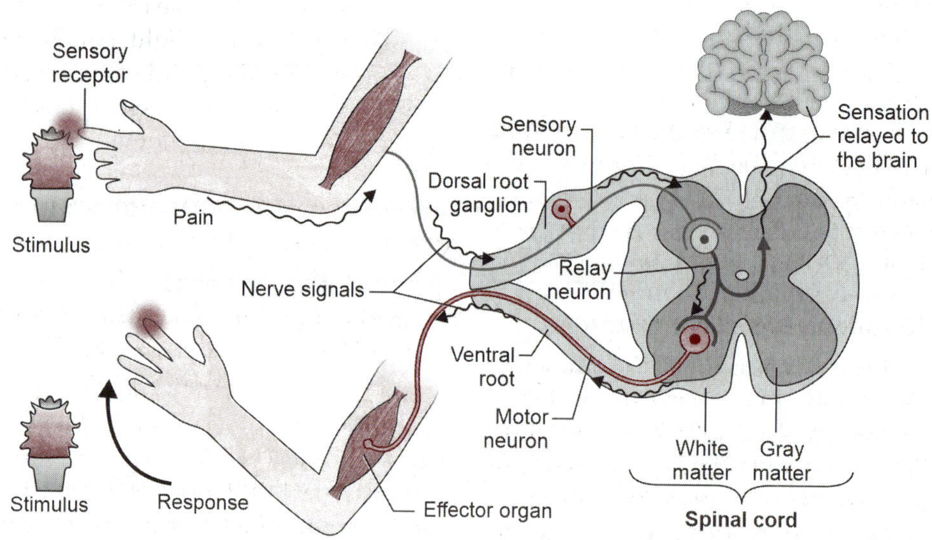

Fig. 6.31: Reflex arc

BAQ: Explain the use of anesthetic injections in the dental practice.

Ans: The inferior alveolar nerve originating from the mandibular branch of the trigeminal nerve contribute to the sensory innervation to the mouth and face. It is desensitised by the anesthetic injection prior to extraction or filling of a specific tooth. The alveolar nerve branches into the mental nerve. An anestetic injection near the mental nerve desensitizes the lower incisor teeth. The teeth in the upper jaw could be desensitised by an anestetic injection near the sphenopalatine ganglion, that blocks a maxillary nerve.

SAQ: Describe the distribution and functions of the vagus nerve.

Ans: The paired vagus nerves are the main autonomic nerves that innervate the visceral organs. These regulate glandular secretions and peristalsis. The vagos nerves are able to convey sensations of hunger, laryngeal movements, abdominal discomfort and abdominal distension.

Objective: To discuss the clinical conditions related to the spinal cord injury.

Spinal Cord Injury

SAQ: Write consequences related to the spinal cord injury.

Ans: The spinal cord injuries can be caused by trauma to the spinal column due to various activities such as stretching, bruising, laceration, falling on the back, etc. The spinal cord may get damaged in accidents. The vertebral bones or intervertebral disks can shatter, causing the spinal cord to become punctured by a sharp fragment of bone. Usually, the victims of the spinal cord injuries suffer from the loss of feeling in certain parts of their body. In milder cases, a victim might only suffer loss of hand or foot function. Severe spinal injuries may result in paraplegia, tetraplegia (quadriplegia), or full body paralysis below the site of injury to the spinal cord.

Meninges (Fig. 6.32)

BAQ: Write a note on the meninges.

Ans: The brain is situated inside the cranium, a bony covering, which protects the brain from injury. The meninges are present between the skull and brain. The meninges consist of three layers of tissue that cover and protect the brain and spinal cord. These layers are as follows: The outermost layer, the dura mater followed by arachnoid and pia mater layers (Fig. 6.32).

The dura mater is made up of two layers of whitish, nonelastic membrane. The outer layer is called the periosteum. An inner layer is called the dura, which lines the inside of the entire skull. The two folds of the dura in the brain are called the falx and the tentorium.

Arachnoid membrane layer is thin and delicate and covers the entire brain. A space between the dura and the arachnoid membranes is called the subdural space. The arachnoid is made up of a delicate elastic tissue and blood vessels.

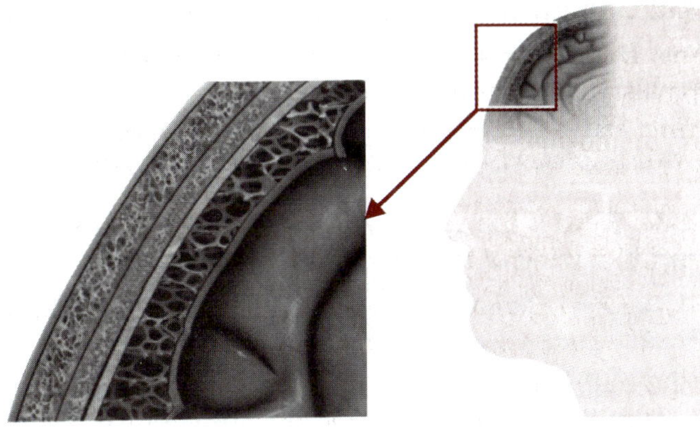

Fig. 6.32: Meninges

The pia mater has many blood vessels that are seen deep in the surface of the brain. The pia membrane covers the entire surface of the brain. The major arteries of the brain provide blood supply to the pia membrane. The space between the arachnoid mater and the pia mater is called the subarachnoid space. The cerebrospinal fluid (CSF) flows within the subarachnoid space. The function of CSF is to protect the optic nerve and the brain from mechanical damage and provide nutrition for to the neurons and remove of toxic metabolites formed in the cellular metabolism.

Objective: To discuss the composition and functions of the cerebrospinal fluid (CSF).

Cerebrospinal Fluid (CSF)

SAQ: What is cerebrospinal fluid?

Ans: The cerebrospinal fluid (CSF) is formed by selective dialysis of plasma by the choroid plexus of the ventricles of the brain. Through the foramina in the fourth ventricle, it then passes into subarachnoidal cisterns at the base of the brain and travels over the surfaces of the cerebral hemispheres. It is finally absorbed into the blood in the cerebral veins and dural sinuses. CSF is present in the cavity that surrounds the brain in the skull and the spinal cord in the spinal column. The volume of CSF (adults) is about 150 ml.

SAQ: Enumerate the functions of CSF.

Ans: CSF performs the following functions.

1. It helps to protect the brain and spinal cord from injury by acting like a fluid buffer.
2. It also acts as a medium for the transfer of substances from the brain tissue and spinal cord to blood.
3 It maintains intracranial pressure.

Normal Composition of CSF

BAQ: Describe the normal composition of CSF.

Ans: It is colourless and clear fluid. pH of CSF is 7.3–7.4 and specific gravity is 1.003–1.008. Protein content of

CSF is 15–45 mg/dl. Glucose content is 40–80 mg/dl and chloride content is 700–750 mg/dl. It also contains minute quantities of urea, uric acid, creatinine and cholesterol. CSF contains few lymphocytes only. Other white blood cells and red blood are not present.

BAQ: What is the clinical significance of routine CSF test in a clinical laboratory?

Ans: CSF examination is carried out in the laboratory mainly for the diagnosis of meningitis. It is inflammation of the meninges, the lining of the skull, and the covering of the brain and spinal column. Meningitis causes disturbance in the central nervous system. The other clinical conditions in which CSF examination may be required are encephalitis, subarachnoid hemorrhage, spinal cord tumor, multiple sclerosis, central nervous system syphilis, etc. CSF examination is also carried out in the treatments of elevated CSF pressure in selected patients with benign intracranial hypertension.

Ventricular System (Fig. 6.33)

BAQ: Write a note on the ventricular system of the brain.

Ans: The ventricular system is formed of four cavities called ventricles, which are connected by a series of holes, called foramen, and tubes. First and second ventricles enclosed in the cerebral hemispheres are called the lateral ventricles. They communicate with the third ventricle through an opening called the foramen of Munro. The third ventricle is in the center of the brain. It connects with the fourth ventricle through a long tube called the aqueduct of Sylvius. CSF flowing through the fourth ventricle, further flows around the brain and the spinal cord.

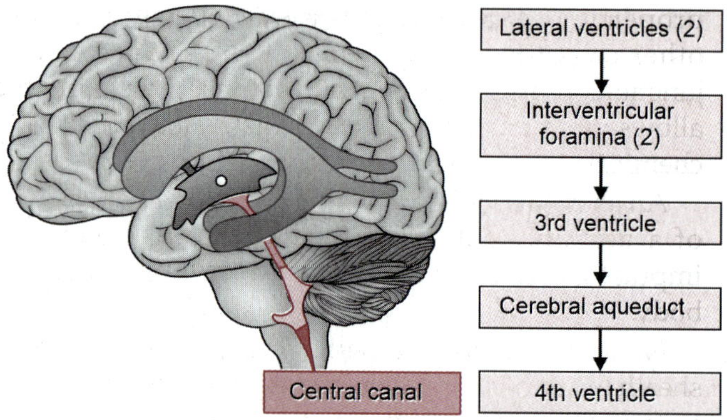

Fig. 6.33: Ventricular system of the brain

Objectives: To describe the anatomical features of the nerves.

NERVE STRUCTURE

LAQ: Write a note on the nerves.

Ans: The nerves are cylindrical bundles of fibers that flow from the brain and central cord, and branch to reach every part of the body. A microscopic examination shows that nerves consist primarily of the axons of neurons, along with a membranes in which these are wrapped. The cell bodies of neurons reside within the brain, central cord, or peripheral ganglia.

Neuron Anatomy (Fig. 6.34)

The basic structure of a neuron can be observed under a microscope. The basic structural components of an average neuron include the following components: The dendrite, cell body, nucleus, node of Ranvier, myelin sheath, Schwann cell, axon and axon terminal.

A dendrite is a branch-like structure, where a neuron receives input from other cells. Most fundamental

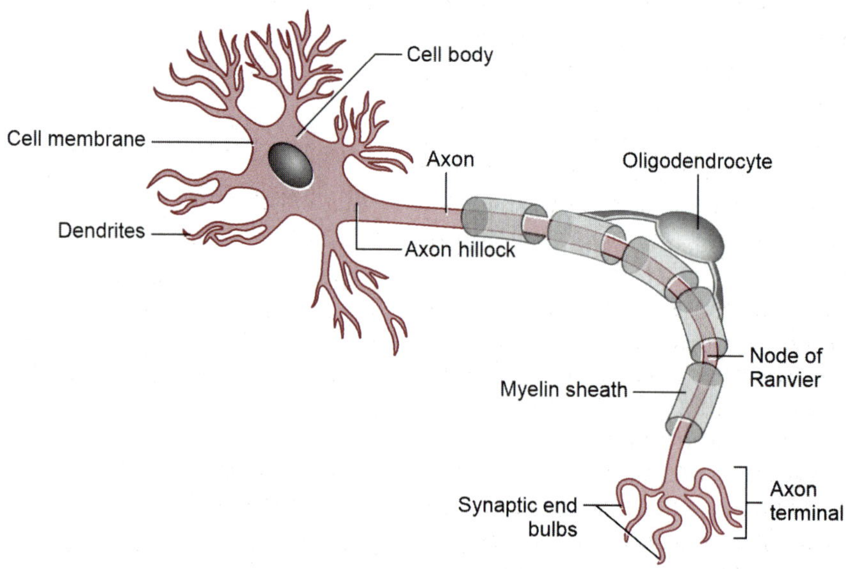

Fig. 6.34: Anatomical feature of a neuron

property of neuron is that they communicate with other cells through synapses (Fig. 6.33), which are junctions containing s specific molecular structure that allows rapid transmission of signals, either electrical or chemical.

An axon (nerve fiber) is a slender and long projection of a neuron. Axon specifically conducts electrical impulses (action potentials), away from the nerve cell body.

Node of Ranvier is a periodic gap in the insulating sheath (myelin) on the axon of certain neurons that serves to facilitate the rapid conduction of nerve impulses. Nodes of Ranvier expose the neuron membrane to the external environment.

Myelin sheaths are covers of fatty tissue that cover and protect nerve cells.

Schwann cells (SCs) are the main glial cells of the peripheral nervous system. SCs wrap around axons of motor and sensory neurons to form the myelin sheath.

SAQ: What are dermatomes? What is the importance of dermatomes?

Ans: A dermatome is a specific area of the skin, innervated by the specific cranial nerves and spinal nerves. Dysfunction of dermatomes provide information about the injury to specific spinal nerve or spinal cord. The pattern of dermatome innervation also provides information on the anesthetising of specific area of the body.

Objective: To describe and discuss various neurotransmitters and their functions.

NEUROTRANSMITTERS

LAQ: Write a note on neurotransmitters.

Ans: Neurotransmitters are chemical messengers secreted by neurons. These help sensory and motor nerve cells (neurons) to communicate with each other to carry out sympathetic and parasympathetic nervous system functions. These functions are regulation of blood pressure, heartbeat, breathing, muscle movements, digestion, thinking, learning, memorising, hormone regulation, response to senses and stress, sleep patterns, etc.

The most neurotransmitters are synthesized from simple precursors such as amino acids. Examples of most common neurotransmitters are acetylcholine, gamma-amino butyric acid (GABA), dopamine, serotonin, norepinephrine and glutamate. Dopamines are synthesized from the amino acid tyrosine. Serotonin is synthesized from the amino acid tryptophan. Acetyl choline is synthesized from choline. Glutamate is a nonessential amino acid and GABA is synthesized from glutamate.

Neurotransmitters are generally stored in the synaptic vesicles. These are accumulated close to the cell membrane at the axon terminal of the presynaptic neuron (Fig. 6.33). Generally, a neurotransmitter is released at the presynaptic terminal in response to an electrical signal called an action potential in the presynaptic neuron. Neurotransmitters are then released and diffuse across the synaptic cleft, where they bind to specific receptors on the membrane of the postsynaptic neuron. The effect of neurotransmitter effect on the target cell is determined by the specific receptor on the postsynaptic neuron. Depending on the receptor, binding of neurotransmitters may cause excitation, inhibition, or modulation of the postsynaptic neuron.

Neurotransmitter influences trans-membrane ion flow either to increase (excitatory) or to decrease (inhibitory) the probability that the cell with which it comes in contact will produce an action potential. Glutamate is an excitatory neurotransmitter.

The levels of neurotransmitters may get disturbed in various clinical conditions. Acetylcholine imbalance is associated with Alzheimer's disease and myasthenia gravis). Dopamine deficiency is observed in Parkinson's disease, Increased levels of glutamate and GABA are associated with epilepsy and seizures, and serotonin imbalance is associated with depression episodes.

SAQ: Write a short note on the roles of glutamate neurotransmitter.

Ans: Glutamate is used at the great majority of fast excitatory synapses in the brain and spinal cord. Excessive glutamate release can overstimulate the brain and lead to excitotoxicity causing cell death resulting in seizures or strokes. Excitotoxicity has been associated with many clinical conditions such as stroke, epilepsy, ischemic stroke, epilepsy, Parkinson's disease Alzheimer's disease and Huntington disease.

SAQ: Write a short note on the roles of GABA neurotransmitter.

Ans: GABA is used at the great majority of fast inhibitory synapses in practically every region of the brain. Many sedative drugs act by increasing the effects of GABA.

SAQ: Write a short note on the roles of acetylcholine neurotransmitter.

Ans: Acetylcholine activates skeletal muscles in the somatic nervous system by either excitatory or inhibitory actions in the autonomic system. It is a transmitter at the neuromuscular junction that connects motor nerves to muscles.

SAQ: Write a short note on the roles of dopamine neurotransmitter.

Ans: Dopamine functions in the brain include, regulation of motor behaviour, pleasures related to motivation and also elevation of emotions. Deficiency of dopamine leads to the Parkinson's disease and high levels of dopamine may lead to schizophrenia.

SAQ: Write a short note on the roles of serotonin neurotransmitter.

Ans: Serotonin is produced in the intestine and the part of it is present in central nervous system neurons. It functions to regulate sleep, learning, behaviour, memory, moods, appetite, temperature, muscle contraction regulation of the endocrine system and cardiovascular system. Low concentrations of serotonin are associated with depression.

Objective: To describe the nerve physiology.

NEURON PHYSIOLOGY

SAQ: What is an action potential (nerve impulse)? What is the importance of an action potential?

Ans: An action potential (nerve impulse) is a short-lasting event in which the electrical membrane potential of a cell rapidly rises and falls (Figs 6.36 and 6.37). In neurons, they play important role in cell-to-cell communication.

Importance of an Nerve Impulse

Sensory neurons transmit nerve impulses from sense organs to the brain. After receiving signals from sense organs, motor neurons from the brain and spinal cord transmit nerve impulses to a specific targeted area of the body for further related action.

BAQ: Describe the mechanism of transmission of an action potential.

Ans: Sensory neurons transmit nerve impulses from sense organs such as skin, eyes, ears, nose, and tongue to the brain. After receiving signals from sense organs, motor neurons from the brain and spinal cord transmit nerve impulses to a specific targeted area of the body for further related action.

Neurotransmitters stored in synaptic knobs, transmit messages from one neuron to another neuron. The nerve impulse travels from the first nerve cell through the axon to the axon terminal and the synaptic knobs. Each synaptic knob communicates with a dendrite or cell body of another neuron. The synapse lies between the synaptic knob and the next cell (Fig. 6.35). For the impulse to continue traveling across the synapse to reach the next cell, the synaptic knobs release the neurotransmitter into that space, and the next nerve cell is stimulated to pick up the impulse and continue it in a structure called the postsynaptic membrane of another nearby neuron. Once the neurotransmitter is picked up by receptors in the postsynaptic membrane, the neurotransmitter is internalized in the neuron and the impulse continues. This process of nerve cell communication is extremely rapid and takes less than a thousandth of a second.

Thus, the nerve impulse ultimately reaches the specific target muscle and a specific action related to touch, smell, noise, heat, etc. is executed.

SAQ: What are the consequences of defective flow of neurotransmitters?

Ans: Once the neurotransmitter is released from the neurotransmitter vesicles of the presynaptic membrane, the normal movement of molecules should be directed to receptor sites located on the postsynaptic membrane. In certain diseases, the flow of the neurotransmitter is defective. For example, in depression, the flow of the inhibitory neurotransmitter serotonin is defective, and molecules flow back to their originating site (the presynaptic membrane) instead of to receptors on the postsynaptic membrane meant to transmit the impulse to a nearby neuron.

Objective: To define and describe action potential (nerve impulse), synapse and synaptic transmission.

Action Potentials (Nerve Impulses)

BAQ: Write a note on action potentials (nerve impulses)

Ans: Nerve impulse or an action potential (Figs 6.35 and 6.36) is a short-lasting event in which the electrical

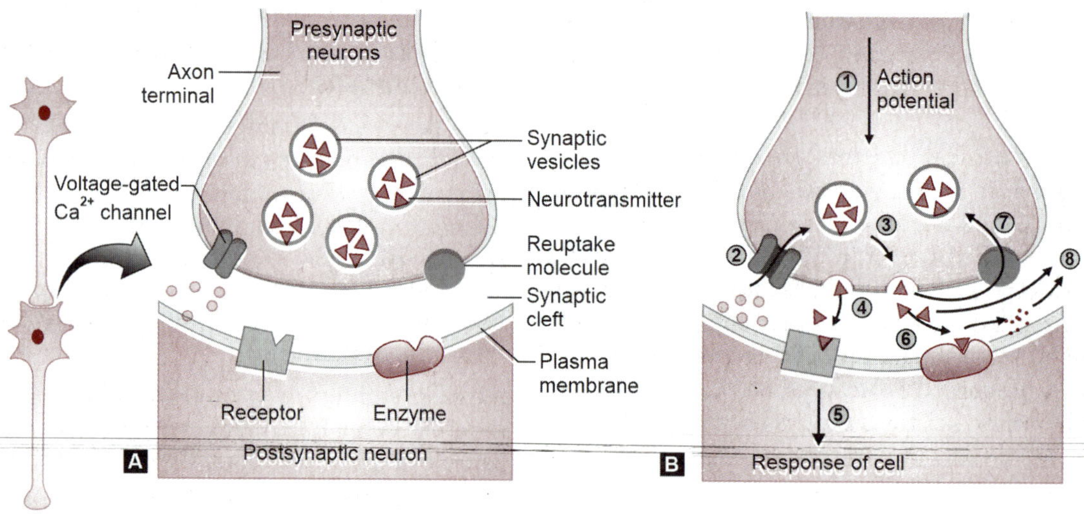

Figs 6.35A and B: (A) Presynaptic neuron (at rest); (B) presynaptic neuron (active)

membrane potential of a cell rapidly rises and falls. In neurons, they play important role in cell-to-cell communication. In other types of cells, their main function is to activate intracellular processes. For example, in muscle cells, an action potential initiates the chain of events leading to muscle contraction. In beta cells of the pancreas, action potential stimulates release of insulin.

Action potentials are generated by special types of voltage-gated ion channels embedded in the plasma membrane of a cell. These channels are shut when the membrane potential is near the resting potential of the cell. However, these channels open due to nerve impulse. This leads to increase in membrane potential to a precisely defined threshold level. When the ion-channels open, they allow an inward flow of sodium ions and outward flow of potassium ions. This event causes more channels to open, producing a greater electric current. The process proceeds explosively until all of the available ion channels are open, resulting in a large upswing in the membrane potential. Once threshold potential is reached, the sodium channels close and sodium ions can no longer enter the neuron, and they are actively transported out of the plasma membrane. Potassium channels are then activated, and there is an inward current of potassium ions, returning the electrochemical gradient to the resting states and prevent an action potential traveling in reverse direction (Fig. 6.36).

Objective: To define and describe resting membrane potential.

SAQ: What is resting membrane potential?

Ans: Neurons have a negative concentration gradient most of the time, meaning there are more positively charged ions outside than inside the cell. This regular state of a negative concentration gradient is called resting membrane potential. During the resting membrane potential there are more sodium ions outside than inside the neuron and more potassium ions inside than outside the neuron. The neuron maintains a fairly consistent negative concentration gradient between –40 to –90 millivolts.

Objective: To describe the chain of events of an action potential.

SAQ: Write briefly on the excitable part of cell membrane.

Ans: Each excitable part of cell membrane has two important levels of membrane potential: The resting potential and the threshold potential. The resting potential is the state the neuronal membrane potential maintained as long as the neuronal cell is not disturbed. The higher value of action potential is called the threshold potential. At the axon hillock of a typical neuron, the resting potential is around –70 millivolts (mV) and the threshold potential is around –55 mV (Fig. 6.37).

Action potentials are triggered when sufficient depolarization causes due to flow of sodium ions inside neuron and the neuron membrane potential increase up to threshold potential level. When an action potential is triggered, the membrane potential abruptly shoots upward reaching as high as +100 mV, then equally abruptly shoots back downward, often ending below the resting level, where it remains for some period of time (Fig. 6.36). In most neurons, the entire process takes place in less than a thousandth of a second.

SAQ: What is depolarisation and repolarization?

Ans: Action potentials are triggered when sodium ions flow inside a neuron, in response to a stimulus

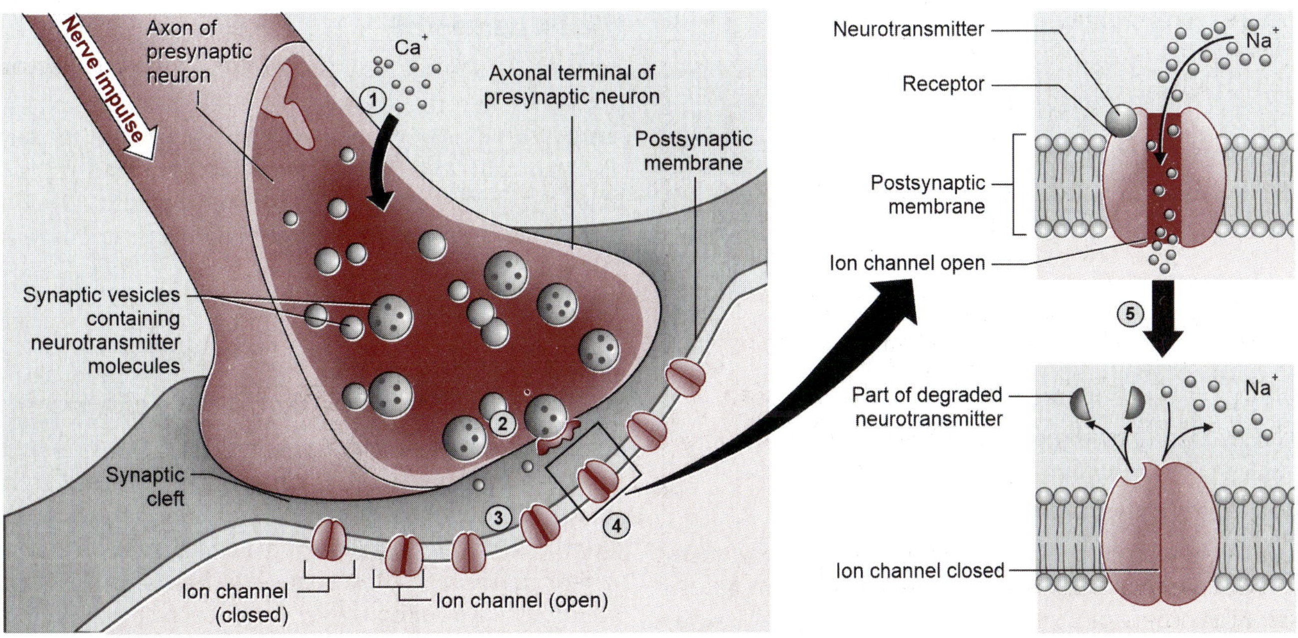

Fig. 6.36: Roles of sodium and potassium ions in initiation of action potential

6 Nervous System

and the neuron membrane potential increase up to threshold potential level. When an action potential is triggered, the membrane potential abruptly shoots upward reaching as high as +100 mV, then equally abruptly shoots back downward, often ending below the resting level, where it remains for some period of time (Fig. 6.37). Repolarization leads the neuron back to resting potential (Fig. 6.38).

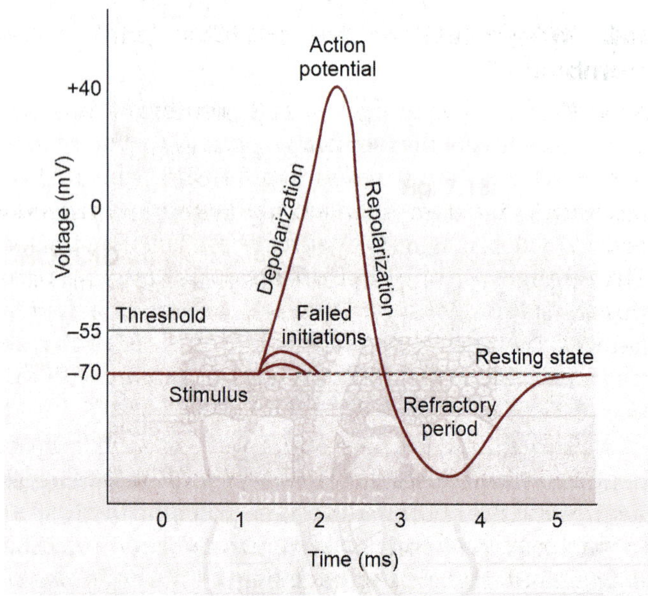

Fig. 6.37: Action potential

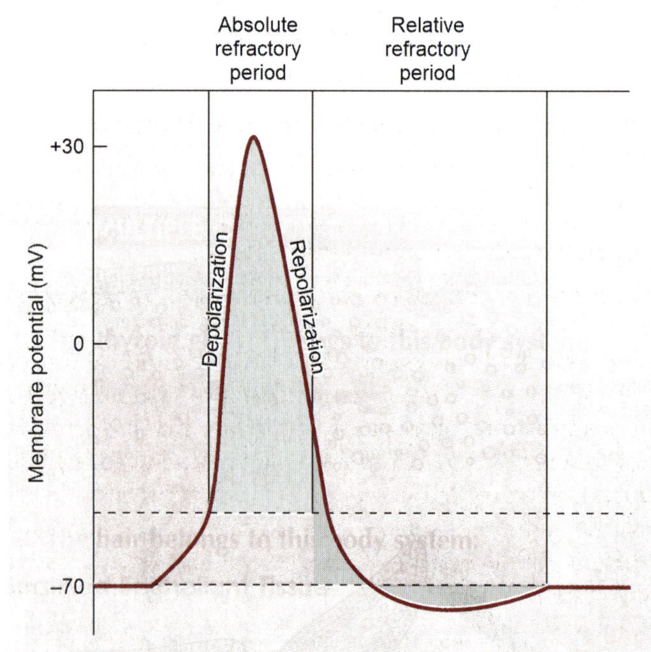

Fig. 6.38: Depolarization and repolarization of neuron membrane

SAQ: What is refractory period?

Ans: A refractory period is the amount of time taken by an excitable membrane to remain ready for a second stimulus once it returns to its resting state following an excitation (Fig. 6.37).

BAQ: Draw a neat labelled diagram of graphical presentation of action potential.

Ans: Refer to Fig. 6.37.

SAQ: Write a brief note on the acetylcholine receptor of a nerve cell.

Ans: The acetylcholine receptor is gated Na^+/K^+ channel. It transitorily opens when acetylcholine binds to it and allows Na^+ to move inside the cell and K^+ out of the cell and the membrane then becomes depolarized. In effect, the nerve impulse moves along the axon by a repeat of the membrane depolarization caused by acetylcholine.

SAQ: What is the action of the venum of Indian cobra on nerve cells?

Ans: The venum of Indian cobra contains a powerful post-synaptic neurotoxin. The toxin acts on the synaptic gaps of the nerves, thereby paralyzing muscles, leading to respiratory failure or cardiac arrest. The venom components include enzymes such as hyaluronidase that cause lysis and increase the spread of the venom.

SAQ: What is the action of the venum of Indian krait?

The Indian krait's venom consists of presynaptic neurotoxins. These neurotoxins generally affect the nerve endings near the synaptic gap of the brain leading to muscle paralysis.

SAQ: What are nerve gases and their action on the nerve cells?

Ans: Nerve gases are a class of organic chemicals that inhibit acetylcholinesterase enzyme, which is necessary to transmit nerve impulses (action potentials) in the nervous system. The action of nerve gases disrupt the action potential; which transfer messages to various organs. This disruption of nerve impulses lead to respiratory failure and subsequent death.

What is dementia?

Ans: In dementia, neurons and their connections may degenerate with advancing age in senior citizens. Progressive loss of neurons in hippocampal region of brain may eventually get destroyed leading to the loss of memory and other important mental functions. Dementia leads to impaired ability in remembering, thinking, and taking decisions. Alzheimer's disease is the most common cause of dementia.

Blood–Brain Barrier

SAQ: Write a note on the blood–brain barrier.

Ans: The blood–brain barrier (Fig. 6.39) is a highly selective semipermeable border of endothelial cells. It prevents solutes in the circulating blood from crossing into the extracellular fluid of the central nervous system where neurons are present. The blood–brain barrier prevents toxins and other adverse compounds from reaching the brain.

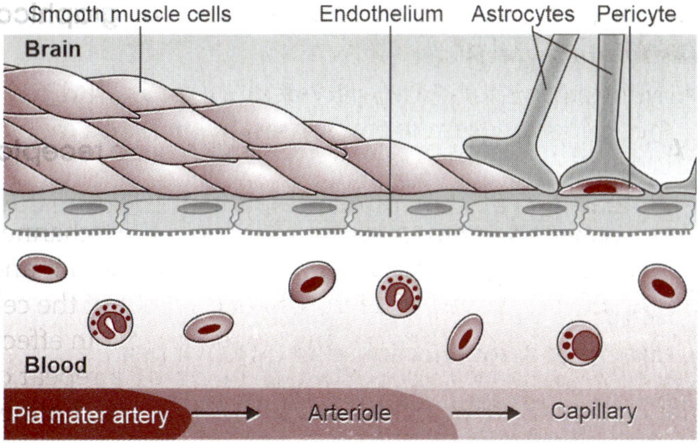

Fig. 6.39: Blood–brain barrier endothelium

> **Objective:** To describe the clinical conditions related to various diseases of the nervous system.

SAQ. Write a note on tetany.

Ans: Tetany is the involuntary contraction of muscles, caused by diseases and other conditions that increase the action potential frequency. Low plasma calcium increases the permeability of neuronal membranes to sodium ions, causing a progressive depolarization. If the plasma calcium level decreases significantly, action potentials may be spontaneously generated, causing significant contraction of peripheral skeletal muscles (Fig. 6.40).

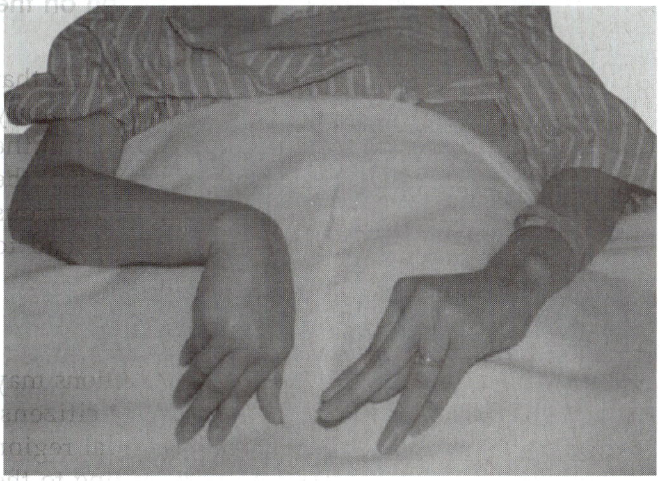

Fig. 6.40: Titany: Spasmed hands

SAQ: Write a note on tetanus.

Ans: Tetanus is an infection caused by a *Clostridium tetani* bacteria. The primary symptoms are caused by tetanospasmin, a neurotoxin produced by the bacteria. This infection generally occurs through wound contamination and often involves a cut or deep puncture wound. As the infection progresses, muscle spasms develop in the jaw (lockjaw) and elsewhere in the body (Fig. 6.41).

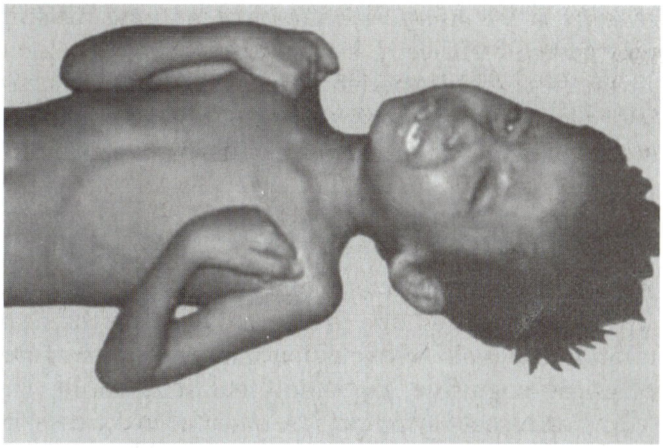

Fig. 6.41: A child suffering from tetanus

BAQ: Describe various changes that occur in the neurological system in an elderly.

Ans: Neuronal cells (neurons) do not regenerate. The following different types of changes occur in the neurological system in an elderly, with the advancing age:

1. Macroscopic changes and 2. Microscopic changes.

1. **Macroscopic changes:** These include—
   - Decreases in the volume and weight of the brain.
   - Thinning of the cortical mantle and white matter tracts.
   - Widening of meningeal thickening, sulci and fissures.
2. **Microscopic changes:** These include—
   - Dendritic and neuronal losses
   - Thinning of axons.
   - Thinning of myelin sheaths.
   - Decrease in the number of receptors.
   - Decrease in the quantities of neurotransmitters.
   - Decrease in the blood supply to nerve tissue.

In addition to these changes, in some cases, the following changes also occur: Presence of neurofibrillary tangles and senile plaques.

Presence of lipofuscin (a pigment) and granulovacuolar organelles (double membrane bodies).

Consequences of macroscopic and microscopic changes: Due to the macroscopic and microscopic changes in the neurological system an elderly individual suffers from decreased recent memory with a decreased ability to process information leading to an increased central motor conduction time. These factors lead to an increase in the learning time, response time and also in the recovery time. Decreased blood supply to neurons is due to the thickening of arteries (by cholesterol plaque deposits). Affected arteries tend to bleed, which may lead to stroke.

BAQ: Write a note on head injury.

Ans: A head injury results in trauma to the skull or brain. Head injuries may cause due to falls, accidents, vehicular accidents, physical assault, or due to any specific sport event. In the case of an open head injury, the skull may get cracked and break leading to bleeding and brain damage. Many neurological changes may occur due to the head injury and these depend on the degree of severity of the injury. An individual, after head injury may vomit, feel sleepy, lose consciousness, develop a severe headache, experience mismatched pupil sizes, and may be unable to move specific parts of the body. Many neurological problems may develop later in life, following a head injury.

SAQ: What is a concussion?

Ans: A concussion is a form of a traumatic brain injury. It is may be caused due to a severe blow on the head of an individual. A concussion may lead to irregular physical, cognitive, and emotional behaviours. The following types of symptoms are observed in concussion: Confusion, nausea, headache, fatigue, and blurry vision. Severity of concussion is measured using various grading systems (Table 6.3).

Table 6.3: Grading scale for cerebral concussions

Grade I	*Grade II*	*Grade III*
Transient confusion	Transient confusion	Any of consciousness
No loss of consciousness	No loss of consciousness	
Symptoms resolve in less than 16 minutes	Symptoms last more than 15 minutes	

Increased Intracranial Pressure

A brain injury or a clinical condition affecting brain may cause increase in pressure inside skull. This condition is called increased intracranial pressure (ICP) which can be harmful to the brain and spinal cord. The immediate sign of ICP is development of headache requires immediate medical attention.

Various Causes of ICP

The following are various reasons that may lead to ICP:

- Head and related brain injury
- Increase in cerebrospinal fluid
- Bleeding in some part of the brain
- Swelling in the brain
- Aneurysm
- Brain tumor
- Infections such as encephalitis or meningitis
- Hydrocephalus
- High blood pressure
- Stroke

The following are the most common symptoms of an ICP:

- Headache
- Blurred vision
- Sleepiness
- Vomiting
- Change in behaviour pattern
- Weakness or problems with moving or talking
- Lack of energy

Diagnosis ICP is done by the physicians on the basis of the following aspects:

- Medical history and physical exam including a neurological exam to test senses, balance and mental status
- Spinal tap (lumbar puncture), which measures the pressure of cerebrospinal fluid
- Computed tomography (CT) scan of the head and brain
- Magnetic resonance imaging (MRI) of head

Increased intracranial pressure is an emergency and treatment aspects include:

- Medicine to reduce swelling
- Draining extra cerebrospinal fluid or bleeding around the brain
- Rarely, craniotomy (removing part of the skull) is performed to decrease swelling
- Treatment on the underlying cause of intracranial pressure, which may due to stroke, high blood pressure, an infection, or tumor
- ICP may lead to serious complications, such as: Neurological damage, stroke, seizures and ultimately death.

NEUROMUSCULAR DISORDERS

SAQ: Write a brief note on neuromuscular disorders.

Ans: Neuromuscular disorders affect the muscles and (or) their nervous control. In general, problems with nervous control can cause either spasticity or some degree of paralysis, depending on the location and the nature of the neuromuscular disorder. Some examples of these disorders include stroke, Parkinson's disease, multiple sclerosis, muscular dystrophy, myasthenia gravis, Huntington's disease, etc.

Symptoms of muscle disease may include muscular weakness, spasticity, rigidity, loss of muscular control, myoclonus (twitching, spasming), and myalgia (muscle pain).

Stroke

SAQ: Write a brief note on stroke.

Ans: A stroke is the rapidly developing loss of brain functions due to disturbance in the blood supply to the brain. This can be due to ischemia caused by blockage (thrombosis, arterial embolism), or by haemorrhage. The affected area of the brain is unable to function, which might result in an inability to move one or more limbs on one side of the body, inability to understand or formulate speech, or an inability to see one side of the visual field.

Risk factors for stroke include old age, hypertension (high blood pressure), high blood cholesterol, cigarette smoking and rapid irregular heart rhythm. The treatment for an ischemic stroke is use of medicines that decrease and dissolve the blood clots and facilitate flow of blood to the brain of the patient.

Parkinson's Disease

SAQ: Write a brief note on Parkinson's disease.

Ans: Parkinson's disease (PD) is a degenerative disorder of the central nervous system. It results from the death of dopamine-containing cells in the substantia nigra, a region of the midbrain. Early in the course of the disease, the most obvious symptoms are movement-related, including shaking, rigidity, slowness of movement and difficulty with walking and gait. Later on cognitive and behavioural problems may arise with dementia. Other symptoms include sleep and emotional problems. PD is more common in the elderly with most cases occurring after the age of 50.

For the management of PD, drugs are used to increase dopamine levels.

SAQ: Define dementia.

Ans: Dementia is the loss of cognitive functioning, i.e. thinking, remembering, and reasoning and eventually, it interferes with a person's daily life and activities.

Alzheimer's Disease (AD)

BAQ: Write a brief note on Alzheimer's disease (AD).

Ans: Alzheimer's disease (AD) is an irreversible, progressive brain disease that slowly destroys memory and thinking skills. Eventually, the ability to carry out the simplest tasks is also lost in AD. In most people with Alzheimer's, symptoms first appear after 60 years of age.

Alzheimer's disease (AD) is the most common form of dementia and damage to the brain begins as many as 10 to 20 years before any significant symptoms are evident. In AD, specific protein tangles begin to develop deep in the brain, in an area called the entorhinal cortex, and plaques form in other areas. As more and more plaques and tangles form in particular brain areas, healthy neurons begin to work less efficiently. Neurons lose their ability to function and communicate with each other, and eventually they die. This damaging process spreads to the hippocampus, which is essential in forming memories. As the death of neurons increases, affected brain regions begin to shrink. By the final stage of AD, damage is widespread and brain tissue becomes shrunk significantly. Alzheimer's disease is the most common cause of dementia among older people. Cholinesterase inhibitors are used for the management of AD.

Myasthenia Gravis (MG)

BAQ: Write a brief note on myasthenia gravis (MG).

Ans: Myasthenia gravis (MG) is an autoimmune neuromuscular disease, which leads to muscle weakness and fatiguability. It is an autoimmune disorder, in which muscle weakness is caused by specific circulating antibodies that block acetylcholine receptors at the postsynaptic neuromuscular junction, inhibiting the stimulative effect of the neurotransmitter acetylcholine. Fatigability is the hallmark of MG. Muscles become progressively weaker during periods of activity and improve after periods of rest. Muscles that control eye and eyelid movement, facial expressions, chewing, talking, and swallowing are especially susceptible. The muscles that control breathing and neck and limb movements can also be affected.

For the management of NG, cholinesterase inhibitors are used. Immunosuppressant drugs such as corticosteroids decrease inflammation and the specific antibodies.

Schizophrenia

SAQ: Write a brief note on schizophrenia.

Ans: Schizophrenia is a mental illness. In schizophrenia, impairment of dopamine-containing neurons in the brain is observed. It is a mental disease marked by disturbances in thinking and emotional reactions. A combination of altered brain dopamine levels, genetics, and specific environment factors have roles in causing this disorder. An individual with schizophrenia may suffer from symptoms such as lak of motivation, slow movements, change in sleep patterns, hallucinations, etc.

Specific antipsychotic drugs are used to decrease the psychotic symptoms present in the acute phase of schizophrenia.

Depression

SAQ: Write a brief note on depression.

Ans: Depression is a common mental disorder. Depression causes feelings of sadness and loss of interest in normal activities. It can lead to a variety of emotional and physical problems. Depression may decrease the ability of a person to function normally at work and also at home.

There are many possible causes of depression. These include, disturbed mood regulation by the brain due to imbalance in serotonin neurotransmitter, genetic factors, certain medicines, stressful life events, and medical problems. Many of these factors together may lead to depression.

Psychological treatments could be useful for depression include. Antidepressant medications also could be used which include selective serotonin reuptake inhibitors.

Objective: To understand and explain the central theme of competency based medical and paramedical education (CBME): Horizontal and vertical integration of subjects.

BAQ: Show horizontal integration of premedical subjects: Physiology and biochemistry, with the following anatomical change: Death of memory cells in hippocampal region of the brain (Alzheimer's disease).

Ans:

Horizontal Integration with Physiology

The neurons lose their ability to function and communicate with each other.

Transmission of nerve impulses from hippocampal region of the brain are affected, leading to loss of mrmory.

Horizontal Integration with Biochemistry

Synthesis of abnormal amyloid beta proteins in the brain tissue. Deficiency of acetyl choline neurotransmitter takes place and related neurotransmission.

BAQ: Show vertical integration of the paramedical subjects: Microbiology, pharmacology and preventive medicine, with the following anatomical change: Death of memory cells in hippocampal region of the brain (Alzheimer's disease).

Ans:

Vertical Integration with Pharmacology

Use of appropriate drug to maintain acetylcholinesterase levels (acetylcholinesterase inhibitors).

BAQ: Show horizontal integration of premedical subjects: Physiology, and Biochemistry, with the following anatomical change: Death of dopamine-containing cells in the substantia nigra, a region of the midbrain (Parkinson's disease).

Ans:

Horizontal Integration with Physiology

Transmission of nerve impulses from the substantia nigra region of the brain are affected, due to deficiency of dopamine neurotransmitter. Normal movements of body parts are affected in the absence of dopamine, which controls body movements and muscle tone.

Horizontal Integration with Biochemistry

Synthesis of dopamine is decreased significantly, due to the loss of cell in the substantia nigra.

BAQ: Show vertical integration of the paramedical subject: Pharmacology, with the following anatomical change: Death of dopamine-containing cells in the substantia nigra, a region of the midbrain (Parkinson's disease).

Ans:

Vertical Integration with Pharmacology

Use of appropriate drug to maintain dopamine level (use of levodopa).

BIBLIOGRAPHY

1. Medical Biochemistry, 1st Edition (2023). Godkar PB, Godkar DP, CBS Publishers, New Delhi, India.
2. Text book of Medical Laboratory Technology, 4th Edition, (2024). Godkar PB, Godkar DP, Bhalani Publishing House, Mumbai, India.
3. Anatomy of the Human Body. 42nd Edition. Henry Gray, Editor-in-chief: Susan Standring, Elsevier (2020).
4. Ross & Wilson Anatomy and Physiology in Health and Illness, 13th Edition, by Allison Wynn Grant, Anne Waugh, and Kathleen J. W. Wilson (2018).
5. Schaum's outline of theory and problems of Human anatomy and Physiology, 2nd Edition (1997), Tata MaGraw-Hill Publishing Company Limited, New Delhi, India.

MULTIPLE CHOICE QUESTIONS (MCQs)

Select the correct option.

1. After the conception, by end of the fourth week, the following part(s) develop(s):

(A) Prosencephalon (forebrain)
(B) Mesencephalon (midbrain)
(C) Rhombencephalon (hindbrain)
(D) All of the above

2. In the third trimester, the cerebrum develops prenatally from the:

(A) Forebrain (prosencephalon)
(B) Cerebral cortex,
(C) Ventral telencephalon
(D) Both (A) and (C)

3. In the third trimester, the dorsal telencephalon develops into:

(A) Forebrain (prosencephalon)
(B) Cerebral cortex
(C) Ventral telencephalon
(D) Both(A) and (C)

4. This part of the brain contains the largest neural integration:

(A) Cerebrum (B) Cerebral cortex
(C) Brain stem (D) Hypothalamus

5. The basal ganglia (basal nuclei) are:

(A) Specialized paired masses of the grey matter
(B) Present superficially on the grey matter
(C) These are made of the corpus stratum
(D) All except B

6. All the following statements about the meninges are correct, *except*:

(A) Made up of two layers of membranes
(B) Made up of three layers of membranes
(C) The inner layer is delicate and called the pia mater
(D) The tough outer layer is called the dura mater

7. The tough outer layer of meninges is called:

(A) Pia mater (B) Arachnoid
(C) Dura mater (D) Gray matter

8. The basal nuclei form all these components, *except*:

(A) Caudate nucleus (B) Putamen
(C) Infundibulum (D) Globus pallidus

9. White matter cell body clusters of brain are referred to as:

(A) Gyri (B) Nuclei
(C) Sulci (D) Ganglia

10. This content of blood is not recorded by the hypothalamus:

(A) Fatty acids (B) Glucose
(C) Amino acids (D) PCO_2

11. This statement related to medulla oblongata is not correct:

(A) It is located within the mesencephalon
(B) It contains special nuclei for specific cranial nerves
(C) It is the site of decussation of many motor and sensory fibers
(D) It controls vasomotor, cardiac and respiratory centers

12. Afferent neurons carry nerve impulses from:

(A) Receptors to CNS
(B) CNS to muscles
(C) CNS to receptors
(D) Effector organs to CNS

13. The third ventricle of the brain is also known as:

(A) Metacoel (B) Rhinocoel
(C) Paracoel (D) Diocoel

14. This is one of the parts of the hindbrain:

(A) Cerebellum (B) Hypothalamus
(C) Corpus callosum (D) Spinal cord

15. The hypothalamus injury is most likely to affect:

(A) Decision-making
(B) Regulation of body temperature
(C) Co-ordination during locomotion
(D) Short-term memory

16. The heartbeat is regulated by this cranial nerve that regulates:

(A) IX (B) X
(C) VIII (D) VII

17. Nissl's granules of the neurons are made up of:

(A) RNA (B) DNA
(C) Protein (D) Ribosome

18. This is a part of the rhombencephalon:

(A) Thalamus (B) Temporal lobe
(C) Medulla (D) Substantia nigra

19. This part of the brain controls the body temperature and eating desire:

(A) Hypothalamus (B) Thalamus
(C) Cerebellum (D) Pons

20. This cranial nerve has the highest number of branches:

(A) Vagus nerve (B) Facial nerve
(C) Trigeminal nerve (D) Both (A) and (C)

21. A neuron that carries information from the peripheral nervous system to the central nervous system is

(A) Efferent neuron (B) Afferent neuron
(C) Either (A) or (B) (D) Both (A) and (B)

22. The correct order of meninges from the inner side:

(A) Durometer – arachnoid mater – pia mater
(B) Pia mater – arachnoid mater – durometer
(C) Pericardium – myocardium – endocardium
(D) Durometer – pia mater – arachnoid mater

23. Space which separates the arachnoid mater and durometer is separated by:

(A) Epidural space (B) Subdural space
(C) Mediastinum space (D) Subarachnoid space

24. These are all the glial cells, *except*:

(A) Ependymal (B) Oligodendrocytes
(C) Astrocytes (D) Lymphocytes

25. This structure at a synapse contains the neuro-transmitter

(A) Schwann cells (B) Synaptic cleft
(C) Synaptic vesicles (D) Synaptic knobs

26. The propagation of action potential of a nerve impulse is due to the movement of:

(A) K^+ ions from intracellular to extracellular fluid
(B) Na^+ ions from extracellular to intracellular fluid
(C) K^+ ions from extracellular to intracellular fluid
(D) Na^+ ions from intracellular to extracellular fluid

27. The falx cerebri that develope from the durometer is present between:

(A) Cerebral hemispheres
(B) Brain and spinal cord
(C) Cerebellar hemispheres
(D) Subdural and epidural space

28. This is the ability of neurons to initiate nerve impulses:

(A) Myelination
(B) Irritability
(C) Conductivity
(D) Neurotransmission

29. Broca's area in the left hemisphere is related to:

(A) Smell sensation
(B) Impulses received from eyes
(C) Reasoning and learning
(D) Speech

30. Cocaine interferes with the reuptake of this neuro-transmitter at synapses:

(A) Epinephrine (B) Acetylcholine
(C) Dopamine (D) Oxygen

31. At neuromuscular junction, the synaptic vesicles discharge this neurotransmitter:

(A) Adrenaline (B) Acetylcholine
(C) Epinephrine (D) None of the above

32. This one is the neurotransmitter between sympathetic postganglionic fibers and the effctor organs:

(A) Acetylcholine
(B) Adrenaline
(C) Norepinephrine
(D) Epinephrine

33. Parasympathetic fibers arise from these sets of cranial nerves:

(A) V, IX, X, XII
(B) IV, V, IX, X
(C) III, VII, IX, X
(D) III, V, IIX, X

34. In this part of the brain, the cell bodies of the preganglionic neurons of sympathetic system are located:

(A) The lateral horn of the grey matter of spinal cord
(B) The sacral and servical region of the spinal cord
(C) The white matter of the spinal cord
(D) The sacral region and the brain

35. The autonomous nervous system is responsible for this function:

(A) Sensory
(B) Motor
(C) Sensory and motor
(D) None of these

36. These receptors are found in the heart:

(A) Nicotine
(B) Beta
(C) Alpha
(D) GABA

37. To treat bronchial asthama, these types of drugs are used:

(A) Adrenergic blockers
(B) Adrenergic
(C) Cholenergi
(D) Anticholinesterase

38. This one is *not* the function of autonomous nervous system:

(A) Conscious control of motor activities
(B) Regulation of vital activities
(C) Innervation of internal organs
(D) Transmission of motor and sensory impulses

39. A ganglion is present:

(A) Inside the brain and the spinal cord
(B) Only in the brain
(C) Only in the spinal cord
(D) Outside the brain and the spinal cord

40. The knee-jerk reflex due to a tap over the patellar ligament is:

(A) A conditional reflux
(B) A polysynaptic reflux
(C) Has reflux center in the spinal cord
(D) Mediated by a three-neuron arc

41. Which cranial nerve is damaged, when a person is unable to walk in a straight line?

(A) The accessory nerve
(B) The hypoglossal nerve
(C) The vestibulocochlear nerve
(D) The trochlear nerve

42. The eyeball turns in the horizontal direction by the rectus eye muscle. It is innervated by this nerve:

(A) The abducens nerve
(B) The optic nerve
(C) The facial nerve
(D) The oculomotor nerve

43. This cranial nerve mediates taste sensation:

(A) Facial and trigeminal
(B) Facial and glossopharyngeal
(C) Abducens and trochlear
(D) Trigeminal and glossopharyngeal

44. Autonomous nervous system innervates:

(A) The heart
(B) The glands
(C) The smooth muscle
(D) All of the above

45. Dysfunction of these leads to motor disorders and Parkinson's disease death of dopamine-containing cells in the substantia nigra, a region of the midbrain:

(A) Dopamine-containing cells in the substantia nigra
(B) Pons
(C) Thalamus
(D) Parietal lobe

46. Parkinson's disease results from the deficiency of:

(A) Dopamine
(B) Acetyl choline
(C) Glutamate
(D) Aspartic acid

47. Alzheimer's disease results from the deficiency of:

(A) Dopamine
(B) Acetylcholine
(C) Glutamate
(D) Aspartic acid

48. Myasthenia gravis (MG) is an autoimmune disorder, in which muscle weakness is caused by:

(A) Antibodies that block dopamine receptors at the presynaptic neuromuscular junction
(B) Antibodies that block acetylcholine receptors at the postsynaptic neuromuscular junction
(C) Antibodies that block glutamate receptors at the postsynaptic neuromuscular junction
(D) Both (A) and (C)

49. In schizophrenia, impairment of neurons containing which neurotransmitter in the brain is observed?

(A) Dopamine (B) Acetylcholine

(C) Glutamate (D) Aspartic acid

50. Depression may cause due to:

(A) Imbalance in serotonin neurotransmitter

(B) Genetic factors

(C) Stressful life events

(D) All of the above

ANSWERS

1. D	2. A	3. B	4. B	5. D	6. A	7. C
8. C	9. B	10. D	11. A	12. A	13. D	14. A
15. B	16. B	17. D	18. C	19. A	20. C	21. A
22. A	23. B	24. D	25. C	26. B	27. A	28. C
29. D	30. C	31. B	32. C	33. C	34. A	35. C
36. B	37. B	38. A	39. D	40. C	41. C	42. A
43. B	44. D	45. A	46. A	47. B	48. B	49. A
50. D						

MATCH THE COLUMNS

I	II
1. Hypothalamus	A. Cutaneous nerves
2. Thalamus	B. Bipolar nerves
3. Pons	C. Taste, smell, balance
4. Pineal glands	D. Conduct impulses to muscles
5. Choroid plexus	E. Controls osmotic concentration of blood
6. Medulla oblongata	F. Responds to intense pain
7. Motor nerves	G. Apneustic center
8. Dermatome	H. Secretion of melanin
9. Sensory nerves	I. CSF production
10. Olfactory nerve	J. Area of decussation

ANSWERES

1. E	2. F	3. G	4. H	5. I	6. J	7. D
8. A	9. C	10. B				

CHAPTER

7

Sense Organs

SAQ: Short answer question: Marks: 2
BAQ: Brief answer question: Marks: 4 or 5
LAQ: Long answer question: Marks: 9 or 10
MCQs: Multiple choice questions: Marks: 0.5 each
Match the columns: Marks: 0.5 each
Draw a labelled diagram: Marks: 5

Objective: To describe the term sensory organs and their related specific senses.

INTRODUCTION

BAQ: Write a note on the sense organs.

Ans: The sense organs consist of the eye, ear, nose, and skin. These sense organs contain specific receptors that relay information through sensory neurons to the appropriate parts of the body, with respect to a specific physical stimulus. The basic working of a sense organ is as follow:

A sensory organ contains a group of interrelated sensory cells. These cells respond to a specific physical stimulus. The nerves of the central system (CNS) and peripheral nervous systems (PNS) relay stimulus related sensory information to the brain and from the brain to the related different types of sensory receptor cells in sensory organs. The sensory information from these organs passes to the central nervous system and finally, the sensory information arrive at the sensory cortices in the brain. From the brain, sensory signals are processed and interpreted for the specific actions from the body parts.

The sensory cortex in the brain performs processing of sensory inputs. Five main sensory cortices are, visual, auditory, gustatory (related to the sense of taste), somatosensory (related to the sense of sensation) and olfactory (related to the sense of smell). The system of senses is divided into the following two types: (1) External sensory systems and (2) internal sensory systems.

1. External sensory system is based on the functions of sensory organs such as the eyes, ears, skin, nose, mouth and the vestibular system.
2. Internal sensation system detects stimuli from internal organs and tissues. Internal senses include nociception (pain), spatial orientation and proprioception (body position). Internal sense system is responsible for the signals produced that lead to the feelings such as nausea, thirst, hunger, vomiting, etc.

SKIN

For the information on skin, refer to the integumentary system (Chapter 3, page 47).

Objective: To describe the anatomy of eye and important functions of anatomical parts of the eye.

EYE (Fig. 7.1)

The eye is a complex optical system. Two eyes collect light from the surrounding environment and regulate light through various specialized parts to brain. The brain through complex neuronal processes prepares real image of the environment and various objects in front of the eyes.

Eye Socket (Fig. 7.1)

BAQ: Write a note on the eye socket.

Ans: The eye has a diameter of about one inch in adults. The eye is enclosed in a socket which is made up of portions of many bones of the skull to form a four-sided pyramid.

Function: The socket of bone protects eyes from mechanical injury (Fig. 7.1).

BAQ: Draw a neat labelled figure of an eye socket and the related bones.

Ans: Refer to Fig. 7.1.

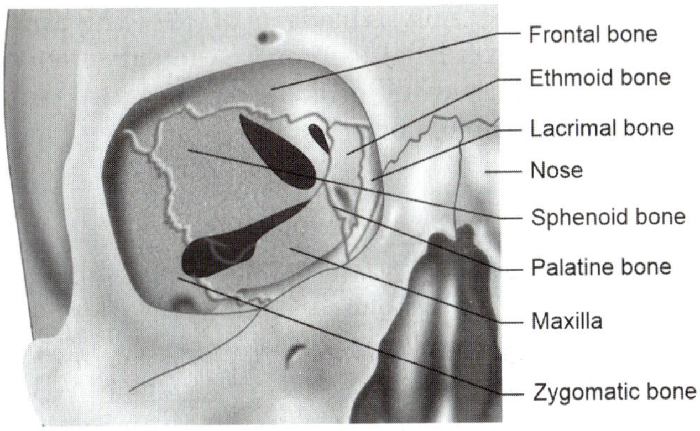

Fig. 7.1: Eye socket and related bones that protect eyes

Floor of Eye Orbit and Related Functions (Fig. 7.1)

BAQ: Write a note on the floor of eye orbit and related functions.

Ans: The floor of the eye orbit is made up of parts of the maxilla, zygomatic, and palatine bones. The roof of eye orbit is made up of the orbital plate of the frontal bone and, behind this is part of the sphenoid bone (Fig. 7.1).

Functions:

1. The optic foramen (foramen means open hole) is the opening through which the optic nerve passes to the brain (Fig. 7.2).
2. The large ophthalmic artery enters the orbit at the nasal side.
3. Large veins and nerves pass through the superior orbital fissure (fissure means a slit). These nerves carry nonvisual sensory messages like pain and motor nerves control the muscles of the eye. Since, vision is the dominant sense, about 70% of all sensory receptors are present in the eyes (Fig. 7.2).

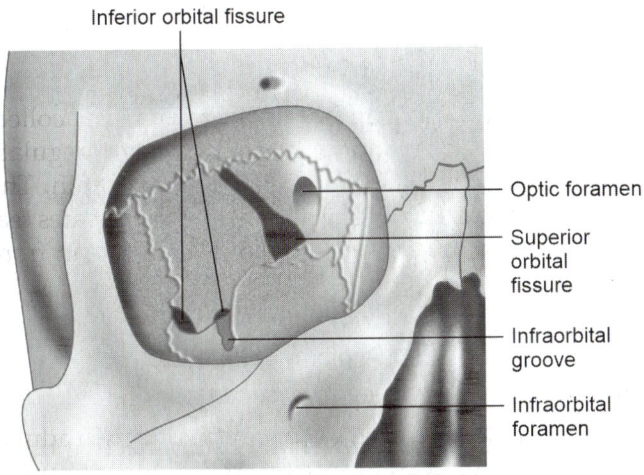

Fig. 7.2: Foramens, grooves (deep slits) and fissures of eye

Eye Coats (Fig. 7.3)

BAQ: Write a note on the eye coats.

Ans: The eye is made up of the following three coats: The outer coat, middle coat and inner coat.

The outermost coat is made up of the cornea and the sclera. Aqueous humour is the clear fluid that fill the space in the front of the eyeball between the lens and the cornea.

The middle coat contains the main blood supply to the eye and consists of the choroid, the ciliary body, and the iris.

The inner part of the eyeball contains the lens and the vitreous body and it is divided into the anterior and the posterior chamber.

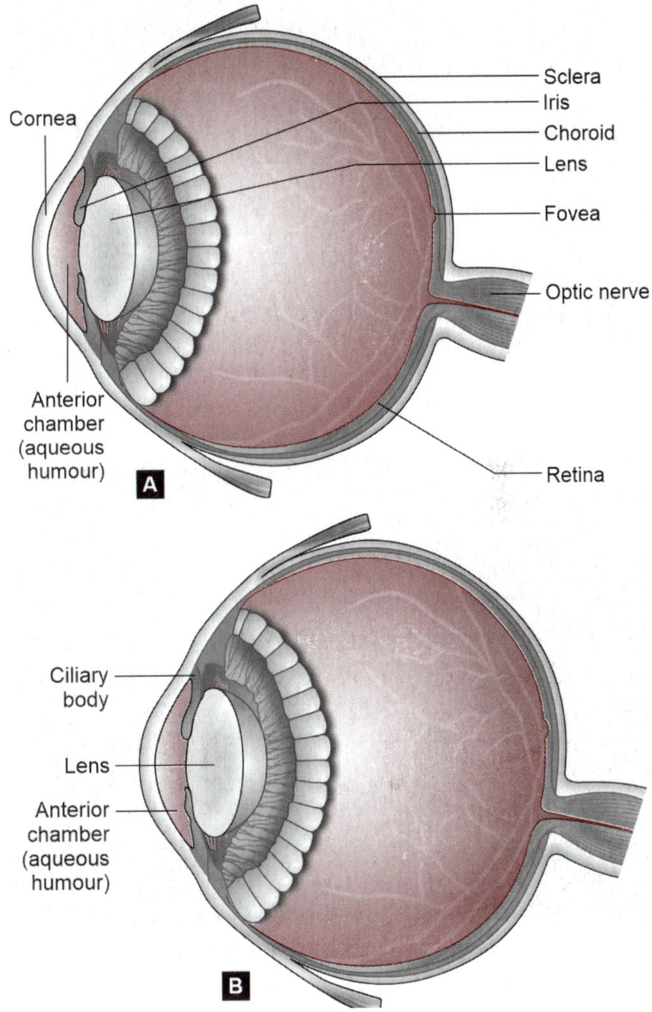

Figs 7.3A and B: Anatomy of eye coats

Objective: To describe the accessory structures of the eye and their respective functions.

ACCESSORY STRUCTURES OF THE EYE

LAQ. Describe the accessory structures of the eye.

Ans: The various accessory structures of an eye include the following parts: (1) Eyebrow, (2) eyelids, (3) lacrimal apparatus, (4) eye muscles and (5) conjunctiva.

Eyebrows (Fig. 7.4)

Eyebrows are short coarse hairs that overlayer the supraorbital margins of the skull (Fig. 7.5).

Eyebrows, prevent perspiration from passing into the eyes and also protect the eyes from direct sunlight.

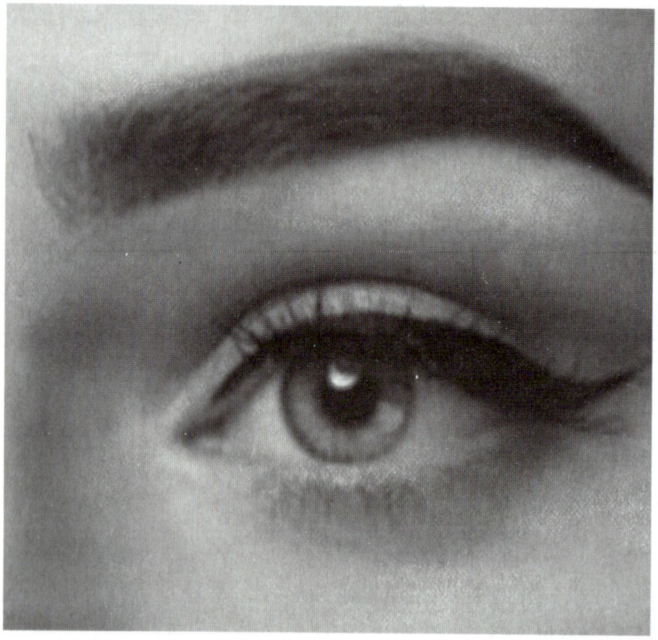

Fig. 7.4: Eyebrow

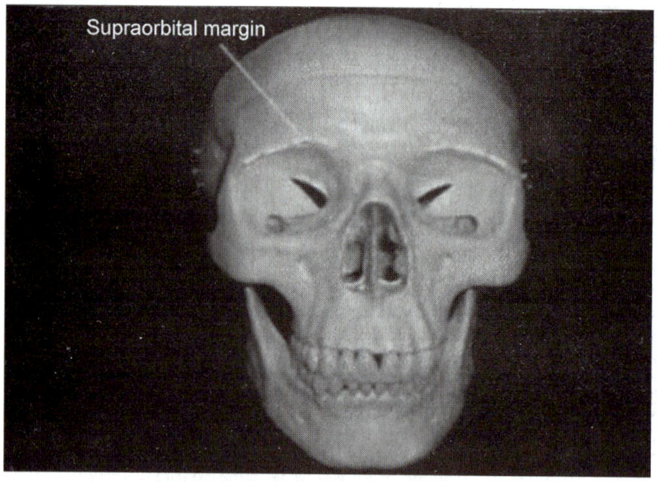

Fig. 7.5: Supraorbital margin

Eyelids and Eyelid Layers (Fig. 7.6)

Eyelids are movable tissues, mainly consist of skin and muscle, that shields and protects the eyeball from mechanical injury. Eyelids also help to provide moist chambers, which are required for the normal functioning of the internal parts of the eyes.

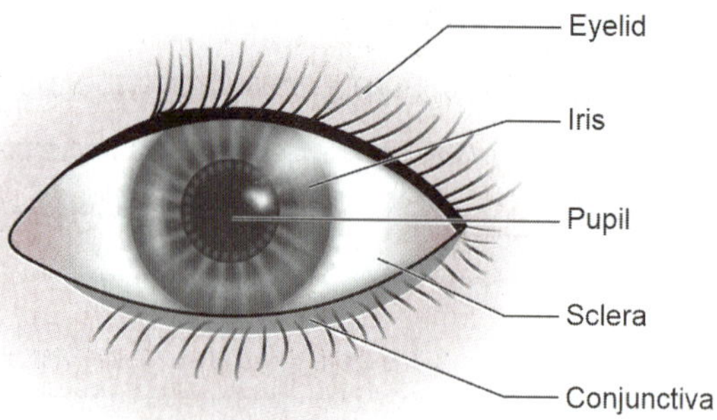

Fig. 7.6A: Eyelid, conjunctiva, sclera, pupil and iris (parts of an eye)

The eyelid (Fig. 7.6A) is made up of following various layers (from superficial to deep): Skin, subcutaneous tissue, orbicularis oculi, orbital septum, tarsal plates, and palpebral conjunctiva (Fig. 7.6C).

Eyelid

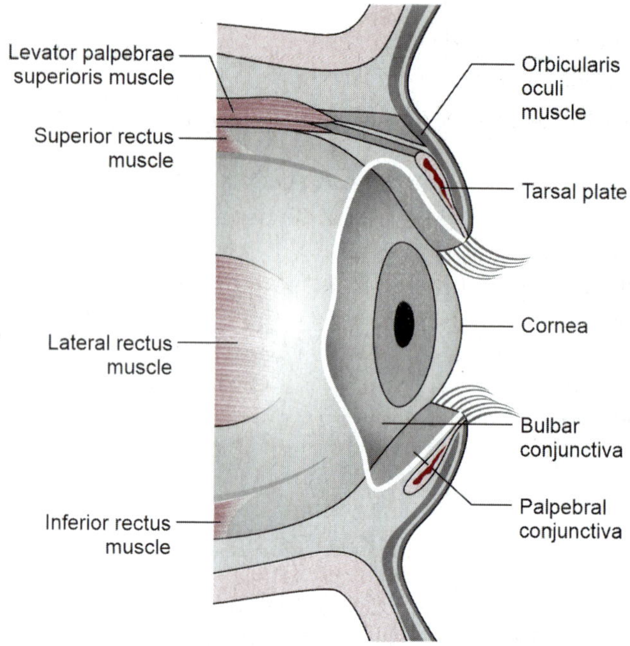

Fig. 7.6B: Eyelid muscle layers

BAQ: Draw a labelled figure of the eyelid muscle layers.
Ans: Refer to Fig. 7.6B

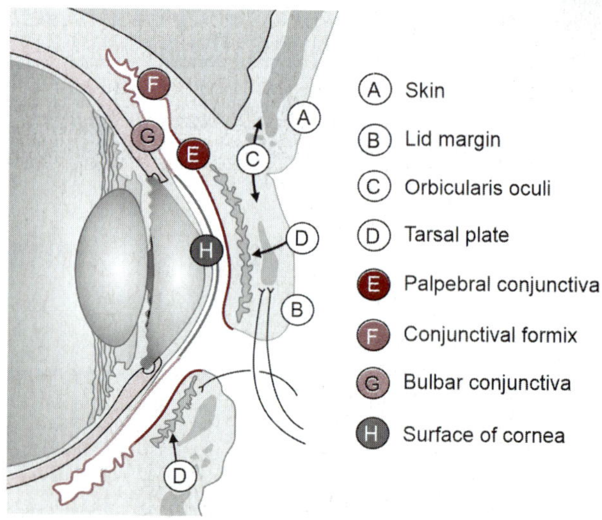

Fig. 7.6C: Anatomy of the eyelid

Eye Muscles

Eyelids are supported internally by connective tissue sheets called tarsal plates (Figs 7.6B and C). The levator palpebrae superioris muscle raises the superior eyelid to open the eye, and the orbicularis oculi muscle brings the eyelids together and to shut the eye (Figs 7.6B and C). These muscles are activated to cause eye blinking after every 3–7 seconds. Eye blinking prevents dehydration of the eye. With every blink, accessory structure secretions are spread across the eye. These muscles are also activated when the eye is exposed to foreign objects (Table 7.1).

Table 7.1: Extrinsic eye muscles

Muscle	Action	Controlling cranial nerve
Inferior oblique	Elevation of eye, lateral eye rotation	Oculomotor III
Superior oblique	Depresses eye, lateral eye rotation	Trochlear IV
Inferior rectus	Depresses eye, medial rotation of eye	Oculomotor III
Lateral rectus	Lateral movement of eye	Abducens VI
Superior rectus	Elevates eye, medial rotation of eye	Oculomotor III
Medial rectus	Medial movement of eye	Oculomotor III

Eye lashes project from the edge of each eyelid. These are richly innervated, hence, eye-touch triggers blinking. Meibomian glands (tarsal glands) are located in the tarsal plates (Fig. 7.7). Their ducts open behind the eyelashes. Meibomian glands produce a lubricating oily secretion called meibum. The conjunctiva is a transparent mucous membrane that lines the anterior surface of the eye, as well as the insides of the eyelid.

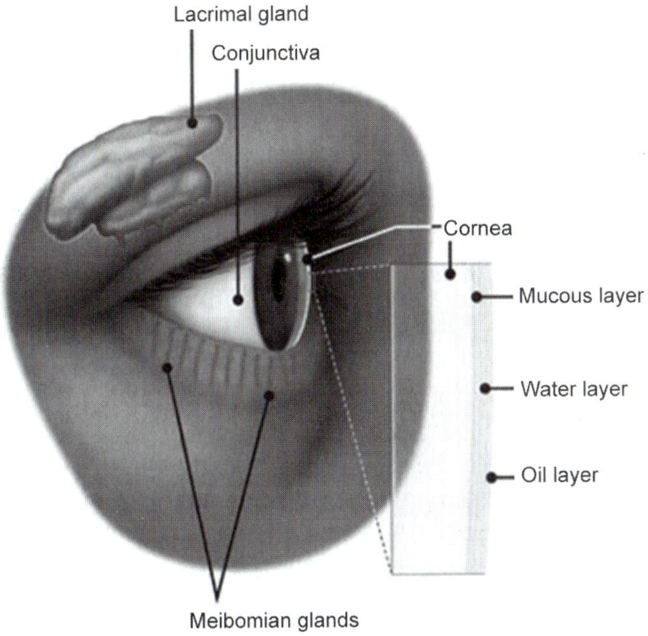

Fig. 7.7: Meibomian glands and lacrimal gland

Lacrimal Glands (Fig. 7.7)

The lacrimal gland is a bilobed, tear-shaped gland. It is situated in the anterior, superotemporal orbit within the lacrimal fossa of the frontal bone. The primary function of lacrimal glands is to secrete the aqueous part of the tears. Tears keep the eyes moist and protect the eyes from dust and microorganisms.

Conjunctiva (Fig. 7.7)

The conjunctiva is a transparent membrane made up of loose connective tissue. It covers the surface of the eyeball. It is composed of nonkeratinized, stratified squamous epithelium containing goblet cells, stratified columnar epithelium and stratified cuboidal epithelium (at some layers).

The conjunctiva secret mucus and protect the eyes with the help of a lubricating fluid formed by the combination of mucus, tears (from lacrimal glands) and meibum (from the meibomian glands). The major function of the conjunctiva is to prevent the eyes from becoming dry using the lubrication fluid.

Eye Canthi (Fig. 7.7)

BAQ: Write a brief note on the eye canthi and their functions.

Ans: The canthi (singular: Canthus) are present at the corner of the eyes where the upper and lower eyelids meet. The eye has two canthi, the medial canthus and the lateral canthus (Fig. 7.7).

Function: The eye canthi provide anchor points that enable the eyelids to close completely over the eye.

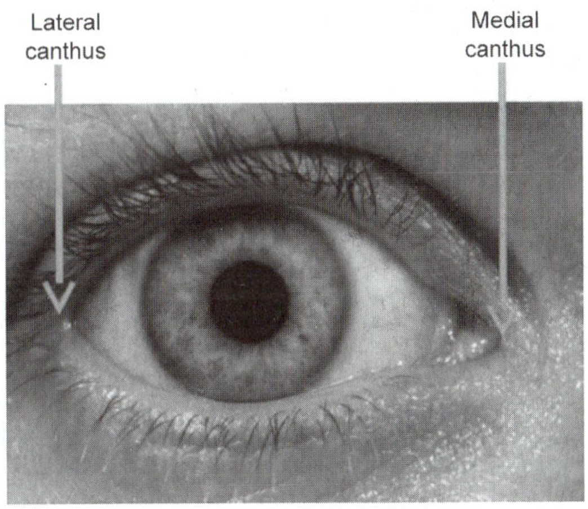

Fig. 7.7A: Eye canthi

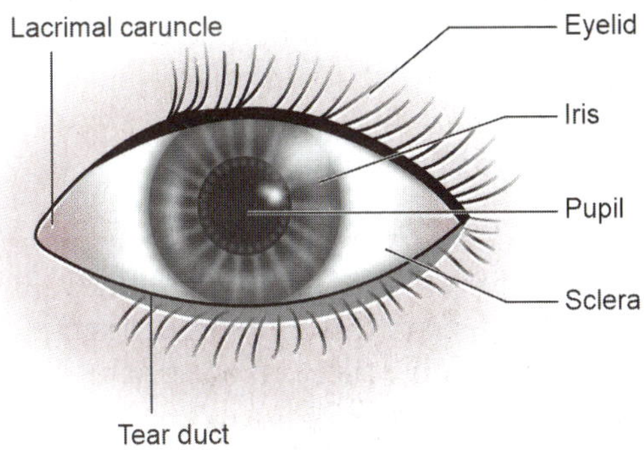

Fig. 7.7B: Lacrimal caruncle near the medial canthus

SAQ: What is lacrimal caruncle and its function?

Ans: The lacrimal caruncle is a slightly elevated part present next to the medial canthus (Fig. 7.7B). It contains sebaceous and sweat glands. These glands produce a whitish oily secretion, known as "eye boogers". The eye boogers means accumulation of mucus in the eyes. The combination of mucus, tears (from lacrimal glands) and meibum (from the meibomian glands) prevent the eyes from becoming dry.

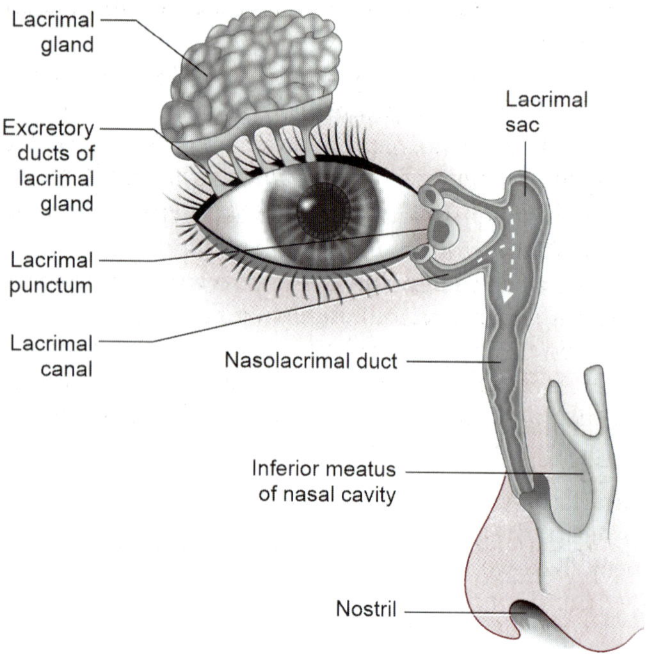

Fig. 7.8: Lacrimal secretion (tears) passage into nasal cavity

BAQ: Write importance of the lacrimal apparatus in the eye.

Ans: The lacrimal apparatus consists of the lacrimal gland and a series of ducts. The tears travel through excretory ducts and on the surface of the eye. Blinking spreads the tears in the eyes, where they enter the lacrimal canaliculi through two small holes called lacrimal punctum (Fig. 7.8). Tears empty through the lacrimal canaliculi to the lacrimal sac and to the nasolacrimal duct and then into the nasal cavity (Fig. 7.8). Tears lubricate, moisten and cleanse the surface of the eye. Tears contain antibodies and lysozyme enzyme that kill bacteria.

Objective: To describe the muscles of the eye and their respective functions.

EYE MUSCLES

BAQ: Write a note on eye muscles.

Ans: There are two types of eye muscles: (1) Extrinsic eye muscles that control eye movement and position, and (2) intrinsic muscles that control near focusing and control of light entering in the eye.

Extrinsic Eye Muscles (Fig. 7.9A)

Extrinsic eye muscles are skeletal muscles. Extrinsic muscles hold the eye in the orbit. These muscles precisely and rapidly control muscles of the eyes. Extrinsic muscles originate from the walls of the orbit and insert into the outer surface of the eyeball. The eye is moved by six extrinsic eye muscles (extraocular muscles). These muscles help the eye to move up and down, to move from side to side, and also to help eyes to rotate around These muscles allow the eyes to maintain its shape and also help to follow a moving object.

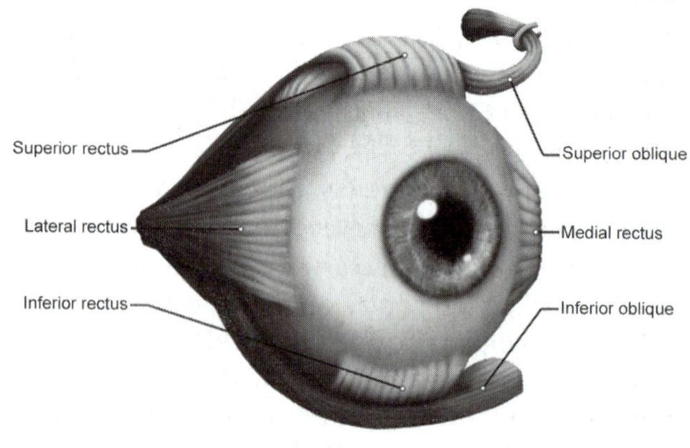

Fig. 7.9A: Extrinsic eye muscles

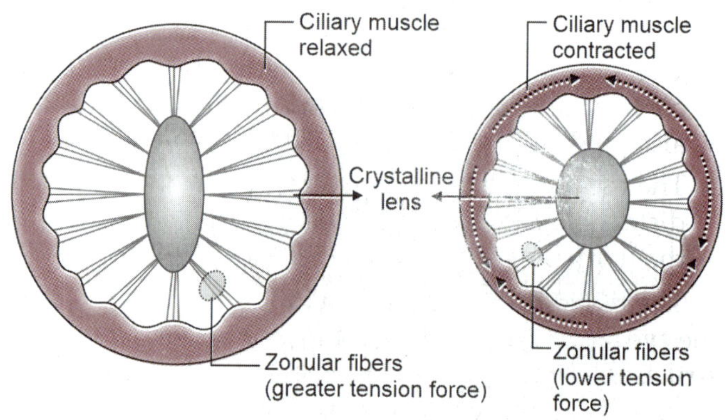

Fig. 7.9B: Intrinsic muscle, ciliary body actions

The extrinsic eye muscles include four rectus muscles: Superior, inferior, lateral, and medial and two oblique muscles: Superior and inferior (Fig. 7.9A, Table 7.1).

Intrinsic Eye Muscles

The following are the intrinsic eye muscles: The ciliary muscle, iris sphincter and radial pupil dilator muscles. The intrinsic eye muscles are innervated by branches of autonomic nervous system and these are controlled by reflex action.

Functions: The function of intrinsic eye muscles is to focus the eye, and control the iris by means of which only controlled amount of light to enter the eye (Fig. 7.9B).

ANATOMICAL STRUCTURE OF THE EYEBALL (Fig. 7.10)

LAQ: Describe anatomical structure of the eyeball under the following headings: (A) applied anatomy, (B) the eye muscles are related functions, (C) innervation of the eyeball and (D) blood supply of the eye ball.

Ans: (A) The eye is made up of the following three layers (from superficial to deep side):

1. The outer layer called the fibrous tunic layer. It consists of the cornea and the sclera.

The cornea plays an important role as the outermost lens of the eye. Cornea controls and focuses the entry of light inside the eye.

The sclera acts as a protective layer of the eyeball. It maintains shape of the eye and protects it from the injuries.

2. The middle layer known as uvea. It is also known as the vascular tunic layer and it consists of the iris, the choroid, and the ciliary body. The iris controls the amount of light reaching the retina.

   The choroid plays important role in the thermoregulation of the posterior eye, the drainage of aqueous humor from the anterior chamber, the modulation of intraocular pressure. The choroid also acts to provide nourishment and oxygen to the outer retina.

   The ciliary body is located behind the iris that alters the shape of the lens during focusing and produces the aqueous humour that bathes the anterior chamber. The uvea layer contains blood vessels that carry blood, which provide nourishment to the eye.

3. The inner layer consists of lens, nervous tissue containing photoreceptors and neurons. Inner layer also contains the retina (Fig. 7.10).

   The lens allows the eye to focus on objects at varying distances. It is located behind the iris and in front of the vitreous body.

The retina is a thin layer of tissue. It lines the back of the eye and it is located near the optic nerve. When light strikes the retina, it initiates a cascade of chemical and electrical events that trigger nerve impulses. The nerve impulses are sent to various visual centres of the brain through the fibres of the optic nerve. The nerve impulses pass on to the brain for visual recognition.

B. **Muscles of the eye:** There are two types of eye muscles: (1) Extrinsic eye muscles that control eye movement and position, and (2) intrinsic muscles that control near focusing and control of light entering in the eye.

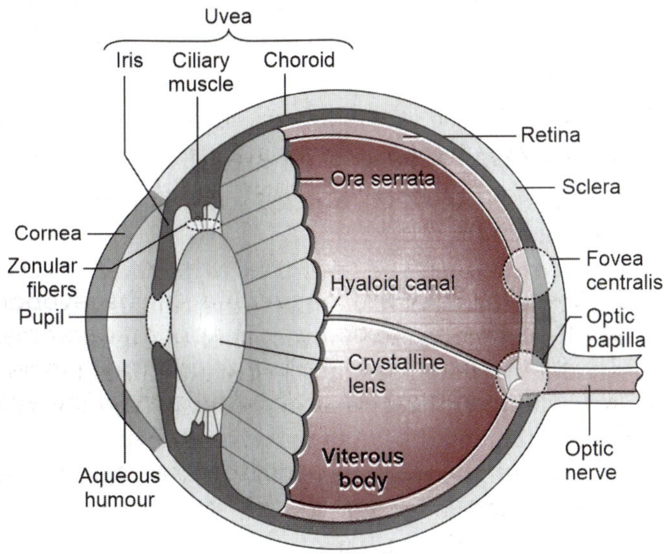

Fig. 7.10: Anatomical structure of the eyeball

The extrinsic eye muscles include four rectus muscles: Superior, inferior, lateral, and medial and two oblique muscles: Superior and inferior.

The following are the intrinsic eye muscles: The ciliary muscle, iris sphincter and radial pupil dilator muscles.

C. **Innervation of the eyeball:** The following cranial nerves innervate motor, sensory, and autonomic structures in the eyes: The facial nerve (CN VII), The trigeminal nerve (CN V), oculomotor nerve (CN III), trochlear nerve (CN IV), abducens nerve (CN VI), and the optic nerve (CN II).

D. **Blood supply of the eye:** An ophthalmic artery and a central retinal artery (that branches off of the ophthalmic artery) provide blood to each eye. Similarly, ophthalmic veins and a central retinal vein drain blood from the eye. These blood vessels enter and leave through the back of the eye (Fig. 7.23).

BAQ: Draw a labelled figure of the anatomical structure of the eyeball.

Ans: Refer to the Fig. 7.10.

SAQ: What is vitreous humour and its function?

Ans: Most part of the eyeball is filled with a transparent gel-like material, called the vitreous humour. It helps to maintain the spheroidal shape of eyeball.

CORNEA (Fig. 7.10)

BAQ: Describe the cornea of an eye under the following heads: (A) Description and applied anatomy, (B) blood supply, (C) nerve supply and (D) functions.

Ans: Description and applied anatomy: The cornea is the front part of the eye. It is transparent and it covers the iris, pupil, and anterior chamber of eye. The cornea refracts two-third of total light that passes through it on retina.

Anatomy of Cornea (Fig. 7.11)

The cornea is comprised of the following five layers: (1) Epithelium, (2) Bowman's layer, (3) stroma, (4) Descemet's membrane, and (5) endothelium.

1. The epithelium is a layer of cells that covers the cornea.

   It contains five to seven cell layers consisting of superficial squamous cells, middle wing cells and inner basal cells. The epithelium absorbs nutrients and oxygen from tears and passes it to other parts of the cornea.

2. Bowman's layer is an acellular condensation of the anterior stroma of the cornea. This layer acts as a physical barrier to protect the subepithelial nerves.

3. *Stroma:* It contains 200–250 distinct lamellae (plates of tissues). The stroma makes up largest portion of the

corneal structure. The unique properties necessary for the functions of cornea such as avascularity, transparency and the mechanical properties necessary for strength, and the maintenance of shape are due to the stroma layer.

4. *Descemet's membrane:* It is a thick, dense, and relatively transparent and cell-free matrix. It separates the posterior corneal stroma from the underlying endothelium.

   Descemet's membrane maintains corneal structure transparency and homeostasis. It facilitates the entry of the fluid nutrients into the corneal stroma.

5. *Endothelium:* The endothelium is a monolayer of cells on the posterior corneal surface. It facilitates the transport of water from the stroma into the anterior chamber of the eye.

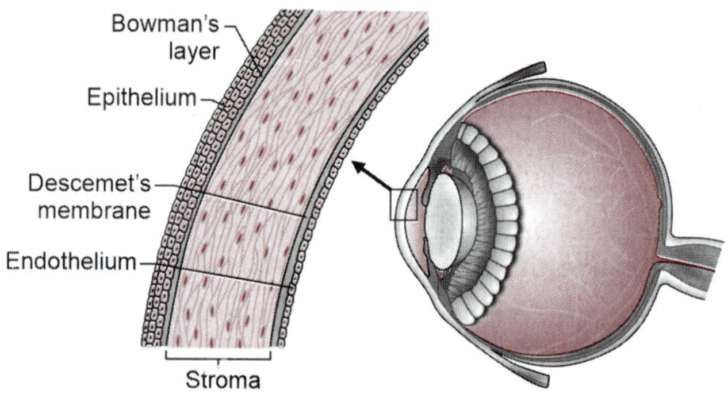

Fig. 7.11: Anatomy of the cornea

C. **Blood supply:** The cornea is primarily avascular and does not contain blood vessels and lymphatic vessels. The blood supply is by very small vessels at the outer edge of the cornea. The aqueous humour provides nutrients to the cornea.

D. **Nerve supply:** The cornea contains unmyelinated nerve endings. These nerve endings are sensitive to touch, chemicals and temperature. A touch to the cornea causes an involuntary reflex, which closes the eyelid.

E. **Functions:** (a) Protection of the inside structures of the eye, (b) contribution to the refractive power of the eye, and (c) controlled focusing of light rays on the retina.

SAQ: What are the functions of tears?

Ans: The following are the various functions of tears: Tear contains oxygen, water, glucose, sodium, potassium, urea, mucin, lipids, lysozyme, albumin and immunoglobulins. Tears contain lysozyme and immunoglobulins that protect against microbial infections. Tears contents diffuse in the entire cornea to keep it in healthy condition.

BAQ: Draw a neat and labelled figure of the eye cornea.

Ans: Refer to Fig. 7.11.

IRIS (Fig. 7.12)

The iris is a coloured tissue at the front side of the eye. It contains the pupil in the center. The iris controls the size of the pupil so that amount of light could be controlled according to the intensity of light.

Anatomy of Iris (Fig. 7.12)

The iris consists of the following two layers: (1) The front pigmented fibrovascular layer known as a stroma and (2) pigmented epithelial cells beneath the stroma.

1. The stroma connects to sphincter pupillae muscle which contracts the pupil in a circular motion, and dilator pupillae muscles, which pull the iris radially to increase the diameter of the pupil (Figs 7.12 and 7.13).
2. The pigmented epithelial cells beneath the stroma: These cell play important role in the restriction of the light that reaches the retina.

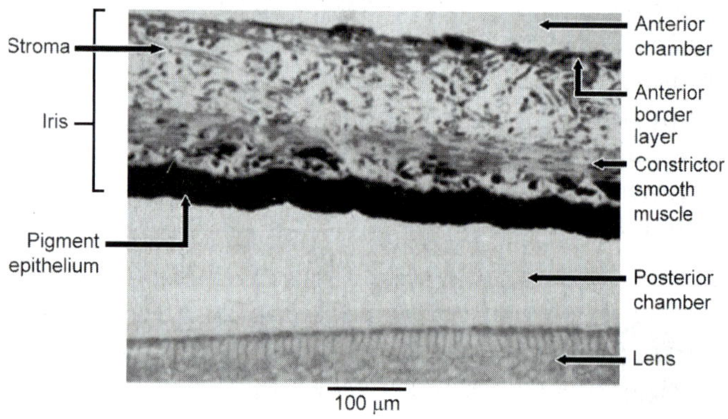

Fig. 7.12: Anatomy of iris

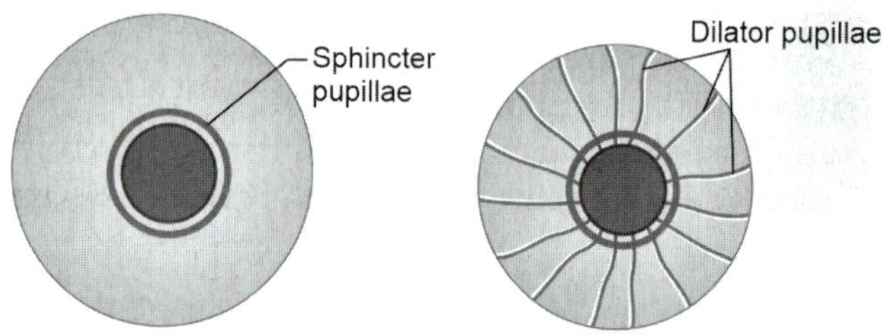

Fig. 7.13: Sphincter and dilator muscles of iris

Uvea

SAQ: Describe the uvea of an eye.

Ans: The uvea of an eye has the following three main parts (Fig. 7.14):

1. Choroid: It is a tissue layer filled with blood vessels
2. Ciliary body: It is a ring of tissue that contains muscles capable of changing the shape of the lens. It also secretes aqueous humour, a clear fluid that fills the space between the cornea and the iris. The aqueous humour maintains the shape of the eyeball and keeps the cornea moist. It also provides nutrition to the central cornea and lens, as they do not have direct access to blood.
3. Iris (as described above).

Objective: To describe how an eye is able to focus on objects at various distances.

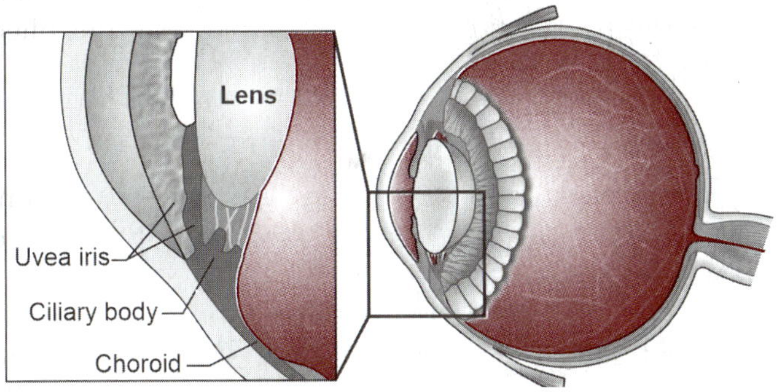

Fig. 7.14: Anatomy of the uvea

PUPIL (Fig. 7.15)

BAQ: Describe the pupil of the eye and its function.

Ans: Pupil is the opening within the iris through which light passes to lens and then light is focused onto the retina. The size of the opening is governed by the muscles of the iris. Muscle of iris rapidly constrict the pupil when exposed to bright light and expand (dilate) the pupil in dim light. This muscular action of iris is known as the photopupillary accommodation reflex action (Fig. 7.15).

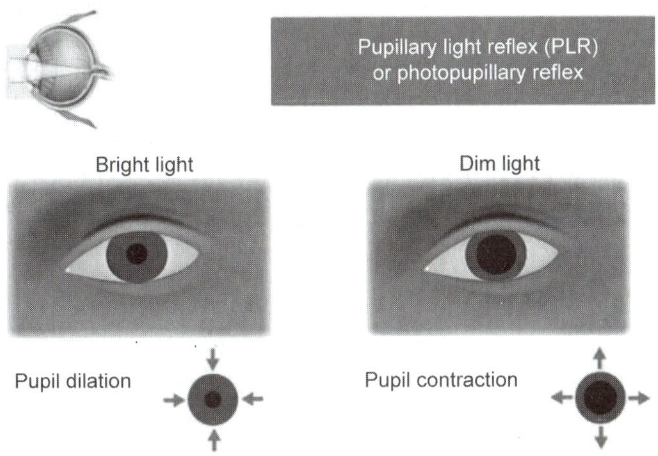

Fig. 7.15: Photopupillary accommodation refex action

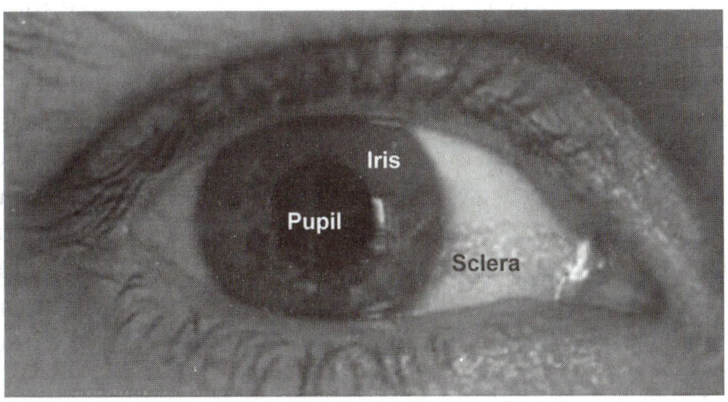

Fig. 7.16: Sclera part of the eye

SCLERA (Fig. 7.16)

LAQ: Describe the sclera of the eye under the following heads: (A) Description, (B) applied anatomy, (C) innervation, (D) blood supply and (E) functions.

Ans:

A. **Description:** The sclera is the white dense connective tissue of the eyeball. The sclera is connected with the stroma layer of the cornea. The junction between the sclera and the cornea is called the limbus (Fig. 7.15). The limbus contains the pathways of aqueous humour to flow out. It is very important site of surgical incisions for operations of cataract and glaucoma (refer page no. 169).

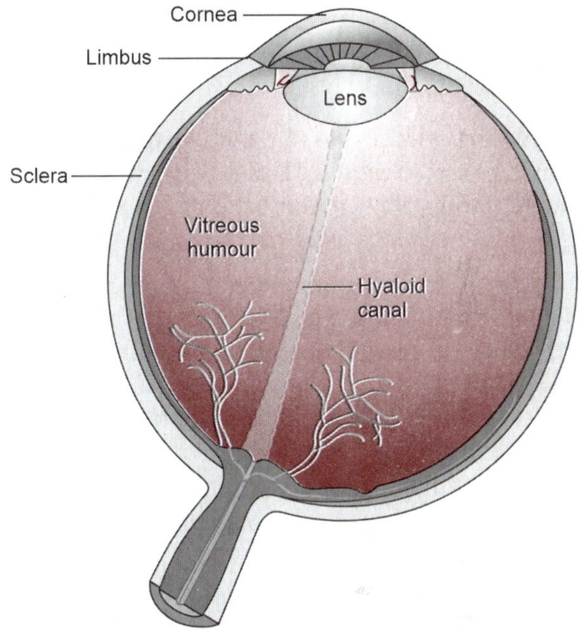

Fig. 7.17: Limbus and other parts of the eye

B. **Applied anatomy:** The sclera is composed of small fibers of collagen. These collagen fibers are arranged in irregular and interlacing bundles. This type of arrangement and interweaving of connective tissue give strength and flexibility to the eyeball.
The sclera is composed of the following four layers from external to internal side: Episclera, stroma, lamina fusca, and endothelium.

C. **Innervation:** Sensory innervation to the anterior sclera is supplied by the long posterior ciliary nerves, which is derived from the ophthalmic nerve. The posterior sclera is innervated by the short posterior ciliary nerves.

D. **Blood supply:** The arterial blood supply is derived from the anterior and posterior ciliary arteries. These arise from the ophthalmic artery.

E. **Functions:** The following are the various functions of sclera:
   1. It maintains the shape of the eyeball.
   2. It protects the eye from serious injuries from external trauma.
   3. It provides a sturdy attachment for the extraocular muscles that control the movement of the eyes.

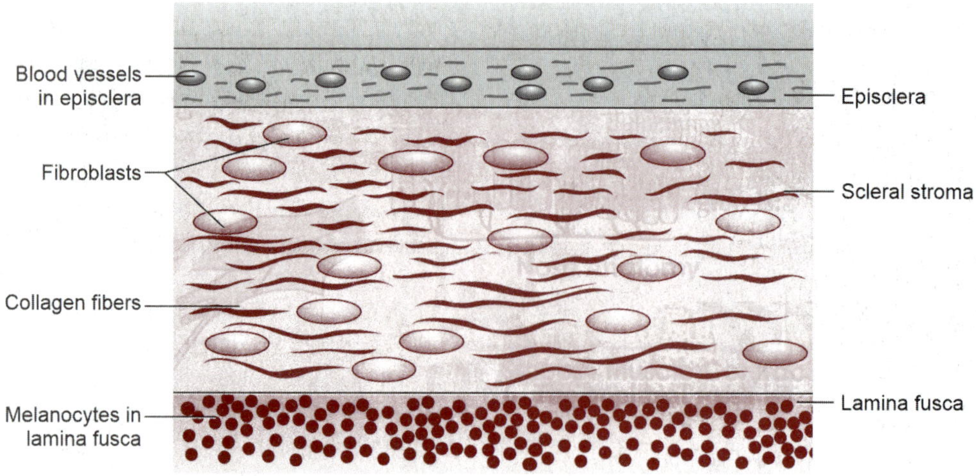

Fig. 7.18: Episclera layer of sclera with blood vessels

CHOROID (Fig. 7.10)

LAQ: Write a note on the choroid of an eye with respect to the following points: (A) Description, (B) applied anatomy, (C) innervation, (D) blood supply and (E) functions.

Ans:

A. **Description:** The choroid is a thin layer of tissue that is part of the middle layer of the wall of the eye. It is present between the sclera and the retina. The choroid is part of the uvea, which consists of the iris and the ciliary body (Figs 7.10 and 7.19). The choriod is filled with blood vessels that bring oxygen and nutrients to the eye.

B. **Applies anatomy:** The choroid is made up of following four different layers:
   1. Bruch's membrane: It is a thin layer of tissue located on the innermost part of the choroid.
   2. Choriocapillaris: It is made up of blood capillaries.
   3. Sattler's layer: It is made up of medium blood vessels.
   4. Haller's layer: It is outermost layer of the choroid that contains large blood vessels.

C. **Innervation:** The choroid is innervated by parasympathetic, sympathetic and trigeminal sensory nerve fibers.

D. **Blood supply:** The choroid is supplied by the long and short posterior ciliary arteries and the anterior ciliary arteries.

E. **Functions:** The following are the functions of he choroid:
   1. Choroidal blood circulation is responsible for nearly 85% of blood flow within the eye. Clear vision of eyes depends on sufficient blood supply.
   2. Choroid blood circulation is responsible for supply of nutrients to the retina, macula and optic nerve.
   3. It regulates the temperature of the retina.
   4. Choroid is also plays important role in fluid pressure control within the eye.
   5. Choroid also plays important role in absorbing light and limiting reflections within the eye, which could harm vision.

CILIARY BODY (Fig. 7.19)

BAQ: Describe the ciliary body of an eye under the following heads: (A) Description, (B) applied anatomy and (C) functions.

Ans:

A. **Description:** The ciliary body is a ring of tissue that surrounds the iris and connects it to the choroid (Fig. 7.19).

B. **Applied anatomy:** The ciliary body contains the ciliary muscle and secretory epithelial cells. The lens is attached to the ciliary body by radiating suspensory ligaments (Fig. 7.19).

C. **Functions:** Contraction and relaxation of the ciliary muscle fibers determine the size and thickness of the lens. The cells of ciliary epithelium cells produce the aqueous humour in the eye that control eye pressure and provise nourishment to the cornea.

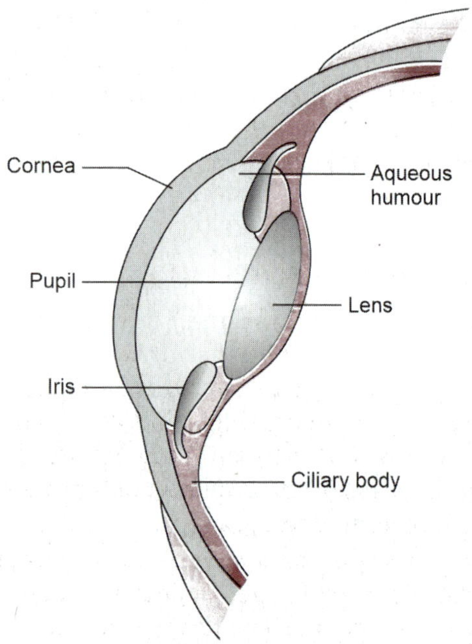

Fig. 7.19: Ciliary body

BAQ. Draw a labelled diagram of the ciliary body.

Ans: Refer to Fig. 7.19.

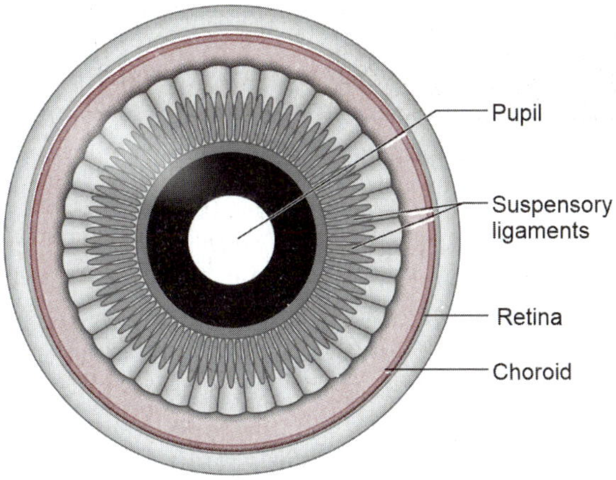

Fig. 7.20: Radiating suspensory ligaments

SAQ: Enumerate the functions of the ciliary body.

Ans: The following are three main functions of the ciliary body: (1) Accommodation, (2) holding the lens in place and (3) production of aqueous fluid.

SAQ: Define the word "accommodation" ability of the eye.

Ans: Accommodation means the ability of the eye that automatically increases its focusing power to enable the eye to see near objects clearly. This action depends on the ciliary muscle.

SAQ: Mention a clinical condition in which circulation of aqueous humour becomes disturbed.

Ans: A clinical condition "glaucoma" arises, if normal formation and circulation of aqueous humour fluid is disturbed, leading to ocular hypertension.

SAQ: Define presbyopia.

Ans: Presbyopia is the gradual loss of ability of eyes to focus on nearby objects. It is a natural part of aging. Presbyopia usually becomes noticeable mainly between the 40–50 years of age. Eye examination confirms presbyopia. It can be corrected using appropriate spectacles or contact lenses.

EYE LENS

BAQ: Write a note on the eye lens.

Ans: The lens is a transparent ellipsoid biconvex structure. The lens is suspended in place by the suspensory ligament (fibrous tissue) of the lens and connects to ciliary muscle (Fig. 7.17). Aqueous humour on anterior side and vitreous body on posterior side bathes the lens. Iris, which is in front of the lens regulates the amount of light entering into the eye.

Along with the cornea, lens is responsible for refraction of light, which gets focused on the retina. By changing the shape, the lens change the focal length of the eye so that it can focus on objects at various distances. This action allows a sharp real image of the object to form on the retina. This adjustment of the lens is known as accommodation (Fig. 7.21).

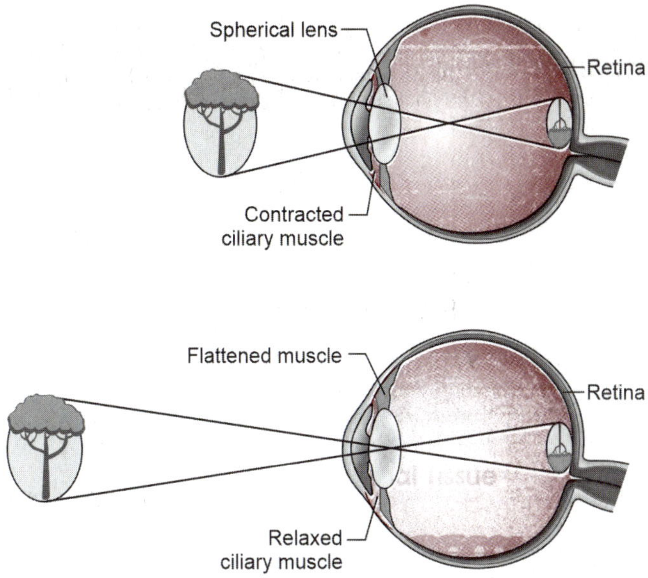

Fig. 7.21: Mechanism of eye accommodation

BAQ: Draw a labelled diagram of the mechanism of eye accommodation.

Ans: Refer to figure 7.21.

ANATOMY OF LENS

BAQ: Write a note on the anatomy of the eye.

Ans: The lens is formed of following three main parts: (1) lens capsule, (2) lens epithelium and (3) lens fibers.

1. **The lens capsule** forms the outermost layer of the lens and the lens fibers form the bulk of the interior of the lens. The lens does not contain connective tissue, nerves, and blood vessels.

   The lens capsule surrounds the lens. The capsule is smooth and elastic transparent basement membrane. It is composed of collagen and synthesized by the lens epithelium.
2. **The lens epithelium:** It is a simple cuboidal epithelium. The cells of the lens epithelium regulate most of the homeostatic functions of the lens by the control of various ions, nutrients, and liquid that enter the lens from the aqueous humour.
3. **Lens fibers:** These are arranged in interlocking layers (Fig. 7.8). These fibers stretch from the equatorial region to the anterior and posterior poles of the lens.

RETINA (Fig. 7.22)

BAQ: Write a note on the retina of the eye with respect to the description and gross anatomy.

Ans: Description: The retina is the innermost layer of tissue of the eye (Fig. 7.10). It is a light-sensitive part of the eye and creates electrical impulses that are sent through the optic nerve to the brain for the processing of the image of an article.

Anatomy of retina (Figs 7.20 and 7.21): Grossly, the retina consists of following parts: (1) Iridial part of retina, (2) ciliary part of retina, (3) optic part of retina, (4) macula (Fig. 7.22).

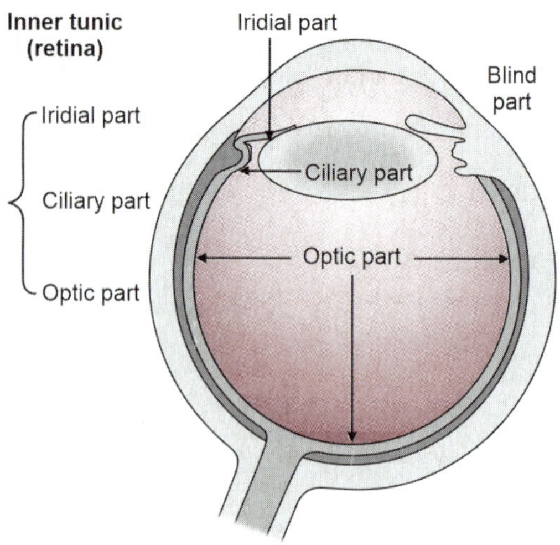

Fig. 7.22: Gross anatomy of retina

1. The iridial part of retina is located on the posterior face of the iris. It is composed of a double layer of pigmented cuboidal epithelium.
2. ***Ciliary part of retina:*** It is located on the posterior face of the ciliary body. It is composed of a simple layer of pigmented cuboidal epithelium.
3. The optic part of retina is the retinal portion sensitive to light. The optic part of retina receives the visual light rays. Optical part is further divided into following two parts, The pigmented epithelium part and the neural (nervous) part (neural retina).
4. The macula is the pigmented part of the retina located in the center of the retina. In the center of the macula is the fovea. The fovea contains a large amount of photoreceptor cells known as cones, which are responsible for clear vision (vision with high acuity).

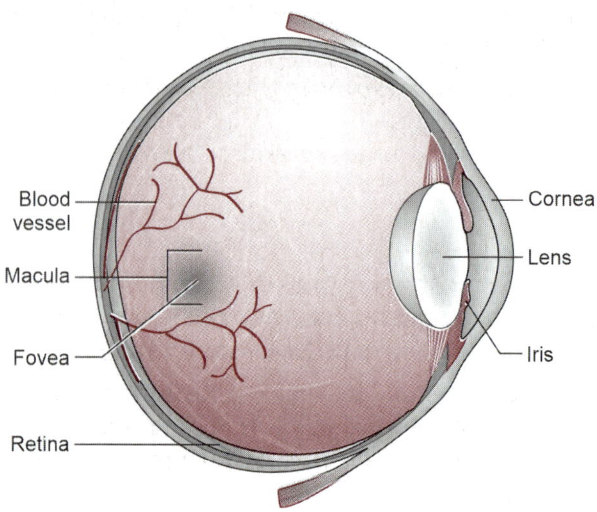

Fig. 7.23A: Macula

Anatomy of Neural Retina (Fig. 7.24)

LAQ: Describe the neural retina under the following heads: (A) Anatomy, (B) Function, (C) Blood supply and (D) Innervation.

Ans:

A. **Anatomy:** The neural retina consists of several layers of neurons interconnected by synapses. The neural retina is composed of two layers: (1) The thin pigmented layer and (2) the nervous layer.
   1. The thin pigmented layer is retinal pigment epithelium (RPE). It is in contact with the choroid and outer thick nervous layer in the visual portion. The RPE is the pigmented cell layer just outside the neurosensory retina. It provides nourishment to retinal visual cells. It is firmly attached to the underlying choroid and overlying retinal visual cells.
   2. The nervous layer contains the following three types of cells: Rods, cones and ganglion neurons. The optic nerve consists of the axons merged from the ganglion neurons. The rods, cones and ganglion cells are the primary light-sensing cells in the retina. Rods function mainly in low intensity of light and provide black-and-white vision. Cones function in good quality of light conditions and these are responsible for the differentiation of colour. The cones are also responsible for vision required for reading. The ganglion cells play important role in the determination and modification of circadian rhythms and reflexive responses such as the pupillary light reflex. The pupillary light reflex is an autonomic reflex that constricts the pupil in response to light and adjusting the amount of light that falls on the retina.

      More than 100 million rods are present in each eye and these are present in large number on the

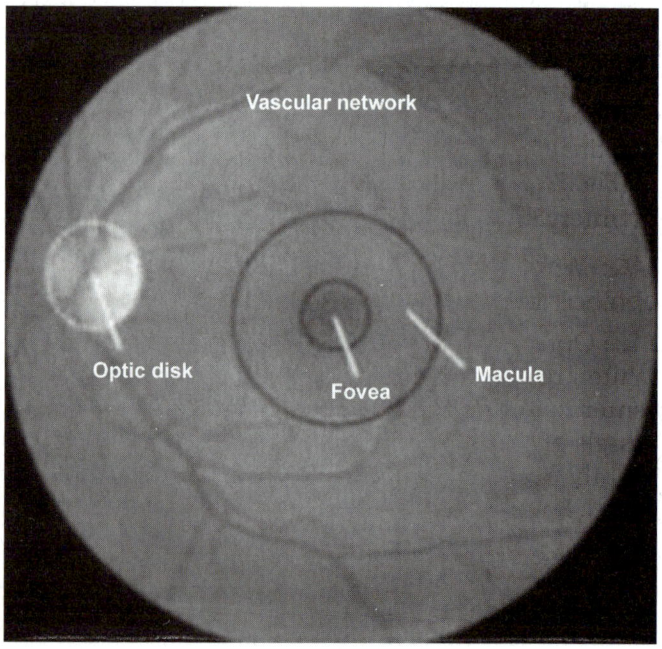

7.23B: Fovea of retina

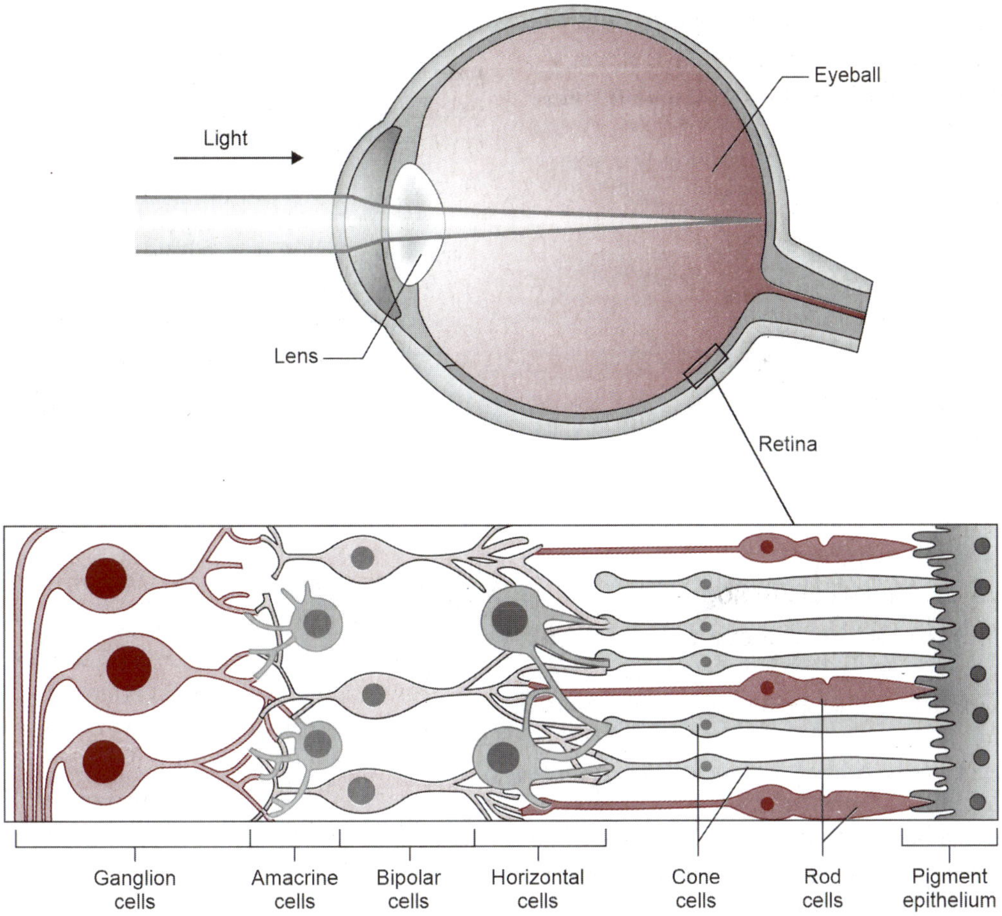

Fig. 7.24: Anatomy of neural retina

periphery of the retina. Number of cones is about 7 million in each eye and these are present mainly in the macular region of the eye.

B. **Function:** When light strikes the retina, it initiates a cascade of chemical and electrical events that trigger nerve impulses. Nerve impulses are sent to various visual centres of the brain through the fibres of the optic nerve. Neural signals from the rods and cones undergo processing of the image of an object by other neurons in the form of action potentials in retinal ganglion cells whose axons form the optic nerve.

C. **Blood supply:** The retina is supplied by the central retinal artery and the short posterior ciliary arteries (Fig. 7.26).

D. **Innervation:** By optic nerve CN II.

SAQ: What view of the retina is observed by the ophthalmologist through the slit-lamp bimicroscope?

Ans: Optic nerve is in the center of the retina as a oval white area measuring (about 1.5 × 2 mm). From the center of the optic nerve the radiating major blood vessels of the retina. On the left side "fovea", which is slightly oval-shaped reddish spot and free from blood vessel. Fovea is at the center of the macula (Fig. 7.25).

BAQ: Draw a neat and lalelled figure of the anatomical features of neural retina

Ans: Refer to Fig. 7.24.

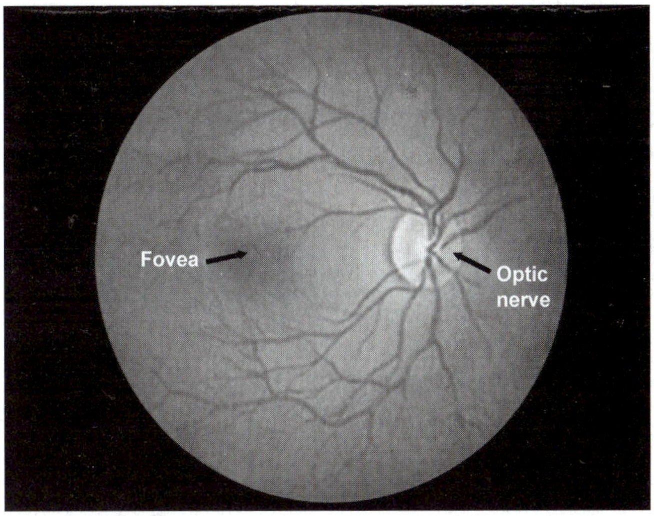

Fig. 7.25: Retina as observed by the ophthalmologist

BLOOD SUPPLY OF THE EYE

SAQ: Write a note on the blood supply of an eye.

Ans: An ophthalmic artery and a central retinal artery (that branches off of the ophthalmic artery) provide blood to each eye. Similarly, ophthalmic veins and a central retinal vein drain blood from the eye (Fig. 7.26). These blood vessels enter and leave through the back of the eye.

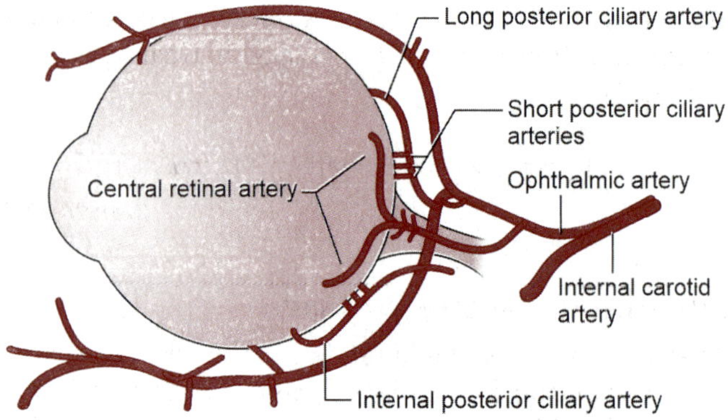

Fig. 7.26: Blood supply to the eye

Objective: To describe the physiology of eyes.

EYE PHYSIOLOGY

BAQ: Write a note on the eye physiology.

Ans: The transparent lens of the eye focuses light on cone cells in fovea region of the retina. The cone cells, which are present in fovea region of retina, are sensitive to colour. The rod cells present around fovea region are not sensitive to colour, but they have greater sensitivity to light than the cone cells. These rod cells are responsible for peripheral vision and night vision. The eye is connected to the brain through the optic nerve. The occipital lobe of the brain maps the visual input from the eyes. The brain combines the input of two eyes into a three-dimensional image. Although, the image on the retina is upside-down because of the focusing action of the lens, the brain compensates and provides the right-side-up perception (Fig. 7.27). In the dark, photopigments produced by the rod cells increase the sensitivity of the eye. Hence, it is possible to see objects in very dim light. In strong light, the iris contracts and the size of the aperture gets reduced and light entering into the eye get reduced.

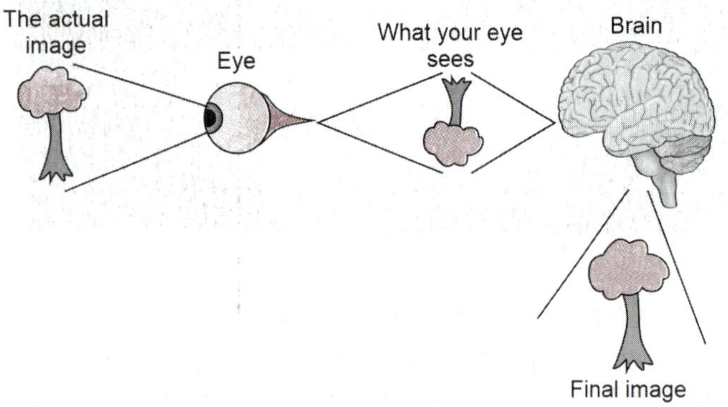

Fig. 7.27: Image of an object produced on the retina and the final image

SAQ: What is blind spot?

Ans: The light-sensitive cells are not present at the spot where optic nerve connects to retina. That specific spot on retina is called "blind spot", which cannot see the object (Fig. 7.28).

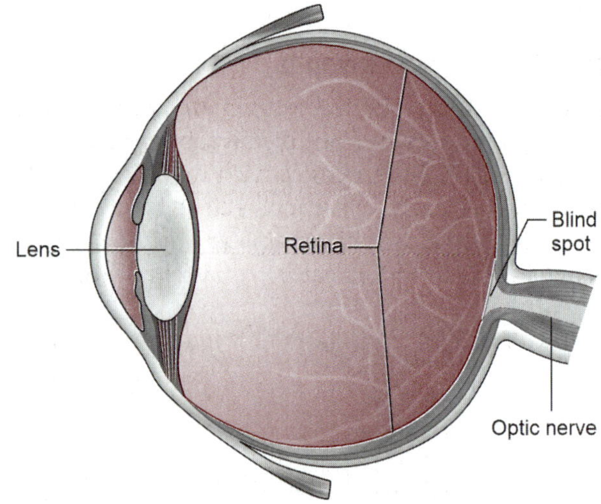

Fig. 7.28: Blind spot

SAQ: Which spectral range is recorded and processed by the eyes?

Ans: A human eye can see and differentiate visible spectrum range from the red colour to the violet colour. A normal eye cannot see lower electromagnetic frequencies in the infrared light. However, these can be sensed as heat. Ultraviolet light also cannot be seen. The human eye is also not sensitive to the polarized light.

Objective: To identify and explain the refractory errors of the eye.

REFRACTORY ERRORS (REFRACTIVE ERRORS) OF THE EYE

BAQ: Write a note on the refractory errors of the eye.

Ans: Refractive disorders are observed when the shape of the eye prevents light from focusing directly on the retina. This results in blurred vision (Fig. 7.29).

The most common types of refractive disorders include: Myopia (near-sightedness), hyperopia (far-sightedness), astigmatism, which lead to make far-away and nearby objects look blurry or distorted and presbyopia is an age-related condition in which the lens of eye can no longer change shape appropriately to allow the eye to focus clearly. Refractive disorders can be corrected with eyeglasses, contact lenses, or by using refractive surgery methods.

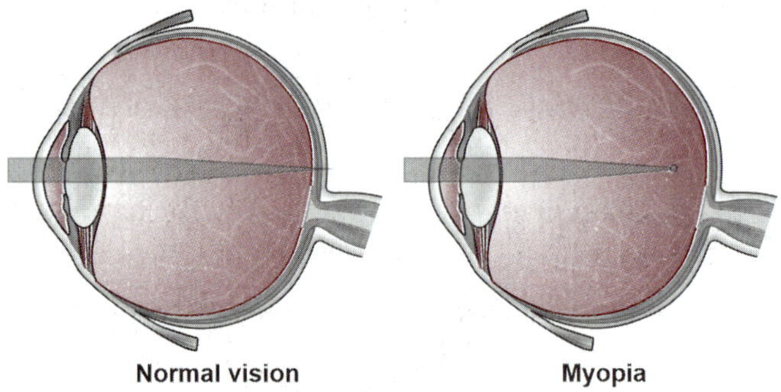

Fig. 7.29: Myopia

Myopia

BAQ: Write a note on myopia.

Ans: Myopia (near-sightedness) is an eye disorder, in which, light focuses in front of the retina instead of on the retina (Fig. 7.30). A person with myopia cannot see distant objects clearly. Distant objects in myopia appear blurry. However, close objects appear normal in myopia. Concave lens is used to treat myopia (Fig. 7.30).

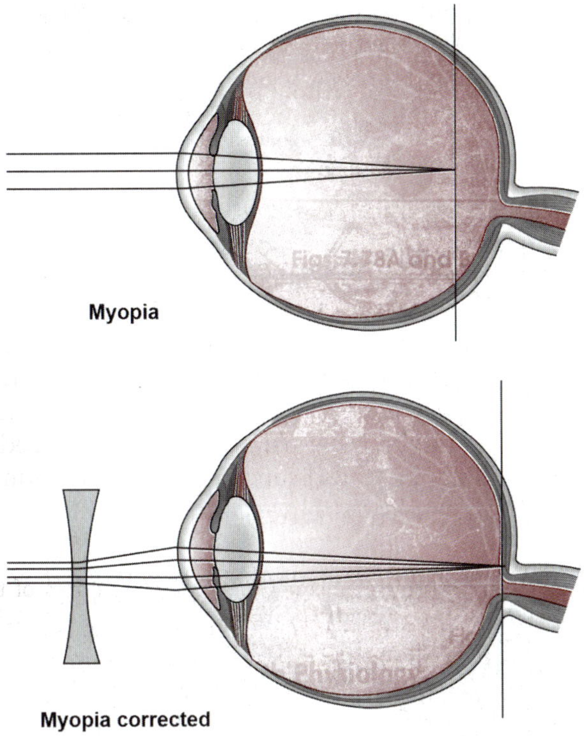

Fig. 7.30: Myopia corrected using concave lens

Hyperopia

BAQ: Write a note on hyperopia.

Ans: Hyperopia (far-sightedness) is an eye disorder, in which, light focuses beyond the retina instead of on the retina (Fig. 7.31). Hyperopia is caused due to insufficient accommodation. Convex lens is used to treat hyperopia (Fig. 7.31).

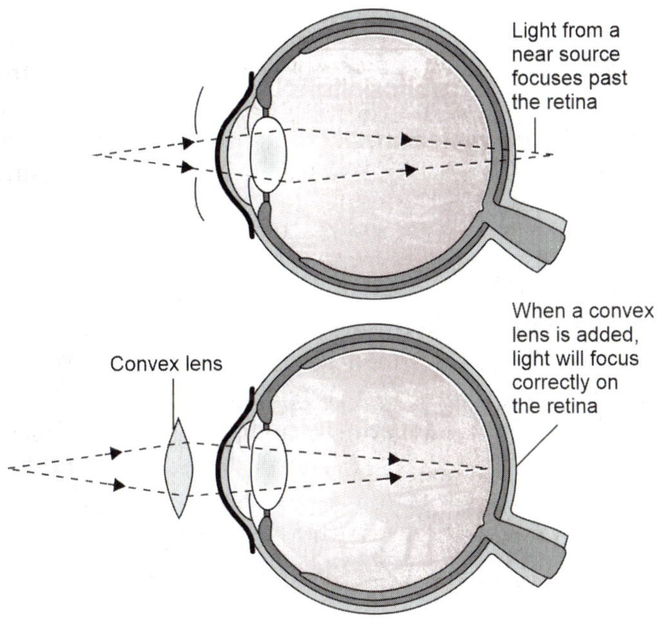

Fig. 7.31: Hyperopia and correction by convex lens

Objective: To explain the formation of eye colours.

EYE COLOURS (Fig. 7.32)

BAQ: Write a note on eye colours.

Ans: The colour of eye is related to the iris. It depends on the amount of melanin pigment distributed in eye and on the ratio of eumelanin to pheomelanin. Eye colours have been divided into nine categories. There are 16 genes associated with eye-colour determination. The following are three types of naturally occurring melanins: Eumelanin, pheomelanin and neuromelanin.

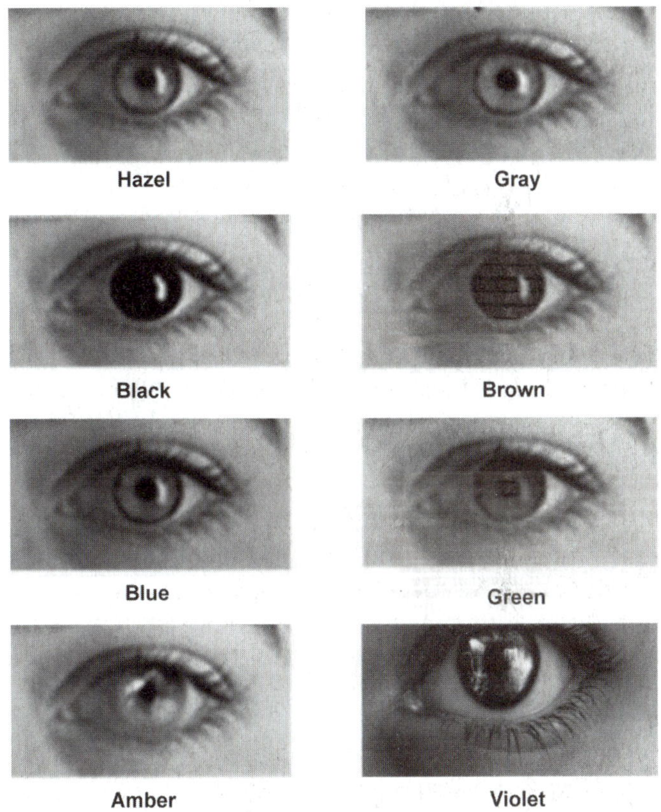

Fig. 7.32: Eye colours

Objective: To explain the importance of the visual field.

Visual Field

BAQ: Write a note on the visual field.

Ans: The visual field is the total area in which objects can be seen in the side (peripheral) vision when focus of eyes are on a central point. Central vision is needed for seeing objects clearly and for common daily tasks such as reading and driving. Macula provides central vision. Central vision is useful to focus on the details of the object and peripheral vision is useful to gather information about the surroundings.

The anterior position of eyes allow an overall field of vision about 1800. Within the field of vision, the following are three visual fields: (1) Macular field, (2) binocular field and (3) monocular fields.

The macular field is the area of sharp vision obtained as central vision, since, light rays from this area activate phosphoreceptors in fovea and macula regions.

The binocular field can be viewed from both eyes, however, it is not as sharp as macular field (Fig. 7.33).

The monocular field is viewed by only one eye and it is hazy peripheral vision (Fig. 7.34).

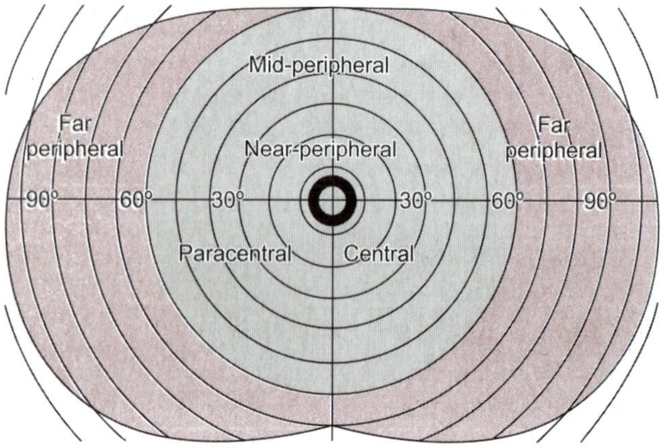

Fig. 7.33: Central vision and macular field

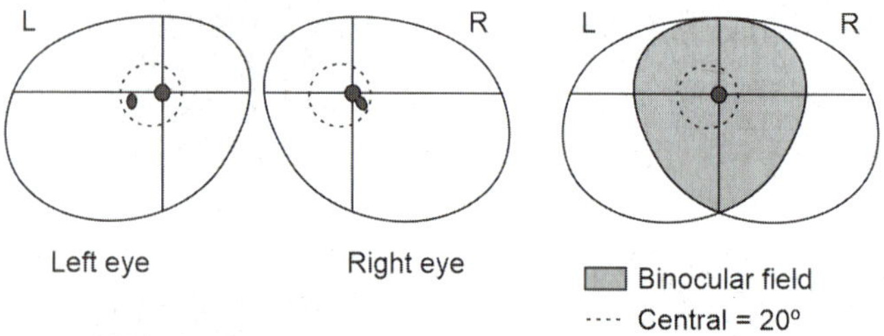

Fig. 7.34: Monocular and binocular fields

EYE DISORDERS

Objective: To describe various eye disorders and diseases.

Night Blindness (Nyctalopia)

BAQ: Write a note on night blindness.

Ans: Night blindness is a clinical condition, which leads to inability to see clearly in darkness. Night blindness may be caused by the following main reasons: (1) Genetic deficiency of specific proteins in the rods since birth as a congenital clinical condition. (2) Vitamin A deficiency. Vitamin A is necessary for process of the visual cycle performed by the rods that involve rhodopsin, a light sensitive protein. Presently there is no treatment on the congenital night blindness, however, vitamin A deficiency could be corrected by appropriate food supplements containing vitamin A.

Colour Blindness

BAQ: Write a note on colour blindness.

Ans: Colour blindness is the decreased ability to see differences in colour. It can impair tasks such reading traffic lights and selecting coloured substances such as fruits and clothes, etc. The most common cause of colour blindness is an inherited defects in cone cells, which differentiate colour. More men are affected than female.

Colour blindness can also result from physical or chemical damage to internal part of eye, the optic nerve, and specific part of the brain related to vision.

Inherited colour blindness cannot be treated. However, if colour blindness is caused by other treatable clinical condition, appropriate treatment may be effective in treating colour blindness.

Macular Degeneration

BAQ: Write a note on macular degeneration.

Ans: Macular degeneration leads to failure of eyes to see sharp and central vision (Fig. 7.35). Macular degeneration causes loss in the centre of the field of vision. There are two types of macular degenerations: Dry macular degeneration and wet macular degeneration. In dry macular degeneration deterioration of center of retina takes place. In wet macular degeneration, blood vessels under the retina leak blood. Macular degeneration usually occurs in older persons.

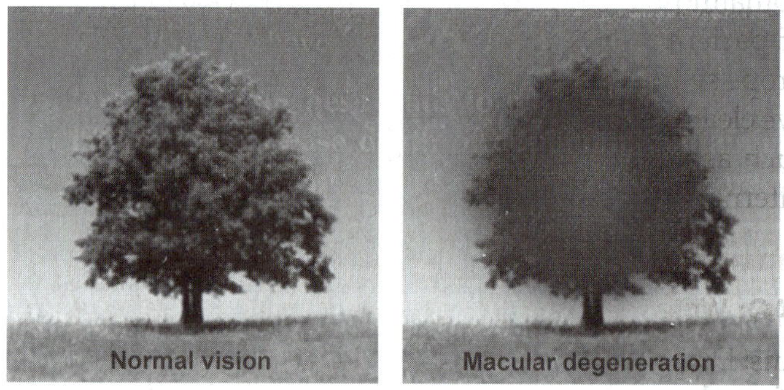

Fig. 7.35: Images seen by normal vision and in macular degeneration

Cataract (Fig. 7.36)

BAQ: Write a note on cataract.

Ans: A cataract is a clouding of the lens of the eye (Fig. 7.36). Lens of the normal eye is clear. Most cataracts develop slowly in several years. Activities such as reading and driving become difficult with advancing cataract. Cataracts develop slowly and do not disturb eyesight during earlier years. However, once cataract develops further with significant proportion, it will eventually interfere with normal vision.

Most cataracts develop with advancing age and also due to injury to the lens tissue Proteins and fibers in the lens slowly break down, leading to development of cataract. A cataract scatters and blocks the light that passes through the lens, and prevents formation of a sharp defined image on retina, leading to blurred vision.

Prolonged untreated diabetes mellitus may lead to early development of cataract. Similarly, certain inherited genetic disorders also can increase risk of cataracts.

The only treatment for cataracts is surgical replacement of lens affected by cataract with an artificial intraocular lens. It is very safe and effective treatment to treat cataract.

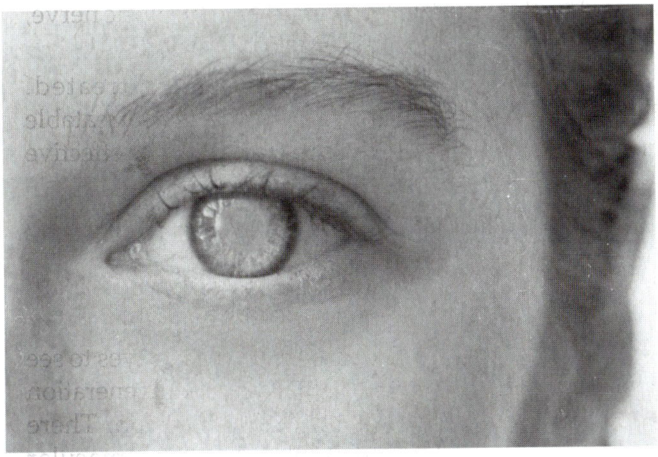

Fig. 7.36: Cataract

SAQ: What is fundoscopy?

Ans: The fundus of eye is made up of the retina, macula, optic disc, fovea and blood vessels in retina (Fig. 7.25). In fundoscopy, ophthalmologists use an instrument opthalmoscope to check the fundus of the eye. The pupils of patient are dilated (enlarged) with medicated eye drops so that the doctor can see the fundus region of an eye clearly. Fundoscopy is used to check for eye disorders such as macular degeneration, cataract, glaucoma and internal eye injury.

Diabetic Retinopathy (DR) (Fig. 7.37)

BAQ: Write a note on diabetic retinopathy.

Ans: Diabetic retinopathy (DR) is a common complication of prolonged uncontrolled diabetes mellitus. It is characterized by progressive damage to the blood vessels and nerves of the retina caused by high blood sugar, and related increased cholesterol and sorbitol (Fig. 7.34).

Early symptoms include floaters, blurriness, dark areas of vision and difficulty perceiving colours. Diabetic retinopathy may lead to blindness, if diabetes is not managed appropriately.

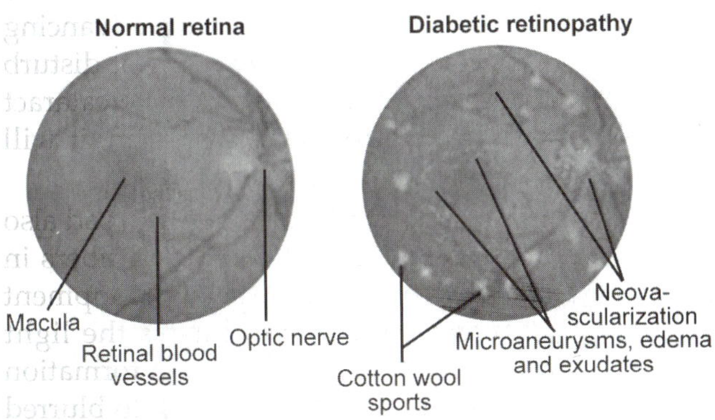

Fig. 7.37: Normal retina and diabetic retinopathy

Glaucoma

BAQ: Write a note on glaucoma.

Ans: Glaucoma is an eye disease that damages optic nerve of eye. Optic nerve damage leads to vision loss and blindness. Glaucoma occurs when the normal fluid pressure inside the eyes increases significantly. Glaucoma is a leading cause of blindness for persons over the age of 60 years. However, blindness from glaucoma can often be prevented using early treatment.

Eye constantly makes aqueous humour. When newly formed aqueous flows into the eye, same amount of aqueous humour drain out. The fluid drains out through the drainage angle in the eye (Fig. 7.38). This process of normal circulation of aqueous humour keeps intraocular pressure in the eye stable. However, defect caused in the drainage angle leads to increase in fluid and pressure inside the eye rises. The rise in the eye pressure leads to the optic nerve damage.

Following are two major categories of glaucoma: (1) Open angle glaucoma and (2) closed angle glaucoma.

1. Open angle glaucoma is a slow progressing chronic condition. It progresses over long period of time and patient may not notice vision loss until the disease reaches advanced stage. Various reasons for this clinical condition are advanced age, uncontrolled diabetes mellitus, high blood pressure and congenital reasons.
2. Closed angle glaucoma may appear suddenly and it is a painful clinical condition. Visual loss in this condition progresses very fast. Various reasons for closed angle glaucoma may be due to malignancy, accident, unknown severe diabetes, and hypertension, etc. (Fig. 7.39).

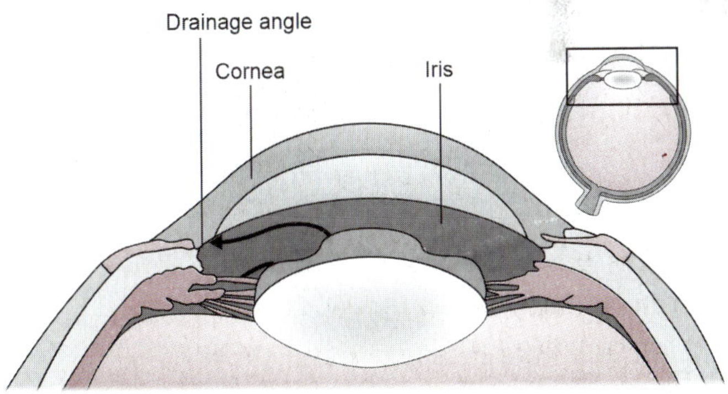

Fig. 7.38: Fluid drainage angle in the eye

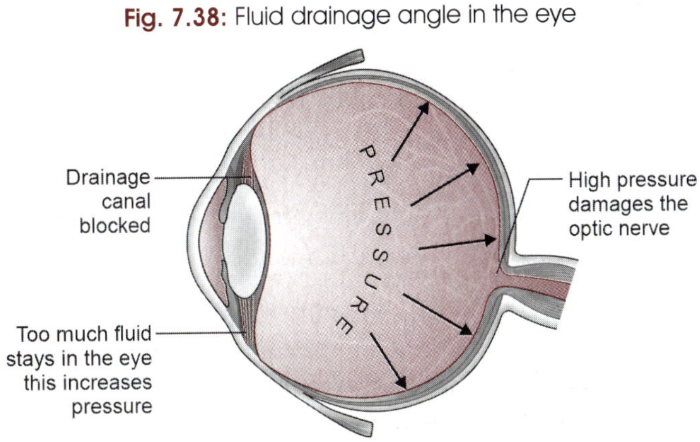

Fig. 7.39: Blocked fluid drainage canal leading to glaucoma

Amblyopia (Lazy Eye) (Fig. 7.40)

BAQ: Write a note on amblyopia (lazy eye).

Ans: Amblyopia (lazy eye) is a disorder of sight. In amblyopia the brain fails to fully process inputs from one eye, which results in the decrease in the vision in this eye. However, inputs from other eye are processed by the brain and vision is normal in the other eye. Amblyopia is the most common cause of decreased vision in a single eye among children (Fig. 7.40).

Amblyopia can occur from the following reasons: (1) Poor alignment of the eyes (strabismic), (2) irregular shape of an eye, leading to difficulty in focussing and (3) one eye more farsighted or nearsighted than the other eye (refractive), (4) clouding of the lens of an eye.

Amblyopia is difficult to diagnose, since, affected eye looks normal. Hence, eye examination is recommended for all young children. After the diagnosis of underlying cause, appropriate glasses may be useful in the large number of cases.

If amblyopia is not treated in early childhood, it usually persists into adulthood, and is the most common cause of permanent one-eye vision impairment.

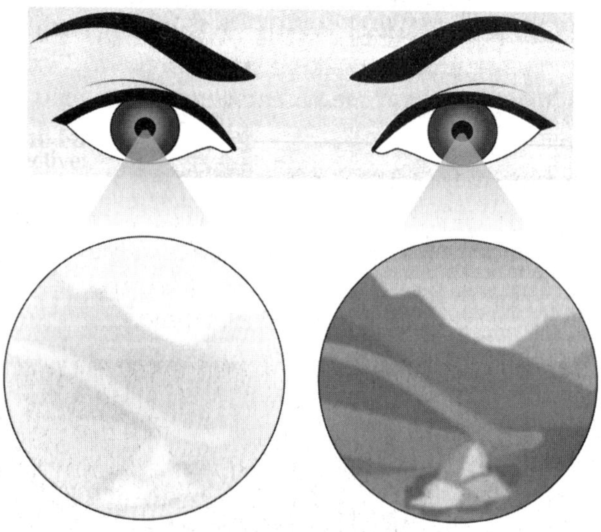

Fig. 7.40: Amblyopia

Strabismus (Fig. 7.41)

BAQ: Write a note on strabismus.

Ans: Strabismus is an imbalance in the positioning of the two eyes. Strabismus is caused by a lack of coordination between the eyes. Hence, the eyes look in different directions and do not focus simultaneously at a single point. When the two eyes fail to focus on the same image, there is reduced depth perception and the brain may tend to ignore the input from one eye, causing permanent vision loss in that eye.

Strabismus may be present since birth of a child or it may occur in later age due to nerve injury, infections or dysfunction of the muscles controlling the affected eye.

Following are various types of strabismus:

1. Esotropia, when the eyes are crossed (cross eyed)
2. Exotropia, when the eyes look diverge (lazy eyed) and
3. Hypertropia or Hypotropia when they are vertically misaligned (Figs 7.41 and 7.42).

Early treatment on strabismus is recommended to prevent vision loss and treatment depends on the type of strabismus and the underlying cause. Treatment may include the use of appropriate glasses and surgery.

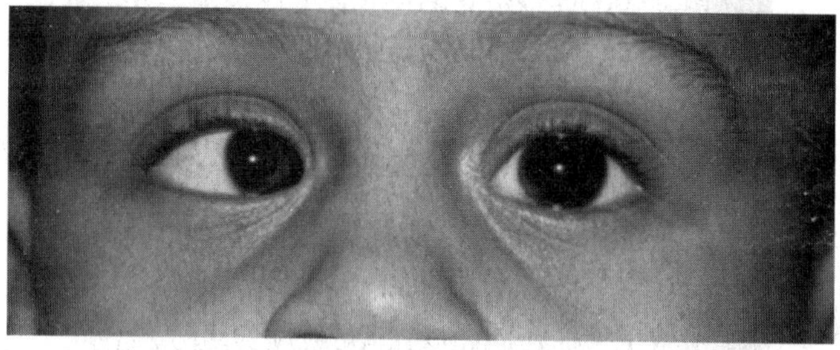

Fig. 7.41: Strabismus (crossed eyes)

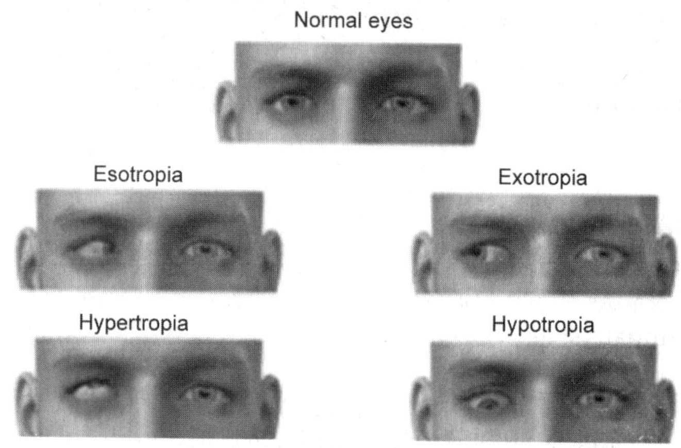

Fig. 7.42: Various types of strabismus

EYE INFECTIONS

SAQ: Write a note on eye infections.

Ans: Eye infections are caused by microorganisms such as viruses, bacteria, fungi and parasites. Eye infections lead to red eyes, pain, blurred vision, excessive formation of tears, eye discharge, increased sensitivity to light, and itching of eyes. It is necessary to diagnose and treat eye infections early to prevent complications and serious damages to eyes.

Conjunctivitis is the most common eye infection. However, it rarely causes vision loss. Corneal infection (keratitis) and endophthalmitis (inflammation of eye) are less common eye infections. However, these infections pose a serious risk to vision.

Conjunctivitis (Pink Eye) (Fig. 7.43)

BAQ: Write a note on conjunctivitis (pink eye).

Ans: Conjunctivitis is inflammation of the outermost layer of the white part of the eye and the inner surface of the eyelid. The eyes appear pink or reddish when person suffers from conjunctivitis.

Viral conjunctivitis is the most common cause of infectious conjunctivitis. Bacterial conjunctivitis is a less frequent cause of conjunctivitis. It is more common in children. Conjunctivitis caused by bacteria or virus

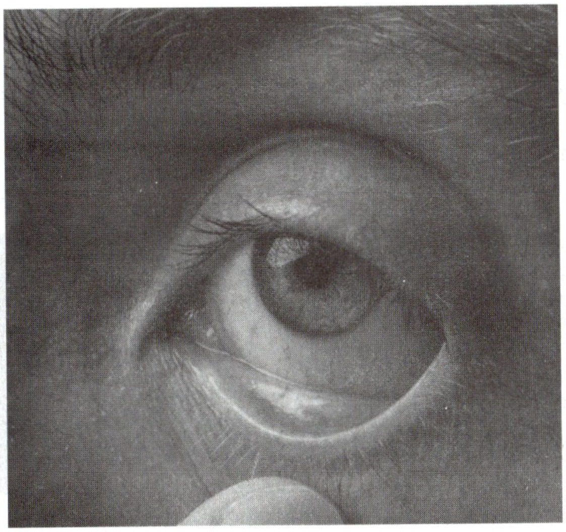

Fig. 7.43: Conjunctivitis

is highly contagious. Certain allergens also may cause conjunctivitis.

Infectious Keratitis (Fig. 7.44)

SAQ: What is infectious keratitis?

Ans: Infections of the cornea are called infectious keratitis. Infectious keratitis results from bacterial, viral, fungal, or parasitic infections.

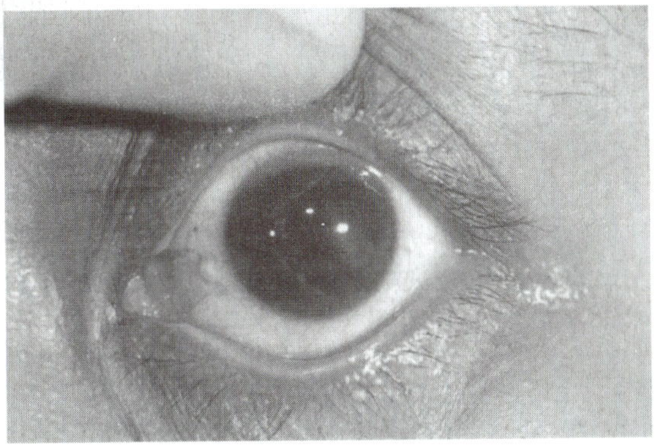

Fig. 7.44: Infectious keratitis

Endophthalmitis (Fig. 7.45)

SAQ: Write a note on endophthalmitis.

Ans: Endophthalmitis is severe inflammation of the inside of eye resulting from a bacterial or fungal

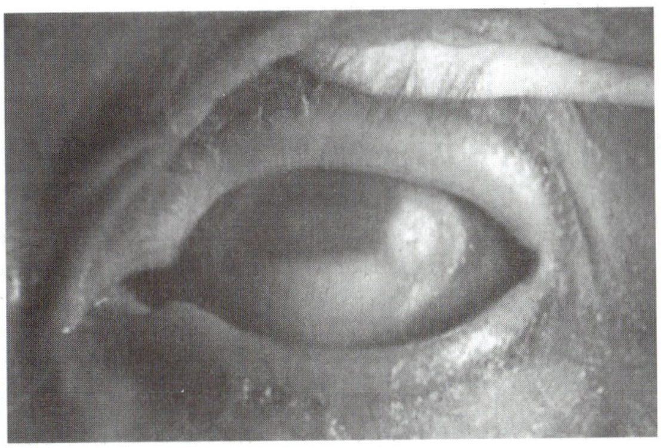

Fig. 7.45: Endophthalmitis

infection. Fungal infections (e.g. candida) are the most common cause of endophthalmitis.

Endophthalmitis may occur after certain eye surgeries, such as cataract surgery, which is very rare.

Blepharitis (Fig. 7.46)

SAQ: Write a note on blepharitis.

Ans: Blepharitis is an inflammation of eyelid. It is usually caused by clogging of the oil glands inside the eyelid skin at the base of eyelashes. Blepharitis may be caused by bacterial infection.

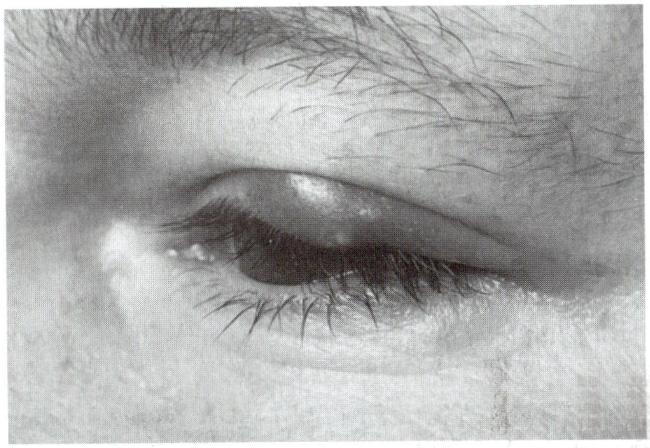

Fig. 7.46: Blepharitis

Stye (Fig. 7.47)

BAQ: Write a note on a style.

Ans: A stye is a red and painful lump near the edge of the eyelid. It looks like a pimple or boil. A stye may develop when the small glands that line the eyelid get blocked. A stye can form on the inner part of the eyelid.

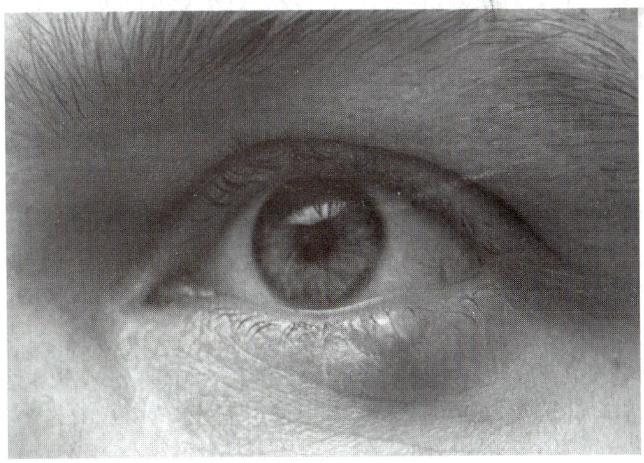

Fig. 7.47: A stye

Trachoma (Fig. 7.48)

BAQ: Write a note on tracoma.

Ans: Trachoma is an infectious disease caused by *Chlamydia trachomatis* bacteria. Trachoma is a contagious eye disease. It spreads by means of contact with the eyes, nose or throat secretions of the infected persons. Repeated or untreated trachoma infections may lead to permanent blindness.

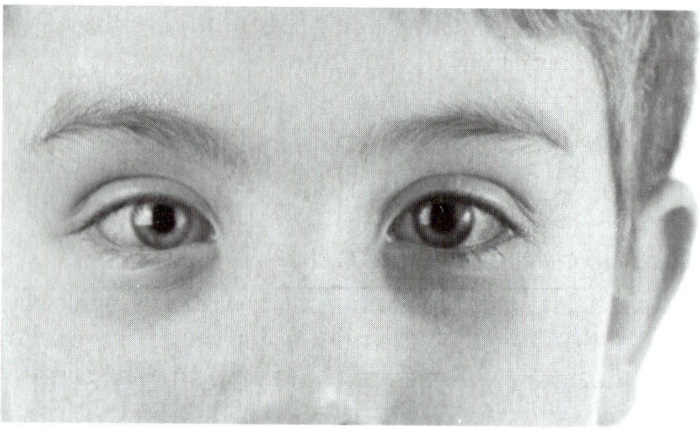

Fig. 7.48: Trachoma infection

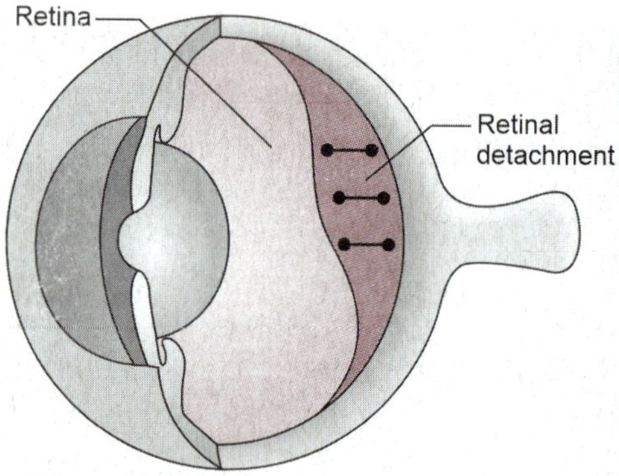

Fig. 7.50: Retinal detachment

Corneal Ulcer (Fig. 7.49)

BAQ: Write a note on corneal ulcer.

Ans: A corneal ulcer is an open sore of the cornea. Various factors responsible for corneal ulcer are: Viral, bacterial, fungal, and parasitic infections, physical and chemical trauma. Persons who wear contact lenses are also likely to get corneal ulcers. Corneal ulcers are serious eye problems and if not treated in time, may lead to loss of vision.

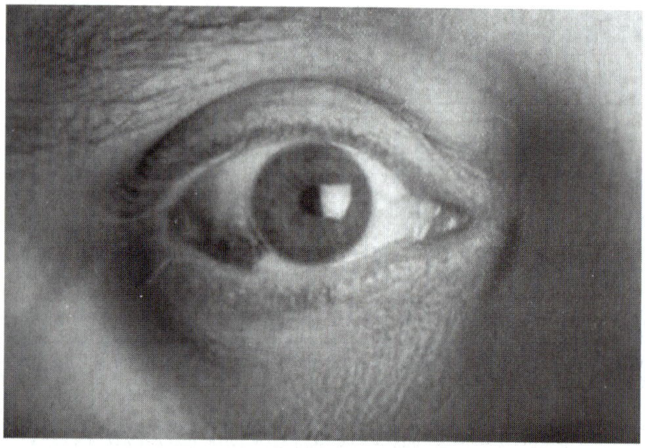

Fig. 7.49: Corneal ulcer

Retinal Detachment (Fig. 7.50)

BAQ: Write a note on retinal detachment (Fig. 7.50).

Ans: Retinal detachment means the retina pulls away from its normal position. Retinal detachment leads to separation of the retinal cells from the layer of blood vessels that provides nourishment and oxygen. Untreated retinal detachment increases risk of permanent vision loss of the affected eye.

Retinitis Pigmentosa (Fig. 7.51)

BAQ: Write a note on retinitis pigmentosa.

Ans: Retinitis pigmentosa is a rare, inherited degenerative eye disease that leads to vision impairment. Symptoms of retinitis pigmentosa often begin in childhood. The symptoms include decreased vision in low light and loss of side vision. There is no effective treatment for retinitis pigmentosa.

EYE CANCERS

BAQ: Write a note on eye cancers.

Ans: Eye cancer is a general term used to describe tumor present in any part of the eye. Tumour formation takes place when normal cells in the eye change and grow uncontrollably leading to formation of a tumour. The tumour can be cancerous or noncancerous (benign). Most eye tumours are caused by cancer cells that spread from one part of the body to another part.

A tumour of melanin-forming cells is called a melanoma. Most eye melanomas occur in the choroid, which is located between the retina and the sclera. Choroidal melanoma is the most common primary malignant intraocular tumour (Fig. 7.52).

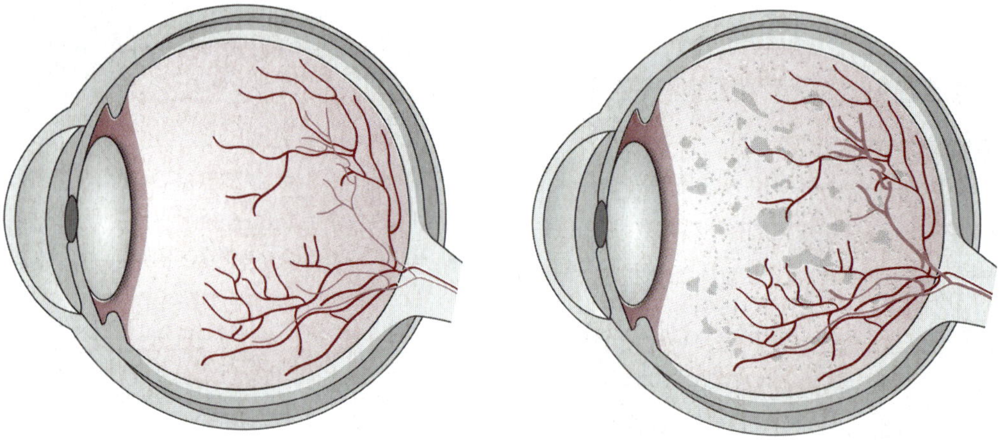

Fig. 7.51: Retinitis pigmentosa

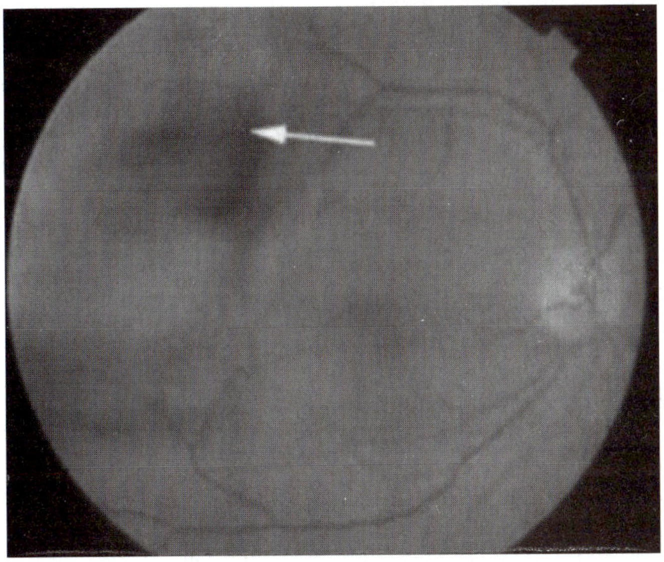

Fig. 7.52: Choroidal malignant melanoma

Retinoblastoma is a type of primary intraocular tumour (Fig. 7.53). Eyelid carcinoma, conjunctival melanoma, and lacrimal gland tumor are some rare types of eye cancers.

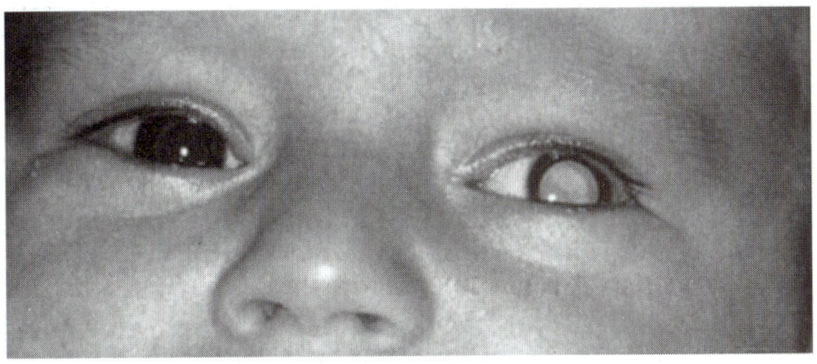

Fig. 7.53: Retinoblastoma

Objective: To describe the anatomy of ear and important functions of anatomical parts of an ear.

EAR (Fig. 7.55)

The ear is the organ of hearing and balance.

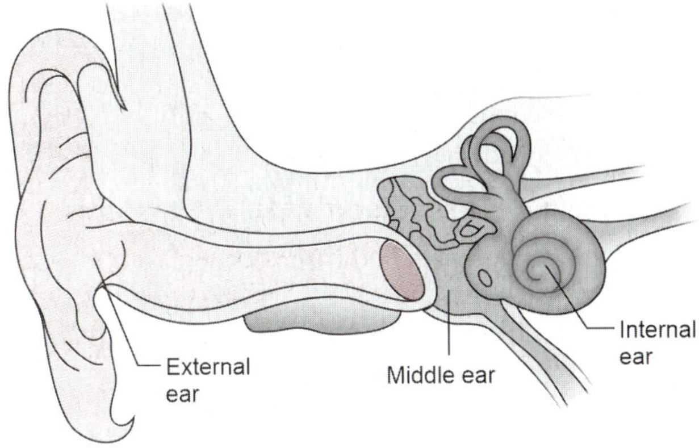

Fig. 7.54: Three main parts of ear

Anatomy of the Ear (Fig. 7.54)

SAQ: What are the main parts of ear?

Ans: Ear can be divided into the following three main parts: (1) the outer ear, (2) the middle ear, and (3) the inner ear. The outer ear and middle ear collect sound and amplify it. The inner ear converts sound waves to messages that are sent to the brain (Fig. 7.54).

BAQ: Draw a neat and labelled figure of main parts of ear.

Ans: Refer to Fig. 7.54.

Outer Ear (Figs 7.55A and B)

BAQ: Write a note on the outer ear.

Ans: The auricle (pinna) is the visible portion of the outer ear. The outer ear appears in different types of shapes and sizes. Outer ears give each individual unique appearance. It is made up of skin and cartilage. Following are three main parts to the outer ear: The tragus, helix and the lobule. The ear canal begins at the outer ear and ends at the ear drum.

Nerve Supply to External Ear

BAQ: Write a note on the nerve supply to the ears.

Ans: Sensory innervation to the external ear is supplied by cranial and spinal nerves. Cranial nerves are branches

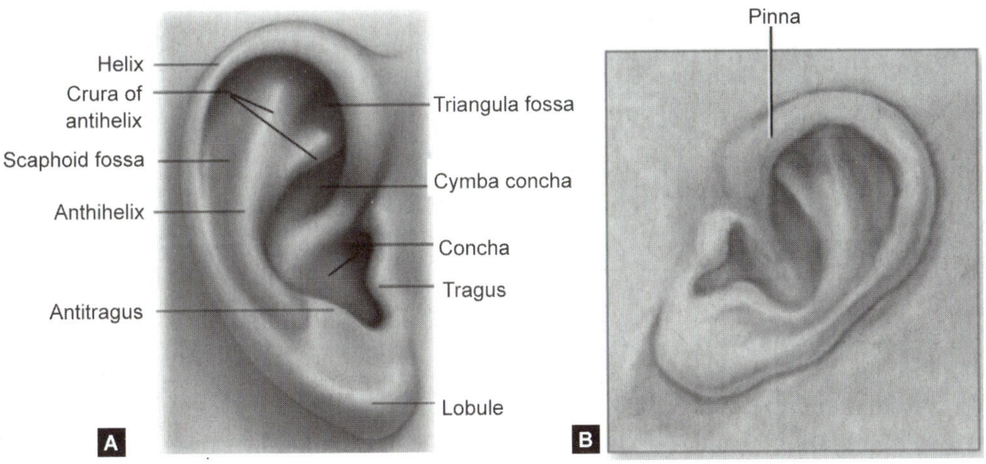

Figs 7.55A and B: Outer ear (pinna) parts

of the trigeminal, facial, and vagus nerves (CN V, VII, X) and the spinal nerves are lesser occipital (C2, C3) and greater auricular (C2, C3) nerves.

Blood Supply of Ears (Fig. 7.56)

BAQ: Write a note on blood supply to the ears.

Ans: The ear receives blood from a branch of the external carotid artery. The external carotid artery extends a branch called the posterior auricular artery to the ear.

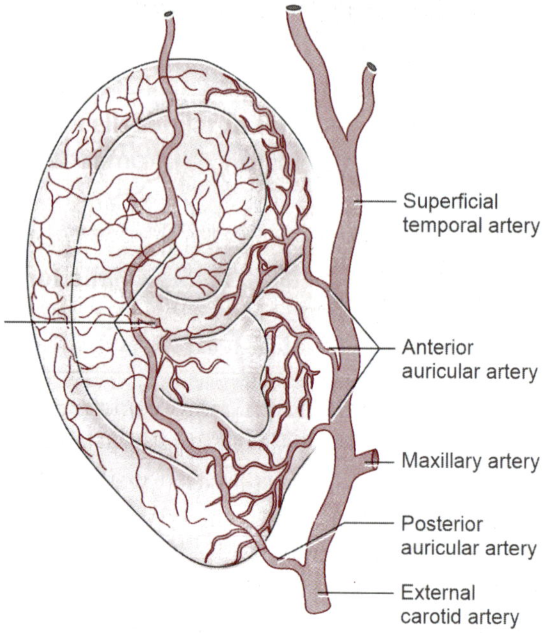

Fig. 7.56: Blood supply of ear

Middle Ear

BAQ: Write a note on the middle ear, using a labelled figure.

Ans: Middle ear is divided into the following main parts:

1. **Tympanic cavity** (Figs 7.58A and B): It contains three small bones called as the auditory ossicles. These small bones are, the malleus, incus and stapes. They transmit sound vibrations through the middle ear.

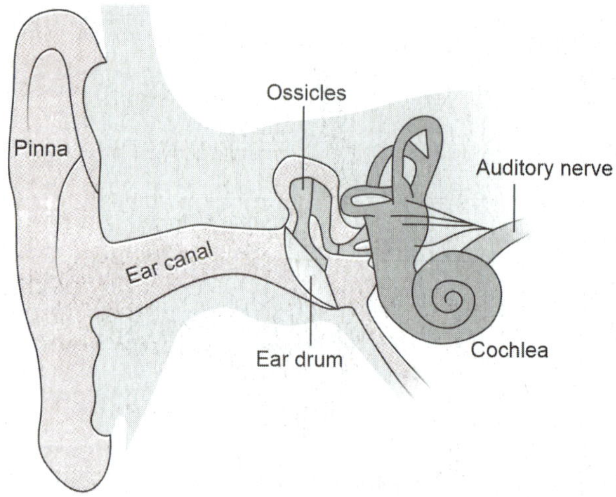

Fig. 7.57: Ear drum and other anatomical parts in the ear canal

2. **Epitympanic recess:** The malleus and incus bones partially extend upwards into the epitympanic recess.

Ear drum is present in the tympanic cavity (Fig. 7.57). It is also called as tympanic membrane or myringa. It is a thin, cone-shaped membrane that separates the external ear from the middle ear. The function of ear drum is to transmit sound from the air to the ossicles inside the middle ear, and then to the fluid-filled cochlea. Ear drum is responsible to convert and amplify vibrations in air and vibration in cochlear fluid. Three ossicles transfer the vibrations of the eardrum into waves in the fluid and membranes of the inner ear (Fig. 7.57).

> ***Note:*** Perforation or rupture of the eardrum can lead to hearing loss. Retraction of the eardrum can cause conductive hearing loss.

Mastoid Air Cells

SAQ: What are mastoid cells and their functions?

Ans: The mastoid air cells are a collection of air-filled spaces in the mastoid process of the temporal bone (Fig. 7.55B). These air cells are located within a cavity

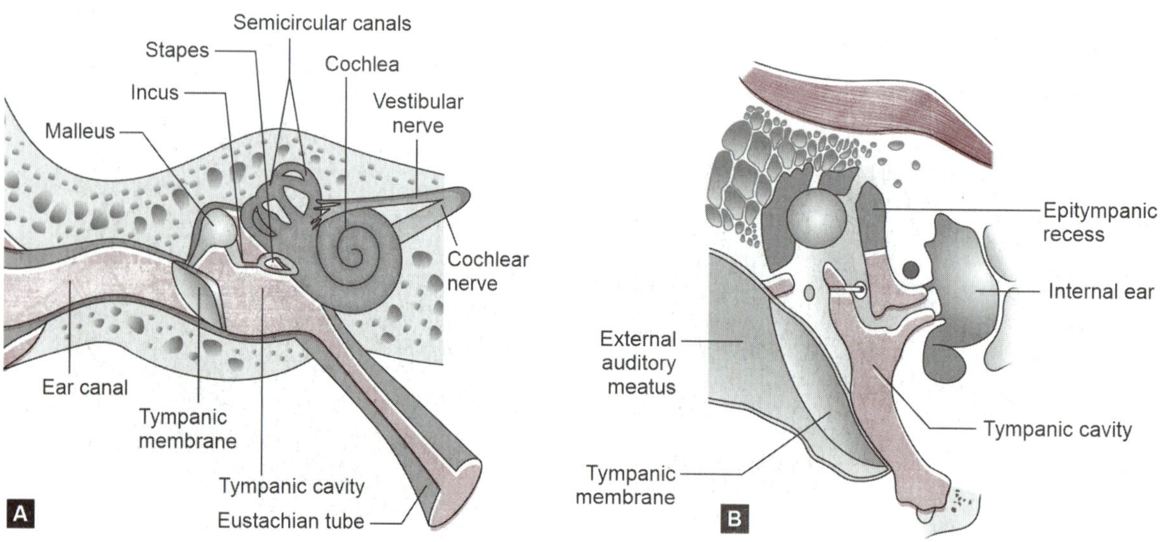

Figs 7.58A and B: (A) Middle ear anatomy-1; (B) middle ear anatomy-2

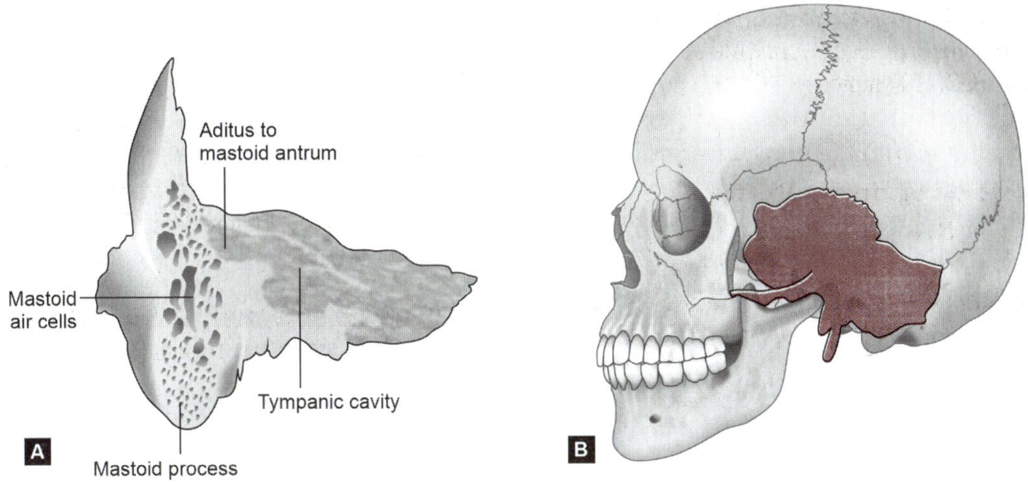

Figs 7.59A and B: (A) Mastoid antrum and mastoid cells; (B) temporal bone

called the mastoid antrum. The function of mastoid cells is to regulate pressure in the middle ear and protection of the inner ear. The mastoid antrum communicates with the middle ear through the aditus to the mastoid antrum (large irregular aperture) (Fig. 7.59A).

Eustachian Tube (Figs 7.57 and 7.58)

BAQ: Write a note on the Eustachian tube.

Ans: The Eustachian tube is a cartilaginous and bony tube. It connects the middle ear to the nasopharynx. The Eustachian tube performs the following three primary functions: (1) Maintenance of normal ventilation of the middle ear by facilitating adjustment of equal pressure around it and middle ear pressure. (2) protection of the middle ear from bacterial flora and reflux of nasopharyngeal secretions and (3) normal maintenance of drainage of secretions from the middle ear into the nasopharynx.

Muscles of Middle Ear (Fig. 7.60)

BAQ: Write a note on the muscles of middle ear.

Ans: The following two muscles give protection to the middle ear: The tensor tympani muscle and stapedius muscle. They contract in response to loud noise and inhibit the vibrations of the malleus, incus and stapes. They also reduce the transmission of sound to the inner ear.

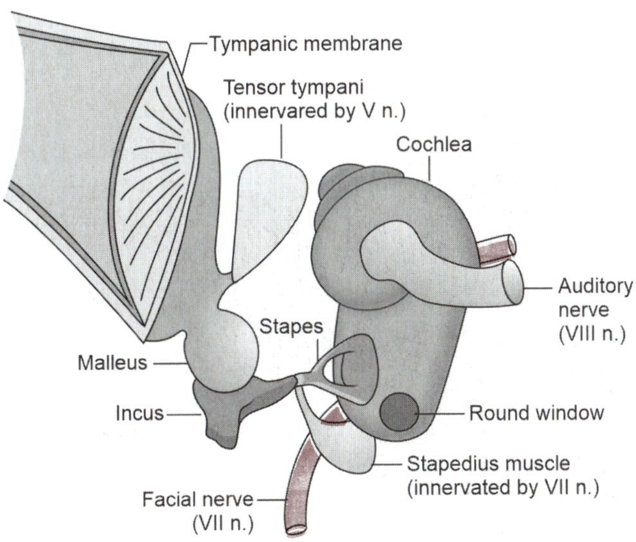

Fig. 7.60: Muscles of middle ear

Inner Ear

BAQ: Write a note on the main parts of the inner ear.

Ans: The inner ear is at the end of the ear tubes. It is present in a small cavity in the skull bones. The inner ear is located within the temporal bone of skull (Fig. 7.59B). The inner ear has two main components: (1) The bony labyrinth and (2) membranous labyrinth (Figs 7.61 and 7.62).

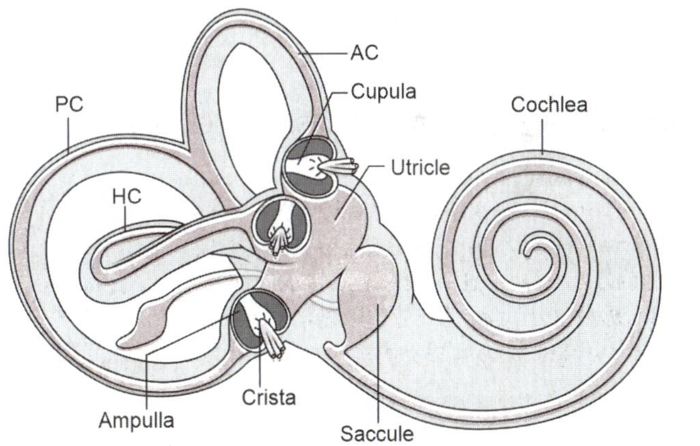

Fig. 7.61: Bony labyrinth (yellow) and membranous labyrinth (blue)

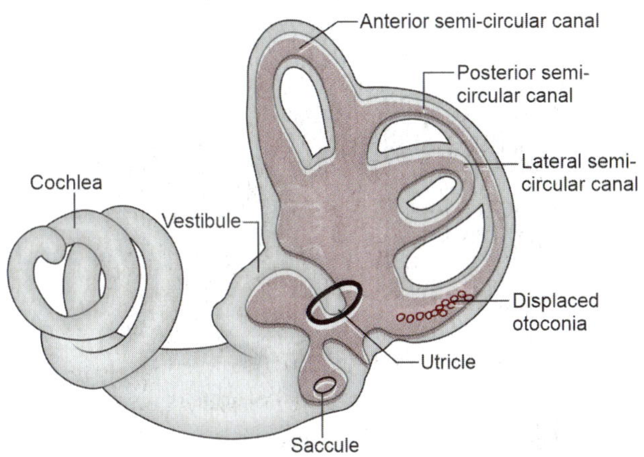

Fig. 7.62: Bony labyrinth

Bony labyrinth is composed of the cochlea, vestibule and three semi-circular canals. The membranous labyrinth is composed of a group of ducts and chambers filled with endolymphatic fluid. The membranous labyrinth is located within the bony labyrinth. It can be subdivided into the cochlear labyrinth and vestibular labyrinth. The vestibular labyrinth contains two sac like structures, utricle and saccule and three semicircular canals. All these structures contain a fluid called perilymph (Fig. 7.63).

BAQ: Draw a neat and labelled figure of the main parts of an inner ear.

Ans: Refer to Fig. 7.61.

Cochlea

SAQ: Write a note on the cochlea of the inner ear.

Ans: The cochlea is a hollow, spiral-shaped bone found in the inner ear (Fig. 7.62). The cochlea is made up of the following three compartments: (1) Scala tympani, (2) Scala media, and (3) scala vestibuli. These compartments are separated from each other by two membranes, basilar membrane and Reissner's membrane (Fig. 7.63). A tiny organ called the **organ of Corti** is present on the top of the basilar membrane (Fig. 7.64).

Cochlea plays very important role in the sense of hearing. Sound waves are passed onto the cochlea that contains. The organ of Corti, the organ meant for hearing. It consists of tiny hair cells that line the cochlea. These cells translate sound waves into electrical impulses that are carried to the brain by sensory nerves (Fig. 7.64).

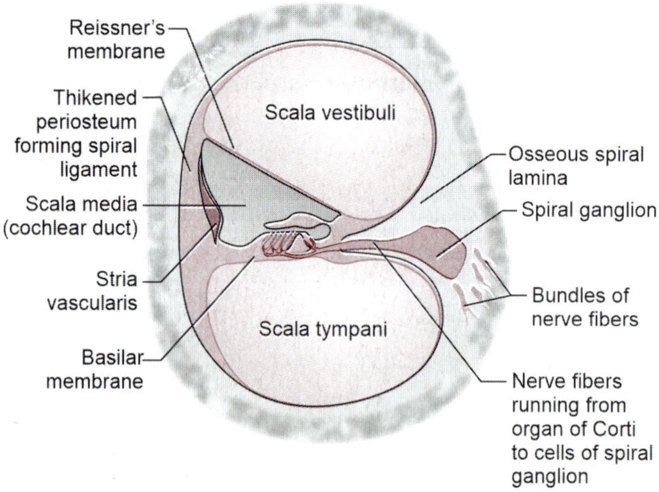

Fig. 7.63: Compartments of cochlea

BAQ: Draw a neat and labelled figure of the organ of Corti of the inner ear.

Ans: Refer to Fig. 7.64.

Vestibule (Fig. 7.62)

BAQ: Write a note on the vestibule of the inner ear.

Ans: The vestibule is the central part of the bony labyrinth in the inner ear. The main function of vestibule is to detect changes in gravity and linear acceleration. The vestibule is responsible for the realization of standing up straight position or an upside down position. The vestibule also helps one to sense the actions such as going up or down while walking. The vestibule also determines the tilt of head when eyes of a person are closed.

Semi-circular Canals (Fig. 7.65)

LAQ: Write a note on the semi-circular canals of inner ear.

Ans: There are three semi-circular canals: anterior, lateral and posterior. They contain the semi-circular ducts, which are responsible for balance (along with the utricle and saccule).

Membranous Labyrinth (Fig. 7.61)

BAQ: Write a note on the membranous labyrinth of the inner ear.

Ans: The membranous labyrinth lies within the bony labyrinth. It consists of the cochlear duct, semi-circular ducts, utricle and the saccule. The membranous labyrinth is filled with fluid called endolymph.

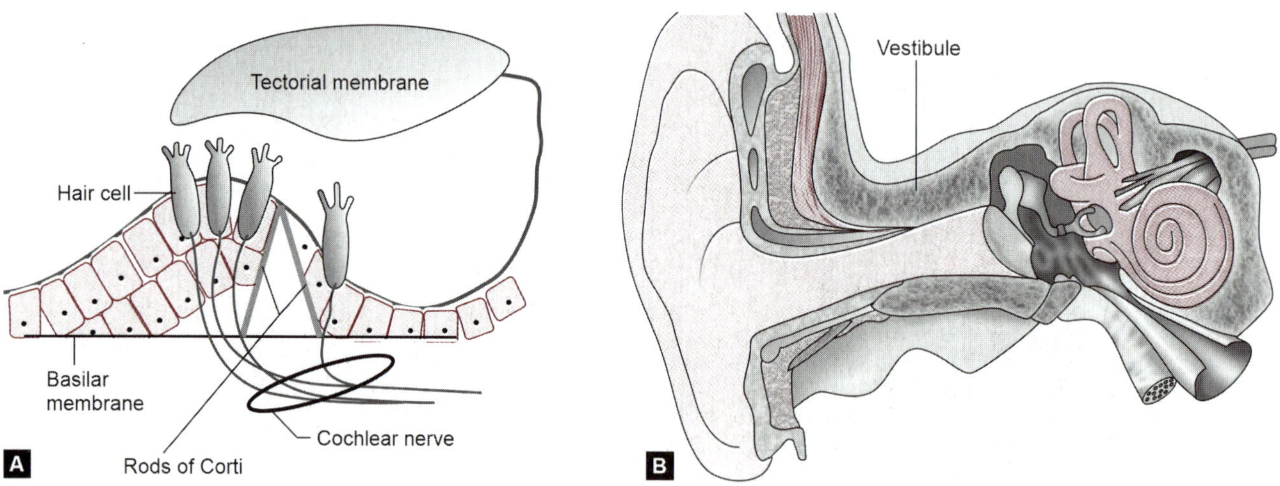

Figs 7.64A and B: (A) Organ of Corti; (B) vestibule

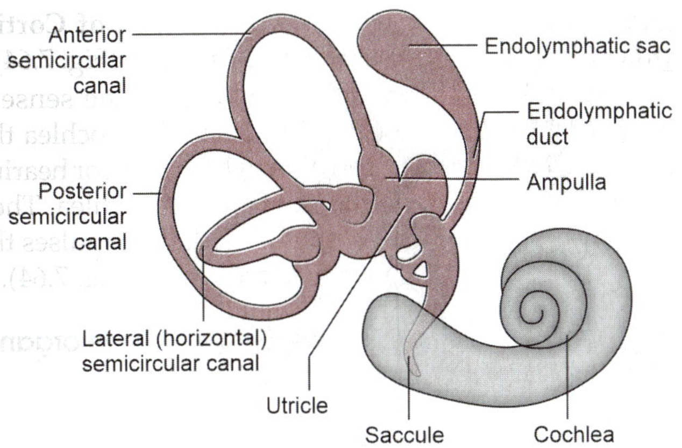

Fig. 7.65: Semi-circular canals

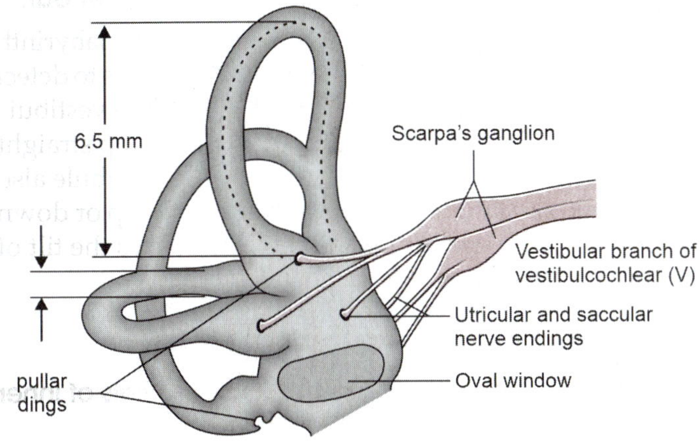

Fig. 7.66: Nerves of semi-circular canal

The membranous labyrinth is a collection of fluid filled tubes and chambers which contain the receptors, which are responsible for the senses of equilibrium and hearing.

BAQ: Draw a neat and labelled figure of the semi-circular canal of the inner ear.

Ans: Refer to the Fig. 7.65.

Objective: To describe ear physiology.

EAR PHYSIOLOGY

BAQ: Write a note on ear physiology.

Ans: Hearing starts with the outer ear in the following way:

1. When a sound is made outside the outer ear, the sound waves, or vibrations, travel down the external auditory canal and strike the eardrum (tympanic membrane). The eardrum vibrates. The vibrations are then passed to the ossicles (tiny bones in the middle ear). The ossicles amplify the sound. They send the sound waves to the inner ear and into the fluid-filled hearing organ (cochlea).
2. Once the sound waves reach the inner ear, they are converted into electrical impulses. The vestibulo-cochlear nerve transmits these impulses to the auditory nuclei in medulla of brain (Figs 7.66 and 7.67). The brain then translates these electrical impulses as sound.

The determination of the motion, acceleration, direction and distance of sound the following points are important:

1. The brain combines the input of two ears to determine the direction and distance of sounds. The vestibular system of inner ear formed by three semicircular canals are approximately at right angles to each other. These are responsible for the sense of balance and spatial orientation.

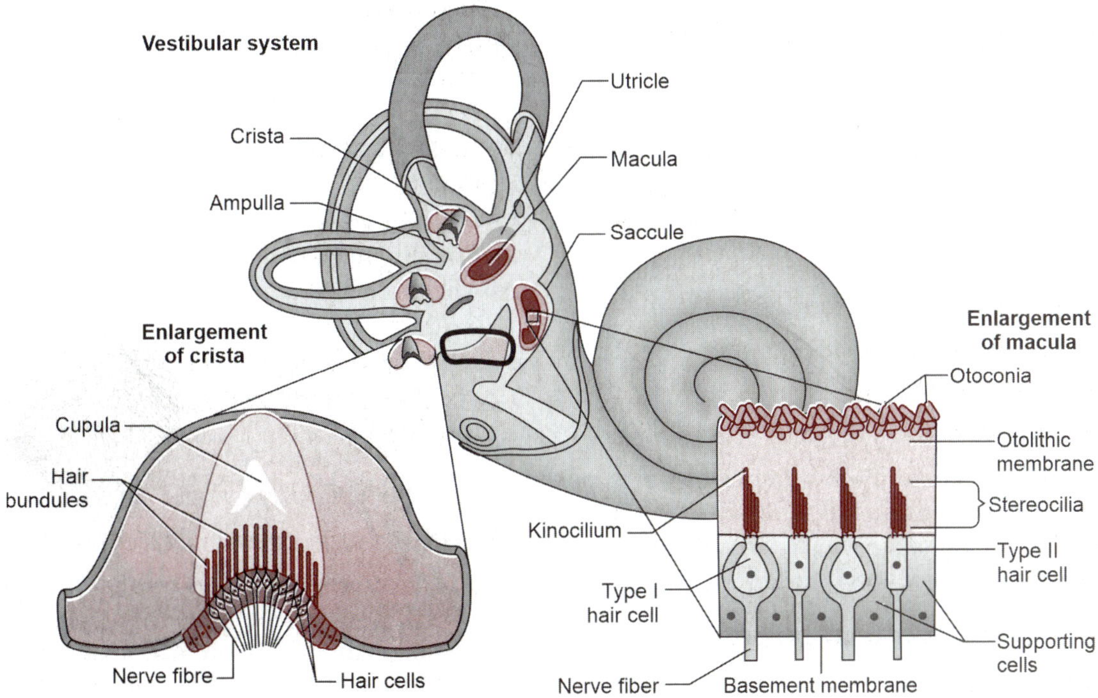

Fig. 7.67: Macula and crista anatomy

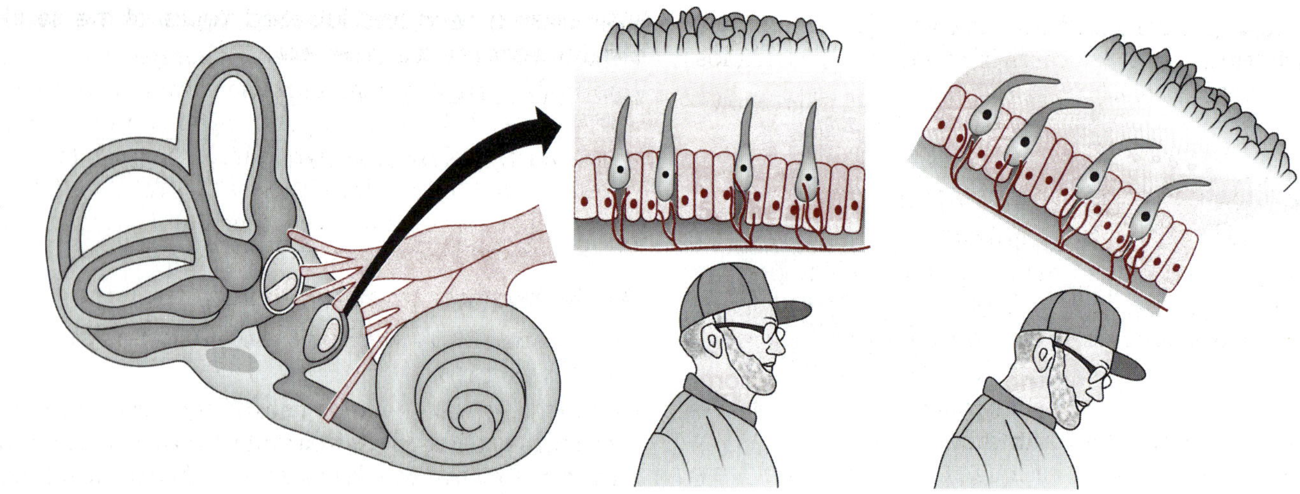

Fig. 7.68: Response of Macula to change of head position. In the semi-circular canals of the ear, receptors are located, which provide input on rotatory movements. The utricle and saccule parts of semi-circular canal generate information on linear acceleration and the influence of gravitational pull. This information is relayed by the vestibular fibres. The bipolar cell bodies present in the vestibular fibers are located in the vestibular Scarpa ganglion (Fig. 7.67). The central processes of these neurons exit the temporal bone and enter the brainstem alongside the facial nerve.

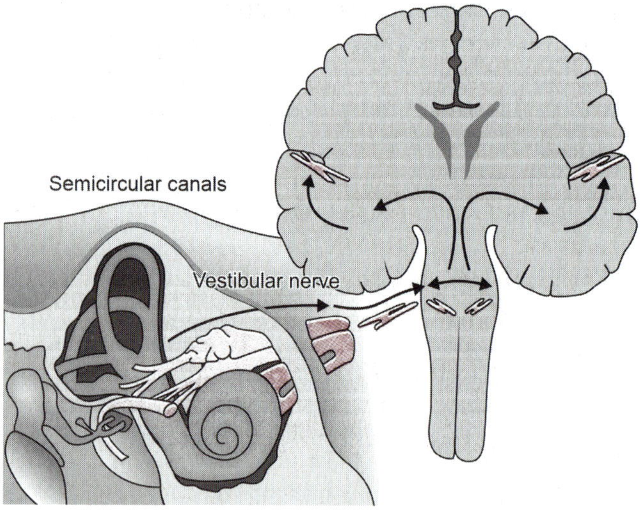

Fig. 7.69: Vestibular Scarpa ganglion connection to brain

2. The inner ear chambers are filled with a viscous fluid and small particles (otoliths) containing calcium carbonate. The movement of these particles over small hair cells in the inner ear sends signals to the brain that are interpreted as motion and acceleration (Figs 7.68 and 7.69).

SAQ: How sound moves are measured?

Ans: Sound moves through a medium (air or water as waves. It is measured in terms of frequency and amplitude.

SAQ: What is the frequency or pitch of a sound?

Ans: Frequency or pitch is the number of times per second that a sound pressure wave repeats itself. The lower frequency means less oscillations. High frequencies produce more oscillations.

SAQ: Write a note on frequency of sound.

Ans: The unit of frequency is called hertz (Hz). Humans with normal hearing ability can hear sounds between 20 Hz and 20,000 Hz. Frequencies above 20,000 Hz are known as ultrasound. The human ear can detect very small pitch changes.

SAQ: Write a note on the amplitude of sound.

Ans: Amplitude is the relative strength of sound waves which we perceive as loudness. Amplitude is measured in decibels (dB).

Decibels is sound pressure level or intensity. The lower threshold of human hearing is 0 dB at 1 kHz. Moderate levels of sound (a normal conversation voice) are under 60 dB. Noise above 70 dB over a prolonged period of time may cause damage to hearing. Loud noise above 120 dB can cause serious harm to the ears.

Objective: To describe ear disorders and dideases.

DISORDERS OF THE EAR

SAQ: Describe hearing impairment. Enumerate classes of hearing loss.

Ans: Hearing impairment is mainly due to disease or abnormality of the outer, middle, or inner ear. Hearing loss can be classified as following three types:

1. **Conductive,** which involves outer or middle ear
2. **Sensorineural,** which involves inner ear
3. **Mixed,** which may be combination of the above two categories.

Conductive Hearing Loss

SAQ: Write a note on conductive hearing loss.

Ans: Conductive hearing loss results when there is defect in delivering sound energy to hearing component in the inner ear. Common reasons of conductive hearing loss include blockage of ear canal, defects created in three small bones in ear (Fig. 7.58A), or fluid accumulation in the space between eardrum and cochlea or formation of hole in eardrum. Most cases of conductive hearing loss can be treated well.

Sensorineural Hearing Loss (SNHL)

SAQ: Write a note on sensoneural hearing loss.

Ans: Sensorineural hearing loss (SNHL) is caused by damage to the structures in the inner ear or auditory nerve of inner ear. The tiny hairs (Figs 7.64 and 7.65) in cochlea get damaged due to prolonged exposure to sounds louder than 85 decibels.

In adults, it is the main cause of hearing loss. Common causes of SNHL include natural aging process, exposure to loud noises and genetic factors. SNHL can range from mild hearing loss to complete hearing loss, which depends on the degree of the damage to the inner ear components.

Presbycusis

SAQ: Write a note on presbycusis.

Ans: Presbycusis refers to age-related, sensorineural hearing impairment in elderly persons. Presbycusis involves bilateral high-frequency hearing loss first, associated with difficulty in speech discrimination and central auditory processing of information. Later on, with advancing age, low frequency hearing loss also takes place.

Otosclerosis

SAQ: Write a note on otoslerosis.

Ans: Otosclerosis is caused when the stapes bone (Fig. 7.58A) in internal ear is unable to vibrate due to specific anatomical changes. Thus, sound is unable to travel through the ear and hearing becomes impaired. It is usually a hereditary and observed more in female compared to male.

Serous Otitis Media

SAQ: Write a note on serous otitis media.

Ans: The middle ear is usually ventilated three to four times a minute as the Eustachian tube opens during swallowing process, and oxygen is absorbed in blood in the blood vessels of the middle ear mucous membrane. If the opening of the Eustachian tube is impaired, a relative negative pressure develops within the middle ear, leading to fluid accumulation. This fluid may cause hearing loss.

Serous otitis media may also result from prolonged accumulation of effusion; in the middle ear from an upper respiratory tract infection or due to obstruction of auditory tube due to pharyngeal swelling.

Meniere's Disease

SAQ: Write a note on Meniere's disease.

Ans: Increase in the endolymph of the membranous labyrinth leads to Meniere's disease. The main reasons for the imbalance caused in the endolymph may be due to hereditary reasons, specific allergies leading to abnormal immune system response, viral infections, or head injuries. It is an inner-ear clinical condition that causes vertigo, ringing in ear (tinnitus), and a feeling of pressure in the ear. Usually, only one ear is affected, however, another ear also may get affected. The hearing loss eventually may become permanent.

INFECTIONS OF EAR

SAQ: Write a note on ear infections.

Ans: Ear infections may be caused by bacterial, viral or fungal infections. These ear infections may occur in outer, middle ear, or in the inner ear. The ear infections can be chronic or acute. Acute ear infections are of short in duration and chronic ear infections are of prolonged duration and may recur many times. Prolonged ear infections can cause damage to the middle and inner ear.

External Otitis

SAQ: Write a note on external otitis.

Ans: External otitis (otitis externa) is inflammation of the ear canal due to microbial infections or due to autoimmune disorders. It usually presents with swelling of the ear canal, ear pain and occasionally associated with decreased hearing.

Acute Otitis Media (AOM)

SAQ: Write a note on acute otitis media (AOM).

Ans: Acute otitis media is an ear infection of the middle ear. It may be caused by upper respiratory tract infections. Children are more likely to get acute otitis media than adults. Swelling and irritation of adenoids (part of lymphatic system) is also responsible for acute middle ear infections in children (Fig. 7.70).

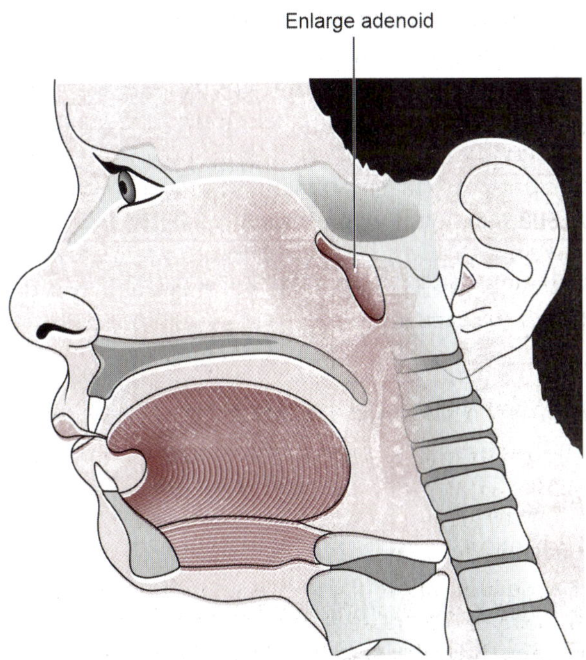

Fig. 7.70: Increased adenoid due to infection

Sense Organs 7

Chronic Otitis Media (COM)

SAQ: Write a note on chronic otitis media (COM).

Ans: Chronic otitis media is an ear disease in which patient suffers from chronic infection of the middle ear, caused by viruses or bacteria. In chronic otitis media chronic inflammation of the middle ear and mastoid cavity is observed. When dysfunction of the Eustachian tube occurs, the pressure equilibration in the middle ear is impaired, leading to the specific symptoms of chronic otitis media. Symptoms generally associated with chronic ear disease include otorrhea (drainage of liquid from the ear), hearing loss, sensation of ear blocking, and vertigo.

Labyrinthitis

SAQ: What is labyrinthitis?

Ans: Inner ear contains the labyrinth (Fig. 7.61). It controls hearing and body balance. An viral or bacterial infection of labyrinth may lead to loss of hearing and vertigo.

Motion Sickness

SAQ: Write a note on motion sickness.

Ans: Motion sickness is induced by air, car or boat travel. Symptoms of motion sickness include vomiting, dizziness, fatigue, and uneasiness. When motion stops, motion sickness usually goes away.

The inner ear contains sensors for rotational and linear motion. Airsickness occurs when the central nervous system receives conflicting messages from the inner ear, eyes and muscles affecting balance and equilibrium. Airsickness is usually caused by spatial disorientation.

SAQ. What is spatial disorientation?

Ans: Spatial disorientation means the inability of a person to determine his true body position, motion, and altitude relative to the earth or his surroundings.
Spatial orientation is natural ability to maintain body orientation and posture in relation to the surrounding environment at rest and during motion. It is possible to maintain spatial orientation on the ground. However, the three-dimensional environment of flight is unfamiliar to the human body. Hence motion in air creates sensory conflicts and illusions that make spatial orientation difficult to maintain.

Objective: To describe the anatomy of the nose and important functions of related anatomical parts.

NOSE

Introduction

The nose is an organ that helps an individual to breathe and to smell. The nose brings warm humidified air into the lungs. It facilitates filtering out particles in inspired air. It also serves to provide first-line immunologic defence by bringing inspired air in contact with mucous-coated membranes that contain immunoglobulins. Inspired air comes in contact with the olfactory nerves of nose and provides the sense of smell, which is associated with the taste sensation. Nasal dysfunction leads to nasal congestion, sinus infections, postnasal drainage, headache, facial pressure and headache.

Nose Anatomy

SAQ: Write a note on nose anatomy.

Ans: The nose has two holes called nostrils (Fig. 7.71). The internal nose is divided into the left and right nasal cavities by the nasal septum (Fig. 7.72). The septum is made of very thin pieces of bone. Each nostril is connected with nasal cavity. Each nasal cavity contains a roof, floor, medial wall, and lateral wall. Each nasal cavity has the following three regions: (1) Nasal vestibule, (2) respiratory region, and (3) olfactory region (Fig. 7.74). Three sections, the medial crus, the middle crus, and the lateral crus contribute to the outer shape of the nasal tip (Fig. 7.73).

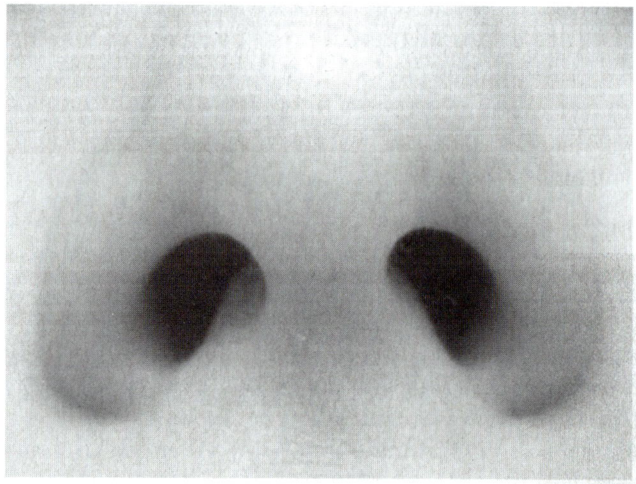

Fig. 7.71: Nostrils

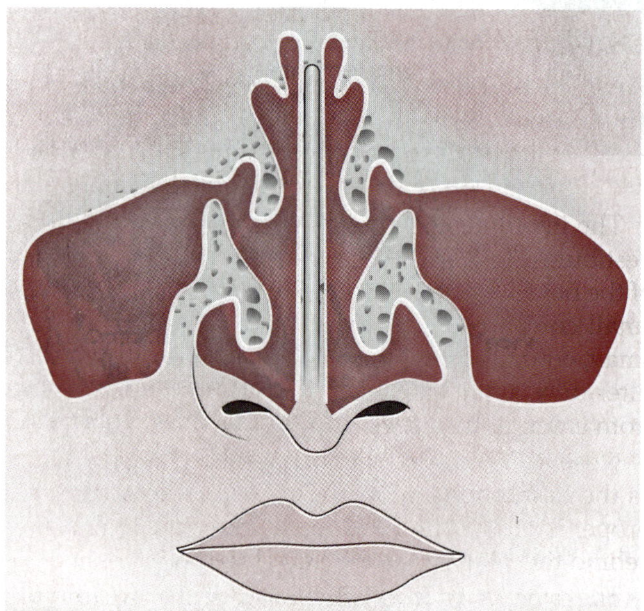

Fig. 7.72: Nasal septum and other anatomical parts of the nose

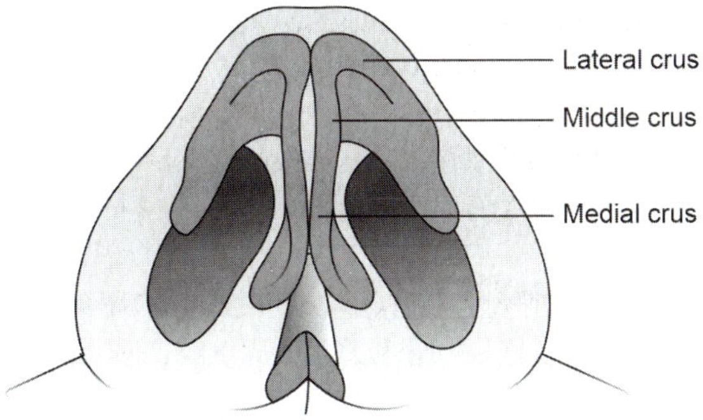

Fig. 7.73: Medial crus, the middle crus, and the lateral crus

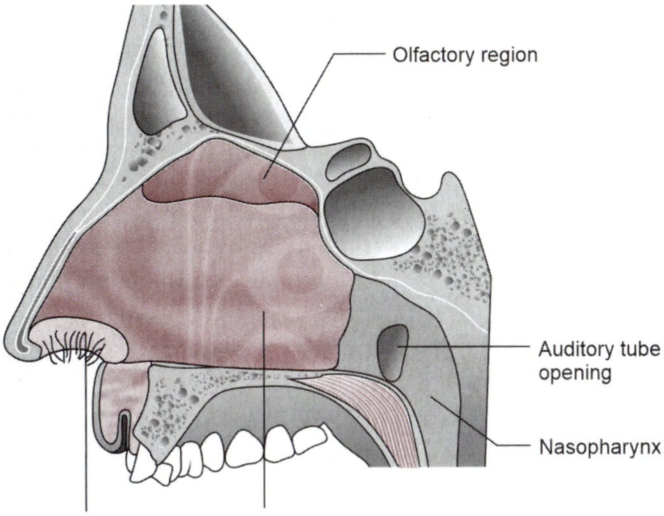

Fig. 7.74: Nasal vestibule, respiratory region, and olfactory region

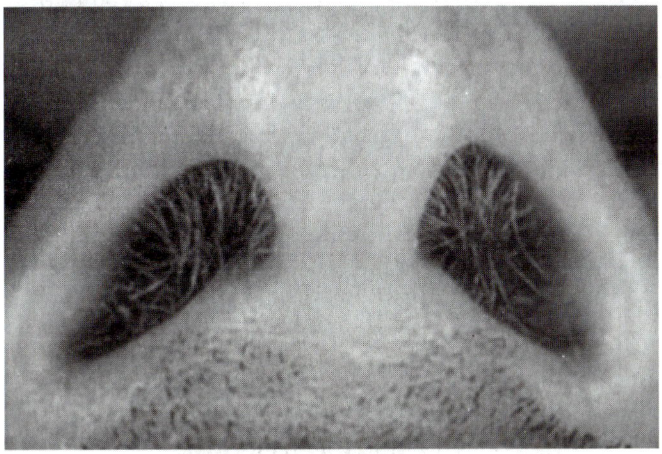

Fig. 7.75: Nose hairs (course)

The internal nose consists of a region known as the vestibule (Fig. 7.74), which is supported by the cartilage of the nose. Vestibule is a skin-lined part, which contain small course hair and lined with tissue that contains small, course hairs (Fig. 7.75). These hairs are useful to filter dust, sand, and other particles and to keep these from entering the lungs.

Nose also contains the mucosa-lined region known as the nasal cavity proper (Fig. 7.72). The nasal cavity proper is a large, air-filled space. It is present above and behind the nose and at the middle of the face.

The cavity of the nose is lined with mucous membranes that have smell receptors connected to the olfactory nerve (Fig. 7.76). The smell receptors are sensitive to seven types of sensations such as flower, mint, ether, musk, and acrid or putrid. The smell receptors interact with the molecules of these sensations and transmit the sensations to the brain. The sense of smell is sometimes temporarily lost when a person has a respiratory tract infection such as COVID-19.

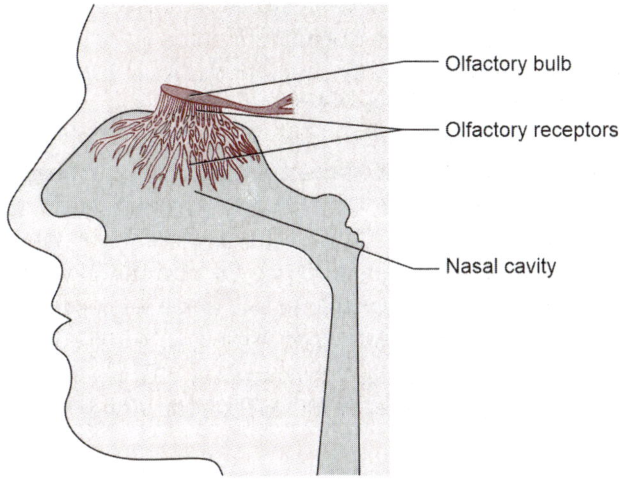

Fig. 7.76: Smell receptors of nose

Objective: To describe the physiology of smell. To identify neural pathways and receptors for the sense of smell.

PHYSIOLOGY OF SMELL

SAQ. Write a note on the physiology of smell.

Ans: Olfaction is the capacity of smelling. Several thousand odors can be distinguished by the sense of smell. A trained human can recognize several classes of compounds, such as aromatic (camphor, menthol), balsamic (violet, vanilla), empyreumatic (tar, coffee), ethereal (wine), alliaceous (garlic, iodine), ambrosial (amber, musk), nauseous (putrefaction). hircinnic (sweat), repulsive (pyridine, opium), etc.

Odor molecules are detected by the olfactory sensory neurons (olfactory receptors), the sustentacular or supporting cells, and the basal epithelial or stem cells. These cells relay signals to the olfactory bulb, a structure in the forebrain where initial odor processing occurs.

SAQ: Write a note on anosmia.

Ans: Anosmia is loss of sense of smell. Anosmia is observed in nose infections by viral infections and it was an important observation in COVID-19 pandemic.

Temporary loss of smell is the main neurological symptom and one of the earliest and most commonly reported indicators of COVID-19. It has been observed that anosmia better predicts the disease than other known symptoms such as fever and cough.

An international team of researchers led by neuroscientists at Harvard Medical School has identified the olfactory cell types in the upper nasal cavity the most vulnerable to infection by COVID-19.

COVID-19

SAQ: Write a brief note on COVID-19.

Ans: Corona viruses cause respiratory tract infections. COVID-9 is a disease caused by SARS-CoV-2 that causes respiratory tract infection. COVID-19 affects upper respiratory tract including nose, sinuses, and throat and may spread to lower respiratory tract including windpipe and lungs.

SAQ: What is sensory adaptation?

Ans: Sensory adaptation takes place when the body's sensory receptors are exposed to particular stimuli such as strong scents (and also loud noise and high temperature) for long time. The respective receptors then decrease their sensitivity to the stimuli. Hence an individual unable to sense smell when exposed to a particular smell for prolonged time.

Objective: To describe the anatomical features of the sinuses.

SINUSES

BAQ: Write a note on the sinuses.

Ans: The sinuses are air-filled pockets, near the nasal passage (Fig. 7.77). The sinuses are lined with mucous membranes. The cells of mucous membrane secret mucous to keep nose moist. The following are 4 different types of sinuses:

1. **Ethmoid sinuses:** These are found in the ethmoid bone in the upper part of the nose between the eyes (Fig. 7.77).
2. **Maxillary sinuses:** These sinuses are the largest and are located inside the face, around the area of the cheeks (Fig. 7.77).
3. **Frontal sinuses:** These sinuses are located in the area of the forehead (Fig. 7.77).
4. **Sphenoid sinuses:** These sinuses are located deep in the face, behind the nose (Fig. 7.77).

Sinusitis

BAQ: Write a note on sinusitis using a labelled figure.

Ans: Sinusitis is a clinical condition in which the membrane of sinus cavities around the nasal passages becomes inflamed. Symptoms of sinusitis include nasal congestion, runny nose, headache, facial pain.

Sinusitis can be of following two types: (1) Acute sinusitis and (2) chronic sinusitis.

Acute sinusitis may suddenly occur due to microbial infections, cold or due to allergies. Acute sinusitis could be treated by appropriate treatment. Chronic sinusitis may be caused by an microbial infection. Symptoms of chronic sinusitis are similar to acute sinusitis. Chronic sinusitis may take long time to resolve.

Objective: To describe the anatomy of throat and important functions of anatomical parts of a throat. To describe the anatomy of tongue and important functions of anatomical parts of a tongue. To identify neural pathways and receptors for the sense of taste.

THROAT (Figs 7.78A and B)

BAQ: Write a note on the anatomical features and related functions of throat.

Ans: The throat is a ring-like muscular tube. It is the passageway for air, food, and liquid. It also helps in forming speech. The throat contains larynx, epiglottis, tonsils and adenoids.

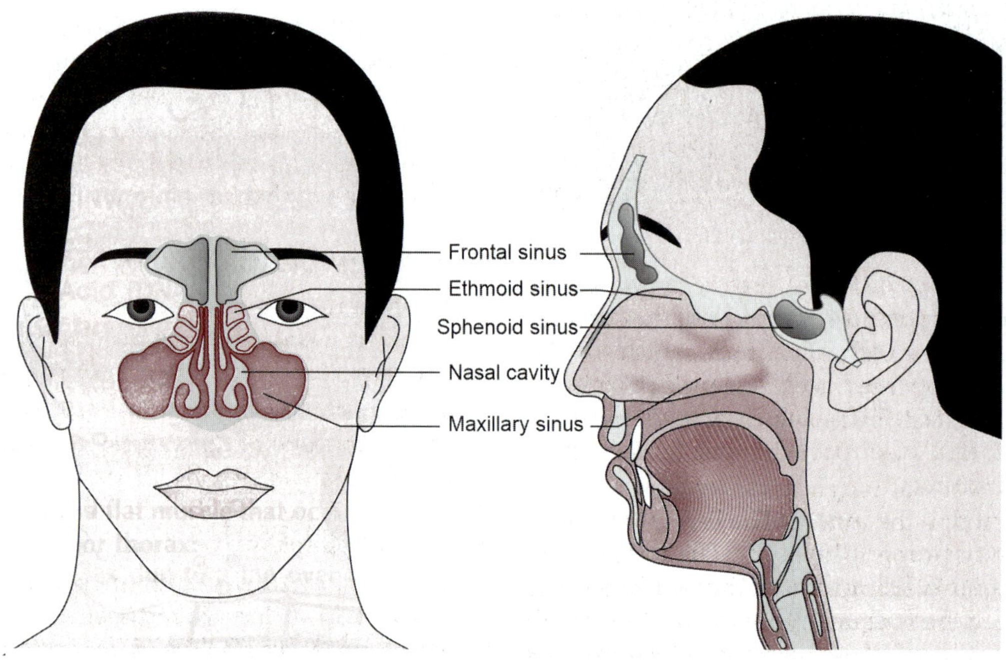

Fig. 7.77: Sinuses

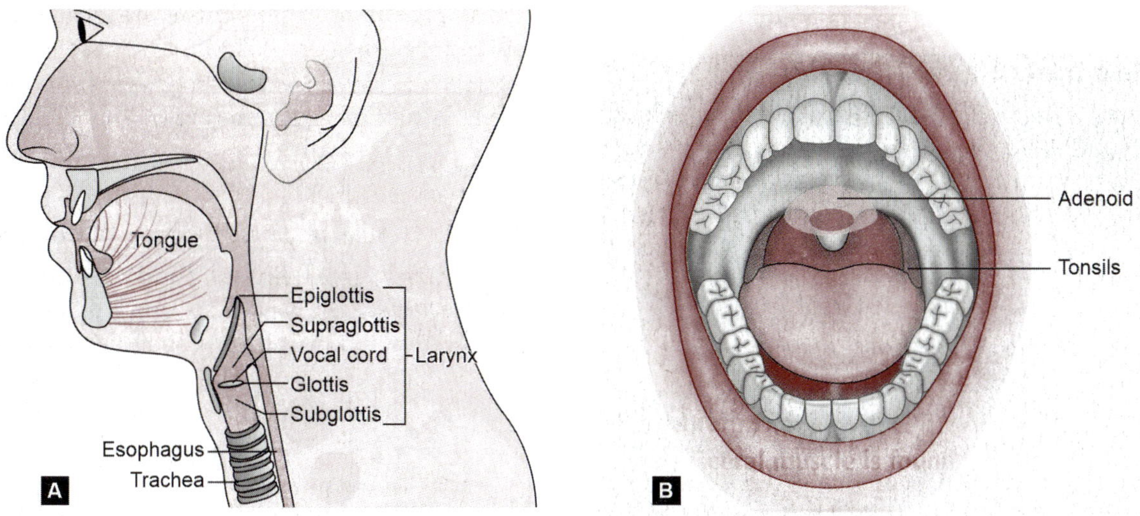

Figs 7.78A and B: (A) Anatomy of the larynx; (B) adenoids and tonsil

Voice box (larynx): It is a cylindrical group of cartilages, muscles, and soft tissue that contains the vocal cords. The vocal cords are the upper opening into the windpipe (trachea), the passageway to the lungs (Fig. 7.78). Sound is produced when the air that passes through the vocal cords; causes vibrations and creates sound waves in the pharynx, mouth and nose.

Epiglottis: It is a flap of soft tissue located just above the vocal cords. The epiglottis folds down over the vocal cords, while eating, to prevent food and irritants from entering the lungs.

Tonsils and adenoids: These are made up of lymph tissue and are located at the back and the sides of the mouth. Function of tonsils and adenoids is to protect against infections.

TONGUE

BAQ: Write a note on the tongue and related anatomical features.

Ans: Tongue is a flexible muscular organ in the mouth. The functions of tongue are to mix food by moving food around and to detect taste of food. Tongue also modifies the flow of air from the lungs in order to produce different sounds in speech.

Anatomy of the Tongue (Fig. 7.79)

The tongue is mainly composed of muscles. It is covered with a mucous membrane. Small nodules of tissue, called papillae, cover the upper surface of the tongue. Between the papillae are the taste buds, which provide the sense of taste (Fig. 7.79).

By means of webs of tough tissue and mucosa, the tongue is anchored to the mouth. The lingual frenulum is a mucous membrane fold found underneath the tongue (Fig. 7.80). It extends from the midline of the ventral surface of the tongue to the floor of the mouth. The lingual frenulum helps the tongue to move and perform tongue functions such as speech, swallowing and feeding. The tongue is anchored into the hyoid bone in the back of mouth.

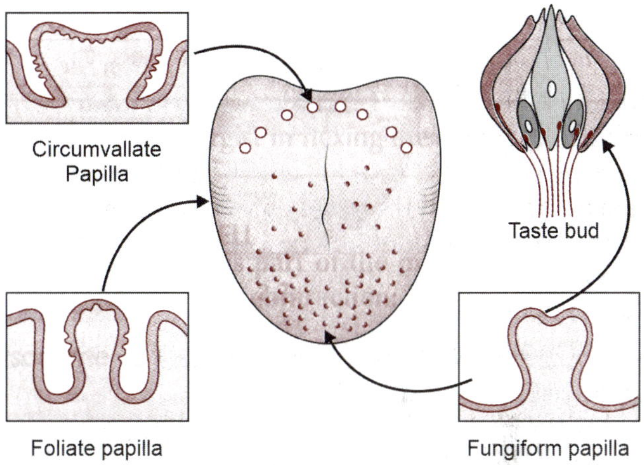

Fig. 7.79: Papillae and taste buds of tongue

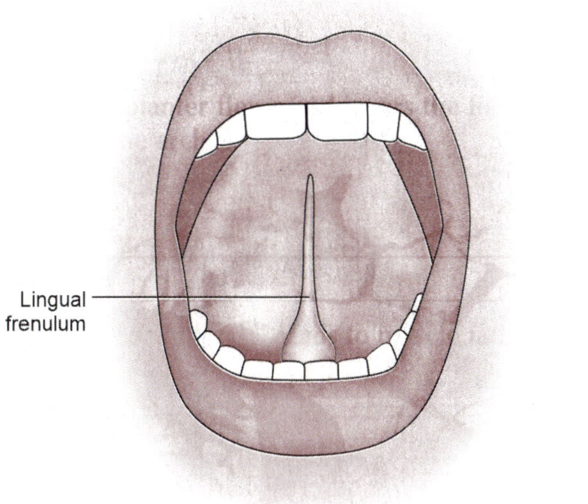

Fig. 7.80: Lingual frenulum mucous membrane of the tongue

Parts of the Tongue (Figs 7.81A and B)

BAQ: Describe the various parts of the tongue.

Ans: The following are the various parts of tongue:

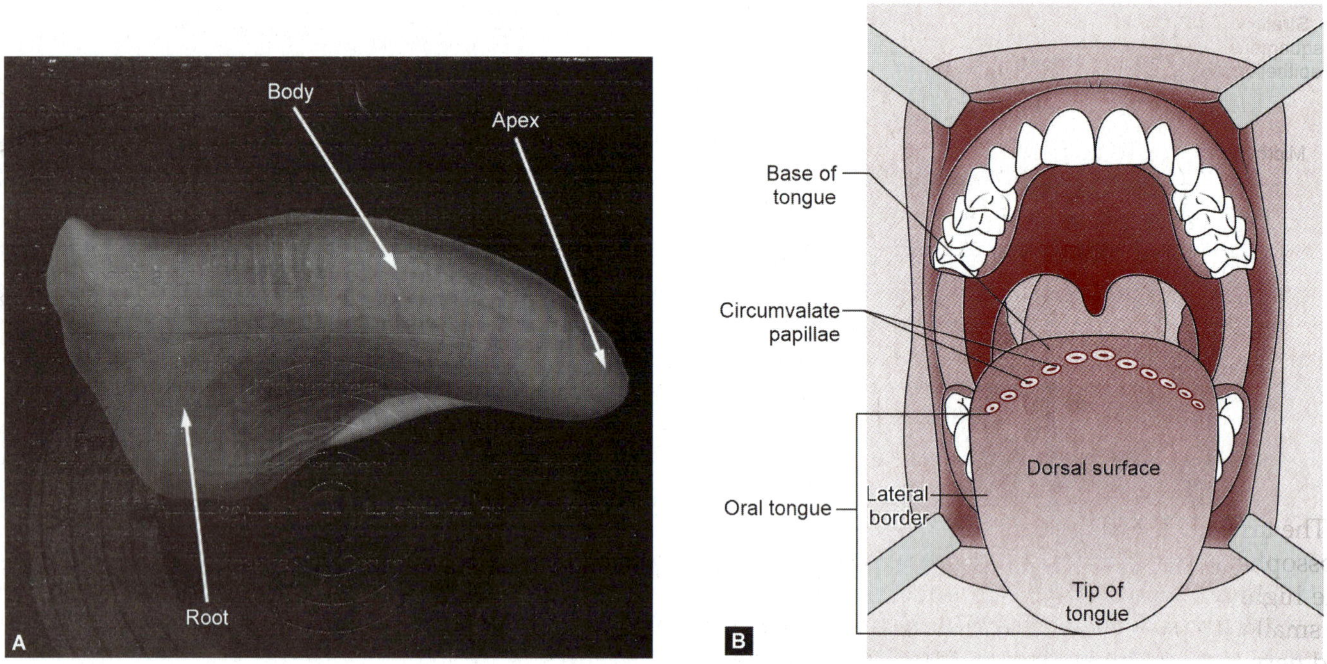

Figs 7.81A and B: Parts of tongue

Root: This is about 30% of back part of the tongue

Body: It is the rest of the tongue, means, the forward 70% that lie in the front side.

Apex: This a pointed portion. It is the tip of the tongue.

Dorsum: This is the curved upper surface of the tongue.

Taste Buds of Tongue and Physiology of Taste

(Figs 7.79 and 7.82)

BAQ: Describe the taste buds of tongue and physiologyof taste.

Ans: The taste buds are receptors for taste. These are situated chiefly in the tongue, and they are also located in the roof of the mouth and near the pharynx. They are able to detect four basic tastes: Salty, sweet, bitter, and sour. The tongue also can detect "umami" taste from taste receptors sensitive to amino acids. The umami taste is a meaty and broth-like taste. The taste buds near the tip of the tongue are sensitive to sweet tastes, while, taste buds in the back of the tongue are sensitive to bitter taste. The taste buds on top and on the side of the tongue are sensitive to sour and salty sour tastes.

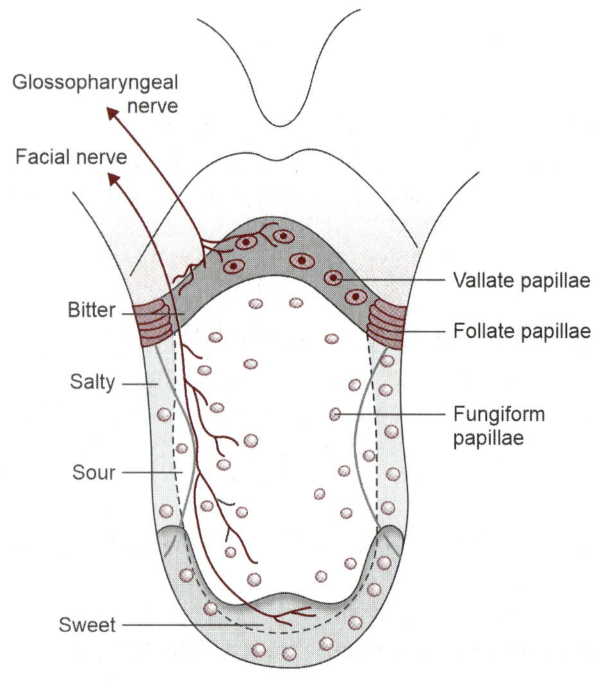

Fig. 7.82: Taste buds of tongue

BAQ: Draw a labelled diagram of taste buds of the tongue.

Ans: Refer to Fig. 7.82.

BAQ: Describe physiology of taste.

Ans: At the base of each taste bud of a tongue, a nerve is present. It sends the taste sensations to the brain (Figs 7.83 and 7.84). The sense of taste functions in coordination with the sense of smell. The tongue is covered with the papillae which give the tongue a rough texture.

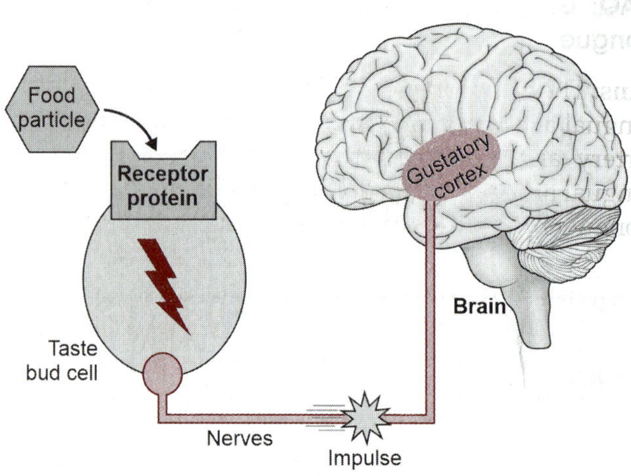

Fig. 7.83: Taste link from tongue to the brain

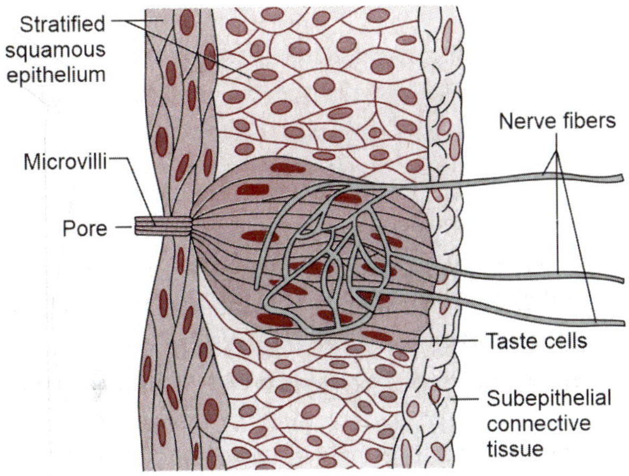

Fig. 7.84: Taste bud nerve fibers

The taste buds contain sensory nerve endings of the glossopharyngeal, facial and vagus nerves (Fig. 7.85). The highly sensitive sensory receptors are stimulated by small amounts of food chemicals dissolved in saliva and nerve impulses are generated; and taste is noted in the parietal lobe of cerebral cortex.

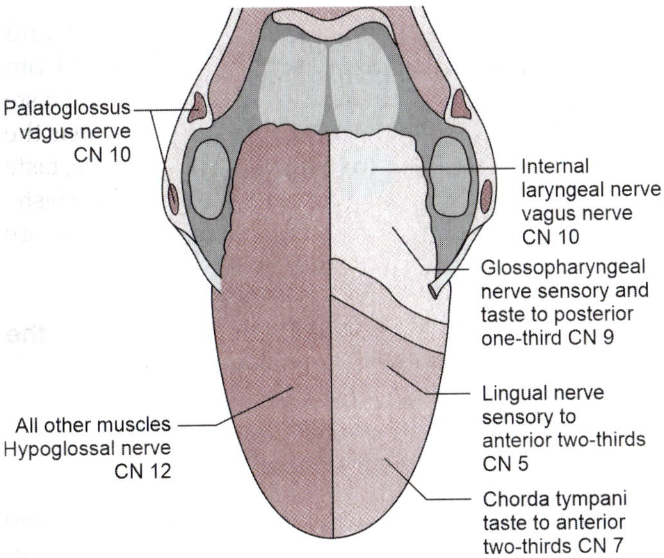

Fig. 7.85: Nerve supply of the tongue

Tongue Blood Supply (Fig. 7.86)

SAQ: Give information on the blood supply of the tongue.

Ans: The tongue receives blood supply mainly from the lingual artery, which is a branch of the external carotid artery and also from the lingual artery and dorsal lingual artery. The deep lingual veins drain blood from tongue into the internal jugular vein.

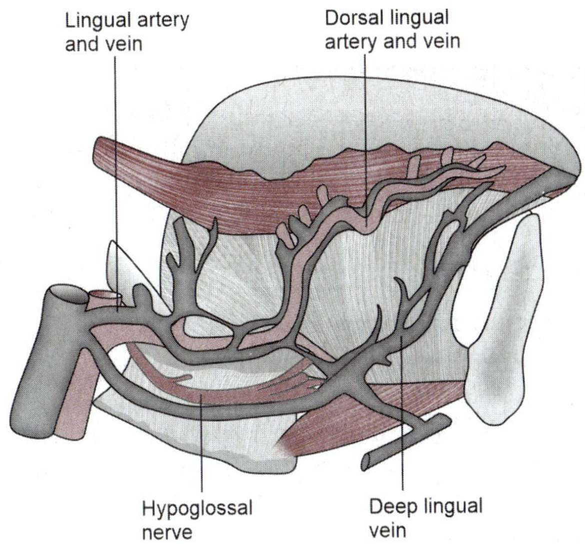

Fig. 7.86: Tongue blood supply

Objective: To describe various tongue diseases.

TONGUE DISEASES

Candidiasis (Thrush)

SAQ: What is candidiasis (thrush)?

Ans: Candida infection leads to candidiasis and it is caused by *Candida albicans* fungus, which grows over the surface of the tongue and surface of mouth. Thrush may occur in persons with suppressed immune systems. Candida infection is treated using antifungal medicines.

Oral Cancer

SAQ: Write a short note on oral cancer.

Ans: Mouth cancer develops in any of the following parts of the oral cavity: Gums, tongue, lips, cheeks, roof of mouth and floor of mouth. The signs and symptoms of mouth cancer may include: A reddish or white patch in the oral cavity for very long duration, a non-healing lip or mouth sore, prolonged mouth and ear pain, and difficulty in swallowing.

Oral cancer is more common in people who are alcoholic and smoke regularly. Oral cancer is treated using surgical methods to remove the cancerous growth, followed chemotherapy and radiation therapy.

Big Tongue (Macroglossia)

SAQ: What is big tongue (macroglossia)?

Ans: Big tongue (macroglossia) may occur due to congenital, cancerous, inflammatory and traumatic reasons.

Geographic Tongue

SAQ: What is geographic tongue?

Ans: In the case of geographic tongue, ridges and coloured spots migrate over the surface of the tongue and these periodically change its appearance. The patches appear like a map, hence this condition is called geographic tongue. The patches often appear in one area and then move to a different part of the tongue. Geographic tongue is an inflammatory condition. Geographic tongue may be a clinical condition takes place due to prolonged vitamin B complex deficiency, or deficiencies in iron, vitamin D, and zinc.

Bald Tongue

SAQ: What is bald tongue?

Ans: The tongue appears without bumpy texture. Complete atrophy of the lingual papillae leads to bald tongue. It may be due to prolonged vitamin B complex deficiency, or deficiencies in iron, vitamin D, and zinc.

Oral Leukoplakia

SAQ: What is oral leukoplakia?

Ans: In this clinical condition, white patches appear on the tongue, which cannot be scraped off. It has been observed that the long-term irritation from the use of tobacco may lead to oral leucoplakia. This clinical condition may be benign, or it may progress to oral cancer.

Oral Lichen Planus

SAQ: What is oral lichen planus?

Ans: Oral lichen planus is an inflammatory condition that most often affects mucous membranes of oral cavity. It may appear as white patches or swollen red sores. These lesions may cause pain and burning. Oral lichen planus may be caused due to the immune system disorder, in which, immune system attacks the skin and lining of the mouth.

> **Objective:** To understand and explain the central theme of competency based medical and paramedical education (CBME): Horizontal and vertical integration of subjects.

LAQ: Explain horizontal integration of the following eye diseases, with other pre-medical subjects such as physiology, biochemistry and nutrition.

Ans: Eye diseases: (1) Diabetic neuropathy, (2) cataract, and (3) glaucoma.

Horizontal Integration

1. Diabetic neuropathy

Anatomical change: Retinal nerve damage.

Physiological change: Progressive damage of the blood vessels in the eyes due to deposition of lipids on the arteries (uncontrolled diabetes mellitus).

Biochemical change: High levels of circulating blood glucose.

Nutrition: Suggested nutritional plan: Diet free from high glycemic sugars.

2. Cataract

Anatomical change: Eye lens damage

Physiological change: Light is not able to pass through the lens.

Biochemical change: Lens protein degeneration, making it cloudy. It may be due to aging or due to effects of increased sorbitol (in uncontrolled diabetes mellitus).

Nutrition: Suggested nutritional plan: Sugar free diet, if the person is diabetic.

3. Glaucoma

Anatomical change: Optic nerve damage

Physiological change: Light is not able to pass to the brain.

Biochemical change: Fluid accumulation in the eyes leading to increase in the eye pressure.

Nutritional plan: Normal diet containing multivitamins.

BAQ: (A) Explain horizontal integration of "nose infection" by COVID-19" with other pre-medical subjects such as physiology and biochemistry.

(B) Explain vertical integration of "nose infection" by COVID-19" with paramedical subjects such as microbiology and preventive medicine.

Ans:

A. Horizontal Integration

Anatomical change: Inflammation of mucus membrane of the nose and destruction of the cells in the olfactory region by SARS CoV-2 virus.

Physiological change: Neuronal transmissions from the olfactory cells to the brain are affected. Loss of smell.

Biochemical change: Synthesis of inflammatory markers such as prostaglandins, leukotrienes, C-reactive protein leding to initiation of inflammatory reactions.

B. Vertical Integration

Microbiology: Study of infectious organism.

Preventive medicine: Suggestion of appropriate vaccine to prevent COVID-19.

BIBLIOGRAPHY

1. Medical Biochemistry, 1st Edition (2023). Godkar PB, Godkar DP, CBS Publishers, New Delhi, India.
2. Text book of Medical Laboratory Technology, 4th Edition, (2024). Godkar PB, Godkar DP, Bhalani Publishing House, Mumbai, India.
3. Anatomy of the Human Body. 42nd Edition. Henry Gray, Editor-in-chief: Susan Standring, Elsevier (2020).
4. Ross and Wilson Anatomy and Physiology in Health and Illness, 13th Edition, by Allison Wynn Grant, Anne Waugh, and Kathleen J. W. Wilson (2018).
5. Schaum's outline of theory and problems of Human anatomy and Physiology, 2nd Edition (1997), Tata MaGraw- Hill Publishing Company Limited, New Delhi, India.

MULTIPLE CHOICE QUESTIONS (MCQs)

Select the correct option.

1. This part of an eye provides covering to sclera and incoming light falls first on it:

(A) Pupil (B) Bulbular conjunctiva
(C) Iris (D) Pupil

2. The tympanic membrane is directly in contact with:

(A) Basal membrane (B) Ciliary body
(C) Macula lutea (D) Suspensory ligament

3. **This muscle facilitates superolateral movement of the eye:**

(A) Superior oblique (B) Superior rectus
(C) Inferior oblique (D) Lateral rectus

4. **When light is processed by the eye, this property of light is not processed:**

(A) Accommodation (B) Refraction
(C) Inversion (D) Dispersion

5. **This part of the eye does not contain refractive medium:**

(A) Cornea (B) Pupil
(C) Lens (D) Aqueous humour

6. **The aqueous humour is drained from the eye through:**

(A) Scleral venous sinus (B) Nasal lacrimal gland
(C) Optic canal (D) Tarsal duct

7. **The main function of the cornea:**

(A) Structural support to the eye
(B) Changes the shape of the lens enabling image to be focused on the retina
(C) Contains rod cells at the correct orientation
(D) Bends light before it reaches the lens

8. **The type of cells found in retina are:**

(A) Schwann cells (B) Purkinje cells
(C) Amacrine cells (D) Neuroglial cells

9. **In myopia, the image of a distant object will be formed:**

(A) On the blind spot (B) Behind the retina
(C) In front of the retina (D) None of these

10. **In hyperopia, the image of a distant object will be formed:**

(A) Behind retina (B) In front of the retina
(C) On the blind spot (D) None of these

11. **A cornea transplant is never rejected since:**

(A) It does not have blood supply and no antibody formation
(B) It consists of nucleated cells
(C) It is a non-living layer
(D) Both (B) and (C)

12. **This is an incorrect statement**

(A) Retinal is a derivative of vitamin A
(B) Retinal is a derivative of vitamin C
(C) Retinal is the light-absorbing part of visual photo-pigments
(D) Rhodopsin is the purplish-red protein situated in rods only

13. **The fovea is the mammalian eye is the centre of the visual field in which:**

(A) More cones than rods are found
(B) No rods are present
(C) No cones and no rods are present
(D) Only rods are found

14. **The photosensitive compound in the eye is composed of:**

(A) Opsin and retinal
(B) Guanosine and retinol
(C) Transducin and retinene
(D) Opsin and retinol

15. **The nature of eye lens is:**

(A) Biconcave (B) Concave
(C) Biconvex (D) Convex

16. **The persistence of vision for the eye is:**

(A) 1/16th of a second (B) 1/10th of a second
(C) 1/18th of a second (D) 1/6th of a second

17. **The function of the tapetum lucidum in the eye is:**

(A) To give the coloured appearance
(B) To give transparent appearance to vitreous humour
(C) To make the lens hazy
(D) To give night vision

18. **The innermost layer of the eyeball in which the photoreceptors are located:**

(A) Cornea (B) Choroid
(C) Retina (D) Sclera

19. **This part of the eye dilates and contracts according to the intensity of light:**

(A) Pupil (B) Cornea
(C) Lens (D) Sclera

20. **The lens in the eye is stabilised by:**

(A) The ligaments attached to the ciliary body
(B) The ligaments attached to the iris
(C) The smooth muscles attached to the iris
(D) The smooth muscles attached to the ciliary body

21. **This colour least scattered by fog or dust is:**

(A) Blue (B) Yellow
(C) Green (D) Red

22. **This one is the basic functional unit of hearing:**

(A) Semicircular unit (B) Auricle
(C) Spiral organ (D) Auricle

23. **Through the inner ear, transmission of sound waves occurs through:**

(A) A solid medium containing wax
(B) A fluid medium containing perilymph
(C) Nerve fibers
(D) Auditory ossicles

24. **This portion of the cochlea responds to low frequency sound:**

(A) Middle portion (B) Initial portion
(C) End portion (D) Both (A) and (B)

25. **Support for the hair cells in the spiral organ is obtained by:**

(A) Vestibule (B) Tectorial membrane
(C) Cochlear plate (D) Basilar membrane

26. Conduction deafness may be caused due to the damage in:

(A) Cochlea
(B) Inner ear
(C) Outer ear and the middle ear parts
(D) All of the above

27. This part of the ear does not play a role in hearing:

(A) Eustachian tube (B) Vestibular apparatus
(C) Ear ossicles (D) Organ of Corti

28. This part of ear receives sound vibration and passes to the eardrum:

(A) Middle ear (B) Inner ear
(C) Outer ear (D) Eustachian tube

29. The border between the middle and inner ear is formed by:

(A) Pinnae (B) Tympanic membrane
(C) Incus (D) Oval window

30. The organ of Corti is present in:

(A) The scala media (B) The scala tympani
(C) The scala vestibuli (D) None of these

31. The membranous labyrinth contains:

(A) Perilymph (B) Endolymph
(C) Hemolymph (D) Both (A) and (C)

32. The Eustachian tube:

(A) Equalises pressure between middle ear and outer atmosphere
(B) Connects middle ear to pharynx
(C) Connects internal ear to external ear
(D) Both (A) and (B)

33. This statement is correct about the inner ear:

(A) In it the membranous labyrinth encloses bony labyrinth
(B) The endolymph surrounds membranous labyrinth
(C) It is made up of bony and membranous segments
(D) It contains air-filled inner segment

34. The incorrect match is:

(A) Cristae—perform hearing function
(B) Middle ear—amplifies sound waves
(C) Hair cells—present on basilar membrane
(D) Saccule and utricle—maintain static equilibrium

35. The basilar membrane is present between

(A) Scala vestibule and scala media
(B) Scala vestibule and scala tympani
(C) Scala media and scala tympani
(D) None of these

36. The correct match of ear part and its function?

(A) Semicircular canal—equalizes the pressure on either sides of the eardrum
(B) Eustachian tube—maintains body balance and posture
(C) Organ of Corti—increases the efficiency of sound waves
(D) Tectorial membrane—determines patterns of sensitivity and vibration of sound waves

37. Odor molecules are detected by:

(A) The olfactory sensory neurons
(B) The sustentacular or supporting cells,
(C) The basal epithelial or stem cells
(D) All of the above

38. Vestibule is a:

(A) Skin-lined part of nose
(B) Part of nose that contain small course hair.
(C) Part of nose that keeps dust and microbs from entering the lungs.
(D) All of the above

39. Muscle (or muscles) that help the tongue to move and perform tongue functions such as speech, swallowing and feeding:

(A) Genioglossus muscle
(B) Lingual frenulum
(C) Styloglossus muscle
(D) Both (A) and (C)

40. The tongue is anchored into the:

(A) Ethmoid bone (B) Hyoid bone
(C) Temporal bone (D) Sphenoid bone

41. This muscle protrudes the tongue:

(A) Genioglossus muscle
(B) Styloglossus muscle
(C) Hyoglossus muscle
(D) None of these

42. The taste buds near the tip of the tongue are sensitive to:

(A) Bitter taste (B) Sour taste
(C) Salty taste (D) Sweet taste

43. The taste buds at the back of the tongue are sensitive to:

(A) Bitter taste (B) Sour taste
(C) Salty taste (D) Sweet taste

44. The taste buds on the side of the tongue are sensitive to:

(A) Bitter taste (B) Sour taste
(C) Salty taste (D) Sweet taste

ANSWERS

1. B	2. A	3. C	4. D	5. B	6. A	7. D
8. C	9. C	10. A	11. A	12. B	13. B	14. A
15. C	16. A	17. D	18. C	19. A	20. A	21. D
22. C	23. B	24. C	25. D	26. C	27. B	28. C
29. D	30. A	31. B	32. B	33. C	34. A	35. C
36. D	37. D	38. D	39. B	40. B	41. A	42. D
43. A	44. C					

MATCH THE COLUMNS

I	II
1. Inferior oblique	A. Contain sweat glands
2. Lacrimal glands	B. Secrete oily substance
3. Superior oblique	C. Equalization of air pressure
4. Lacrimal caruncle	D. Tears
5. Tarsal gland	E. Responsible for sharp image
6. Basilar membrane	F. Elevation of eye
7. Ciliary body	G. Refraction of light
8. Auditory tube	H. Attaches to lens capsule
9. Fovea centralis	I. Secretes ear wax
10. Cornea	J. Depression of eye
11. Suspensory ligament	K. Secretion of aqueous humour
12. Ceruminous gland	L. Vibration by sound waves

ANSWERS

1. F 2. D 3. J 4. A 5. B 6. L 7. K
8. C 9. E 10. G 11. H 12. I

CHAPTER

8

Cardiovascular System

SAQ: Short answer question: Marks: 2	**MCQs:** Multiple Choice Questions: Marks: 0.5 each
BAQ: Brief answer question: Marks: 4 or 5	**Match the columns:** Marks: 0.5 each
LAQ: Long answer question: Marks: 9 or 10	**Draw a labelled diagram:** Marks: 5

Objective: To describe the circulatory system.

INTRODUCTION (Fig. 8.1)

BAQ: Write a note on the cardiovascular system.

Ans: The cardiovascular system (circulatory system) is an organ system, which is involved in the circulation of blood to the various organs, tissues and cells of the body. By normal blood circulation, nutrients, oxygen, carbon dioxide, hormones, and blood cells are circulated to various parts of the body. The circulated blood provides nourishment to the cells of the body organs in the form of glucose, amino acids, fatty acids, vitamins, etc. The circulated blood also removes harmful substances such as ammonia, urea, creatinine, etc. formed in the cells during metabolic activities. The circulatory system plays important role in the protection of an individual from various infectious diseases with the help of specific white blood cells such as neutrophils, lymphocytes, monocytes, etc. and antibodies in blood circulation. Normal blood circulation is also important to stabilizing pH of blood, body temperature and in the maintenance of the homeostasis.

The cardiovascular system is made up of blood vessels that carry blood away from heart and from the various organs towards the heart. **Arteries** carry blood away from the heart to various organs and cells and veins carry blood from the cells and organs back to the heart (Fig. 8.1). **Arterioles** are very small blood vessels that branch off from the arteries and carry blood away from the heart to tissues and organs. **Venules** are the smallest veins and receive blood from capillaries. Venules play important role in the exchange of oxygen and nutrients from the cells. The **capillaries** are very small blood vessels that connect the arteries and veins to facilitate the exchange of essential components such as nutrients, waste products, etc., between blood and tissues (Fig. 8.2).

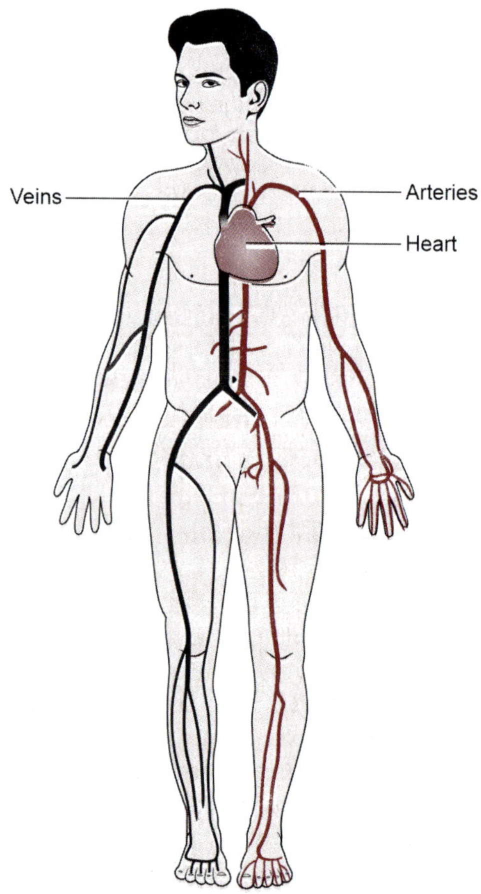

Fig. 8.1: Cardiovascular system

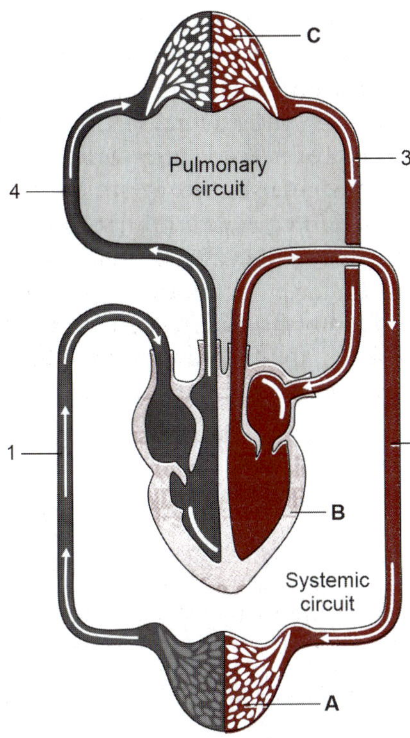

Fig. 8.2: Main components of cardiovacular system with pulmonary and systemic blood circulations. 1. Deoxygenated blood collected from the body to the heart (by Vena cava vein). 2. Oxygenated blood supply to the body by the heart pumping (by aorta artery). 3. Oxygenated blood from the lungs to the heart (by pulmonary vein). 4. Deoxygenated blood pumped by the heart to the lungs for the purification (by Pulmonary artery). A. Body organ blood capillaries. B. Heart. C. Lung blood capillaries

Objective: To describe the major components of the circulatory system.

Components of the Cardiovascular System (Fig. 8.2)

BAQ: Describe the major components of the cardiovascular system.

Ans: The following are the four major components of the cardiovascular system:

1. **Heart:** It is an organ that works like a pump to circulate blood to all parts of the body and cells. The size of heart is about a clenched fist. It lies in the front and middle of chest. It is located behind breastbone and slightly to the left side of breast bone. By consistent pumping action, the heart maintains continuous working of the cardiovascular system.
2. **Arteries:** Arteries carry oxygen-rich blood from the heart to various organs and cells.
3. **Veins:** Veins carry deoxygenated blood from various organs to the heart. From the heart, deoxygenated blood is directed to the lungs to receive oxygen.
4. **Blood:** Blood is a type of connective tissue, made up of plasma and cells. Blood plasma is pale yellow in colour and makes up about 55% of the total blood volume of the body. Plasma contains, water, protein, other organic substances such as glucose, urea, uric acid, creatinine and inorganic substances such as sidium, potassium, chlorides, bicarbonate, calcium, inorganic phosphorus, etc. Blood cells are the red blood cells, white blood cells and platelets.

Objective: To differentiate the types of blood circulation.

Blood Circulation

SAQ: What are the three main types of blood circulations?

Ans: There are the following three different types of blood circulations that occur in the body continuously:

Pulmonary circulation: This blood circulation carries deoxygenated blood (oxygen-depleted blood) away from the heart, to the lungs, and back to the heart, with oxygenated blood (oxygen-rich blood).

Systemic circulation: This blood circulation carries oxygenated blood away from the heart to various organs of the body and collects deoxygenated blood from various organs to the heart.

Coronary circulation: This blood circulation provides oxygenated blood to the heart.

BAQ: Draw a labelled line diagram of pulmonary and systemic blood circulation.

Ans: Ref. Fig. 8.2.

Objective: To locate and describe the anatomical features of the heart.

ANATOMY OF THE HEART (Figs 8.3–8.6)

BAQ: Write a note on the applied anatomy of the heart.

Ans: The heart is made up of the following four chambers: Upper two chambers known as the left atrium and right atrium and lower two chambers are known as the left and right ventricles. It also contains the following four valves: The tricuspid, pulmonary, mitral and aortic valves (Fig. 8.3).

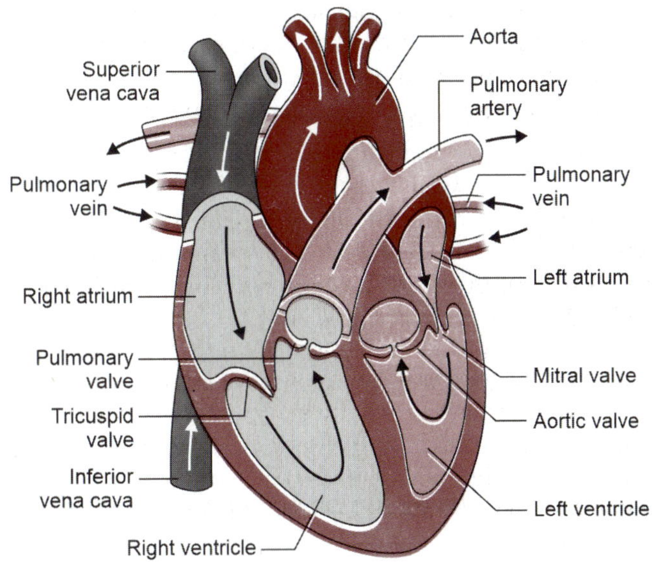

Fig. 8.3: Anatomy of heart

Right atrium: It is a thin-walled chamber that receives blood from body tissues and pumps it into the right ventricle (Fig. 8.3).

Right ventricle: The right ventricle pumps blood from the right atrium to the to the lungs through the pulmonary arteries. Right ventricular wall is thinner than the left ventricular wall (Fig. 8.3).

Left atrium: This thin-walled chamber receives oxygenated blood from the lungs and then pumps it to the left ventricle (Fig. 8.3).

Left ventricle: The thickest of all the chambers, the left ventricle is the hardest working part of the heart as it pumps blood to the entire body (Fig. 8.3).

To keep this continually blood flowing process moving in the right direction, the heart contains following four valves to prevent the backflow of blood:

Tricuspid valve: This valve is located between the right atrium and right ventricle. It is also called the right atrioventricular (AV) valve. The tricuspid valve has three flaps that open and close and allow blood to flow from the right atrium to the right ventricle in the heart and prevents blood from flowing backward (Fig. 8.3).

Pulmonary valve: It lies between the right ventricle and the pulmonary artery and has three cusps (folds). The pulmonic valve is a one-way valve. Blood cannot flow back into the heart through it. The valve is opened by the increased blood pressure of the ventricular contraction. Blood is pushed out of the heart and into the pulmonary artery. Pulmonary valve closes when the blood pressure drops inside the heart. The pulmonary valve is the checkpoint where deoxygenated blood leaves the right ventricle to the lungs (Fig. 8.3).

Mitral valve (the bicuspid valve): The mitral valve is located between the left atrium and left ventricle. It is also called the left atrioventricular (AV) valve. It has two cusps (flaps). Blood flows through an open mitral valve during the contraction of the left atrium and the mitral valve closes during the contraction of the left ventricle. Thus, blood passes in one direction from left atrium to left ventricle and backflow of blood is prevented by mitral valve (Fig. 8.3).

Aortic valve: The aortic valve is located between the left ventricle and the aorta (the largest artery in the body). Through this valve oxygen-rich blood pumps out of the left ventricle to the entire body. The aortic valve opens when the left ventricle contracts to pump out blood, and closes in between heart beats to keep blood from going backward into the heart (Fig. 8.3).

Objective: To describe the blood supply of the heart.

Blood Supply of the Heart

BAQ: Write a note on the blood supply of the heart.

Ans: Right and left coronary arteries supply blood to the myocardium (Fig. 8.4). The left coronary artery gives rise to its major branches, the anterior interventricular artery and circumflex artery. Right coronary artery gives rise to the posterior interventricular artery and marginal artery. The great cardiac vein and the middle cardiac vein return blood from the myocardial capillaries to the coronary sinus (Fig. 8.4) which then returns directly into the right atrium.

The right and left coronary arteries are the first to leave the aorta. These then divide into smaller arteries which encircle the heart and supply blood to all parts of the organ. The blood which returns from the heart is collected mainly by the coronary sinus which later on returns directly into the right atrium (Fig. 8.4).

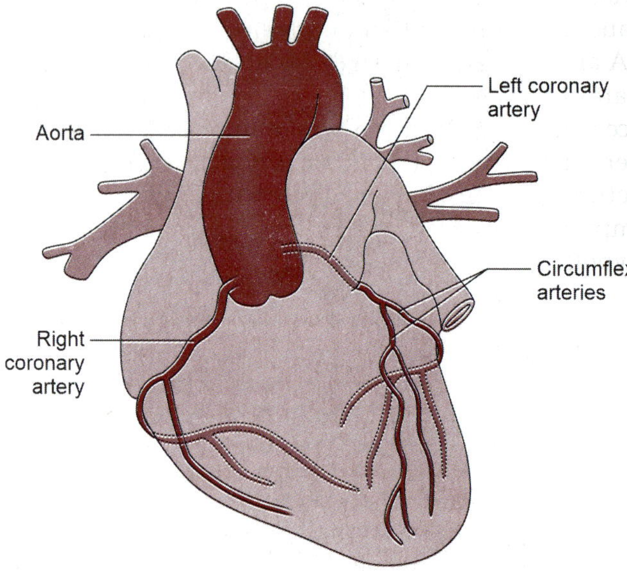

Fig. 8.4: Blood supply of the heart

Objective: To describe the nerve supply of the heart.

Nerve Supply of the Heart

BAQ: Write a note on the innervation of the heart and the related functions.

Ans: The heart is innervated by the sympathetic and parasympathetic nerve fibres from the autonomic branch of the peripheral nervous system. The cardiac plexus is the network of nerves that supply the heart.

The rhythmic rate of contraction of heart is modified by impulses reaching it from the vagus and sympathetic nerves. Branches from these sympathetic nerves pass to the sinoatrial node (SA node), which is a small mass of specialized cells present in the wall of the right atrium (Fig. 8.5). It initiates impulses more rapidly than other groups of neuromuscular cells; hence, it is often described as the pacemaker of the heart. SA depolarizes spontaneously at the rate of 70–80 times per minute, causing the atria to contract.

Due to the specific internal system, the cardiac muscle is automatically stimulated to contract without the need for a nerve supply from the brain. However, the internal system can be stimulated or depressed by nerve impulses initiated in the brain and by circulating chemicals including hormones. The specialized neuromuscular cells in the myocardium initiate and conduct impulses causing coordinated and synchronized contraction of the heart muscle. Atrioventricular (AV) node is a small mass of neuromuscular tissue situated near the atrioventricular valve, is also capable of initiating impulses that cause contraction (Fig. 8.5). The action of the heart is slowed (or inhibited) by the control of vagus nerve (which is a part of the parasympathetic or autonomic system).

Impulses from the SA node pass to the atrioventricular node (AV node), atrioventricular bundle (bundle of His), and finally to the small fibers known as conduction myofibers (Purkinje fibers) within the ventricular walls. Stimulation of the conduction of myofibers causes the ventricles to contract simultaneously. The SA and AV nodes are innervated by sympathetic and parasympathetic nerve fibres. Sympathetic impulses accelerate heart action through the cardiac accelerator nerves and parasympathetic impulses decelerate heart action through the vagus nerve. These autonomic impulses are regulated by the cardiac centers in the hypothalamus and medulla oblongata.

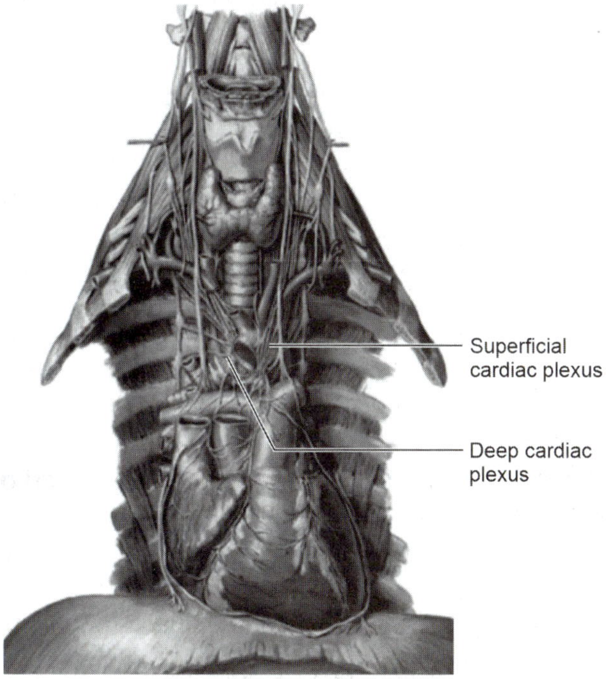

Fig. 8.5A: Cardiac plexus

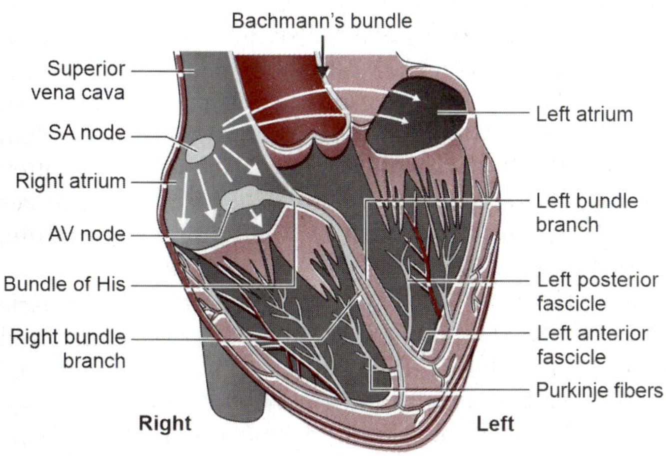

Fig. 8.5B: Electrical conduction of the heart

Objective: To describe the blood circulation function of the heart.

Blood Circulation by the Heart

BAQ: Write a note on the blood circulation function of the heart.

Ans: The heart pumps blood with a rhythm by the pacemaker cells in the sinoatrial node (SA node, Figs 8.5 and 8.6). This action generates an electric current that causes the heart to contract. The electrical current travels through the atrioventricular node (AV node, Figs 8.5 and 8.6) and along the conduction system of the heart. The electrical stimulus causes the chambers of the heart to contract and pump out blood as follows:

Pulmonary Circulation

Deoxygenated blood enters the heart through the right atrium from the superior and inferior vena cava and passes to the right ventricle (Fig.8.3).

Tricuspid valve is located between the right atrium and right ventricle (Fig. 8.3). The tricuspid valve has three flaps; that open and close and allow blood to flow from the right atrium to the right ventricle in the heart and prevents blood from flowing backward. When the right ventricle is full, it squeezes and from the right ventricle, blood is pumped into the pulmonary circulation to the lungs.

Pulmonary valve lies between the right ventricle and the pulmonary artery and has three cusps (folds) (Fig. 8.3). The pulmonic valve is a one-way valve. Blood cannot flow back into the heart through it. The valve is opened by the increased blood pressure of the ventricular contraction. Blood is pushed out of the heart and into the pulmonary artery. Pulmonary valve closes when the blood pressure drops inside the heart. The pulmonary valve is the checkpoint where deoxygenated blood

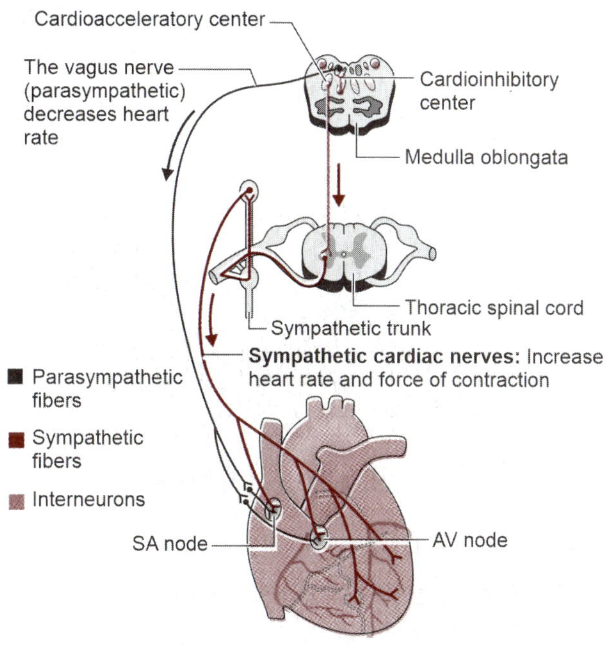

Fig. 8.6: External innervation of the heart

leaves the right ventricle and passes to the lungs where it receives oxygen and gives off carbon dioxide.

Systemic Circulation

Oxygenated blood then returns to the left atrium through the pulmonary veins. From the left atrium blood passes through to the left ventricle.

Mitral valve (the bicuspid valve) is located between the left atrium and left ventricle. It has two cusps (flaps). Blood flows through an open mitral valve during the contraction of the left atrium and the mitral valve closes during the contraction of the left ventricle. Thus, blood passes in one direction from left atrium to left ventricle and backflow of blood is prevented by mitral valve.

The aortic valve is located between the left ventricle and the aorta (the largest artery in the body). When the left ventricle is full, it contracts. Through the aortic valve oxygen-rich blood pumps out of the left ventricle to the entire body.

The aortic valve opens when the left ventricle contracts to pump out blood, and closes in between heart beats to keep blood from going backward into the heart. The blood is then pumped out through the aorta into systemic circulation.

Oxygenated blood then passes through the arteries, arterioles, and capillaries. The nutrients, other organic and inorganic substances and excretory substances are exchanged between the capillaries and the cells.

Coronary Sinus

SAQ: Write a note on the coronary sinus.

Ans: The coronary sinus is a collection of smaller veins that merge together to form the sinus (Fig. 8.7). It is located along the posterior surface of the heart between the left ventricle and left atrium. The coronary sinus collects the majority of the venous blood in the heart. It receives the blood from the myocardium and facilitates the flow of the blood into the right atrium.

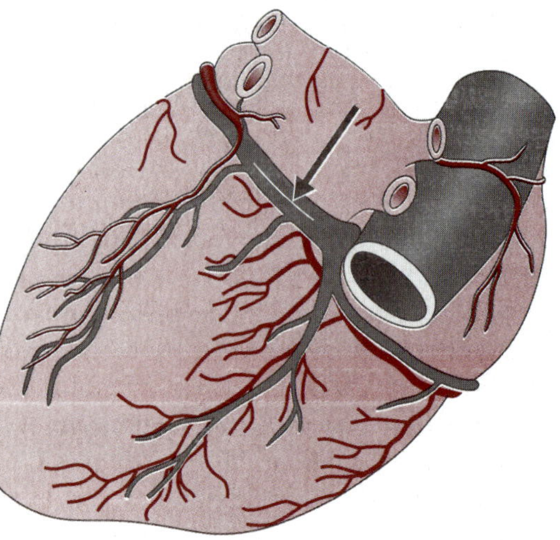

Fig. 8.7: Coronary sinus

Objective: To describe the development of embryonic heart.

Fetal Blood Circulation

SAQ: Write a brief note on the blood circulation in a fetus.

Ans: The fetus is linked to the placenta in the womb of mother by the umbilical cord. The heart development of the fetus begins at the 3rd week of gestation. The lungs are not functional. The fetus gets oxygen, water and all the nutrition through the blood vessels in the umbilical cord. Carbon dioxide and waste products produced during the cellular metabolism of the fetus are passed through the umbilical cord and placenta to the blood circulation of mother for excretion.

BAQ: Write a note on the blood circulation inside the fetus heart.

Ans: The fetus is linked to the placenta in the womb of mother by the umbilical cord. The heart development of the fetus begins at the 3rd week of gestation. The lungs are not functional. The fetus gets oxygen, water and all the nutrition through the blood vessels in the umbilical cord. The umbilical cord is attached to umbilical vein that carries oxygenated blood to the fetus heart and two umbilical arteries that return deoxygenated blood to the placenta.

The following are the various modes of blood circulation inside the fetal heart:

1. Inside the fetal heart, blood enters the right atrium. Most of the blood flows to the left side through the foramen ovale, which is a specific fetal opening between the left and right atria. Part of the blood that enters the right atrium does not flow through the foramen ovale. It remains in the right side of the heart and subsequently, passes into the pulmonary artery.
2. Blood then passes into the left ventricle and passes to the aorta.
3. From the aorta, oxygenated blood is passed to the fetus body.
4. Fetus body cells get oxygen, water and nutrients. Waste products are passed to blood, which becomes deoxygenated.
5. The deoxygenated blood then returns to the right atrium of the heart through the superior and inferior vena cava.

Since, the placenta performs the function of exchanging of oxygen and carbon dioxide through the blood circulation of the mother, the fetal lungs (which are non-functional) are not used for breathing. The fetal blood circulation bypasses most of the blood away from the lungs. The blood is shunted from the pulmonary artery to the aorta through the ductus arteriosus, a specific linked blood vessel.

After birth, the lungs become functional. When the baby takes first breaths of air the fetal circulation changes. A larger amount of blood is then passed to the lungs to become oxygenated. The ductus arteriosus is not needed. It may remain open in premature babies for a longer period. Later on, the ductus arteriosus withers and subsequently closes off.

The blood circulation in the lungs of the newborn increases and more blood flows into the left atrium of the heart. The increased blood pressure causes the foramen ovale to close. Circulation of blood then takes place in a normal way.

Objective: To locate and describe the anatomical features and functions of the pericardium.

PERICARDIUM

SAQ: Write a note on the pericardium.

Ans: The pericardium is a double-walled thin sac that surrounds the heart (Fig. 8.8). The outer layer of the pericardium surrounds the roots of major blood vessels of the heart and the inner layer is attached to the heart muscle. The pericardium is made up of an outer single connective tissue fibrous layer. It is made up of collagen and known as fibrous pericardium. The inner layer is a serous layer, made up of two layers and known as serous pericardium. The two layers of serous pericardium are called visceral pericardium and parietal pericardium. These are separated by the pericardial cavity, which contains about 20 to 60 ml of the plasma ultrafiltrate, known as pericardial fluid.

Function: The pericardium gives mechanical protection to the heart and the major blood vessels. The pericardial fluid provides lubrication to reduce friction between the heart and the surrounding structures. Mesothelial cells in pericardial fluid play important role in providing non-adhesive protective surface to the pericardium.

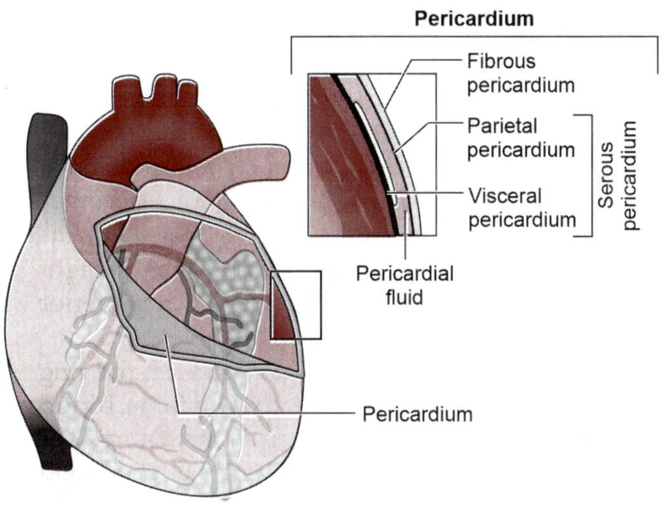

Fig. 8.8A: Pericardium

BAQ: Write a note on pericardial fluid.

Ans: The pericardial sac contains 20–50 ml of clear, straw-coloured fluid (Fig. 8.8A). It is plasma ultrafiltrate. The pericardial fluid provides lubrication to reduce friction between the heart and the surrounding

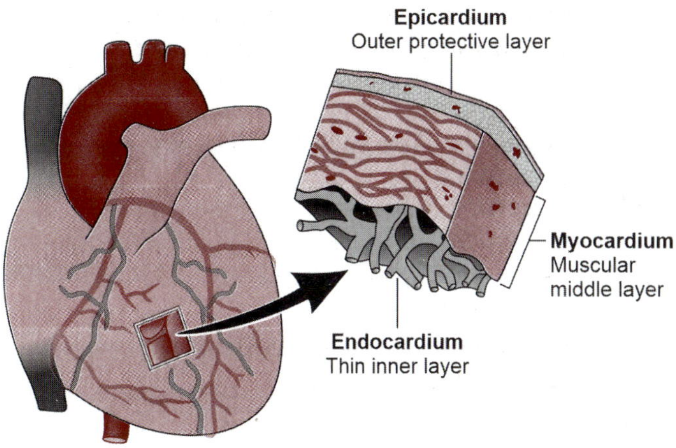

Fig. 8.8B: Heart wall layers

structures. In various clinical conditions related to heart, various changes are observed in the pericardial fluid. By examining the pericardial fluid in a clinical laboratory, it is possible to diagnose a specific clinical condition rlated to the heart. The following are the various changes observed in the pericardial fluid and the related clinical conditions:

1. Increased amounts of normal appearing pericardial fluid may be observed in the inflammation of the heart wall, congestive heart failure and in pericarditis.
2. Change to cloudy appearance may be associated with bacterial infection, rheumatic inflammation and in post-myocardial infarction.
3. Grossly blood containing fluid may be seen in, tuberculosis, bacterial pericarditis. Systemic lupus erythematosus, leaking aortic syndrome and in post-myocardial infarction syndrome.

Objective: To describe the anatomical features of the heart wall.

BAQ: Write a note on the anatomy of the heart wall.

Ans: The wall of the heart separates into the following layers: (1) Epicardium, (2) myocardium, and, (3) endocardium (Fig. 8.8B).

1. The epicardium is the outermost layer of the heart. It is composed of connective tissue mesothelial cells, and fat. The epicardium contains blood vessels and it provides nourishes to the heart walls.
2. The myocardium is a contractile muscle, similar to skeletal muscle. It is involuntary and striated muscle. Each cell of the myocardium has one nucleus and one or two branches and these are interconnected with other myocardial cells. When a impulse is initiated, it spreads over the complete sheet of myocardial muscle. The myocardium performs coordinated contractions that allow heart to pump blood through the circulatory system (Refer to Figs 2.56 and 8.8B).
3. The endocardium is the innermost layer of the heart. It is made up of flattened epithelial cells. The endocardium lines the heart chambers and extends over the valves, and the blood vessels. The atrial endocardium is thicker than that of the ventricles.

The function of the endocardial cell layer is to provide a physical barrier to protect the inner cardiac tissue against the blood driving force of the heart.

Objectives: To identify and describe the structures and functions of arteries, capillaries and veins. To describe the clinical conditions associated with arteries, capillaries and veins.

BLOOD VESSELS

BAQ: Write a note on the blood vessels.

Ans: The blood vessels consist of arteries, arterioles, capillaries, venules and veins. All blood in the body is carried in these vessels. Blood travels from the heart from arteries, which branch into smaller vessels, and become arterioles. Arterioles connect with still smaller blood vessels called capillaries. Oxygen and nutrients pass through the thin walls of the capillaries, from blood into tissues and then to cells (Fig. 8.9). Waste products from cells pass into blood. From the capillaries, blood passes into venules, and then into veins to return to the heart (Fig. 8.9).

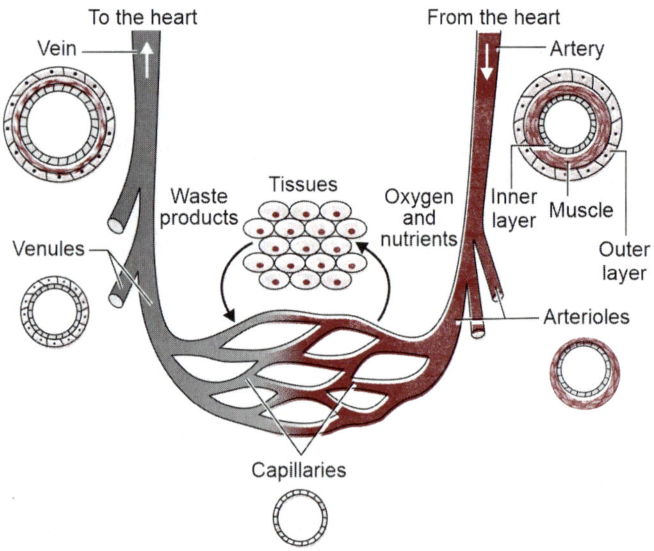

Fig. 8.9: Oxygen and nutrient supply to tissue and cells by blood vessels

Arteries and arterioles have relatively thick muscular walls, since, blood pressure in them is high. Arteries and arterioles are able to adjust their diameter to maintain blood pressure and to control blood flow. Compared to arteries and arterioles, veins and venules have much thinner and less muscular walls, since, the pressure in veins and venules is comparatively low. The veins are able to dilate to accommodate increased blood volume.

Arteries (Fig. 8.10)

BAQ: Write a note on the arteries.

Ans: Oxygenated blood enters the systemic circulation while leaving the left ventricle, through the aortic semilunar valve. Aorta is a massive and thick-walled artery, which receives blood from the heart. The aorta is the first part of the systemic circulation. The aorta arches and gives branches and supply blood to the upper part of the body. Then after passing through the aortic opening of the diaphragm at the level of thoracic ten (T10) vertebra, it enters the abdomen. Later it descends down and supplies branches to abdomen, lower limbs, pelvis and perineum (the region between the thighs) (Fig. 8.10).

The walls of aorta are elastic to maintain the blood pressure throughout the body. Arteries do not contain valves to prevent backflow of blood.

SAQ: Describe the main four divisions of the aorta.

Ans: The aorta can be divided into the four parts: (1) Ascending aorta, (2) aortic arch, (3) thoracic (descending) aorta and, (4) abdominal aorta. The aorta terminates at the level of L4 and bifurcates into the right and left common iliac arteries (Figs 8.10 and 8.11).

SAQ: Describe the ascending aorta and its branches.

Ans: The ascending aorta is a part that commences at the upper part of the base of the left ventricle. It is on a level with the lower border of the third costal cartilage behind the left half of the sternum. The following are the branches of the ascending aorta: Two coronary arteries that supply blood to the heart.

SAQ: Describe the aortic arch.

Ans: The aortic arch is the portion of the aorta that connects at the ascending aorta with the descending aorta. The following are the major arteries that branch from the arch: (1) The brachiocephalic artery, (2) left carotid artery and (3) left subclavian artery (Fig. 8.11).

SAQ: Describe the brachiocephalic trunk.

Ans: The brachiocephalic trunk is the first branch of the aortic arch. It supplies blood to the right arm and right head and the neck.

SAQ: Describe the carotid arteries.

Ans: The common carotid arteries travel from the upper chest to the skull. There two common carotid arteries, the left common carotid artery and the right common carotid artery. Each divides further into two branches. The carotid arteries supply oxygenated blood and nutrients to organs and tissues in the head, brain and the neck (Fig. 8.10).

SAQ: Describe the subclavian arteries.

Ans: The subclavian arteries lie just below the clavicles. These arteries provide oxygenated blood to the bilateral upper extremities including the head and the neck. The left subclavian artery originates directly from the aortic arch and the right subclavian artery derives from the brachiocephalic trunk (Fig. 8.10).

SAQ: Name the arteries that arise from the abdominal aorta and supply oxygenated blood to diaphragm, stomach, liver, pancreas, duodenum and spleen.

Ans: Fig. 8.10; Tables 8.1 and 8.2.

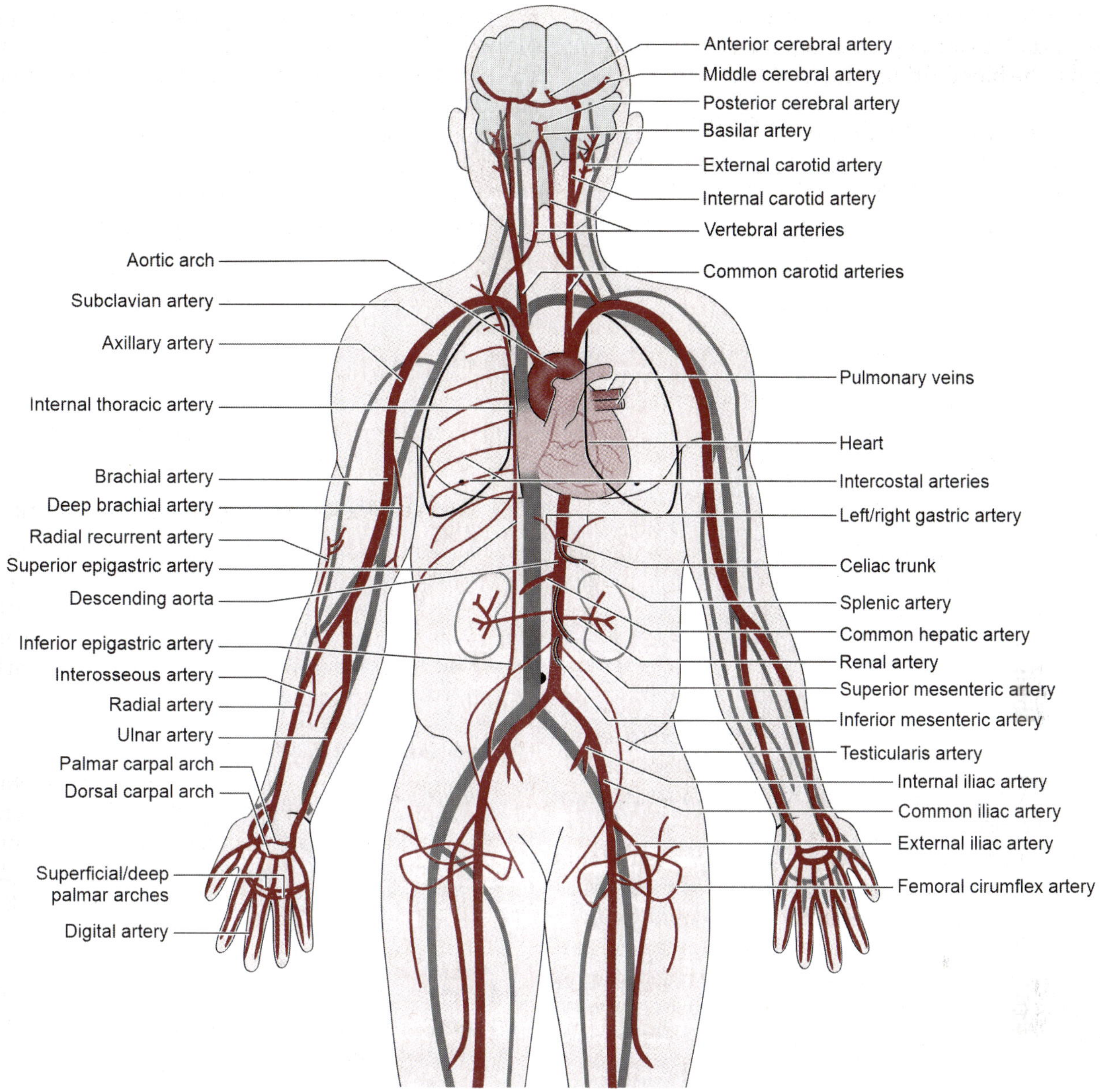

Fig. 8.10: Major arteries of the body

Table 8.1: Abdominal aorta arteries and supply of oxygenated blood (Part-1)

Oxygenated blood supply to	*Name of the artery*
Diaphragm	Inferior frenic arteries
Duodenum, liver, pancreas	Hepatic artery
Stomach, pancreas, spleen	Splenic artery
Esophagus, stomach	Left gastric artery

Table 8.2: Abdominal aorta arteries and supply of oxygenated blood (Part-2)

Oxygenated blood supply to	*Name of the artery*
Lower extremities	External iliac artery
Reproductive organs	Internal iliac artery
Small intestine, pancreas, colon, cecum	Superior mesenteric artery
Adrenal glands	Suprarenal arteries
Kidneys	Renal arteries
Testes and ovaries	Gonadal arteries
Sigmoid colon, rectum	Inferior mesenteric artery

BAQ: Write a note on an aneurysm.

Ans: An aneurysm is an abnormal swelling or bulge in the wall of a bigger blood vessels such as an aorta and arteries that supply blood to the brain, intestine, spleen, and the knee, etc. The following are the various reasons that may lead to an aneurysm:

1. Prolonged hypertension that may result in the weakening of blood vessel leading to swelling in the vessel.
2. Congenital aneurysm present from birth.
3. Arteriosclerosis and/or atherosclerosis leading to a weakness of the vessel wall.
4. Trauma in the specific part of the body, affecting arteries in that region.
5. Chronic infection that may infect arterial wall. Example, syphilis (the sexually transmitted infection), that targets the aorta, causing weakness in the wall of the vessel.

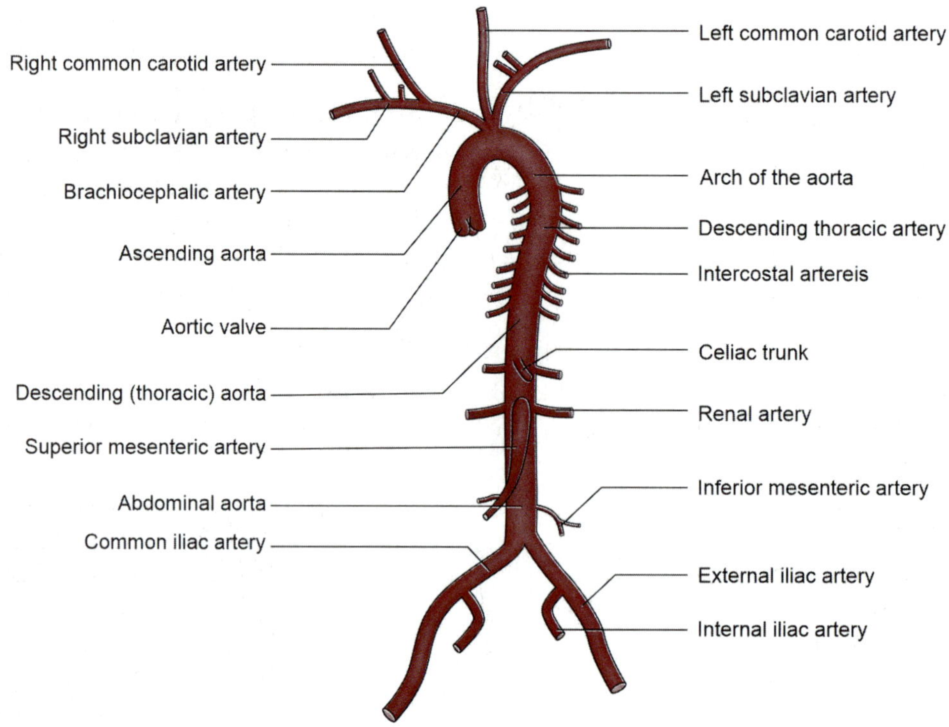

Fig. 8.11: Aortic arch and related branches

The following are the various types of aneurysms: Cerebral aneurysms (in the brain), thoracic aortic aneurysms (in the chest) and abdominal aortic aneurysms (in the abdomen).

Aneurysms does not indicate any symptoms until they get ruptured. A ruptured aneurysm may result in the internal bleeding and stroke and could be fatal. Prolonged pain in a specific part of the body may indicate the presence of an aneurysm and the following tests may give appropriate diagnosis: Ultrasound scans, computed tomography (CT) scans, or CT angiograms and magnetic resonance imaging (MRI) or MR angiograms.

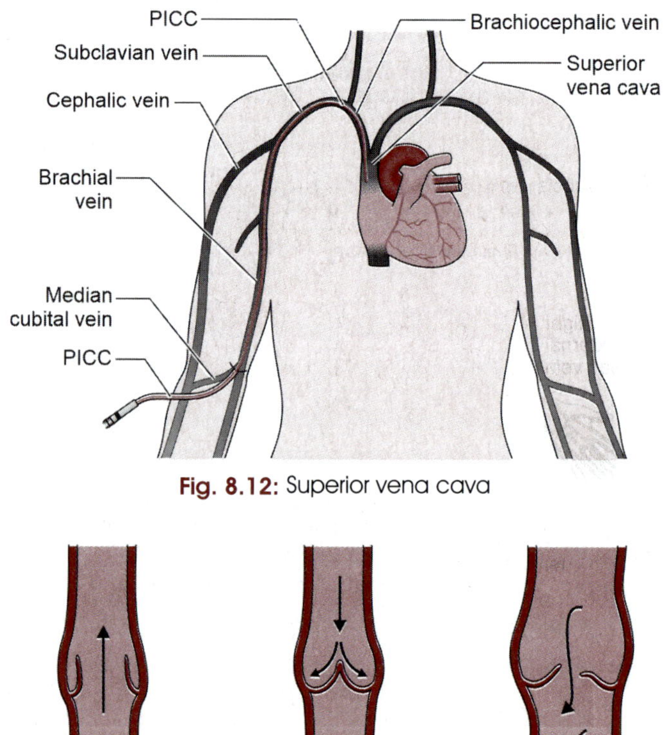

Fig. 8.12: Superior vena cava

Veins (Fig. 8.12)

SAQ: Write a brief note on the veins and the venous system.

Ans: The capillaries merge into venules, which merge into veins. The venous system divides into the two major veins: (1) The superior vena cava which mainly drains tissues above the heart (Fig. 8.12) and (2) the inferior vena cava which mainly drains tissues below the heart (Fig. 8.13). These two large veins empty into the right atrium of the heart. The venous system carries deoxygenated blood to the heart. The veins have valve-like flaps that allow blood to pass only towards the heart (Fig. 8.13). They are able to pass the blood by overcoming the difference in height from the legs to the heart.

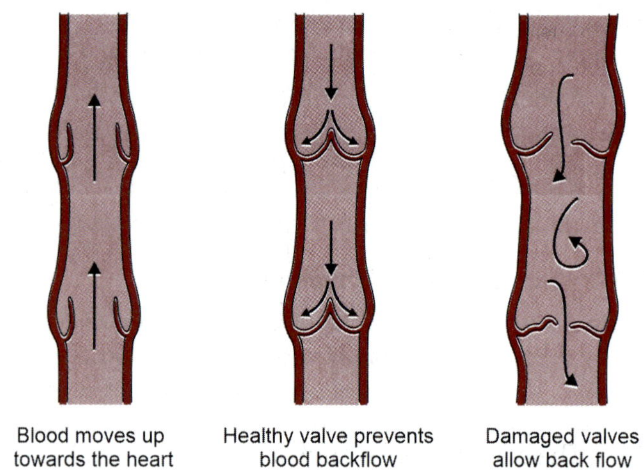

Fig. 8.13A: Valves in the vein

SAQ: What are superficial veins and deep veins?

Ans: Superficial veins are present very close to the surface of the body (Fig. 8.13B). Deep veins are present deep inside the body (Fig. 8.13C). These are thicker than superficial veins. The important function of deep veins is to receive blood from the superficial veins and then to pump it to the heart.

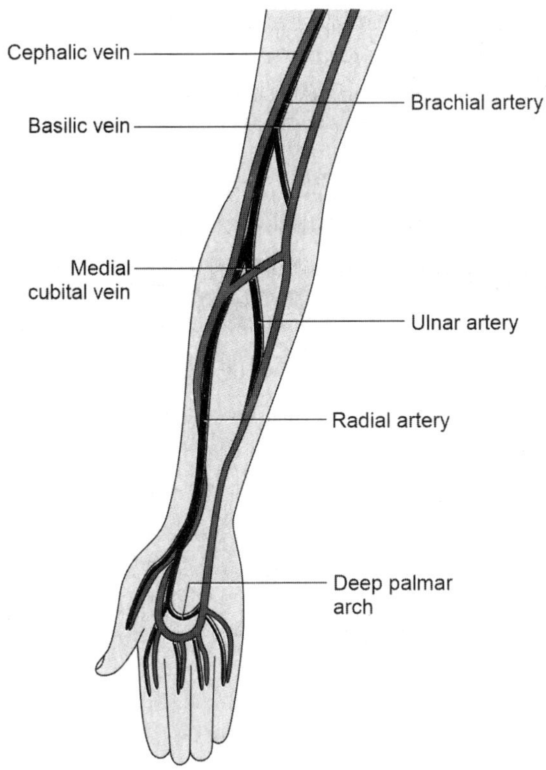

Fig. 8.13B: Superficial veins

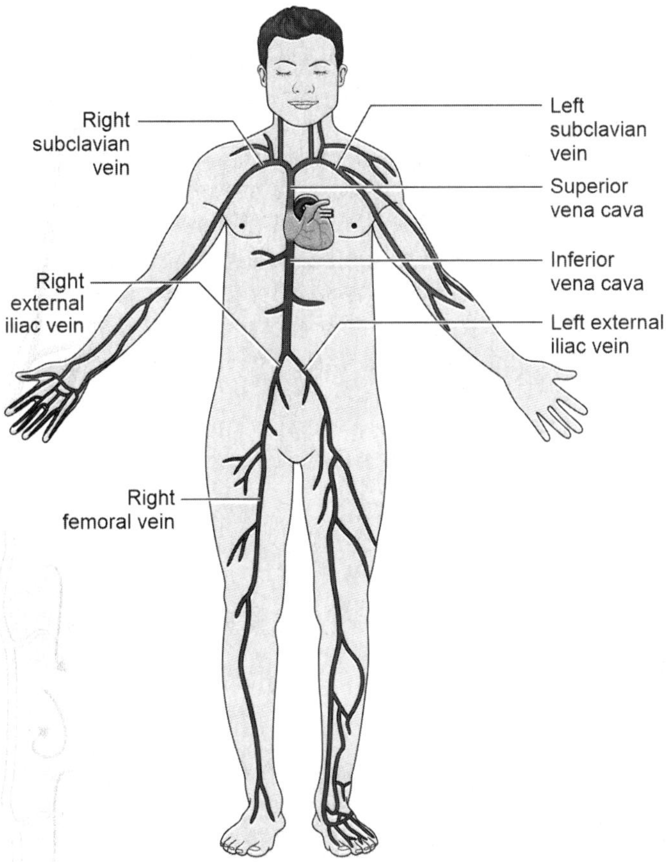

Fig. 8.13C: Deep veins

The examples of superficial veins are, cephalic vein, median cubital vein and basilic vein. For performing blood tests in a clinical laboratory, blood is collected using a syringe and needle, from the median cubital vein. The examples of deep veins are, the deep cerebral vein, internal thoracic vein, common femoral, anterior tibial vein, tibial vein, gastrocnemial vein, etc.

SAQ: What is deep vein thrombosis?

Ans: Deep venous thrombosis (Fig. 8.13D), occurs in the legs, due to formation of clots in the veins of the legs. Deep venous thrombosis is observed mainly in persons that suffer from prolonged diabetes mellitus and also when a person has profession to remains stationary for a long time (job like a traffic police). It is necessary to treat deep vein thrombosis to avoid further complications. The clots formed in the veins may pass to another location in the body by blood circulation and may lead to stroke and pulmonary obstruction.

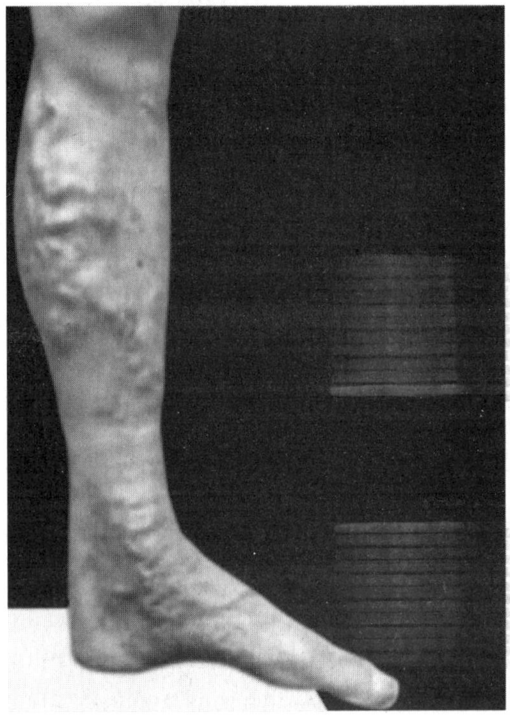

Fig. 8.13D: Varicosed veins

BAQ: Draw labelled figures of superficial and deep veins.

Ans: Refer Figs 8.13B and C.

BAQ: Write a note on varicosed veins.

Ans: Varicosed veins mean enlarged, dilated and coiled veins (Fig. 8.13D). Blood in the legs passes towards the heart against gravity. Due to long periods of pronged standing work, accumulation of blood takes place in the leg veins, leading to deterioration of the valves in the leg veins (Fig. 8.13A) and accumulation of blood, leading to increase in the size of the veins. Other risk factors of varicose veins are old age, obesity, pregnancy and family history. The symptoms of varicose veins include pain and swelling in the legs. In severe cases, blood clots may form in the veins, leading to deep vein thrombosis. Treatment on varicose vein may be supportive or surgical and it depends on the specific nature of varicose veins.

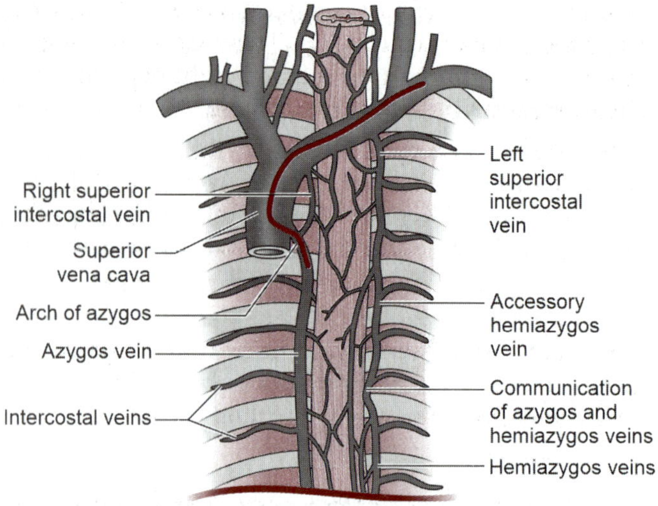

Fig. 8.14: Superior vena cava and its branches

Objective: To identify the principal systemic veins and describe the related functions.

BAQ: Write a note on the superior vena cava.

Ans: The superior vena cava is a large vein that return deoxygenated blood from the systemic circulation to the right atrium of the heart. It receives deoxygenated venous blood from above the diaphragm (Figs 8.12 and 8.14).

The superior vena cava is formed by the right and left brachiocephalic veins, which receive blood from the head, neck and upper limbs. It passes down vertically, behind the first intercostal space and connects the azygos vein before it passes through the fibrous pericardium. It terminates in the upper and posterior part of the sinus venarum of the right atrium, at the upper right front portion of the heart.

BAQ: Write a note on the inferior vena cava.

Ans: The inferior vena cava is a large vein. It carries the deoxygenated blood from the lower and middle part of the body into the right atrium of the heart. It is formed by the joining of the left and right common iliac veins at the level of the fifth lumbar vertebra (Fig. 8.15). Inferior vena cava lies posterior to the abdominal cavity and passes along the right side of the vertebral column. It enters the right auricle of the heart at the lower right and at the back side.

Table 8.3 depicts various veins enter the inferior vena cava and the related specific levels.

Table 8.3: Branches of inferior vena cava, the specific levels and functions

Veins	*Level*	*Deoxygenated blood collected from*
Hepatic veins, inferior phrenic veins	T8	Liver, diphragm
Right suprarenal vein, renal veins	L1	Kidneys, adrenal glands
Right gonadal vein	L2	Gonads
Lumbar vertebral veins	L1–L5	Vertebral column
Right and left common iliac veins	L5	Lower part of the body

Hepatic Portal System and the Portal Circulation

BAQ: Write a brief note on the hepatic portal system and portal circulation.

Ans: The hepatic portal system is comprised of veins that carry out transport of blood containing digested nutrients from the gastrointestinal tract to the liver. It consists of the hepatic portal vein and other veins that drain into the hepatic portal vein, such as the splenic vein, the superior mesenteric vein, and the inferior mesenteric vein (Figs 8.16 and 8.17).

The hepatic portal vein branches into blood capillary system in the liver. This blood circulation is called portal circulation. Portal vein breaks into interlobular veins and then into sinusoids (larger in size than capillaries) (Fig. 8.18). From the sinusoids exchange of nutrients takes place with the liver cells. The sinusoids enable the liver cells to metabolise the nutrients and remove

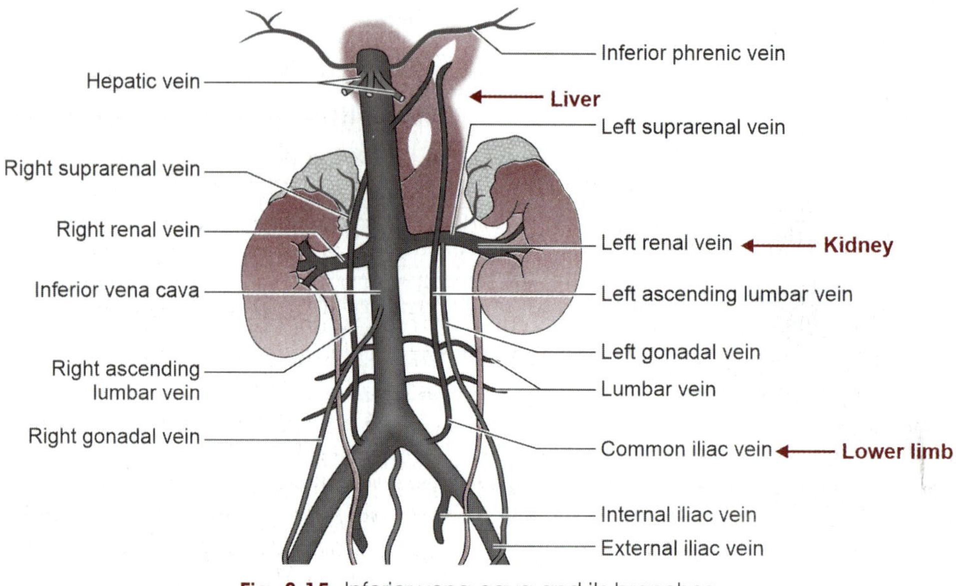

Fig. 8.15: Inferior vena cava and its branches

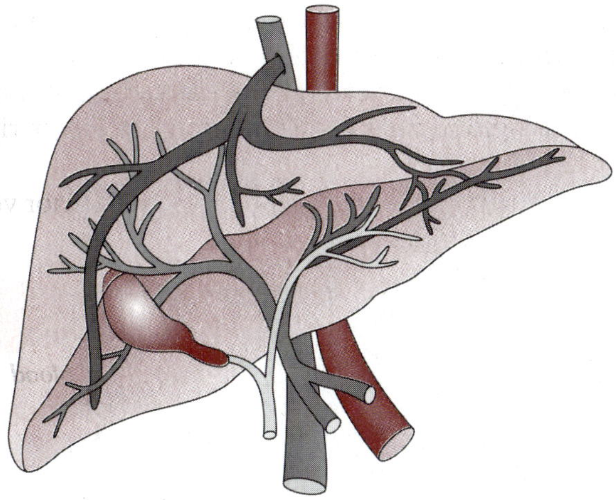

Fig. 8.16: Blood supply to liver

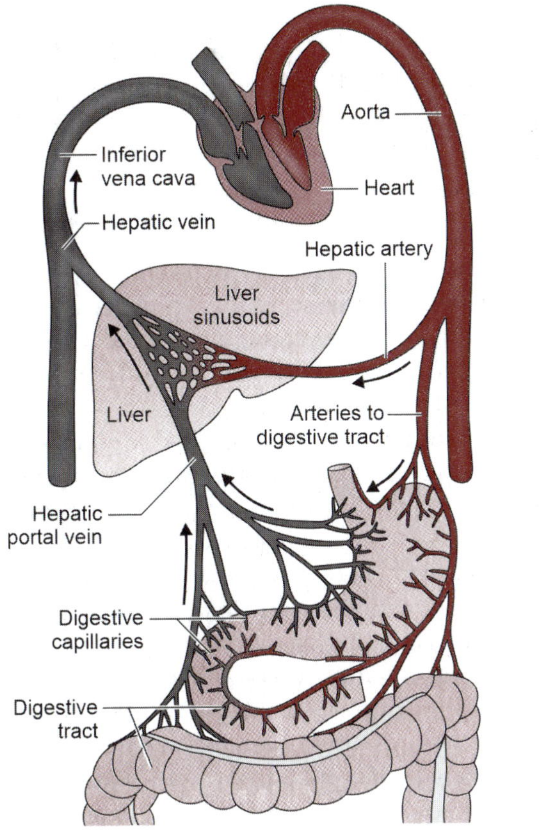

Fig. 8.17: Hepatic portal vein, aorta and inferior vena cava

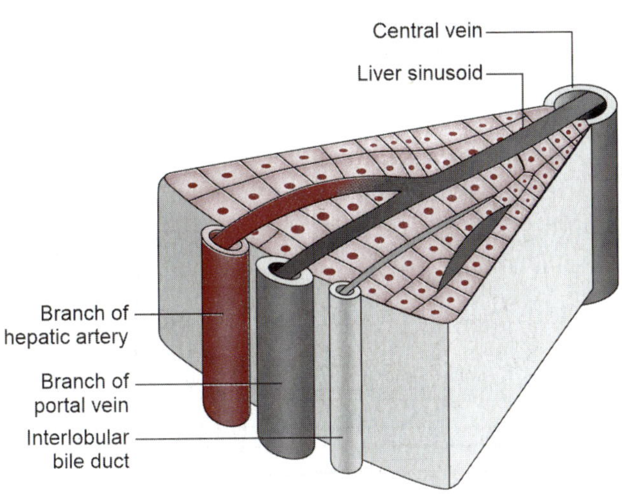

Fig. 8.18: Liver sinusoid

toxic and harmful substances from the blood, before it enters the systemic circulation. The venous drainage is from the liver through the left and right hepatic veins, which enter into inferior vena cava near the right atrium of the heart.

Objective: To describe the difference between the pulmonary and systemic blood circulations.

Pulmonary and Systemic Circulation

Systemic circulation means transportation of oxygenated blood from the heart to the entire body. Pulmonary circulation brings deoxygenated blood back to the heart.

Systemic Circulation

Systemic circulation carries oxygenated blood from the left ventricle of the heart, and passes through the arteries to the blood capillaries in the tissues of the body. The deoxygenated blood returns through the tissue capillaries, to a system of the veins to the right atrium of the heart.

Pulmonary Circulation

In the pulmonary circulation, deoxygenated blood returned from the body to the right atrium of the heart is pumped out from the right ventricle to the lungs. In the lungs, the blood becomes oxygenated and returns to the left atrium to complete the pulmonary circulation circuit.

Objective: To describe the blood circulation of the brain.

Blood Circulation to the Brain

BAQ: Write a brief note on the blood circulation to the brain.

Ans: The brain gets blood supply from arteries at its front side (anterior) and at back side (posterior). The anterior circulation is from the internal carotid arteries and the posterior circulation is from the vertebral arteries. The circulation from the front and the back join together at the circle of Willis (Fig. 8.19).

BAQ: Write a note on stroke.

Ans: Stroke is a clinical condition which takes place when the blood supply to a specific part of the brain is decreased or blocked, due to a blood clot or atherosclerotic plaque. Decreased blood supply prevents the brain tissue from getting oxygen and nutrients. The underlying cause of an ischemic stroke is mainly the blockage of carotid arteries that supply oxygenated blood to the brain Figs 8.10 and 8.19). A hemorrhagic stroke is also may occur, if an artery in or on the surface of the brain gets ruptured leading to bleeding and damage to the specific brain part.

A stroke is a medical emergency and requires immediate treatment to dissolve the formed clot. The specific symptoms of a stroke include, severe headache, confusion, loss of coordination, trouble in speaking, slur words, drooping of mouth, blurred vision in one or both the eyes, paralysis on the face, arm or leg. The patient

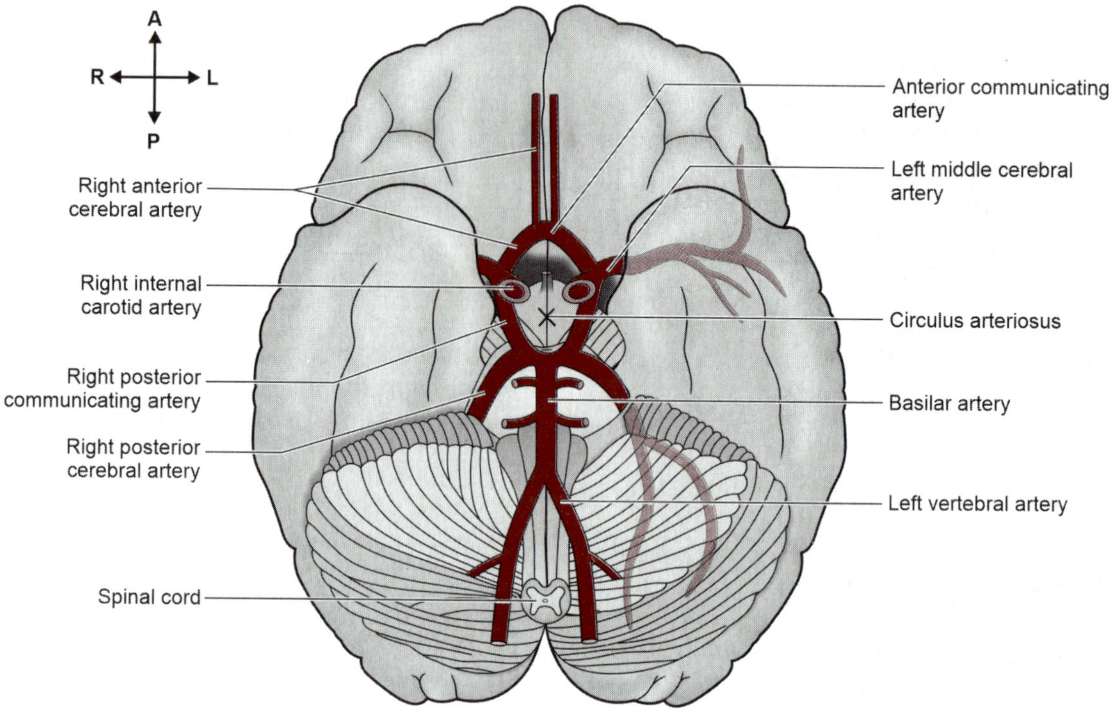

Fig. 8.19: Circle of Willis and its main branches to the brain

may not be able to raise one of the hands. The patient recovers, if treated within 2–3 hours.

Objective: To describe the blood circulation to the kidneys.

Blood Supply to the Kidneys (Fig. 8.15)

BAQ: Write a note on the blood supply to the kidneys.

Ans: Blood flows into the kidney through the renal artery. The renal artery branches into smaller blood vessels that reach the nephrons of the kidneys. In the nephron, the blood is filtered by the tiny blood vessels of the glomeruli and then the filtered blood flows out of the kidney through the renal vein, which joins the inferior vena cava, leading to the heart.

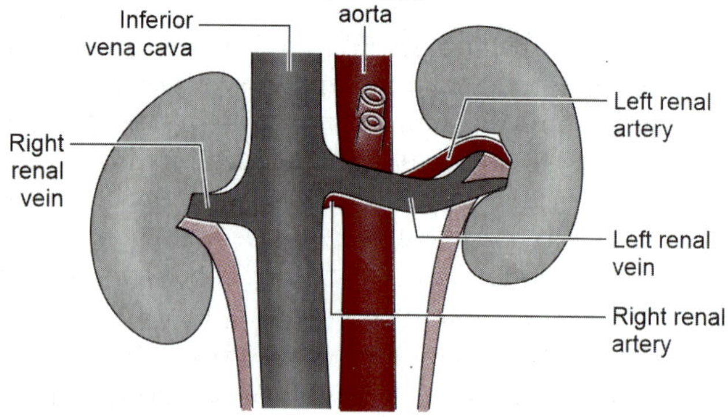

Fig. 8.20: Blood supply of the kidneys

Objective: To describe the anatomical layers (tunics) of blood vessel.

BAQ: Write a note on the anatomical layers (tunicae) of blood vessel.

Ans: A blood vessel is made up of the following three layers: (1) Tunica externa, the outer most layer, (2) tunica media, the intermediate layer and, (3) tunica intima, the innermost layer (Fig. 8.21).

1. The tunica externa is composed of collagen fibers and elastic tissue. The function of the tunica externa is to provide basic structural support to the blood vessels. It prevents a vessel from expanding very large due to the internal blood pressure.
2. The tunica media is made up of smooth muscle cells, elastic tissue (connective tissue proper) and collagen fibres. It is a thicker layer. The function of the tunica media is to provide support to the blood vessel. It also changes blood vessel diameter appropriately to regulate proper blood flow and blood pressure.
3. The tunica intima is in direct contact with the flow of blood. This layer is mainly made up of endothelial cells and a supporting layer of elastin rich collagen. The function of the tunica intima is to provide smooth surface for the blood flow. The elastic tissue of this

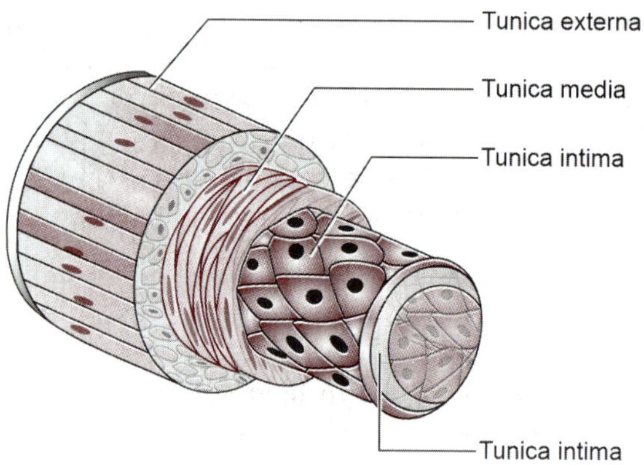

Fig. 8.21: Layers (tunicae) of blood vessel

Table 8.4: Comparative presentation of artery, arteriole, capillary and vein		
Blood vessel	***Anatomical structure***	***Functions***
Artery	Strong structure made up of tunica externa, tunica media and tunica interna Smaller lumen, no valves	Basic support, smooth blood flow Carries oxygenated blood from the heart to various organs, tissues Blood flow is faster
Arterioles	Made up of tunica externa tunica media and tunica externa. Tunica media is thicker	Able to alter diameter to control flow of blood
Capillary	Wall composed of tunica interna only	Facilitates exchange of fluids nutrients and gases with the interstitial fluids
Vein	Thin and elastic structure made up of tunica externa, tunica media and tunica interna Lumen is bigger, valves are present	Carries deoxygenated blood from various tissues to the heart Blood flow is slow

Table 8.5: Comparison of arteries and veins	
Arteries	***Veins***
1. Supply oxygenated blood from heart to various organs and tissues	1. Supply deoxygenated blood from various organs and tissues to the heart
2. Artery walls are thick	2. Venous walls are thin
3. Valves are not present	3. Valves are present
4. Blood flow is rapid	4. Blood flow is slow
5. These are more elastic	5. These are less elastic

layer allows the artery to bend and fit well through the various parts in the body.

SAQ: What is lumen of a blood vessel?

Ans: The hollow internal cavity of blood vessel in which the blood flows is called the lumen.

BAQ: Give comparative presentation of blood vessels such as artery, arteriole, capillary and vein on the basis of anatomical structure and functions.

Ans: Refer to Table 8.4.

BAQ: Write five main differences between arteries and veins.

Ans: The following are five main differences between arteries and veins (Table 8.5).

BAQ. What are sinusoids?

Ans: Sinusoids are vessels slightly larger than capillaries (Fig. 8.18B). The sinusoids have large gaps between endothelial cells present in their walls. Hence, sinusoids are considerably more permeable for nutrient exchange with the cells of the organs in which these are present. The sinusoids are present in the various organs such as liver, spleen, bone marrow and adrenal gland. The macrophages of hepatic sinusoids have phagocytic functions.

OBJECTIVES

- To describe the conduction system of the heart.
- To describe the cardiac cycle.
- To understand the ECG change related to arrhythmias.

CARDIAC CYCLE

BAQ: Write a note on the cardiac cycle.

Ans: The function of the heart is to maintain a constant circulation of blood throughout the body. The heart acts as a pump and the events which occur in the heart during the circulation of the blood are called the cardiac cycle. It consists of the following two periods: During the first period the heart, muscle relaxes and refills with blood and during the second period, contraction of heart takes place and blood is pumped out. The action of contraction of heart is called systole and the action of relaxation is called diastole.

Every single heartbeat is comprised of the following three major stages: Atrial systole, ventricular systole, and complete cardiac diastole. Atrial systole is the contraction of the atria that leads to ventricular filling. Ventricular systole is the contraction of the ventricles in which blood is ejected into the aorta and complete cardiac diastole occurs after systole. The cardiac cycle remains continuous as the blood chambers of the heart relax and fill with blood again.

The action of the heartbeat originates in the sinoatrial node (SA node), and then to the atrioventricular node (AV node), atrioventricular bundle (bundle of His), and finally to Purkinje fibers within the ventricular walls. The SA and AV nodes are innervated by sympathetic and parasympathetic nerve fibres. Sympathetic impulses accelerate heart action through the cardiac accelerator nerves and parasympathetic impulses decelerate heart action through the vagus nerve. These autonomic impulses are regulated by the cardiac centers in the hypothalamus and medulla oblongata.

Electrical Changes in the Heart

BAQ: How the electrical activity within the heart is detected? Give information on the heart rate and electrocardiogram (ECG) and electrocardiograph.

Ans: The electrical activity within the heart can be detected by attaching electrodes to the surface of the body (Fig. 8.22). Electrocardiogram (ECG) means tracing of electrical activity of a heart. An ECG machine is used to determine electrocardiogram.

The pattern of electrical activity is displayed on an oscilloscope screen or traced on a paper as an electrocardiograph. The normal ECG shows five waves P, Q, R, S and T (conventional names) (Fig. 8.23). The ECG originates from the SA node and is known as sinus rhythm. The rate of sinus rhythm is 60–100 beats per minute. A faster heart rate is called tachycardia and a slower heat rate is called bradycardia.

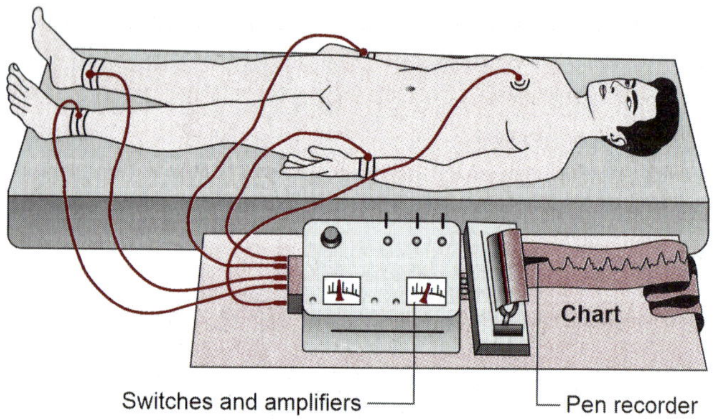

Fig. 8.22: ECG test

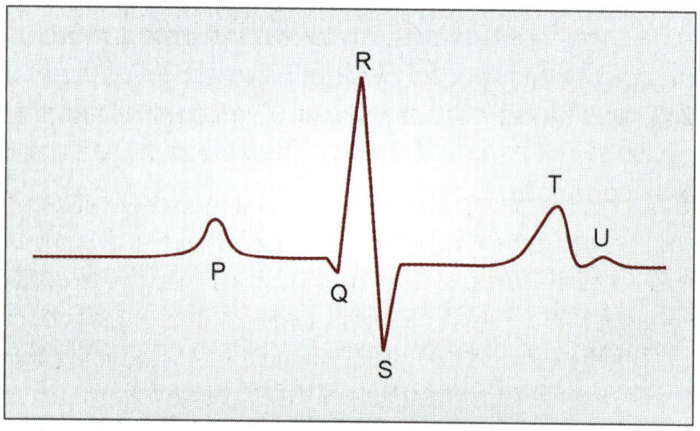

Fig. 8.23: Normal electrocardiogram (ECG)

BAQ: Enumerate the factors that affect the heart rate.

Ans: The following factors affect the heart rate:

- Disturbances in autonomic nervous system
- Circulating chemicals and hormones (such as catecholamines, epinephrine, norepinephrine, thyroxine, etc.)
- Exercise
- Emotional status
- Temperature
- Gender
- Age

BAQ: Draw and describe a normal ECG cardiograph.

Ans: Refer to Fig. 8.23. The various waves of ECG cardiograph indicate the following actions of the heart: The P wave indicates depolarization (electrical excitation) of the atria. Atrial contraction takes place.

1. The QRS complex indicates depolarization (electrical excitation) of ventricles: Ventricular contraction takes place.
2. The T wave indicates repolarization of the ventricles: No electrical excitement.
3. The short segment between S and T indicates refractory state of the ventricular myocardium: It is unable to pass impulses for that short duration.
4. The segment between P and Q indicates nonconductive phase of AV node: In this phase atrial systole gets completed.

SAQ: What is asystole?

Ans: Asystole is a clinical sign observed when the electrical system of the heart fails completely. The heart stops beating entirely and a flat line is seen in ECG.

Objective: To describe the pumping property of the heart and discuss the related disorders.

Pumping Rate of the Heart

BAQ: Write a note on the pumping rate of the heart.

Ans: In case of a resting person, the heart beats about 70 times a minute and pumps about 70 ml blood each time and the amount of blood pumped each minute is therefore about five liters (70 × 70 ml). The pumping rate of heart varies in health under conditions of living, working, food intake, age and emotions. The pulse rate corresponds with the cardiac cycle. During exercise the heart rate may be 150 per minute and the stroke volume over 150 ml, which makes cardiac output of about 20–25 liters per minute. An exactly equal volume of blood is returned to the heart in the veins each minute.

BAQ: Write a note on blood pressure (BP).

Ans: Blood pressure is the pressure of circulating blood against the walls of blood vessels. BP is defined as the force exerted by the circulating blood per unit area against the inner wall of blood vessels. Normal BP is about 120/80 mm Hg and written as 120/80. 120 is the systolic BP and 80 is the diastolic BP. When BP is expressed, systolic BP is written first, followed by diastolic BP. BP is measured using an equipment known as the sphygmomanometer (refer Chapter 16, page no. 373, Fig. 16.24). BP is higher in systemic arteries than in pulmonary arteries. BP decrease in arterioles and capillaries and it is very low in the veins.

SAQ: What is sinus rhythm? Describe sinus tachycardia and sinus bradycardia.

Ans: Sinus rhythm means setting up of heartbeat by the sinoatrial (SA) node.

Sinus tachycardia takes place in response to stressful conditions. The heart beats more than 100 times per minute, and usually returns to normal after the stressful event gets over. Various events responsible for sinus tachycardia may be, fever, fear, effects of certain drugs, intense exercise, nervousness and dehydration, etc. If these symptoms continue for a longer period, urgent treatment is necessary to treat sinus tachycardia.

The goals of treatment are to control or get rid of fast and irregular heartbeats.

Sinus bradycardia is a heart rhythm when heart beats slower than normal. In sinus bradycardia, the heartbeats are lower than 60 per minute in adults. Sinus bradycardia is common in adults over 65 years of age. The following are the various reasons that may lead to sinus bradycardia: Deficiency of electrolytes, infections, rheumatic fever and rheumatic heart disease, inflammation of heart tissue, etc. The following are the common symptoms of sinus of bradycardia: Heart palpitations, chest pain, shortness of breath, fatigue, etc. Treatment on sinus bradycardia depends on the specific cause that leads to significant decrease in the heart beats.

BAQ: What is baroreceptor reflex system?

Ans: The baroreceptor reflex system consists of baroreceptors in the aortic arch and carotid arteries. The baroreceptors sense changes in arterial blood pressure and send appropriate signals to the brain. As a result, increase or decrease in the heart rate takes place to keep blood pressure in the normal range.

BAQ: What is reflex tachycardia and reflex bradycardia?

Ans: The body has feedback mechanisms to maintain normal blood pressure and adequate blood supply. When blood pressure decreases, the heart beats faster in order to raise it. This is called reflex tachycardia.

When blood pressure increases, by the baroreceptor reflex action, abnormal increase in blood pressure is prevented. This is called reflex bradycardia.

SAQ. Write a note on cardiac (heart) arrhythmia.

Ans: The cardiac arrhythmia means an irregular heartbeat. The pattern of the heartbeat becomes inconsistent. The heart may beat very slow, fast or very fast. The cardiac arrhythmia may feel like a fluttering, pounding or racing heartbeat.

The following are the various types of heart arrhythmia:

1. Tachycardia is a fast heartbeat. The heart rate is greater than 100 beats a minute.
2. Bradycardia is a slow heartbeat. The heart rate is less than 60 beats a minute.

BAQ: Describe the various types of tachycardia.

Ans: The following are the various types of tachycardia:

1. Atrial fibrillation means a rapid, uncoordinated heartbeat. It has been observed following a stroke.
2. Atrial flutter is similar to aerial fibrillation, however, the heartbeats may be more organized. Atrial flutter is observed following a stroke.
3. Supraventricular tachycardia means irregular heartbeats that start above the lower ventricles. Supraventricular tachycardia cause pounding heartbeats that may start and stop suddenly.
4. Ventricular tachycardia means rapid and irregular heartbeats due to defective electrical signals in the ventricles. The ventricles are unable to fill blood properly, due to the rapid heart rate. The heart may not be able to pump sufficient blood to the body. Ventricular tachycardia can be an emergency with persons suffering from heart disease.

BAQ: Describe ventricular fibrillation.

Ans: Ventricular fibrillation (VF) means rapid electrical signals that lead to the contraction of ventricles in a very rapid and uncoordinated manner. Ventricles fail to squeeze in the coordinated way. As a result the heart is unable to pump oxygenated blood to the various parts of the body. Prolonged VF can lead to very low blood pressure, loss of consciousness or death, if not treated urgently.

SAQ: Write a brief note on heart block.

Ans: The heart block refers to any interruption in the electrical system of the heart. These interruptions decrease or completely block the electrical current responsible for the heart beats. The following are the most common causes of heart block: Acute ischemic heart disease, repeated myocardial infarctions, effects of inappropriate use of specific drugs during the treatment of cardiovascular disease.

SAQ: Define arteriosclerosis and related clinical significance.

Ans: Arteriosclerosis means decrease in the elasticity and narrowing of the arteries due to the hardening and increase in the thickness of the walls of the arteries. Increase in the arteriosclerosis leads to decreased rate of blood supply to the various organs. The signs and symptoms of arteriosclerosis are dependent on the affected blood vessel in a specific region of the body. The following are the various risk factors that may increase the rate of arteriosclerosis: High blood pressure, uncontrolled diabetes mellitus, obesity, high lipid diet and prolonged inflammation of unknown reason.

BAQ: Write a note on hypertension.

Ans: Hypertension is persistent elevated systolic BP more than 160 mmHg and diastolic BP more than 95 mmHg. Hypertension can be primary (or essential) or secondary. Identifiable cause may not be observed in the primary hypertension. However, life style changes, atherosclerosis, arteriosclerosis and advancing age may be responsible to develop primary hypertension. Secondary hypertension is due to a underlying disease such as renal disease, adrenal tumors, thyroid disease, hypercalcemia and congenital heart disease. Malignant hypertension is a term used to describe patients with high BP and multiple complications with a poor prognosis.

BAQ: Write a note on hypotension.

Ans: Hypotension means low blood pressure (BP). When systolic BP is less than 90 mmHg and diastolic BP is less than 60 mmHg, hypotension is considered. The following are the symptoms of low BP: Dizziness, lightheaded feeling, blurred vision, confusion, weakness, fainting, low pulse rate, and decreased urine excretion, etc. Low BP may be observed in various clinical conditions related to heart, lungs, central nervous system and in severe autoimmune disorders. Low BP is also observed in dehydration It is necessary to find out the underlying cause of low BP. Low BP is commonly observed in elderly.

BAQ: What is orthostatic hypotension (postural hypotension)?

Ans: Orthostatic hypotension (postural hypotension) is low blood pressure that is observed; when a person tries to suddenly stand after lying down or from a sitting position. The blood supply to the brain suddenly decreases and the patient suffers from dizziness and faints on certain occasions.

Objective: To describe the clinical conditions associated with the heart and the circulatory systems.

SAQ: Define embolism and thrombosis.

Ans: An embolus is formed from tissue debris, micro clots and lipid plaques. It moves with blood flow it may deposit in blood vessels and decrease flow of blood to a specific organ. Deposition of embolus in a blood vessel is called embolism.

Thrombus is a blood clot that may move with the blood flow and block any specific blood vessel. Thrombosis is the formation of a clot in a blood vessel, that may reduce blood flow to any specific tissue or organ.

SAQ: Define infarction and ischemia.

Ans: Infarction means death of a specific part of tissue of an organ due to inadequate blood supply. Ischemia means decreased blood supply to a tissue or an organ..

SAQ: What is myocardial infarction (MI)?

Ans: Myocardial infarction (MI) is the death of specific portion of the heart tissue caused due to decreased or complete cessation of blood flow to a portion of the myocardium. MI is indicated as chest discomfort or pressure that radiate to the neck, jaw, shoulder, and arms of the patient. MI is associated with coronary artery disease and the following are the precipitating factors: High blood pressure, uncontrolled diabetes mellitus, obesity, high lipid diet, smoking, excessive alcohol intake, and lack of exercises.

BAQ: What is heart failure and related clinical conditions and symptoms?

Ans: The blood is pumped through the aorta and an exactly equal volume of blood is returned to the heart in the veins each minute. However, when the venous return is not balanced well and if the ventricles fail to deal with the cardiac output, heart failure occurs. The large veins near the heart becomes distended with blood as the venous pressure rises. Due to the low cardiac output the blood flow to the various organs decreases. The kidneys fail to excrete sodium and water and retention of sodium and water leads to edema, i.e. accumulation of water in the tissue spaces.

Coronary artery disease (CAD) is the most common cause of heart failure. The blockages of the coronary arteries are due to the fatty depositions in the lumen of the blood vessels. This clinical condition is known as atherosclerosis. The atherosclerotic plaques decrease the blood flow due to narrowing of the arteries (Fig. 8.24). Complete blockage of the coronary arteries may lead to heart failure.

The various other factors that may led to heart failure are: Uncontrolled high blood pressure, heart valve disease, inflammation of the heart muscle (myocarditis), and untreated specific congenital heart defects, etc. The common signs of heart attack are, chest pain, fatigue, fainting, irregular heartbeats, and shortness of breath.

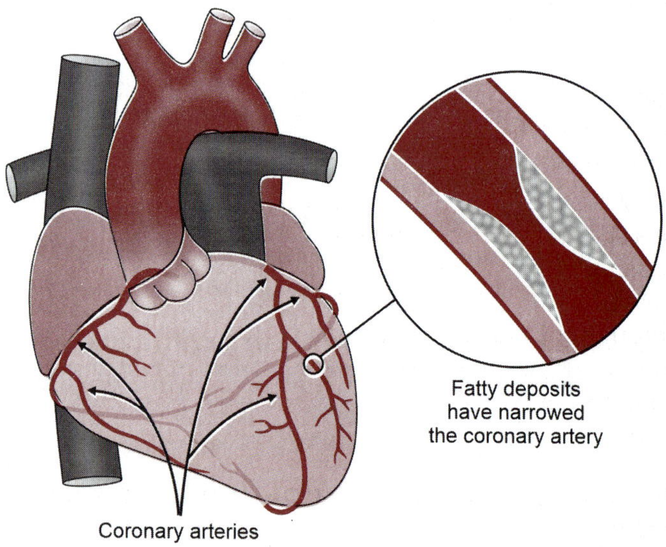

Fig. 8.24: Narrowed coronary artery due to atherosclerosis

BAQ: Write a note on the abnormal ECG changes.

Ans: Abnormal ECG changes (Fig. 8.25) indicate abnormal heart rhythm due to coronary artery disease (CAD), myocardial infarction, heart valve disease, or due to changed size of the heart. The following are the various common types of abnormal ECG changes:

1. Tall T-waves or hyper-acute T waves can be an early sign of ST-elevation in myocardial infarction (Fig. 8.25).

2. An ST-elevation myocardial infarction occurs due to the occlusion of the coronary arteries (Fig. 8.25).
3. Small Q waves indicate a marker of septal ischemia in coronary artery disease (Fig. 8.25). Septal ischemia is observed, when the blood supply to the septum of the heart (the muscular wall that divides the left and right sides of the heart), decreases significantly; mainly due to myocardial infarction.
4. Inverted T waves suggest a severe narrowing of the left anterior descendent coronary artery at a proximal location (Fig. 8.25).

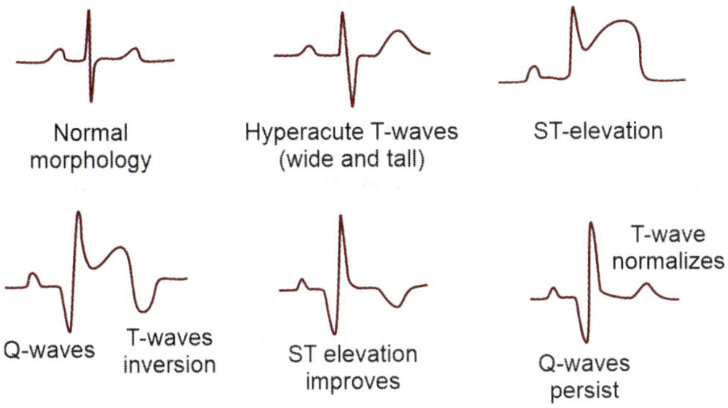

Fig. 8.25: Abnormal ECG changes

BAQ: Write a note on the common heart valve disorders.

Ans: The following are the common heart valve disorders:

1. **Leakage of the valve** may take place, when a specific heart valve does not close completely. This leads to backward flow of blood through the valve, leading to decrease in the forward blood flow. The most common type of heart valve disease is mitral valve regurgitation. The leakage of heart valve can lead to volume overload in the heart.
2. **Narrowing of the valve (stenosis):** When the opening of a specific valve becomes narrow, the flow of blood passing out of the ventricles or atria decreases. The heart has to exert more pressure to pump blood through the narrowed valve.

The most common symptoms of heart valve disease are, fatigue, chest pain, shortness of breath, low of high blood pressure, swelling in the legs, etc.

BAS: Enumerate the common causes of heart valve damages.

Ans: The common causes of heart valve damages are as follows:

1. Changes in the heart valve structure due to aging.
2. Coronary artery disease (CAD).
3. Heart valve infection.
4. Congenital defect related to a specific heart valve.
5. Syphilis (a sexually-transmitted infection), that may cause heart valve damage.

The mitral and aortic valves are most often affected in heart valve disease.

BAQ: What are the various methods used to diagnose a heart valve defect?

Ans: A physician may diagnose the heart valve disease initially using a stethoscope. A characteristic heart murmur could be heard the heart due to disturbed blood flow across the valve. To further find out the type of valve disease and extent of the valve damage, the physician may the following tests: Electrocardiogram (ECG), echocardiogram (echo), transesophageal echocardiogram (TEE), cardiac catheterization, and the magnetic resonance imaging (MRI). Surgery may be needed to repair or replace the defective valve.

SAQ: Briefly describe mitral valve prolapse.

Ans: Mitral valve prolapse is a condition in which the mitral valve between the left atrium and left ventricle does not close properly. Due to mitral valve defect, blood leaks back into the left atrium through the mitral valve.

SAQ: Briefly describe pulmonary stenosis.

Ans: In pulmonary stenosis the blood flowing out of the heart is obstructed at the pulmonary valve. The most common cause of pulmonary stenosis is congenital heart disease. However rheumatic heart disease may also lead to pulmonary stenosis, which can be treated by surgical repair or replacement of the pulmonary valve.

Angina Pectoris

BAQ: What is angina pectoris? Write a note on angina pectoris.

Ans: Angina pectoris is a medical term that describes chest pain or discomfort due to insufficient blood supply to the myocardium during extra physical efforts. The insufficient blood supply to the myocardium may be due to atherosclerotic plaques formed in one or both the coronary arteries.

A narrowed artery may supply sufficient blood to the myocardium to meet its needs during rest but not when increased cardiac output is needed during running or while performing exercises. The increased cardiac output required during the extra physical efforts causes severe ischemic pain in the chest. The pain may radiate to the arms, neck and jaw. The other factors which may precipitate angina include, very cold weather, a heavy meal and strong emotions.

Acute Cardiac Failure

BAQ: Write a note on acute cardiac failure.

Ans: A sudden decrease in the output of blood from both ventricles causes acute reduction in the oxygen supply to all the tissues. The common causes of acute cardiac failure are, ischemia caused by sudden occlusion of one of the larger coronary arteries by atheroma with blood clots, deep vein thrombosis leading to pulmonary embolism (blockage of pulmonary arteries), severe cardiac arrhythmia, severe malignant hypertension, etc. The symptoms of acute cardiac failure are sudden shortness of breath, severe chest pain and dizziness. Death may occur due to anoxia of vital centers in the brain, if acute cardiac failure is not treated urgently.

BAQ: Define shock and enumerate the different types of shock.

Ans: Shock is the response of the body to a sudden drop in blood pressure. Shock may result due to the various clinical conditions such as severe blood loss, septicemia, heat stroke, severe burns, severe allergy, and poisoning, etc.

The following are the main types of shock:

1. Hypovolemic shock, caused due to severe blood loss.
2. Cardiogenic shock, caused due to heart attack.
3. Anaphylactic shock, caused due to severe allergic reactions.
4. Septic shock, caused due to septicemia, i.e. local infection, that spreads all over the body.
5. Neurogenic shock, caused due to damage to the nervous system.

BAQ: Write a note on the hypovolemic shock.

Ans: The hypovolemic shock is caused due to severe blood or body fluid loss. The heart is unable to pump sufficient blood to the body parts leading to failure of various organs. Myocardial infarction, septicemia, severe blood loss during delivery, severe diarrhea, vomiting and severe burns may lead to hypovolemic shock. The hypovolemic shock could be life-threatening. The following are the various symptoms of hypovolemic shock: Shortness of breath, confusion, low blood pressure, low body temperature and pale skin. It is necessary to find out urgently, the etiology of hypovolemic shock to determine blood loss or fluid loss replacement and the related treatment should be carried out as soon as possible to minimize tissue ischemia.

BAQ: Write a note on the cardiogenic shock.

Ans: The cardiogenic shock is most often caused by a severe heart attack. The heart is not able to pump sufficient blood to the various organs of the body. The cardiogenic shock could be life-threatening. The usual immediate measures taken to take care of the patient are, cardiac resuscitation, feeding of isotonic fluids, use of appropriate blood thinning drugs and other drugs to improve blood pumping ability.

BAQ: Write a note on the septic shock.

Ans: The septic shock is caused due to septicemia (or sepsis), means invasion of the bloodstream by pathogenic microorganisms, mainly by bacteria from a localized infection. Sepsis is a life-threatening clinical condition. It may progress to septic shock leading to significant drop in the blood pressure, due to fluid loss through the vessels. Decreased blood pressure may damage various organs such as kidneys, lungs, liver, etc. Sepsis leads to severe immunological reactions against the invading microorganisms. The related symptoms are, confusion, very high temperature, chills, palpitation, rapid heart rate, low blood pressure and decrease in the excretion of urine.

Immediate treatment on septic shock is fluid replacement by intravenous drips, and treatment to decrease high fever and use of appropriate antimicrobial drugs.

BAQ: Write a note on the neurologic shock.

Ans: The neurogenic shock is caused due to the damage to the nervous system after a spinal cord injury, effects of toxins on autonomic nervous system and a specific autoimmune disorder; that attacks the nervous system. When the nerves in the spinal cord are damaged, the nerve impulses are disturbed, which control various functions of the body parts. The specific symptoms of neurological shock are, lack of consciousness, low blood pressure, decreased heart beats, cold skin, etc. Immediate action taken is to keep the patient in a stationary position. Other measures required are, fluid resuscitation, cardiac resuscitation and facilitation of urgent treatment.

BAQ: What is compensated shock?

Ans: The compensated shock means, response of the autonomous nervous system and secretion of specific hormones to maintain homeostasis. The cardiovascular system responds to shock by increasing the heart rate. Increase in myocardial contractility and constriction of peripheral blood vessels are the mechanisms initiated by the direct stimulation through the sympathetic system on the heart and blood vessels by the cardiac and vasomotor centers in the medulla oblongata and lower part of the pons. The cardiac and vasomotor centers modulate heart rate and increase the blood circulation through the sympathetic spinal cord-peripheral nerves. Low blood pressure and increased osmolarity of blood is compensated by increase in ADH secretion, that facilitate increase in water absorption at renal tubular level. Secretion of aldosterone facilitates increase in blood sodium and water and promotes vasoconstriction. The veins also constrict and venous return normalises.

BAQ: What is uncompensated shock?

Ans: In the uncompensated shock, the body mechanisms fail to control the disturbed homeostasis caused by the shock. The patient suffers from severe acidosis, that affect the blood vessels. The fluids from the blood vessels leak in the tissues, leading to further drop in the blood pressure. Various organs including the heart and the brain are deprived of nutrients and oxygen. The common symptoms of the uncompensated shock are low blood pressure, tachycardia, feeble peripheral pulse, increase in the rate of breathing, decrease in urine excretion, etc. Degeneration of cardiovascular system may lead to brain stem damage, followed by death.

Chronic Cardiac Failure

BAQ: Write a note on chronic cardiac failure.

Ans: Chronic cardiac failure condition arises when the capacity of the heart decreases to pump blood normally through the body. It may develop over a long period of time. Symptoms of chronic cardiac failure include chronic fatigue, shortness of breath, swelling on the ancles, feet, and abdomen.

Chronic cardiac failure may develop gradually and the symptoms may not be seen in the early stages. The underlying causes of chronic cardiac failure could be the degenerative changes caused due to old age, chronic hypertension, myocardial fibrosis, heart valve diseases, chronic lung diseases, etc. The supportive treatment is mainly based on appropriate medications, diet and specific exercises.

Pulmonary Hypertension

BAQ: Write a note on pulmonary hypertension.

Ans: Pulmonary hypertension means increase in the blood pressure in pulmonary arteries. Pulmonary blood pressure usually remains low to prevent leakage of capillary fluid into the alveoli. Accumulation of fluid in the alveoli prevents effective exchange of oxygen and carbon dioxide in the lungs. When left ventricle of the heart fails to pump sufficient blood to the lungs, (as seen in the left side heart failure), blood accumulates in the lungs, leading to pulmonary hypertension. In severe lung infections such as COVID-19 also, due to the increase in the permeability of blood capillaries, fluid accumulates in the lungs, leading to pulmonary hypertension. The narrowing of pulmonary arteries due to atherosclerosis and arteriosclerosis also may lead to pulmonary hypertension.

Rheumatic Heart Disease

BAQ: Write a note on rheumatic heart disease.

Ans: Rheumatic heart disease is an autoimmune disease. It occurs following a throat infection caused by *Streptococcus pyogenes* bacteria. The deposition of antigen–antibody complexes may lead to the permanent deterioration of the heart valves. The affected valves are mainly mitral valve and aortic valve. The tricuspid valve also may get damaged. The deteriorated heart valves cause backward flow of blood through the valve, leading to decrease in the forward blood flow. Due to the valve damage, pressure on the heart increases to pump sufficient blood. The most common type of heart valve disease is mitral valve regurgitation.

Infective Endocarditis

BAQ: Write a note on infective endocarditis.

Ans: Infective endocarditis means inflammation of the inner lining of the walls of heart chambers and valves by bacterial or fungal infection. The heart valves may get damaged permanently. The main predisposing factors for infective endocarditis are bacteremia, depressed immune response and congenital heart abnormalities. Infective endocarditis could be treated by appropriate medication and valve surgery.

EFFECTS OF ADVANCING AGE ON CARDIOVASCULAR SYSTEM

LAQ. Write a note on the effects of advancing age on cardiovascular system.

Ans: The following various changes take place in the cardiovascular system due to advancing age:

1. The heart muscle cells degenerate slightly. The thickness of valves inside the heart increases and the valves become stiffer. A heart murmur caused by valve stiffness is common in older people.
2. Some of the pathways of pacemaker system in the heart may develop fibrous tissue and fat deposits. The SA node loses some cells; leading to a slightly slower heart rate.
3. The thickness of heart walls increases; leading to a slight increase in the size of the heart. The capacity of heart chambers to hold blood decreases slightly; in spite of the slight increase in the heart size. The heart may fill blood more slowly.
4. The arterial tree becomes thick and there is a decrease in the flexibility of the arteries leading to increase in systolic blood pressure. Irregular blood pressure (arrhythmias) is more common in older people.
5. The aorta becomes slightly thick, stiff, and decrease its flexibility, due to changes in the connective tissue of the blood vessel walls. This leads to increase in blood pressure and increase the heart work load.
6. The baroreceptors of the arteries; that monitor the blood pressure, become less sensitive. Older persons may develop orthostatic hypotension. In this clinical condition, the blood pressure falls when a person tries to stand from a sleeping position. This may lead to dizziness, since there is less blood flow to the brain.
7. The capillary walls become slightly thick, leading to a slightly slower rate of exchange of nutrients and wastes products.
8. Slight decrease in total body water takes place; leading to slight decrease in blood volume.
9. The regeneration rate of blood cells decreases, leading to a slower response to recovery from the clinical conditions such as anemia and blood loss.
10. Total neutrophils count may decrease, leading to decrease in the immunity.

The common health problems encountered by the elderly are as follows: Shortness of breath, angina, arrhythmias, atherosclerosis, coronary artery disease, anemia, and chronic infections.

Objective: To understand and explain the central theme of competency based medical and paramedical education (CBME): Horizontal and vertical integration of subjects.

BAQ: Explain horizontal integration of the clinical conditions related to the death of part of myocardium (myocardial infarction) with other pre-medical subjects such as physiology, biochemistry and nutrition.

Ans:

Horizontal Integration

Anatomical change: Damage of specific part of the myocardium.

Physiological change: Blood circulation by the heart to the body parts is affected.

Biochemical change: Progressive narrowing of the vessels, due to the deposition of lipids on the arteries, that supply blood to the myocardium.

Nutrition: Suggested nutritional plan: Controlled diet with restricted intake of fats and sugars.

BAQ: Explain horizontal integration of the anatomical changes related to the deep vein thrombosis with other pre-medical subjects such as physiology, biochemistry and nutrition.

Ans:

Horizontal Integration

Anatomical change: Valve damage of the leg veins.

Physiological change: Venous blood circulation to the heart is affected.

Biochemical change: Formation of clots in the veins of the legs.

BIBLIOGRAPHY

1. Medical Biochemistry, 1st Edition (2023). Godkar PB, Godkar DP, CBS Publishers, New Delhi, India.
2. Text book of Medical Laboratory Technology, 4th Edition, (2024). Godkar PB, Godkar DP, Bhalani Publishing House, Mumbai, India.
3. Anatomy of the Human Body. 42nd Edition. Henry Gray, Editor-in-chief: Susan Standring, Elsevier (2020).
4. Ross & Wilson Anatomy and Physiology in Health and Illness, 13th Edition, by Allison Wynn Grant, Anne Waugh, and Kathleen J. W. Wilson (2018).
5. Schaum's outline of theory and problems of Human anatomy and Physiology, 2nd Edition (1997), Tata MaGraw-Hill Publishing Company Limited, New Delhi, India.

MULTIPLE CHOICE QUESTIONS (MCQs)

Select the correct option.

1. During systole:

(A) Atrial relaxation takes place
(B) Atrial filling takes place
(C) Ventricular contraction takes place
(D) Ventricular filling takes place

2. This is not a part of the pulmonary circuit:

(A) Pulmonary semilunar valve
(B) Left atrium
(C) Aortic semilunar valves
(D) Pulmonary veins

3. The prenatal heart begins to function from:

(A) Fourth week
(B) Fifth week
(C) Second week
(D) Eighth week

4. Oxygenated blood of a fetus is carried by:

(A) Umbilical vein
(B) Placental vein
(C) Umbilical artery
(D) Ductus arteriosis

5. The following is the correct sequence of blood that enters through the vena cava and leaves the aorta:

(A) Right atrium, right ventricle, left atrium, right ventricle
(B) Right ventricle, left atrium, right ventricle, right atrium
(C) Left atrium, right ventricle, right atrium, left ventricle
(D) Right ventricle, left atrium, left ventricle, right atrium

6. The following are the major arteries that branch from the aortic arch:

(A) Brachiocephalic artery
(B) Left carotid artery
(C) Left subclavian artery
(D) All of the above

7. The following one is not a superficial vein:

(A) Cephalic vein
(B) Median cubital vein
(C) Common femoral vein
(D) Basilic vein

8. The following one is a superficial vein:

(A) Internal thoracic vein (B) Common femoral
(C) Anterior tibial vein (D) Median cubital vein

9. The action of the heartbeat originates in the following way:

(A) The atrioventricular node (AV node), atrioventricular bundle (bundle of His), and finally to the sinoatrial node (SA node)
(B) Purkinje fibers within the ventricular walls, the sinoatrial node (SA node), and then to the atrioventricular node (AV node) and finally to atrioventricular bundle (bundle of His)
(C) The sinoatrial node (SA node), and then to the atrioventricular node (AV node), atrioventricular bundle (bundle of His), and finally to Purkinje fibers within the ventricular walls

(D) The sinoatrial node (SA node), and then to the atrioventricular node (AV node), to Purkinje fibers within the ventricular walls and finally to the atrioventricular bundle (bundle of His)

10. All these descriptions about the normal direction of the flow of blood are correct, *except*:

(A) Right ventricle to tricuspid valve
(B) Aorta to aortic semilunar valve
(C) Vena cava to right atrium
(D) Lungs to pulmonary artery

11. This is called the pacemaker of the heart:

(A) Atrioventricular node
(B) Sinoatrial node
(C) Diastolic node
(D) Semilunar node

12. This statement is true about the human circulatory system?

(A) Blood flow is slow in capillaries to facilitate the diffusion of nutrients and waste
(B) The right ventricle of the heart does not contain any valve
(C) Veins have thick walls compared to arteries
(D) The arteries contain valves.

13. The ventricular muscles accept impulses directly from:

(A) Purkinje cell system
(B) AV node
(C) Bundle of His
(D) Right and left bundle branches

14. Increase in the carotid sinus pressure leads to:

(A) Reflex hypercapnia (B) Reflex hyperpnea
(C) Reflex tachycardia (D) Reflex bradycardia

15. The location of the neurological activity of the heart is in:

(A) Medulla Oblongata (B) Midbrain
(C) Pons (D) Cerebrum

16. The hormonal regulation of cardiac output is:

(A) Mediated by the adrenal cortex
(B) Mediated by the adrenal medulla
(C) Mediated by thyroid
(D) Mediated by pineal

17. The tricuspid valve is present between:

(A) Ventricle and pulmonary artery
(B) Right auricle and right ventricle
(C) Ventricle and aorta
(D) Left auricle and left ventricle

18. Bundle of His is a network of:

(A) Muscle fibres present only in the ventricle wall
(B) Nerve fibres distributed in right auricle
(C) Muscle fibres distributed in left auricle
(D) Both (B) and (C)

19. At this point, the right ventricle contracts and blood is pumped out:

(A) Pulmonary aorta (B) Superior vena cava
(C) Dorsal aorta (D) Pulmonary veins

20. The middle layer of the heart is:

(A) Pericardium (B) Epicardium
(C) Myocardium (D) Endocardium

21. The outermost layer of the heart is:

(A) Pericardium (B) Epicardium
(C) Myocardium (D) Endocardium

22. The sinoatrial node is placed in this wall:

(A) Left ventricle
(B) Right atrium
(C) Left atrium
(D) Right ventricle

23. The following is not a common causes of heart valve damages:

(A) Changes in the heart valve structure due to aging
(B) Heart valve infection
(C) Birth defect related to a specific heart valve
(D) Persistent low blood pressure

24. The hepatic portal vein drains blood from:

(A) The heart
(B) The intestine
(C) The stomach
(D) The kidneys

25. During this stage, the blood pressure is maximum in the human aorta:

(A) Systole of the left atrium
(B) Diastole of the right atrium
(C) Diastole of the right ventricle
(D) Systole of the left ventricle

26. Systemic circulation in the cardiac system means:

(A) That carries blood from the left ventricle to tissues and organs of the body.
(B) That carries blood to the left side of the heart
(C) That carries oxygenated blood from the lungs to the heart
(D) Both (A) and (B)

27. Oxygenated blood in the cardiac system:

(A) Leaves from the left side of the heart
(B) Leaves from the right side of the heart
(C) Enters lungs from the pulmonary vein
(D) Enters from the hepatic artery

28. Pulmonary circulation means:

(A) That carries blood from the left ventricle to tissues and organs of the body.
(B) That carries deoxygenated blood from the heart to the lungs
(C) Carry oxygenated blood from the lungs to the heart
(D) Both (A) and (B)

ANSWERS

1. C	2. C	3. A	4. A	5. A	6. D	7. C
8. D	9. C	10. D	11. B	12. A	13. A	14. D
15. A	16. B	17. B	18. A	19. A	20. C	21. B
22. B	23. D	24. B	25. D	26. A	27. A	28. B

MATCH THE COLUMNS

I	II
1. Tall T wave of ECG	A. Atrial depolarization
2. Thrombus	B. Tunica externa
3. Normal T wave of ECG	C. Myocardial infarction
4. Normal P wave of ECG	D. Diaphragm
5. Endothelium	E. Rib case muscle
6. Outer layer of blood vessel	F. Formation of clot
7. Superior phrenic artery	G. Between left atrium and left ventricle
8. Intercostal artery	H. Ventricular repolarization
9. QRS complex of ECG	I. Ventricular depolarization
10. Mitral valve	J. Tunica interna

ANSWERS

1. C	2. F	3. H	4. A	5. J	6. B	7. D
8. E	9. I	10. G				

CHAPTER 9

Blood

SAQ: Short answer question: Marks: 2
BAQ: Brief answer question: Marks: 4 or 5
LAQ: Long answer question: Marks: 9 or 10
MCQs: Multiple choice questions: Marks: 0.5 each
Match the columns: Marks: 0.5 each
Draw a labelled diagram: Marks: 5

Objective: To describe the nature and functions of blood as a part of the circulatory system.

INTRODUCTION

Blood may be described as a specialized connective tissue that circulates in a closed system of blood vessels. The circulating blood consists of a suspension of formed elements such as erythrocytes, leukocytes, and platelets in a pale yellow-coloured fluid called plasma. In adults, the total volume of blood comprises about 8% of the body weight or about 5,600 ml in a 70 kg man. The formed elements account for about 46% of total blood volume.

Objective: To describe the composition of blood.

BAQ: Write a brief note on blood.

Ans: Refer to Chapter 2, page no. 40.

BAQ: Enumerate functions of blood.

Ans: The functions of blood are as follows:

1. **Respiration:** Transport of oxygen from the lungs to the tissues and transport of carbon dioxide from tissues to the lungs.
2. **Excretion:** Transport of metabolic wastes to the lungs, kidneys, skin, and intestines for removal from the body.
3. Maintenance of normal acid–base balance.
4. **Nutrition:** Transport of absorbed fatty acids, monosaccharides, and amino acids.
5. Regulation of water balance.
6. Regulation of body temperature.
7. Transport of hormones, vitamins, and salts that contain cations such as sodium, potassium, calcium, etc., and anions such as chlorides, phosphates, sulfates, and carbonates.
8. Transport of various compounds formed during metabolic reactions.
9. Defense against infection by the white cells and the antibodies.
10. **Coagulation of blood:** To stop bleeding by the mechanism of clotting.

Objective: To define and describe the hematopoietic system of the body.

BAQ: Define and describe hematopoiesis?

Ans: Hematopoiesis is production, development, and maturation of cellular elements of blood (Fig. 9.1). It consists of the production of (1) erythrocytes (erythropoiesis), (2) leukocytes (leukopoiesis), and (3) thrombocytes (thrombopoiesis).The development of blood cells takes place through the following three stages: (1) Multiplication of precursor cells, (2) structural and functional maturation, and (3) release into the peripheral circulation. Under normal conditions, the production of blood cells is carried out by the bone marrow (medullary hematopoiesis), while in the fetus, until the bone marrow is matured, the hematopoiesis takes place in the liver and spleen (extramedullary hematopoiesis) takes place.

A totipotent stem cell is a common precursor for all series of cells, i.e. erythrocytes, megakaryocytes, lymphocytes, and granulocytes. The blast cells, through several stages of division and differentiation, develop into mature cells of each series. Vitamin B_{12} and folic acid are necessary for DNA synthesis and hence for the cell division. The deficiency of these two nutrients results in a decrease in the number of mature cells in circulation.

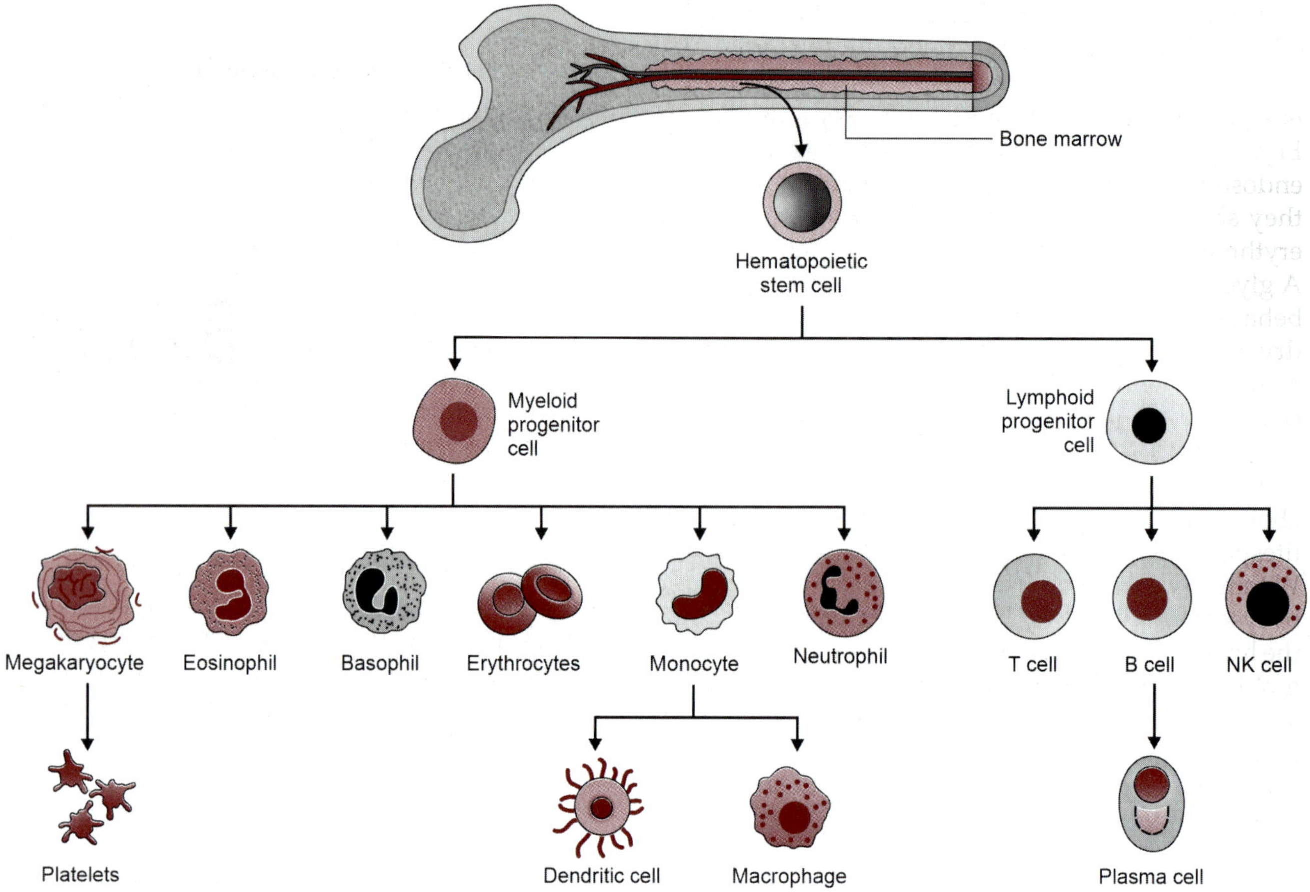

Fig. 9.1: Hematopoiesis

> **Objectives:** To describe the process of erythropoiesis, leukopoiesis and thrombopoiesis. To identify and describe the functions of the various types of red blood cells. To identify and describe the functions of the various types of white blood cells. To identify and describe the functions of the various types of platelets.

ERYTHROPOIESIS

SAQ: What is erythropoiesis?

Ans: The term erythropoiesis means the production of erythrocytes (Fig. 9.1).

BAQ: Write a note on erythropoiesis in fetus.

Ans: The term erythropoiesis means the generation of erythrocytes. Up to the 3rd month of the intrauterine life, erythropoiesis occurs in the mesoderm of the yolk sac. Between the 3rd month and the 5th month of intrauterine life, erythropoiesis occurs in the liver and spleen. This stage is called the 'hepatic stage' of erythropoiesis. From the 5th month, red bone marrow begins to produce erythrocytes. This phase is called 'the 'myeloid phase'.

BAQ: Write a note on erythropoiesis in children and adults.

Ans: The development of a mature erythrocyte takes place through several stages of division and differentiation. A pluripotent stem cell is the most primitive cell, which gives rise to myeloid as well as lymphocytic series cells. The pluripotent stem cell then gives rise to committed stem cells. One type of committed stem cell produces, neutrophils, eosinophils, monocytes, and platelets (cells of the myeloid series) (Fig. 9.1).

ERYTHROCYTES (Fig. 9.2)

LAQ: Write a note on erythrocytes.

Ans: Erythrocytes are red blood cells (RBCs). Normal range of RBCs in male is 4.5–5.5 × 10^6 per microliter of blood and in female it is 4.0–5.0 × 10^6 per microliter of blood.

The erythrocyte is a circular, biconcave cells without a nucleus. It has a diameter of about 7.5 μm and a thickness of 2 μm. It contains hemoglobin and is the heaviest of all the formed elements of blood. Because of the biconcavity, the red blood cell gets a bigger surface area for the diffusion of oxygen. The erythrocyte can also squeeze itself through a capillary more easily. The erythrocyte is devoid of the nucleus and such structures as ribosomes, endoplasmic reticulum, centriole, and mitochondria. It does not have the ability to synthesize protein. In the absence of mitochondria, there is little ability to metabolize fatty acids and amino acids. Energy is generated almost exclusively through the breakdown of glucose. The Embden-Meyerhof pathway is responsible for about 90% of the cell's glucose use. The other pathway is the hexose mono-phosphate shunt.

The internal fluid concentration of the erythrocytes is equivalent to about 0.85% (w/v) sodium chloride. Erythrocytes swell and then rupture in water due to endosmosis, and in concentrated sodium chloride (2%), they shrink due to exosmosis. The cell membrane of erythrocytes is composed of lipid and protein molecules. A glycoprotein present on the outer surface of the cell behaves as a blood group antigen. About 95% of the dry weight of a red blood cell is due to the hemoglobin content. Practically all the functions of the red blood cells are due to hemoglobin, which picks up, carries, and disgorges oxygen as well as carbon dioxide.

The normal red cell (RBC) has a finite lifespan of about 120 + 20 days. The erythrocytes at the end of their lifespan are destroyed in the reticuloendothelial cells. Within the reticuloendothelial cell, the red cell is attacked by lysosomal enzymes. The membrane is disrupted, and the hemoglobin molecule is broken down into heme and globin by the action of the enzyme heme oxygenase. The freed iron is used in the resynthesis of hemoglobin, returned to plasma transferrin, or stored within the reticuloendothelial cell as ferritin and hemosiderin. The protoporphyrin ring is later on converted into bilirubin.

Red cell membrane contains blood group antigens, which are responsible for the human blood group systems.

SAQ: What are the functions of red blood cells?

Ans: Red blood cells contain a specific protein called hemoglobin. It has ability to bind oxygen and carbon dioxide. When blood is circulated to lungs, and air is inspired, hemoglobin in blood captures oxygen.

When blood circulates to the various cells of the body, oxygen is delivered for the cellular oxidation processes, to generate ATP molecules required for cellular activities.

Carbon dioxide produced as an excretory product of cellular activities, is expelled out in expired air, when deoxygenated blood is circulated in the lungs.

Red blood cell membrane contain specific antigens, which determine specific blood groups.

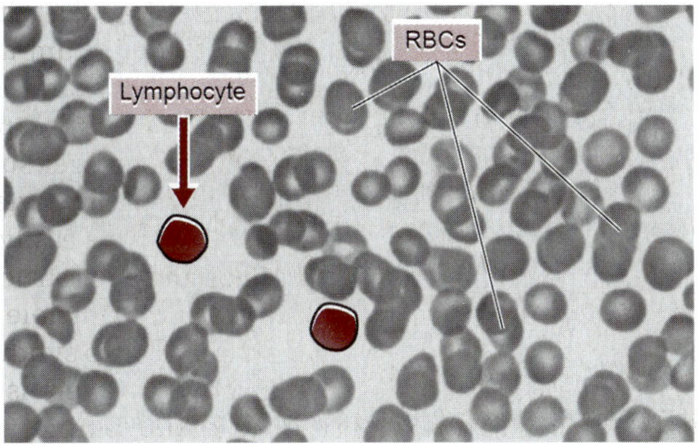

Fig. 9.2: Erythrocytes (as seen under microscope, using a stained blood smear

LEUKOPOIESIS

BAQ: Write a note on leukopoiesis.

Ans: Leukopoiesis is the production of white blood cells. It has three independent series which lead to the formation of (a) granulocytes (b) lymphocytes, and (c) monocytes. The granulocytes are neutrophils, eosinophils and basophils. These are formed in the bone marrow, and the process of maturation is divided into six stages. In this series, the cytoplasm develops specific granules as the cell matures, and the progressive maturation of the nucleus is indicated by segmentation. The stem cell (reticuloendothelial cell) also gives rise to lymphocytes and monocytes, which do not contain granules.

Leukocytes

BAQ: Write a note on the leukocytes (white blood cells).

Ans: The leukocytes or white blood cells (WBc) are nucleated corpuscles. In healthy adults, the number of leukocytes is 5000–10,000 per microliter of blood. The various types of white blood cells found in circulating blood are neutrophils, lymphocytes, eosinophils, monocytes and basophils.

After birth, granulocytes are formed in the bone marrow. Monocytes are produced predominantly in the bone marrow. Monocytes, related to tissue histocytes or macrophages, are present particularly in the spleen, bone marrow, lungs, and liver. Lymphocytes are also produced in the bone marrow. Some lymphocytes undergo subsequent modification in other organs, such as the thymus (T-cells). The majority of lymphocytes are formed outside the bone marrow in lymph nodes, the spleen, and lymphoid collections lining the gastrointestinal tract.

SAQ: How blood hemoglobin concentration and red blood cells of a patient are counted in a clinical laboratory?

Ans: In a practicing clinical laboratory hematology autoanalysers are used for hemoglobin determination, blood cell counting and differentiation of various cells. Blood cells also can be counted using specific glass blood counting plates (Neubauer chamber) (Fig. 16.12A) and autoanalyzers (Fig. 16.17).

SAQ: What is the normal range of red blood cells in blood?

Ans: Normal range of red blood cells is as follows:
Male: 4.5–6.0 × 10^6 per microliter of blood.
Female: 4.0–4.5 × 10^6 per microliter of blood.

BAQ: Draw neat and labelled figures of various white blood cell as seen under high power of a microscope.

Ans: Refer to Fig. 9.3B.

BAQ: Describe the various types of white blood cells.

Ans: Description of various types of white blood cells is as follow:

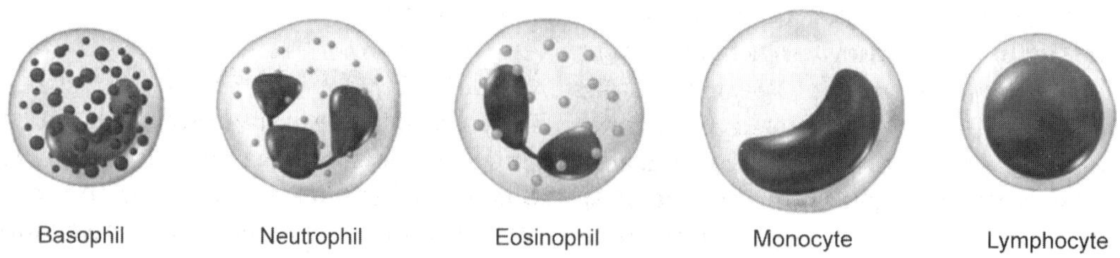

Fig. 9.3A: Various types of white blood cells

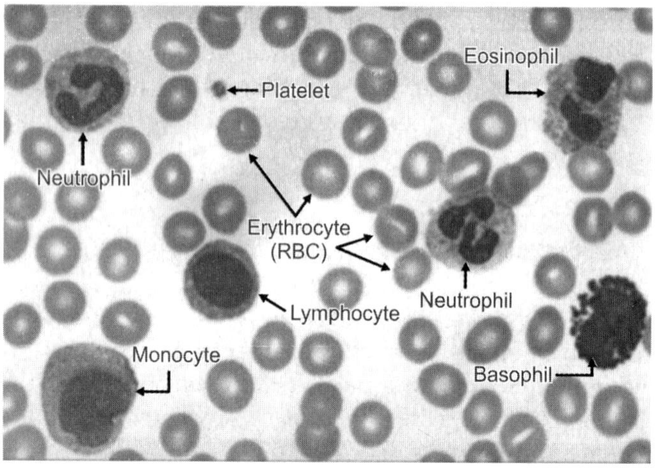

Fig. 9.3B: Various types of white blood cells, RBCs and platelets (as seen under microscope, using a stained blood smear)

1. **Neutrophils:** The diameter of neutrophil ranges between 10 and 14 μm. The nucleus of a neutrophil contains several lobes. The number of lobes increases as the cell grows older. The maximum number of lobes in a neutrophil can be about seven. Neutrophils contain fine cytoplasmic granules (Fig. 9.3A).
2. **Eosinophils:** The diameter of eosipnophils ranges between 10 and 14 μm. The eosinophil nucleus is usually bilobed. It contains very coarse cytoplasmic granules (Fig. 9.3A).
3. **Basophils:** The diameter of basophil ranges between 10 and 14 μm. The basophil nucleus is often 'S' shaped. Basophil also contains very coarse cytoplasmic granules (Fig. 9.3A).
4. **Lymphocytes:** The diameter of lymphocyte ranges between 7–10 μm. A small lymphocyte cell contains a nucleus that almost wholly fills up the cell. The nucleus is not lobed. In large lymphocytes, the amount of cytoplasm is comparatively larger (Fig. 9.3A).
5. **Monocytes:** The diameter of monocyte ranges between 12–20 μm. The monocytes are the biggest of the leukocytes. It contains kidney-shaped nucleus with presence of indentation (Fig. 9.3A).

SAQ: What is the percentage of various white blood cells in the blood and how these are counted?

Ans: The percentage of various white blood cells in the blood is as follows:

Percentage

Neutrophils: 40–75%
Lymphocytes: 20–455
Eosinophils: 1–4%
Monocytes: 2–8%
Basophils: 0–1%

These are counted by using a stained blood smear, using high power and oil immersion lenses of a microscope. In a practicing clinical laboratory hematology autoanalysers are used for hemoglobin determination, blood cell counting and differentiation.

Functions and Properties of Leukocytes

BAQ: Describe the functions of leukocytes.

Ans: Leukocytes are needed by the body for its defense against invading organisms like bacteria, viruses, parasites, and cancer cells. It is mainly the neutrophils and the monocytes that attack and destroy viruses and bacteria in the circulating blood. Although blood monocytes have ability to fight infectious agents, once they enter the tissue, they begin to swell and develop large numbers of lysosomes in the cytoplasm. These cells are called macrophages, which are capable of fighting disease organisms. Plasma cells which are derived from lymphocytes produce immunoglobulins which neutralize the toxins produced by invading organisms.

Functions of Neutrophils

BAQ: Describe he functions of neutrophils.

Ans: When there is an acute infection, the circulating neutrophils adhere to the margins of the blood vessels and come out to protective act by throwing their pseudopodia into the pores in between the endothelial cells of the lining wall of the capillaries. The neutrophils act in the following manner:

1. The neutrophils promptly come to the spot, where invading microorganisms are present.
2. The neutrophils cordon the area, phagocytize the organism and digest them. The lysosomes present in neutrophils carry a large number of proteolytic, amylolytic, lipolytic enzymes and also other enzymes such as nucleotidases and catalases. These enzymes act upon the phagocytized bacteria and hydrolyze the molecules present in the invading organisms.

Functions of Monocytes

BAQ: Describe the functions of monocytes.

Ans: The circulating monocytes leave the intravascular compartment and form tissue macrophages. These macrophages ingest mainly those bacteria which commonly produce chronic infections (e.g. *Mycobacterium tuberculosis* and *Salmonella typhi*). They phagocytize bacteria in acute infections. They also phagocytize tissue debris, organic and inorganic chemicals, and even cancer cells. Giant cells are formed when several macrophages coalesce together.

Functions of Lymphocytes

BAQ: Describe the functions of lymphocytes.

Ans: The lymphocytes are responsible for the normal immunity status of the body. Two types of lymphocytes are present in the blood circulation. T-lymphocytes and B-lymphocytes.

Cellular immunity is produced by T-lymphocytes. These cells combine directly with the bacteria, viruses, and cancer cells and destroy them.

B-lymphocytes are ultimately converted into plasma cells which produce immunoglobulins. These are present in the gamma-globulin fraction of plasma proteins. The immunoglobulins combine with and neutralize bacteria and various toxic materials produced by invading organisms.

Functions of Eosinophils

BAQ: Describe the functions of eosinophils.

Ans: Eosinophils increase in number in allergic disorders and also in parasitic infections. The eosinophils can ingest antigen–antibody complexes, neutralize histamine and dissolve clots. A protein called 'major basic protein' present in the eosinophils destroys the larval parasites.

Functions of Basophils

BAQ: Describe the functions of basophils.

Ans: The basophils of blood contain histamine, serotonin, and heparin. In the tissues, identical mast cells are present. During inflammation, histamine, serotonin, and bradykinin are liberated by the damaged basophils as well as by the mast cells. Histamine and serotonin are powerful vasodilators. By this action, due to increase in the size of the blood vessels at the infection site, blood flow increases and T- and B-lymphocytes, neutrophils and monocytes are able to reach there easily to fight the invading microorganisms.

Life Span of Leukocytes

BAQ: Write a note on the life span of leukocytes.

Ans: Only a fraction of neutrophils, eosinophils, and basophils are present in the general blood circulation. Most of them reside in the bone marrow or in the marginal pool. These cells remain in blood circulation for a couple of hours and then enter the extravascular tissues, where they are destroyed after two days. A large number of neutrophils, after leaving the blood, enter the gastrointestinal tract from where they are lost daily.

Monocytes, after leaving the bone marrow, enter the general blood circulation, and after staying there for about a day, they enter the tissue. In the tissue, they are known as macrophages and constitute the reticuloendothelial system. As a macrophage, the cell has a variable life span.

Lymphocytes circulate through the blood and lymph nodes repeatedly. Each time they spend only a few hours in the blood. By this way, they survey the body for a possible invasion by antigen and maintain their vigil against the antigens. Their life span is variable; some live for two to three days, some others for several months, and yet others may live for many years.

BAQ: What is leukocytosis?

Ans: If the WBC count increases more than 10,000 per microliter of blood, the condition is called leukocytosis. Acute bacterial invasion usually produces leukocytosis with a rise in neutrophils. Parasitic infections also may produce moderate leukocytosis with a sharp rise in the percentage of eosinophils. In some chronic infections, e.g. tuberculosis, the total count of WBC may remain within normal limits, but the differential count of lymphocytes may increase.

BAQ: What is leukopenia?

Ans: Leukopenia is a condition in which a decrease in the total count of WBC (below 5000 per one microliter of blood) is observed. Bone marrow depression leads to leukopenia. Various factors the cause leukopenia are, repeated X-ray exposure, antifolic acid drugs (used against cancer), certain types of leukemia, or idiopathic conditions, produce bone marrow depression.

THROMBOPOIESIS

SAQ: What is thrombopoiesis?

Ans: Thrombopoiesis means the production of platelets.

BAQ: Write a note on thrombopoiesis.

Ans: Thrombopoiesis means the production of platelets. The platelets are produced in the red bone marrow, and the pluripotent stem cell is the most primitive cell responsible for platelet production. The platelets are developed from giant cells called 'megakaryocytes' in the bone marrow (Fig. 9.1). A single megakaryocyte can give rise to about 1000 platelets. Thrombopoietin (TPO) is a polypeptide responsible for the primary regulation of platelet production. It is produced by the liver, kidney, marrow stroma, and other tissues. The thrombopoietin stimulates the production and differentiation of megakaryotic precursor cells.

PLATELETS (Fig. 9.3)

BAQ: Write a note on platelets.

Ans: The platelets are very small non-nucleated bodies. The diameter of platelets is about 3 μm. Platelets contain cytoplasm enclosed within a cell membrane. Golgi apparatus and a scanty amount of mitochondria are found in the cell. Platelets also contain very fine alpha granules, which contain serotonin. Platelets also contain ADP, various clotting factors, and microtubules made up of thrombosthenin, which help the platelets to retract.

The number of circulating platelets (platelet count) is between 100,000 and 450,000 per one microliter of blood. When the platelet count goes below the 'critical count' (<40,000 per one microliter of blood, the patient develops hemorrhagic disorders.

The normal life span of platelets is between 7 and 14 days. About 10% of the circulating platelets are utilized daily for the arrest of minor hemorrhages. Rest of the platelets are destroyed by the macrophages in the spleen.

Functions of Platelets

BAQ: Describe the functions of platelets.

Ans: The main function of platelets or thrombocytes is to assist in hemostasis means prevention of blood loss through various processes as follows:

1. Platelets aggregate and stick to the exposed collagen of a damaged blood vessel. This way, the vent in the blood vessel seals off.
2. The aggregated platelets release vasoactive substances which assist in vasospasm, which lasts for about 30 minutes and helps in the initial process in the arrest of hemorrhage. The platelets also release factor 3 and help in blood coagulation.
3. The platelets can retract and cause clot retraction due to their thrombosthenin content, which is necessary for forming a firm clot.
4. Platelets help in the coagulation of exudate which follows bacterial infection. This coagulation helps to cordon off the bacteria and thus localize the bacterial infection.

SAQ: What is thrombocytopenia?

Ans: Thrombocytopenia is a condition in which the platelet count is very low (less than 40,000 platelets per one microliter of blood. Thrombocytopenia may be observed in bone marrow depression, severe liver disease, severe systemic infections, leukaemia, etc. Thrombocytopenia leads spontaneous bleeding disorders.

SAQ: What is thrombocytosis?

Ans: Thrombocytosis is a condition in which the platelet count is very high (more than 450,000 platelets per one microliter of blood). It is observed in polycythemia vera, chronic myelogenous leukemia and following splenectomy.

Objective: To describe the composition and properties of normal hemoglobin and other various types of hemoglobins.

BAQ: Write a note on hemoglobin.

Ans: Hemoglobin is the major component of red blood cells. It is an iron-containing metalloprotein present in the red blood cells (Fig. 9.4A). It gives red colour to blood. Hemoglobin in the blood carries oxygen from the lungs to the rest of the body tissues, where it releases the oxygen to burn nutrients to provide energy to power the functions of the cells and collects the resultant carbon dioxide to bring it back to the respiratory organs to be expired from the lungs. When fully saturated each gram of hemoglobin holds approximately 1.34 ml of oxygen. It increases the total blood oxygen capacity 70-fold compared to dissolved oxygen in blood. The hemoglobin molecule can bind up to four oxygen molecules. Hemoglobin is involved in the transport of other gases also.

Hemoglobin has a quaternary structure like globular proteins (Fig. 9.4B). A heme group consists of an iron (Fe) ion (charged atom) held in a heterocyclic ring, known as a porphyrin (Fig. 9.4C). This porphyrin ring consists of four pyrrole molecules cyclically linked together (by methene bridges), with the iron ion bound in the center.

SAQ: What are the major types of normal hemoglobin?

Ans: The normally occurring hemoglobins are (1) A (about 96%), (2) A2—a minor component of A (about

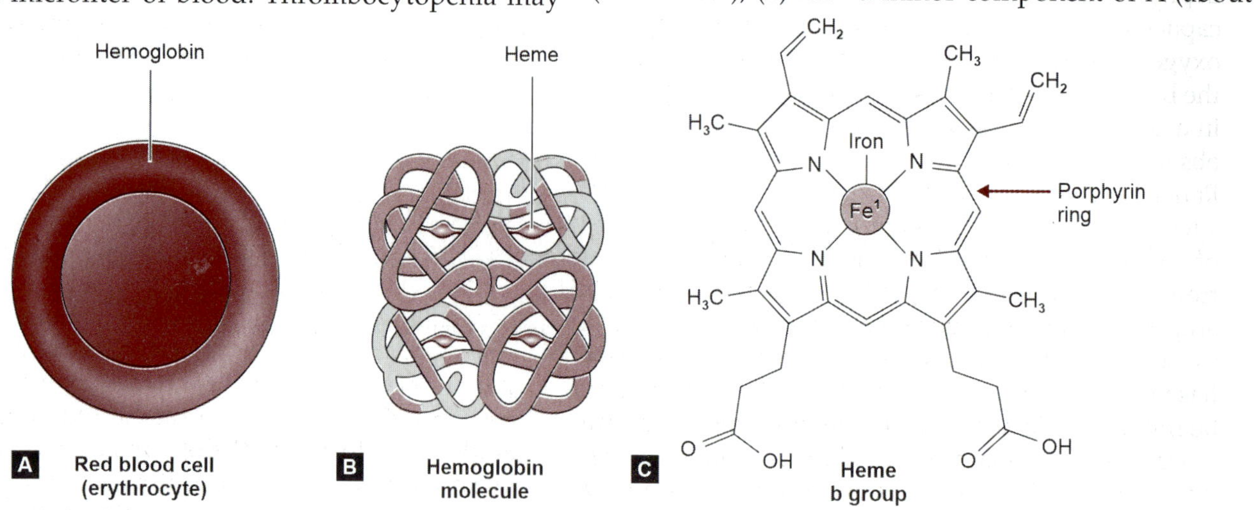

Fig. 9.4: Hemoglobin molecule and porphyrin ring

3%), and (3) fetal hemoglobin (F) (up to 1%). Each molecule of hemoglobin has one globin unit with four heme units.

SAQ: Write four names of hemoglobin derivatives.

Ans: Methemoglobin, sulfemoglobin, oxyhemoglobin and carboxyhemoglobin.

BAQ: What are porphyrins?

Ans: When the iron is removed, porphyrins are obtained with the intact ring of four pyrrole groups (Fig. 9.4). Porphyrins are biologically important heterocyclic compounds of a characteristic chemical structure that includes four pyrrole groups (five-membered organic rings, each containing a nitrogen atom) linked by additional carbon atoms to form a large flat ring. As biological pigments, they are responsible for many of the colours in living organisms. They often occur combined with metal ions and various substituents as coordination complexes. Various examples of porphyrins are uroporphyrin, coproporphyrin and protoporphyrin.

BAQ: Describe porphyrias.

Ans: Porphyrias are mainly a group of inborn errors of metabolism associated with the biosynthesis of heme, leading to the accumulation of porphyrins in blood. The porphyrias are characterized by increased production and excretion of porphyrins and (or) their precursors. The accumulation of porphyrins is toxic to tissues in high concentrations.

Objective: To define and describe "anemia".

ANEMIA

BAQ: Write a note on anemia.

Ans: The term 'anemia' refers to a reduction below normal in the concentration of hemoglobin or red blood cells in blood. In male hemoglobin less than 13 gram% and in female hemoglobin less than 12 gram% is considered a sign of anemia. Anemia may be regarded in physiological term as reduction in oxygen transporting capacity of blood. There is a decrease in the amount of oxygen reaching the tissues and the different organs of the body. This is responsible for many of the symptoms in a person suffering from anemia. Various symptoms observed in anemia are, pallor, dyspnea, palpitation, etc. Patient with severe anemia may experience CNS signs such as headache, vertigo, muscle weakness and lack of concentration. In severe anemia, patient may suffer from glossitis, atrophy of the tongue papillae, stomatitis and fissures at the angles of mouth. Mild fever may be present in many cases of severe anemia. Since anemia has many different causes, before effective treatment can be initiated, it is necessary to diagnose the exact cause. Anemia may be classified in different ways (1) based upon the morphology of the red cell or (2) based upon the etiology (the cause of anemia).

Objective: To identify and describe various blood group systems.

HUMAN BLOOD GROUP SYSTEMS

BAQ: Write a note on human blood groups.

Ans: The ABO and Rh are the major, clinically significant, and most important of all the blood group systems. These are dependent on the presence of A, or B, or O antigens on red blood cells and also on the presence or absence of D antigen on red blood cells.

A person's serum contains naturally occurring ABO group antibodies. The serum contains antibodies for that antigen (or antigens) not represented on his own red cells. Anti-A serum is present in B group people, while Anti-B serum is present in A group people. Anti-A and Anti-B serum is present in O group blood, and persons having AB group, does not contain either Anti-A or Anti-B antibodies in their sera.

All people (with few exceptions) in the ABO system can be divided into 4 major groups in this system, and they are A group, B group, AB group, and O group. This depends on the reactions obtained by mixing their red blood cells with two different reagents, known as anti-A and anti-B. For example, in cell grouping or forward grouping, by using known anti-A and anti-B, the results obtained are as follows (Table 9.1):

Table 9.1: Blood group determination

	Red cell sample	*Reaction*		*Cell group*
1.	Red blood cells +	Anti-A =	Agglutination	A group
	Red blood cells +	Anti-B =	No agglutination	
2.	Red blood cells +	Anti-A =	No agglutination	B group
	Red blood cells +	Anti-B =	Agglutination	
3.	Red blood cells +	Anti-A =	Agglutination	AB group
	Red blood cells +	Anti-B =	Agglutination	
4.	Red blood cells +	Anti-A =	No agglutination	O group
	Red blood cells +	Anti-B =	No agglutination	

Blood from one category person should not be transfused into another category person. Mismatching of blood groups may result in the recipient's death.

RHESUS BLOOD GROUP SYSTEM

Persons whose red cells possess "D" (or Rho) antigen are designated as Rh-positive and persons whose red cells lack "D" (or Rho) are designated as Rh-negative.

The rhesus (Rh) group system is clinically the second most important blood group system in humans, after the ABO system. Rh-positive blood cells are antigenic for Rh-negative individuals, even though their type with respect to the A and B systems of blood groups may be identical. Introduction of such antigenic cells into an Rh-negative person will stimulate the production of antibodies which will agglutinate and hemolyze

Rh-positive cells. Therefore, Rh-negative individuals must be transfused with only Rh-negative cells of the correct blood type.

Example of reporting blood group: A person having A group and Rh positive is reported as follows: Mr. Sanjay Mehta: Blood group A Rho (D): Positive.

Objective: To define and describe the process, hemostasis.

HEMOSTASIS

LAQ: Write a note on hemostasis and thrombosis.

Ans: Hemostasis is a complex process that causes the bleeding process to stop. It refers to the process of keeping blood within a damaged blood vessel. The endothelial cells of intact blood vessels prevent blood coagulation by the secretion of substances like heparin and thrombomodulin and prevent platelet aggregation by the secretion of nitric oxide and prostacyclin. When an endothelial injury occurs, the endothelial cells cease secretion of coagulation and aggregation inhibitors and instead secrete a glycoprotein called von Willebrand factor and tissue thromboplastin, which initiate the maintenance of hemostasis after injury. Thrombosis means clotting of blood.

The hemostasis has three major steps: 1) Vasoconstriction, 2) Temporary blockage of a break by a platelet plug, and 3) Blood coagulation or formation of a clot that seals the hole until tissues are repaired.

Normal hemostasis and thrombosis involve three protein systems and a number of factors, such as platelets, monocytes, and granulocytes. The protein systems are the coagulation protein system, fibrinolytic protein system, and anticoagulant protein system. Each of the three protein systems balances the activities of other protein systems. Blood vessel wall endothelium also plays an important role in the normal hemostasis mechanism.

BAQ: Write a note on zymogens (proenzymes) of the coagulation system.

Ans: Zymogen means inactive form of an enzyme, which becomes active, when it is required for a specific purpose (Table 9.2). The zymogens (proenzymes or inactive enzyme precursors) and various cofactors comprise the proteins of the coagulation system. Zymogens are of the following two types: Phospholipid-bound proenzymes and surface-dependent proenzymes.

The phospholipid-bound proenzymes are physiologically important components of the hemostatic system, which require vitamin K.

The surface-bound proenzymes include coagulation factor XII (Hageman factor); and a protein, called prekallikrein (Fletcher factor and factor XI. These zymogens are known as 'contact systems' since factor XII autoactivates when it gets associated with a negatively charged surface (Table 9.1).

BAQ: What are the main phases of hemostasis and thrombosis?

Ans: The following are the four main phases of hemostasis and thrombosis:

1. Constriction of the injured blood vessel to diminish blood flow.
2. Formation of a loose and temporary platelet aggregate at the site of injury.
3. Formation of a fibrin mesh that binds to the platelet aggregate, which gives to a more stable hemostatic plug or thrombus.
4. Partial or complete dissolution of the hemostatic plug or thrombus by plasmin.

About twelve main coagulation factors (specific proteins) are present in circulating plasma and the tissue surrounding the blood vessels (Table 9.2). These factors are in the inactive (zymogen) form under normal circulating conditions. Whenever bleeding takes place, they are activated, and by their action, blood coagulation takes place.

Table 9.2: Coagulation factors

Factor	*Synonym*
I	Fibrinogen
II	Prothrombin
III	Tissue thromboplastin
IV	Calcium ions
V	Labile factor (proaccelerin)
VI	Accelerin exists in combined with factor 'V' (Va)
VII	Stable factors (proconvertin)
VIII	Antihemophilic factors 'A' (AHF)
IX	Plasma thromboplastin component (PTC) (or antihemophilic factor 'B' or Christmas factor)
X	Stuart (or Peower) factor
XI	Plasma, thromboplastin antecedent
XII	Hageman (or contact) factor
XIII	Fibrin stabilizing factor.
	Other required components: Prekallikrein and high molecular weight kininogen (HMWK).

MECHANISM OF BLOOD COAGULATION: COAGULATION CASCADE (Fig. 9.5)

Intrinsic Pathway (Fig. 9.5)

- The intrinsic pathway involves factors XII, XI, IX, VIII, and X. It also requires prekallikrein, high molecular weight (HMW) kininogen, Ca^{2+}, and platelet phospholipids.
- This pathway commences with the contact phase in which prekallikrein, HMW kininogen, factor XII and factor XI are exposed to a negatively charged activating surface. Collagen on the exposed surface of a blood vessel provides this negative surface.
- Under physiologic conditions *in vivo*, prekallikrein, when assembled on endothelial cells, is first activated then it activates factor XII.

- When the components of the contact phase assemble on the activating surface, factor XII is activated to factor XIIa by the proteolytic action of kallikrein.
- Factor XIIa, once formed, activates factors XI to XIa and also releases bradykinin.
- Factor XIa in the presence of Ca^{2+} activates factors IX to the factor IXa.
- Factor VIII (antihemophilic factor), when activated to factor VIIIa, acts as a cofactor for factor IXa and also activates factor X to form active Xa.

Extrinsic Pathway (Fig. 9.5)

- Factor Xa occurs at the site where the intrinsic and extrinsic pathways converge and lead to the final common pathway of blood coagulation.
- The extrinsic pathway involves tissue factor (TF), factors VII, X, and Ca^{2+} ions.
- It is initiated at the site of tissue injury with the expression of tissue factor.
- TF combines with factor VIIa in the presence of calcium ions, and this complex acts as a cofactor in the activation of factor X to Xa.

Final Common Pathway of Blood Clotting

- In the final common pathway, factor Xa, produced by either the intrinsic or the extrinsic pathway, activates prothrombin (factor II) to thrombin (factor IIa).
- Thrombin converts fibrinogen to fibrin. Calcium ions are necessary for clotting reactions.

The fibrinolytic system is responsible for the dissolution of a blood clot. The deposition of fibrin and its removal are regulated by the fibrinolytic system. By this system, first plasmin forms from plasminogen (circulating inactive precursor) and acts on fibrin, and leads to its dissolution.

SAQ: Describe briefly blood clotting reactions.

Ans: In blood clotting, mainly, the following reactions take place:

$$\text{Prothrombin} \xrightarrow{\text{Xa, Calcium ions}} \text{Thrombin}$$

$$\text{Fibrinogen} \xrightarrow{\text{Thrombin, Calcium ions}} \text{Fibrin}$$

Prothrombin in the blood is converted to thrombin, in the presence of active factor Xa and calcium ions. Thrombin acts on fibrinogen, in the presence of calcium ions and converts it to fibrin clot.

Objective: To distinguish difference between plasma and serum and their respective composition.

BLOOD PLASMA

BAQ: Write a note on blood plasma.

Ans: Blood plasma is a pale amber-coloured liquid component of blood. When blood cells are removed, the fluid part is plasma. It makes up about 55–60% of total blood volume of the body. It contains about 90% of water and dissolved organic and inorganic components. The organic components are, proteins, glucose, urea, uric acid, various hormones, vitamins, fibrinogen, clotting factors, etc. Main proteins present in the plasma are albumin and globulins. Various inorganic ions present in the plasma are, sodium, porassium, chlorides, calcium, inorganic phosphorus, bicarbonate, carbonic acid, etc.

Functions: The main function of plasma is to carry nutrients, hormones, and proteins to various organs, tissues and cells. It carries waste products formed during the metabolic reactions to kidneys for excretion. It maintains acid–base balance by keeping proper ratio of bicarbonate and carbonic acid. The proteins maintain

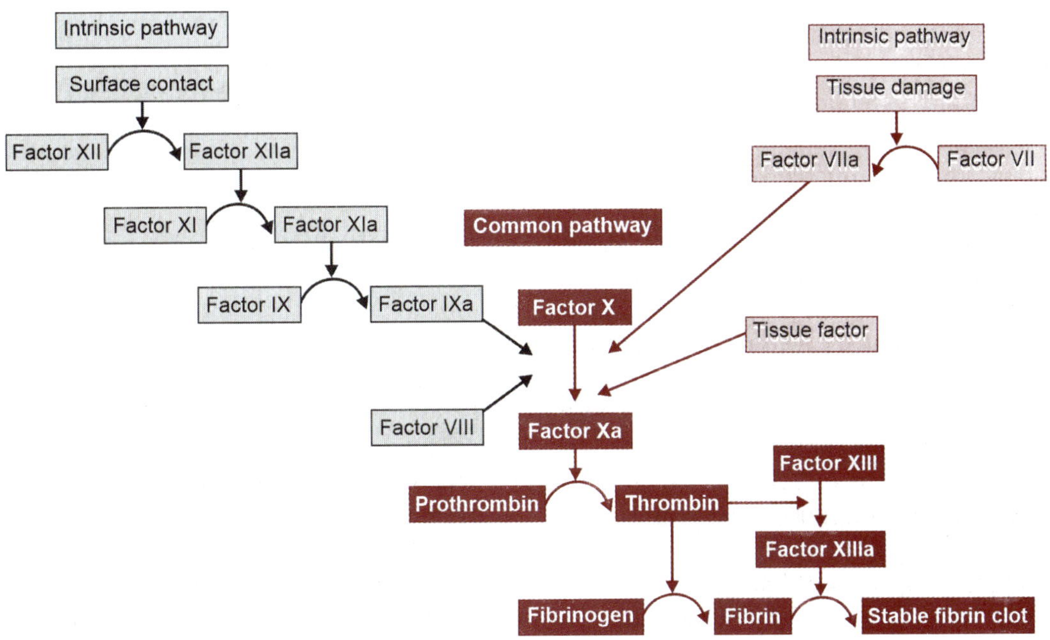

Fig. 9.5: Coagulation cascade

normal osmotic pressure of blood. Immunoglobulins present in plasma, protect body from invading microorganisms.

SAQ: What is an anticoagulant? Give examples of anticoagulants.

Ans: Anticoagulant is a chemical, which prevents blood coagulation by binding with calcium required for clotting, or by acting as antithrombin. Examples of anticoagulants are, ethylenediaminetetraacetic acid (EDTA), heparin, sodium citrate, etc.

SAQ: In which anticoagulant blood is collected for complete blood count (CBC), which includes hemoglobin determination and blood cell morphology?

Ans: Blood is collected in ethylenediaminetetraacetic acid (EDTA) containing tube for CBC test (Fig. 9.6).

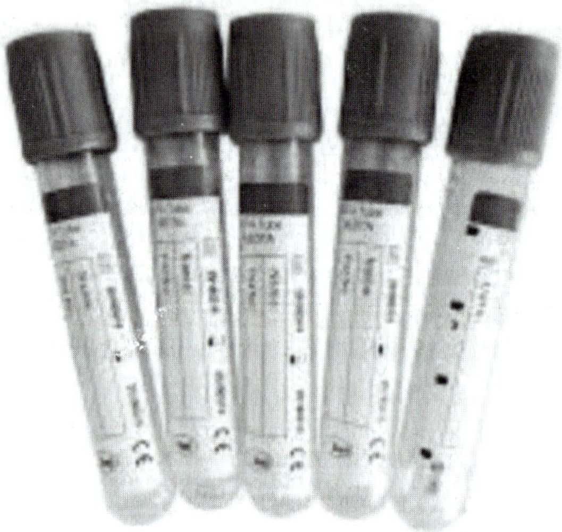

Fig. 9.6: EDTA tubes

SAQ: How to separate plasma from blood?

Ans: Blood is collected in an anticoagulated tube by venipuncture. Anticoagulant used is mainly heparin. After mixing the blood is centrifuge as shown in the Fig. 9.7. After centrifugation, supernatant is plasma, which is removed using a pipette.

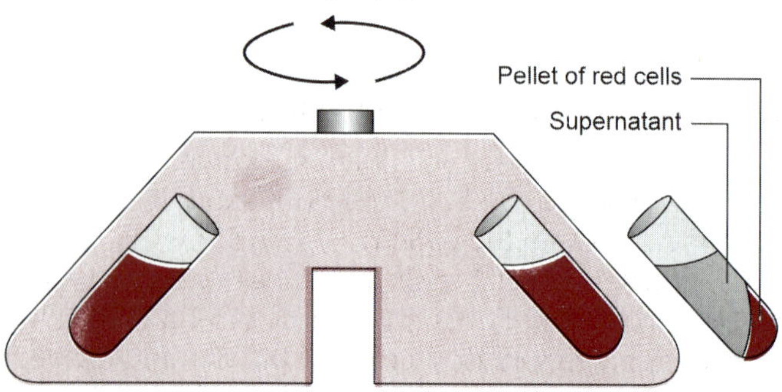

Fig. 9.7: Centrifuged anticoagulated blood

SAQ: What is the difference between plasma and serum?

Ans: Plasma contains fibrinogen and serum does not contain fibrinogen. Otherwise all other components of serum are similar to plasma.

SAQ: How to separate serum from blood?

Ans: Blood is collected in a tube without anticoagulant. This blood allowed to clot for at least 30 minutes. The fluid without clot is serum. This fluid is centrifuged as shown in Fig. 9.7, to get serum free from blood cells and clot fragments.

HEMATOLOGICAL DISORDERS

Iron Deficiency Anemia

BAQ: Write a note on iron deficiency amemia.

Ans: Deficiency of iron leads to iron deficiency anemia (IDA). IDA may develop into following two stages: (1) The progressive depletion and ultimate exhaustion of available tissue iron stores and (2) the development of anemia.

The following are three major factors in the pathogenesis of IDA:

1. In increased physiological demand for iron.
2. Pathological blood loss, and
3. Inadequate iron intake

Increased physiological demand for iron: During the period of growth, there is progressive increase in the number of red cells in the body and consequently in the total amount of hemoglobin. This results in an increased demand for iron.

During the reproductive life of the female, menstruation, pregnancy, parturition and lactation significantly increase the physiological requirements for iron. Each pregnancy requires extra iron for the fetus and to cover blood loss at parturition.

Pathological blood loss: Blood may be lost through gastrointestinal tract or urinary tract due to microbial and worm infections, trauma, ulcers or cancerous growth. The loss of blood to any extent causes lowering of the total body iron, since 60–70% of the total iron content of the body is confined (contained) in the hemoglobin of red cells. The normal adult has tissue iron reserves sufficient to replace between one-third and one-half of the circulating hemoglobin. Once this reserve is exhausted, continued bleeding causes a state of iron deficiency.

Inadequate intake: Inadequate intake may result from either nutritional deficiency or impaired absorption. Nutritional deficiency may be present as a result of an inadequate diet in infants and young children. It may occur in adults due to poor economic circumstances, specific dietary habits or dislikes and anorexia (especially in pregnancy).

A long-standing impairment of iron absorption: A long-standing impairment of iron absorption may result from gastrectomy or gastroenterostomy, tropical sprue or coeliac disease in either children or adults.

Iron deficiecy anemia (IDA) signs and symptoms: Iron deficiency anemia signs and symptoms: Weakness, extreme fatigue, headache, chest pain, dizziness, pale skin, cold hands and feet, brittle nails, loss of appetite.

Diagnosis of iron deficiency anemia (IDA): Complete blood count determination and iron using EDTA—blood is used for the diagnosis of IDA.

Significant decrease in hemoglobin, ferritin and iron, microcytic and hypochromic red cells are the main observations in IDA.

Hemolytic Anemia

BAQ: Write a note on hemolytic anemia.

Ans: Hemolytic anemias result from an increase in the rate of red cell destruction. The lifespan of the normal red cell is 100–120 days. In hemolytic anemias, lifespan of red blood cells is decreased by varying degrees. Anemia, in these cases, develops due to the inability of the bone marrow to compensate for the degree of destruction of red blood cells. Hemolytic anemia may not be seen until the red cell lifespan is less than 30 days.

The hemolytic anemias may be classified into two broad groups:

1. Intracorpuscular or intrinsic abnormality due to a corpuscular defect. These are mainly congenital, and the basic defect may be in any of the following three main components of the cell: The membrane, the hemoglobin molecule, and the enzymes concerned with cell metabolism.

   Examples: Congenital defect in the alpha and beta chains of hemoglobin, leading to alpha- and beta-thalassemia, sickle cell anemia, etc. It may be due to red blood cell membrane defect, as seen in hereditary spherocytosis, elliptocytosis etc. Due to these defects life of red blood cells decreases significantly, leading to hemolytic anemia.
2. Extracorpuscular or extrinsic abnormality due to an abnormal hemolytic mechanism. These disorders are acquired, and hemolysis may result from either an immune or a non-immune mechanism.

   Examples: Hemolytic anemia due to destruction of red blood cells due to burns, direct action of drugs and heave metals like lead, autoantibodies and microbial infections cause by bacteria (brucella) and parasites (malarial parasite).

THALASSEMIAS

SAQ: What are thalassemias?

Ans: The thalassemias are inherited disorders and are characterized by a reduced rate of production of normal hemoglobin due to absent or decreased synthesis of one or more types of globin polypeptide chains (alpha or or chains). This results in the decrease in the amount of hemoglobin in red blood cells. There are two main groups of thalassemia, one affecting the synthesis of alpha-chains (alpha-thalassemia) and the other affecting the synthesis of beta-chains (beta-thalassemia). It is possible to diagnose thalassemias in a clinical laboratory by testing blood.

Beta-thalassemia Minor (Trait)

BAQ: Write a note on beta-thalassemia trait.

Ans: Beta-thalassemia is characterized by a moderate reduction in beta-chain synthesis of hemoglobin as directed by a beta thalassemia gene (inherited from one carrier parent). Clinically, it is a mild disorder with little or no anemia and without any significant symptoms. It is possible to diagnose beta-thalassemia trait in a clinical laboratory by testing blood.

Beta-thalassemia Major

BAQ: Write a note on beta-thalassemia major.

Ans: Beta-thalassemia condition occurs on average in one in four offspring if both parents are carriers of the beta thalassemia trait. In this condition, either small amounts of beta chain are produced or synthesis of beta chain may not take place. In the absence of beta chain, excess alpha chains are synthesized. These precipitate in erythroblasts and in red cells and cause hemolysis, leading to hemolytic anemia. It is possible to diagnose beta-thalassemia major in a clinical laboratory by testing blood by hematological and molecular biology tests.

Sickle Cell Trait (Fig. 9.8)

BAQ: Write a note on sickle cell trait.

Ans: In sickle cell anemia, due to one carrier parent, hemoglobin S is present in the child. Hb-S comprises 35–95% of the total hemoglobin. The other hemoglobins present are Hb-A, Hb-A2, and HbF. The red cell life span is normal since cell do not contain sufficient Hb-S to form sickle shape at deoxygenated state. It is possible to diagnose sickle cell trait in a clinical laboratory by testing blood by hematological and molecular biology tests.

Sickle Cell Disease

BAQ: Write a note on sickle cell disease.

Ans: In sickle-cell disease, the patient receives one Hb-S gene from each parent, both of whom show sickle-cell trait. The red cells of the patient contain sufficient Hb-S for the formation of sickle cells (Fig. 9.8) at deoxygenated state. Nearly, all patients are anemic and sickle-cell crises are a characteristic feature of the disease. Sickle cell crisis means, when the flow of blood is blocked due to sickle form of red blood cells, these get stuck in the blood vessel. The patient can suffer from pain in the chest, arms, and legs. It is possible to diagnose sickle cell disease in a clinical laboratory by hematological and molecular biology tests.

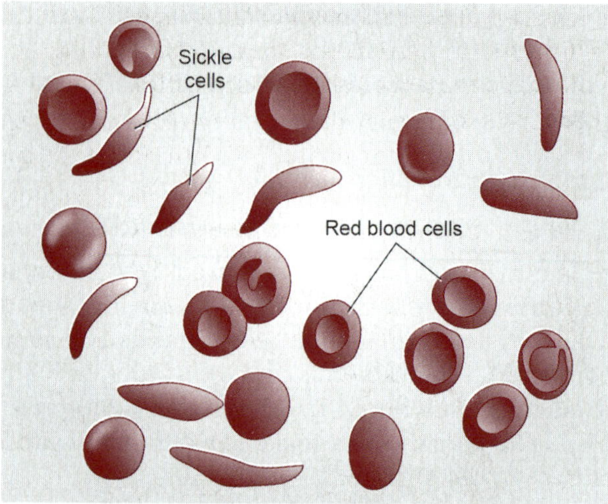

Fig. 9.8: Sickle cells and normal red blood cells

LEUKEMIAS (Fig. 9.9)

Abnormal increase in the growth of myeloid progenitor or lymphoid progenitor cells (related to white blood cells) takes place; due to loss of cell proliferation control. Very high immature white blood cells in the general blood circulation lead to the leukemia, a specific type of cancer. The rate of increase in immature blast cells varies in different types of leukemia. The various types of leukemias are: Acute lymphoblastic leukemia (ALL), acute myelogenous leukemia (AML), chronic lymphocytic leukemia (CLL), chronic myelogenous leukemia, etc. Complete hemogram (CBC) is useful to diagnose leukemia.

BAQ: Write a note on leukemias.

Ans: The leukemias are malignant diseases. The leukemias are diseases in which abnormal increase of hemopoietic cells affects the normal functions of bone marrow. In certain forms of leukemia the lymphatic tissues are particularly affected. Leukemic cells are usually present in the peripheral blood, where the count of cells ranges from very low to very high values. The rate of progression of leukemia varies considerably in different types of leukemia. Leukemia accounts for about four per cent of all deaths from malignant disease. It is possible to diagnose leukemia in a clinical laboratory by hematological blood tests.

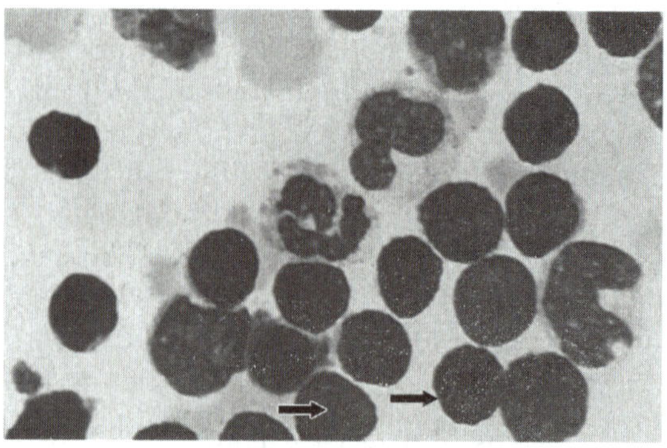

Fig. 9.9: Leukemia cells in a stained blood film. As seen under the microscope (high power lens)

BAQ: Write a note on aplastic anemia.

Ans: Aplastic anemia is caused due to damage to the stem cells in bone marrow of a patient. Stem cells are responsible for the production of blood cells. The main reason is the production of antibodies against the stem cells, which attack stem cells and destroy them. The following are other factors that can injure bone marrow and affect blood cell production: Viral infections (COVID-19, HIV, etc.), exposure to toxic chemicals such as benzene and pesticides, prolonged exposure to X-rays and radiations, chemotherapy treatments, effects of certain drugs and antibiotics. Aplastic anemia can be short-lived, or it can become chronic. Clinical laboratory blood tests could give indication of the status of aplastic anemia.

Hemophilia A

SAQ: What is hemophilia A?

Ans: Hemophilia A is caused due to congenital deficiency of factor XIII. Hemophilia is a sex-linked disorder and males are mainly affected. A person with this disorder suffers from excessive bleeding due to any type of injury. The patient with hemophilia requires life-long therapy of factor VIII.

Hemophilia B

SAQ: What is hemophilia B?

Ans: Hemophilia B is caused due to congenital deficiency of factor IX. It is also an X chromosome-linked disorder. A person with this disorder suffers from excessive bleeding due to any type of injury. The patient with hemophilia requires life-long therapy of factor IX.

> **Objective:** To understand and explain the central theme of competency based medical and paramedical education (CBME): Horizontal and vertical integration of subjects.

BAQ: Show horizontal integration of physiology, and biochemistry with the following anatomical change: Decrease in the size and shapes of red blood cells (as seen in "iron deficiency anemia (IDA)).

Ans:

Horizontal Integration with Physiology

Decrease in oxygen carrying capacity of RBCs.

Horizontal Integration with Biochemistry

Decrease in the circulating serum iron and depletion of iron stores of the body.

Horizontal Integration with Nutrition

Feeding of adequate iron-rich diet and food supplements to improve iron circulation in the body.

BAQ: Show vertical integration of clinical conditions associated with "iron deficiency anemia (IDA), with pharmacology, microbiology and preventive medicine.

Ans:

Vertical Integration with Pharmacology

Study and use of appropriate drugs to treat IDA.

Vertical Integration with Microbiology

Study of gastrointestinal microbial and parasitic infections that may cause intestinal bleeding and related decrease in blood hemoglobin.

Vertical Integration with Preventive Medicine

Suggestion of balance food containing adequate protein and iron.

BAQ: Show horizontal integration of physiology, biochemistry and nutrition with the following anatomical change: increase in the size and shapes of red blood cells (as seen in megaloblastic anemia).

Ans:

Horizontal Integration with Physiology

Increase in the hemolysis of red blood cell, due to decreased life span.

Horizontal Integration with Biochemistry

Deficiency of vitamin B_{12}, required for the normal development of red blood cells.

Horizontal Integration with Nutrition

Feeding of adequate folic acid, vitamin B_{12}-rich diet and protein supplements to manage megaloblastic anemia.

BAQ: Show vertical integration of clinical conditions associate with megaloblastic anemia with pharmacology, microbiology and preventive medicine.

Ans:

Vertical Integration with Pharmacology

Study and use of appropriate drugs to treat megaloblastic anemia.

Vertical Integration with Microbiology

Study of gastrointestinal microbial infections (such as *Helicobacter pylori* infection) that may cause deficiency of vitamin B_{12}.

Vertical Integration with Preventive Medicine

Preventive medicine: Study of education of good food habits and hygiene to prevent vitamin deficiency and microbial infections, respectively.

BIBLIOGRAPHY

1. Medical Biochemistry, 1st Edition (2023). Godkar PB, Godkar DP, CBS Publishers, New Delhi, India.
2. Text book of Medical Laboratory Technology, 4th Edition, (2024). Godkar PB, Godkar DP, Bhalani Publishing House, Mumbai, India.
3. Anatomy of the Human Body. 42nd Edition. Henry Gray, Editor-in-chief: Susan Standring, Elsevier (2020).
4. Ross & Wilson Anatomy and Physiology in Health and Illness, 13th Edition, by Allison Wynn Grant, Anne Waugh, and Kathleen J. W. Wilson (2018).
5. Schaum's outline of theory and problems of Human anatomy and Physiology, 2nd Edition (1997), Tata MaGraw-Hill Publishing Company Limited, New Delhi, India.

MULTIPLE CHOICE QUESTIONS (MCQs)

Select the correct option.

1. **The dietary components needed for normal development of red blood cells:**
   (A) Calcium and phosphorus
   (B) Iron and magnesium
   (C) Vitamin B_{12} and folic acid
   (D) Proteins
2. **Normal life span of red blood cells is about:**
   (A) 120 days (B) 240 days
   (C) 10 days (D) 360 days
3. **This clinical condition is directly related to bone marrow suppression:**
   (A) Aplastic anemia (B) Anemia
   (C) Sickle cell anemia (D) Megaloblastic anemia
4. **This metabolic pathway is responsible for 90% of red blood cell's glucose requirement:**
   (A) HMS (B) Citric acid cycle
   (C) Gluconeogenesis (D) Embden-Mayerhoff
5. **Major regulator of human erythropoiesis is:**
   (A) Vitamin B_{12} (B) Folic acid
   (C) Erythropoietin (D) Vitamin D
6. **These all may lead to bone marrow depression, *except*:**
   (A) X-ray exposure (B) Vitamin A deficiency
   (C) Antifolic acid drugs (D) All of the above
7. **These all are required for the synthesis of hemoglobin, *except*:**
   (A) Amino acids (B) Iron
   (C) Copper (D) Sodium
8. **Percent of normal HBA is about:**
   (A) 96% (B) 50%
   (C) 80% (D) 45%
9. **When fully saturated 1 g of hemoglobin holds approximately:**
   (A) 5.0 ml oxygen (B) 0.5 ml oxygen
   (C) 2.5 ml oxygen (D) 1.34 ml oxygen
10. **All the following statements about red blood cells are correct, *except*:**
    (A) Mature red blood cells lack nuclei
    (B) Red blood cells contain hemoglobin

(C) Internal concentration of red blood cells is not equivalent to normal saline
(D) Red blood cells lack mitochondria

11. Following dietary components are needed for normal development of red blood cells:

(A) Calcium and phosphorus
(B) Sodium, potassium and calcium
(C) Iron, vitamin B_{12} and folic acid
(D) Vitamin A and D

12. The following are the largest cells in the blood that leave the bloodstream to become macrophages:

(A) Eosinophils (B) Monocytes
(C) Basophils (D) Neutrophils

13. A person with eosinophilia is most likely suffering from:

(A) Allergies or internal parasites
(B) Anemia
(C) An autoimmune disease
(D) Viral disease

14. These cells appear first in an acute infection:

(A) Eosinophils (B) Neutrophils
(C) Lymphocytes (D) Monocytes

15. Normal life span of red blood cells is about:

(A) 120 days (B) 240 days
(C) 10 days (D) 360 days

16. These white blood cells do not contain granules:

(A) Neutrophils (B) Eosinophils
(C) Lymphocytes (D) Basophils

17. These white blood cells contain course granules:

(A) Basophils (B) Neutrophils
(C) Monocytes (D) Both (A) and (B)

18. These cells secrete serotonin and heparin:

(A) Neutrophils (B) Eosinophils
(C) Lymphocytes (D) Basophils

19. These cells are ultimately converted into plasma cells which produce immunoglobulins:

(A) T-lymphocytes (B) Neutrophils
(C) Monocytes (D) B-lymphocytes

20. The following one statement is correct:

(A) Anti-A serum is present in A group people
(B) Anti-B serum is present in B group people
(C) Anti-A and Anti-B serum are present in O group blood
(D) Persons having AB group, contain either anti-A or anti-B antibodies in their sera

21. In male, the following blood hemoglobin value (or values) indicates anemia:

(A) 12.3 gram%
(B) 14.5 gram%
(C) 13.5 gram%
(D) Both (A) and (B)

22. In female the following blood hemoglobin value (or values) indicates anemia:

(A) 13.0 gram% (B) 11.5 gram%
(C) 13.5 gram% (D) Both (A) and (B)

23. The lysosomes present in these white blood cell carry a large number of proteolytic, amylolytic, lipolytic enzymes:

(A) Neutrophils (B) Eosinophils
(C) Lymphocytes (D) Basophils

24. Normal percentage of neutrophils is:

(A) 25–45% (B) 40–75%
(C) 2–8% (D) 1–4%

25. Normal percentage of lymphocytes is:

(A) 25–45% (B) 40–75%
(C) 2–8% (D) 1–4%

ANSWERS

1. C	2. A	3. A	4. D	5. C	6. B	7. D
8. A	9. D	10. C	11. C	12. B	13. A	14. B
15. A	16. C	17. A	18. D	19. A	20. C	21. A
22. B	23. A	24. B	25. A			

MATCH THE COLUMNS

I	II
1. Coagulation factor IV	A. Phagocytosis
2. Monocytes	B. Formation of clot
3. Neutrophil	C. Calcium ions
4. Eosinophil	D. Accumulation of blood
5. Coagulation factor IX	E. Macrophages
6. Thrombus	F. Megakaryocyte
7. Hematoma	G. Allergic reactions
8. Platelets	H. Ingestion of parasites
9. Phagocytosis	I. Antihemophilic factor
10. Coagulation factor VIII	J. Christmas factor

ANSWERS

1. C	2. E	3. A	4. G	5. J	6. B	7. D
8. F	9. H	10. I				

CHAPTER

10

Lymphatic System

SAQ: Short answer question: Marks: 2	**MCQs:** Multiple choice questions: Marks: 0.5 each
BAQ: Brief answer question: Marks: 4 or 5	**Match the columns:** Marks: 0.5 each
LAQ: Long answer question: Marks: 9 or 10	**Draw a labelled diagram:** Marks: 5

Objective: To describe the functional relationship between the lymphatic system and the cardiovascular syst.

INTRODUCTION

SAQ: Briefly describe the lymphatic system.

Ans: The lymphatic system is part of the circulatory system and the immune system. It is made up of a large network of lymph, lymphatic vessels, lymph nodes, lymphatic organs, and lymphoid tissues (Fig. 9.1).

BAQ: Draw a labelled diagram of the lymphatic system and its important components.

Ans: Refer to the Fig. 10.1.

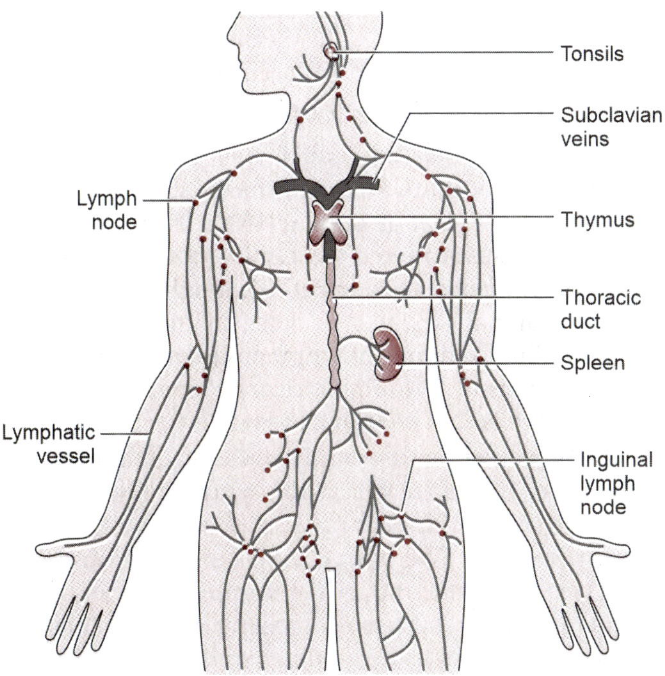

Fig. 10.1: Lymphatic system and its important components

Objective: To describe the composition of lymph and the fluid transport in the lymphatic system.

LYMPH

BAQ: Write a note on the lymph.

Ans: The cardiovascular system is a closed system, however, the lymphatic system is not a closed system. Lymph is formed from blood fluid that passes through the thin walls of blood capillaries into the tissues and cells of body. This fluid contains oxygen, proteins, glucose, amino acids, fatty acids and other nutrients that nourish the tissues. About 90% of this fluid re-enters the blood capillaries and about 3% of it enters the lymphatic vessels as lymph. As lymph further circulates through lymphatic circulation, it contains additional other substances that include damaged cells, cancer cells and foreign invaders like bacteria, viruses, fungi, parasites, etc. Lymph also transports lymphocytes, the white blood cells, that protect the body against foreign microorganisms and cancer cells.

BAQ: Draw a labelled diagram of the connections between the blood capillaries and the lymphatic system.

Ans: Refer to the Fig. 10.2A.

Lymphatic System Functions

BAQ: Write a note on the lymphatic system functions.

Ans: The lymphatic system plays many functions as a part of immune system. It protects body from invading microorganisms such as bacteria, viruses, fungi and parasites. The lymphatic system maintains body fluid levels. It absorbs digested lipids from digestive tract for further processing by body cells and remove cellular waste.

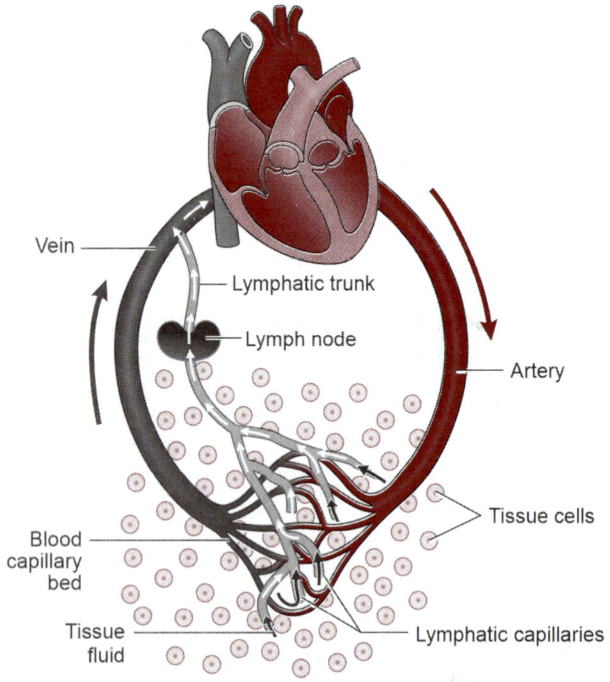

Fig. 10.2A: Connections between the blood capillaries and lymphatic circulation

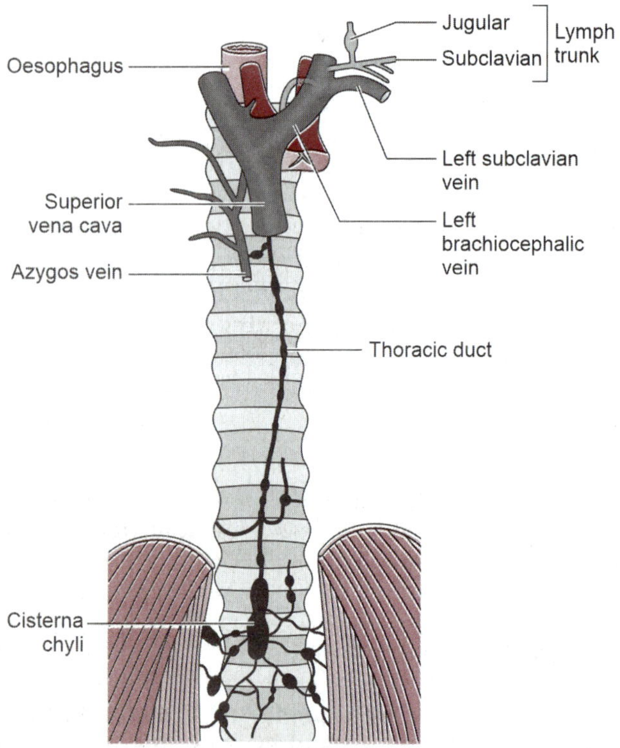

Fig. 10.2B: Cisterna chyli

SAQ: What is the pathway of lymphatic circulation?

Ans: Interstitial fluid enters the lymphatic system through the walls of the lymph capillaries. Lymph then flows from the lower extremities containing the liver and the intestine to the thoracic duct and the right lymphatic duct. These ducts then drain into the left and right subclavian veins (Fig. 10.2B).

SAQ: Describe the cisterna chyli.

Ans: The cisterna chyli is the abdominal origin of the thoracic duct (Fig 10.2B). It is a sac-like enlargement

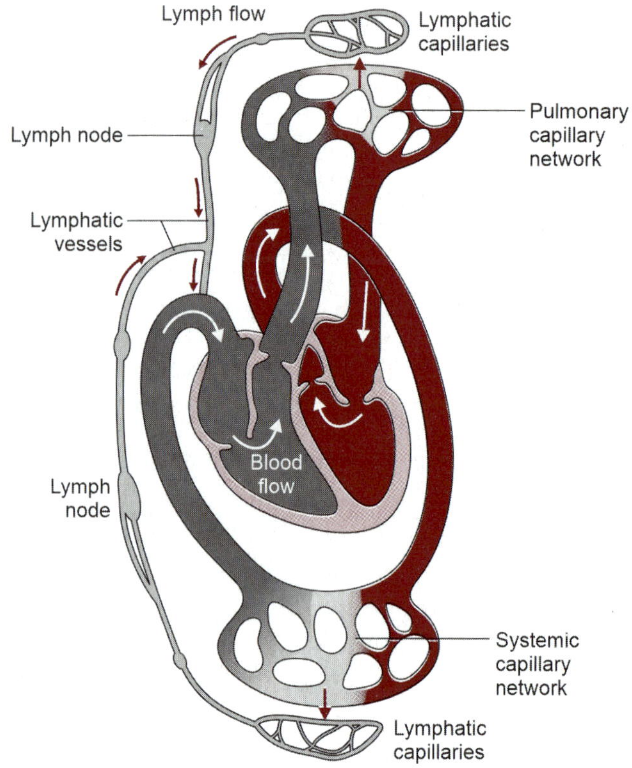

Fig. 10.3: Interrelations between blood circulation and lymphatic system

of the thoracic duct. Lacteals are special type of lymph capillaries in the small intestine. The lacteals transport digested fats through them to the cisterna chyli.

The cisterna chyli receives lymph from the right and left lumbar trunks. The lumbar trunks receive lymph from the kidneys, adrenals, pelvis, and the abdominal wall.

Objective: To describe the distribution and functions of the lymph nodes.

Lymph Nodes (Figs 10.4–10.6)

BAQ: Write a note on the lymph nodes.

Ans: The lymph nodes are bean-shaped glands located in many parts of the body, including the neck, armpit, chest, abdomen (belly), and groin (Fig. 10.4). There are about 600 lymph nodes scattered throughout the human body. Some lymph nodes are present as a single node, while other lymph nodes appear as closely connected chains. More familiar locations of lymph nodes are in the neck, armpit, and groin. Lymph nodes are connected to other lymph nodes by the lymphatic vessels.

As lymph passes through lymph nodes, the lymph nodes monitor and filter the lymph. The lymph nodes filter out the damaged cells, microorganisms and cancer cells. The lymph nodes also produce and store lymphocytes and other immune system cells such as dentritic cells; which are capable of attacking and destroying microorganisms and other harmful substances in the fluid.

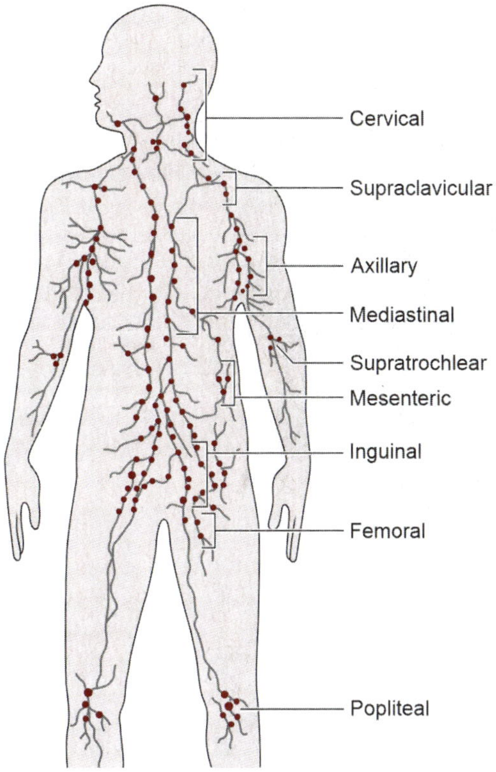

Fig. 10.4: Lymph nodes and vessels

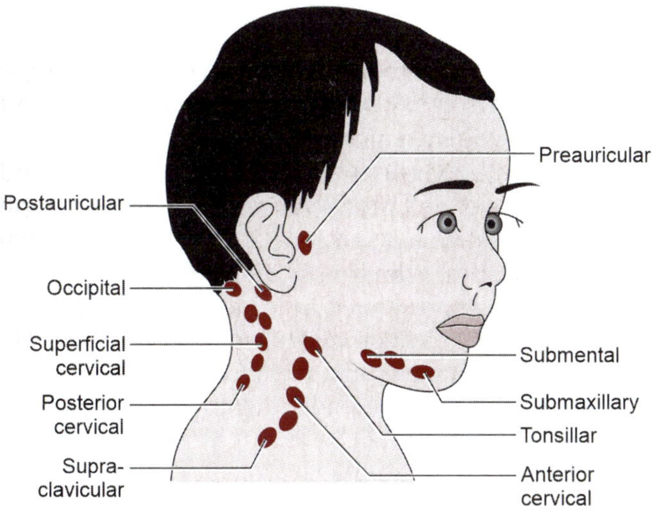

Fig. 10.5: Chains of lymph nodes

BAQ: Draw a labelled diagram of the chains of the lymph nodes.

Ans: Refer to the Fig. 10.4.

Lymphatic Vessels (Figs 10.4 and 10.6)

BAQ: Write a note on the lymphatic vessels.

Ans: The lymphatic vessels are microvessels that form network of capillaries and a large network of tubes located throughout the body. Lymphatic vessels transport lymph away from tissues. Lymphatic vessels collect filtered lymph at the lymph nodes as it continues to move to larger collecting ducts. Lymphatic vessels work like veins. They have a series of valves in them to keep the fluid moving in one direction (Fig. 10.6).

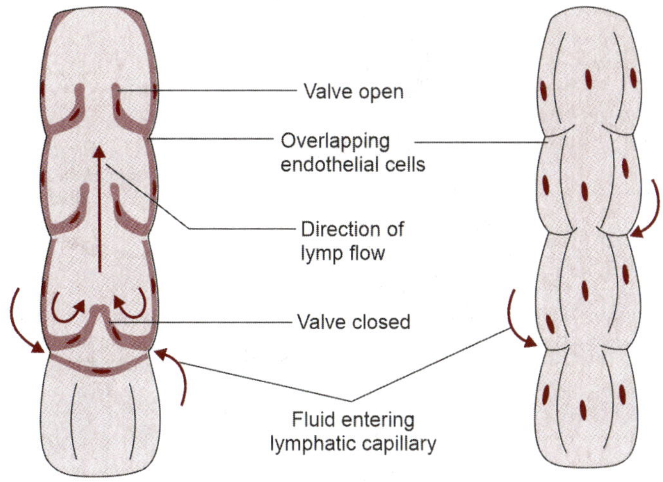

Fig. 10.6: Lymphatic vessels

Lymph Collecting Ducts

BAQ: Write a note on the lymph collecting ducts.

Ans: The lymphatic vessels empty the lymph into the right lymphatic duct and left lymphatic duct known as the thoracic duct. These ducts connect to the subclavian vein, which returns lymph to bloodstream. The subclavian vein is located below the collar bone (Fig. 10.7). Normal blood volume and pressure is maintained by returning lymph to the bloodstream. It also prevents the excess accumulation of fluid around the tissues. Excess fluid that drains from cells and tissue throughout the body is collected by lymphatic system and returns to the bloodstream. It is then recirculated throughout the body (Fig. 10.7).

Objective: To describe the glands associated with the lymphatic system and their distribution in the body.

SPLEEN (Figs 10.8 and 10.9)

LAQ: Write a note on the spleen with respect to the following points: (1) Introduction, (2) applied anatomy and (3) functions.

Ans:

1. **Introduction:** The spleen is purple in colour and the largest lymphatic organ in the body. It is located on the left side of the body, under the ribs and above the stomach. Average weight of normal spleen is about 170 grams (Fig. 10.8).
2. **Anatomy** (Figs 10.8 and 10.9): Spleen is a highly vascular organ. It contains many vessels that carry and circulate fluids in the body. It contains the following two main tissues: White pulp and red pulp.
   The red pulp of the spleen contains venous sinuses, which are cavities filled with blood, and splenic cords made up of connective tissues, which contain red blood cells and white blood cells. White pulp consists of immune lymphocyte cells.
3. **Functions:** The spleen works very closely with blood and lymph systems. It can get affected by

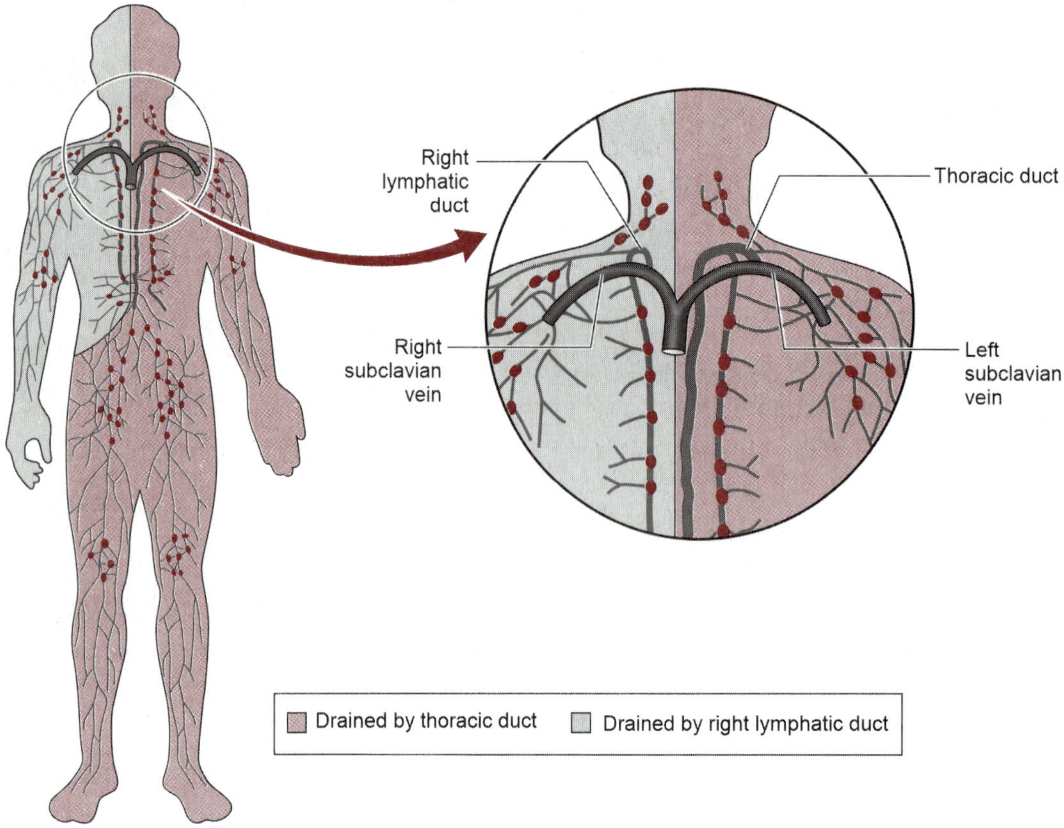

Fig. 10.7: Thoracic duct and subclavian vein connection

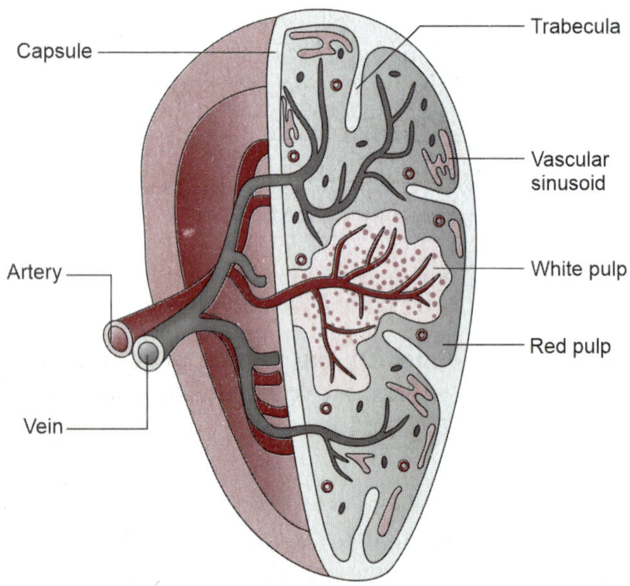

Fig. 10.8: Spleen anatomy

the infections, parasites, liver diseases, and due to spreading cancer cells. The following are the various functions of the spleen:

a. Speen removes old red blood cells and abnormal red blood cells from the blood circulation. Macrophages present in spleen play very important role in the destruction of old red blood cells and abnormal red blood cells.
b. In the white pulp of spleen, antibody-producing lymphocytes and monocytes are present, which remove antibody-coated bacteria and antibody-coated white blood cells by means of blood and lymph node circulation.
c. Spleen metabolizes hemoglobin removed from destroyed red blood cells. The heme released from destructed red blood cells is metabolized to bilirubin, which is subsequently removed in the liver and excreted in urine. The globin part of hemoglobin is degraded to amino acids, which can be used in amino acid metabolism. Similarly, iron separated from degraded hemoglobin is recycled in the body.

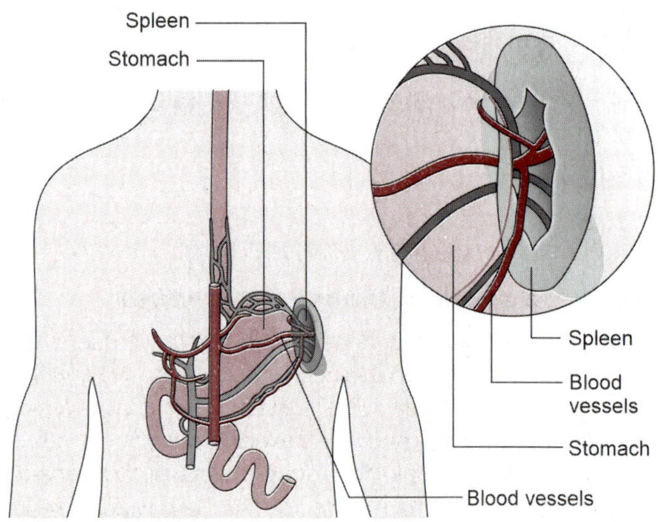

Fig.10.9: Spleen, blood vessels and stomach connections

d. Another important function of spleen is storing of blood. The blood vessels in human spleens are able to get wider or narrower according to the need of the body. When blood vessels are expanded, spleen can hold up significant quantity of reserve blood. In a situation like trauma, when there is loss of blood, spleen can respond by releasing the reserved blood back into blood circulation.

THYMUS GLAND (Fig. 10.10)

BAQ: Write a note on the thymus gland with respect to the following points: (1) Introduction, (2) applied anatomy with blood and nerve supply, and (3) functions.

Ans:

1. **Introduction:** The thymus gland is located in the upper front part of the chest, behind the sternum, and in front of the heart. Normal average size of thymus in adults is about 13 mm and weight is about 15 g. The thymus is a primary lymphoid organ of the immune system (Fig. 10.10).
2. **Applied anatomy, blood and nerve supply:** The thymus gland is made up of two lobes. Each consists of a central medulla and an outer cortex, which is surrounded by a capsule (Fig. 10.11). The arterial supply to the thymus gland is through the anterior intercostal arteries (Fig. 10.12) and small branches from the internal thoracic arteries. Venous blood passes into the left brachiocephalic and internal thoracic veins.

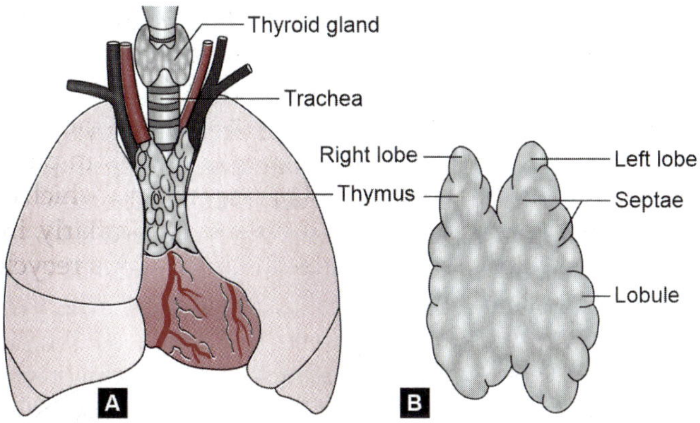

Figs 10.10A and B: Anatomy of thymus gland

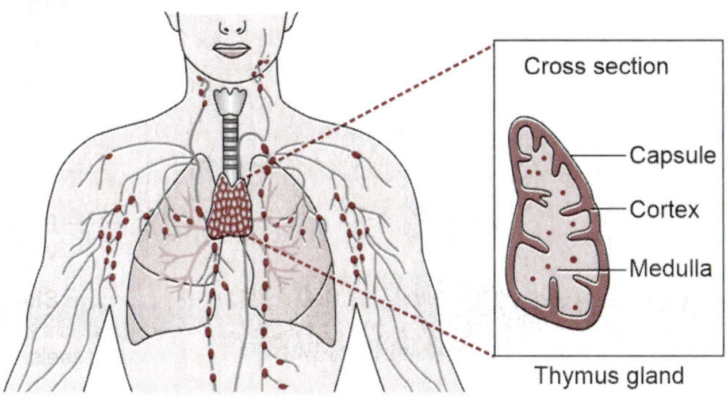

Fig. 10.11: Position of thymus gland in the body

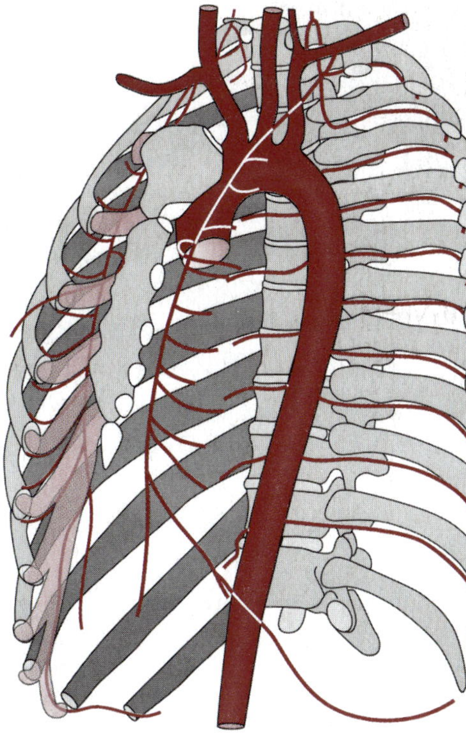

Fig. 10.12: Supply of blood to thymus gland by anterior intercostal arteries

Thymus gland gets nerve branches from the vagus nerve and the cervical sympathetic chain.

3. **Functions:** The thymus gland is a specialized organ for the maturation of specific lymphocytes, known as T cells (since they pass through thymus gland). T cells play very important role in the protection of the body from invading microorganisms and also protection against abnormal cells.

SAQ: What is thymus involution?

Ans: Thymus involution is an important characteristics of thymus gland. The thymus involution leads to the shrinking of the thymus gland with age. It decreases the tissue mass of thymus gland. As a result, the capacity of thymus gland to produce T cell decreases, leading to decrease in the immunity of an elderly individual.

Tonsils and Adenoid (Fig. 10.13)

BAQ: Write a note on tonsils and adenoids.

Ans: The tonsils are a set of lymphoid organs known as Waldeyer's tonsillar ring (Fig. 10.14), which consists of the adenoid tonsil, two tubal tonsils, two palatine tonsils, and the lingual tonsils. These are soft tissue masses and the tissue is similar to lymph nodes.

The tonsils are part of the immune system. These play important role to protect the body from infectious diseases. Tonsils trap bacteria and viruses that may enter body through the nose by inspired air or through food in the mouth.

Objective: To describe the role of bone marrow in the production of T cells.

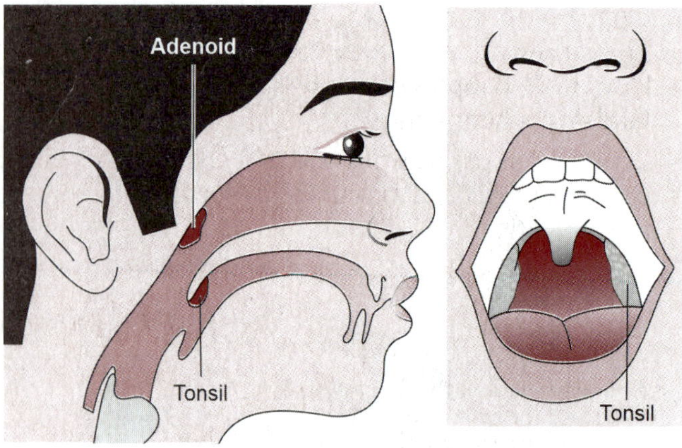

Fig. 10.13: Tonsils and adenoids

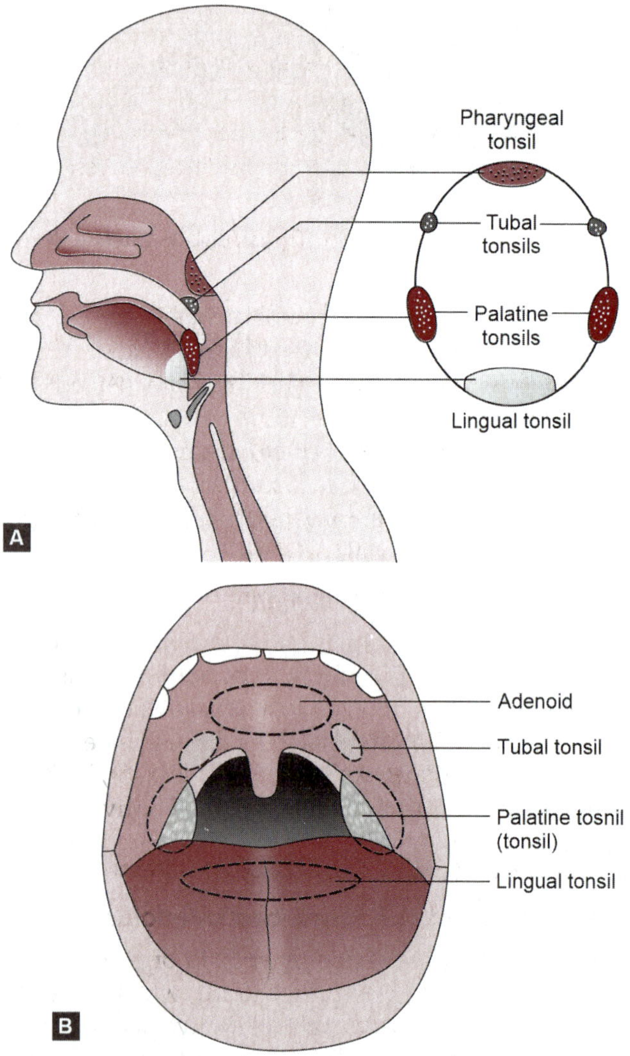

Figs 10.14A and B: Waldeyer ring of lymphoid tissues

SAQ: What is the role of the bone marrow in the production of T cells?

Ans: The bone marrow is soft, spongy tissue inside bones, such as the breast bone and the hip bone. White blood cells, red blood cells, and platelets are made in the bone marrow. As a part of the lymphatic system, it plays very important in the production of T lymphocytes, which protect body from invasion of microorganisms and also from abnormal cells (Fig. 10.15).

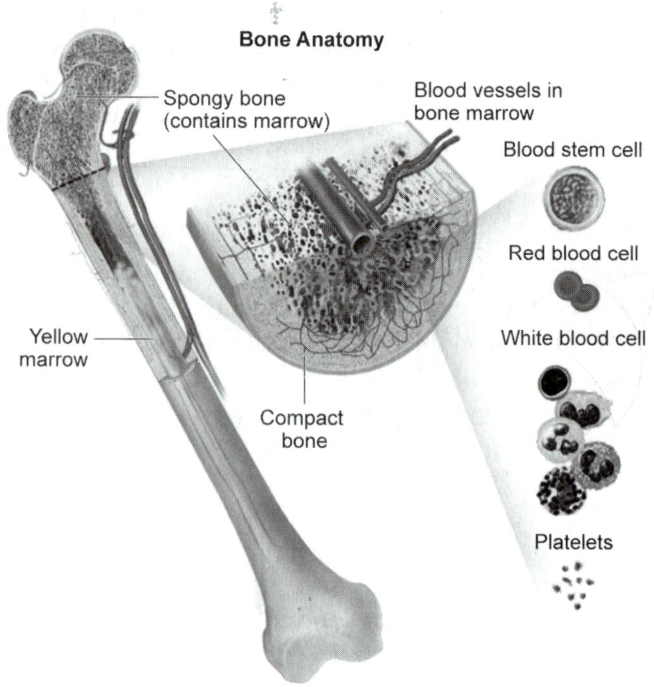

Fig. 10.15: Bone marrow and bone anatomy

Peyer's Patches

BAQ: Write a note on the Payer's patches.

Ans: The Payer's patches are small masses of lymphatic tissue in the mucous membrane that lines ileum part of small intestine.

Peyer's patches contain immune cells such as T cells, B cells, macrophages and dendritic cells and microfold (M) cells. The M cells are located in the epithelium covering of the Peyer's patches. The M cells actively transport antigens to the underlying lymphoid follicles, which contain the macrophages and dendritic cells (Fig. 10.16). The macrophages and dendritic cells then in turn introduce these antigens to T cells and B cells, which determine whether the antigen is harmful or safe for body cells. If they recognize the antigen as a harmful antigen, the T cells and B cells in Peyer's patches signal immune system to destroy it.

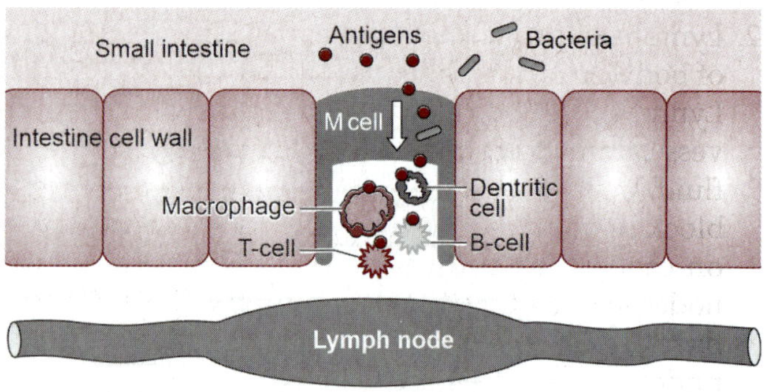

Fig. 10.16: Peyer's patches

APPENDIX (Fig. 10.17)

BAQ: Write a note on lymphoid tissue of appendix.

Ans: The appendix is a thin and normal average four inch long tube. It is a part of gastrointestinal tract. Appendix is a pouch of tissue that is attached to the large intestine. It is located in the lower-right area of the abdomen. Appendix contains lymphoid tissue that may play important role in the protection from bacteria.

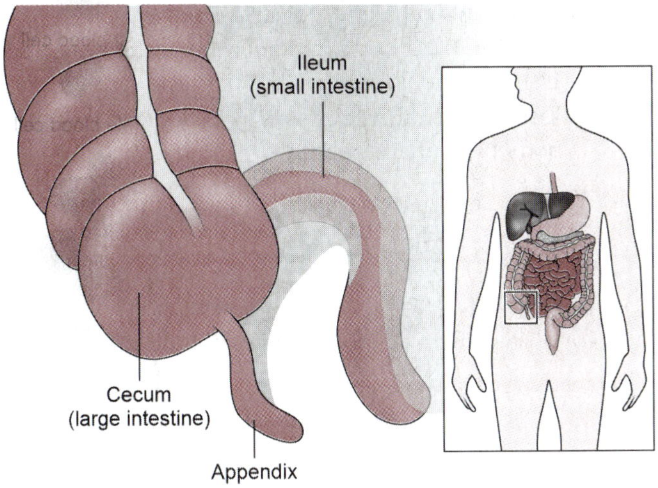

Fig. 10.17: Appendix

> **Objective:** To describe the various clinical conditions associated with lymphatic system.

LYMPHATIC DISEASES

LAQ: Write a note on lymphatic diseases.

Ans: Lymphatic diseases affect the lymphatic system. Lymphatic disease may be caused by microbial infections, blockage of lymph ducts and also due to circulating cancer cells. In lymphatic disease, fluid builds in tissues and causes swelling. The following are various clinical conditions related to lymphatic diseases:

1. Lymphadenopathy means enlarged lymph nodes. Generalized lymphadenopathy may be caused due to microbial infections, malignancies, drug reactions, autoimmune diseases, etc. Examples of various types of infectious diseases that may cause generalized lymphadenopathy are, tuberculosis, HIV infection, toxoplasmosis, secondary syphilis, etc.
2. Lymphedema means localized swelling of the parts of body due to an abnormal accumulation of lymph. Lymphedema occurs by the blockage of the lymph vessels, which are not able to adequately drain lymph fluid, mainly from an arm or leg. Cancer cells may block lymph vessels. Similarly, radiation treatment on cancer also can cause inflammation of lymph nodes leading to lymphedema. The infection caused by filaria worms also lead to clogging of the lymph nodes. Lymphedema may also be observed after specific surgical procedures. Lymphedema is usually observed in the feet or lower legs.
3. Lymphoma is a cancer of the lymphatic system. The following are the main subtypes of lymphoma: Hodgkin's lymphoma (Hodgkin's disease) and non-Hodgkin's lymphoma.
4. Lymphadenitis: Lymphadenitis is an infection of the lymph nodes usually caused by bacteria, virus, or fungi.
5. Lymphangitis is an inflammation of the lymph vessels.

Diseases of Spleen

BAQ: Write a note on splenomegaly.

Ans: The spleen may enlarge, when affected by specific diseases. Enlargement of the spleen is called splenomegaly. The following are some of the causes of splenomegaly:

1. **Cirrhosis of the liver:** In this clinical condition, increase in the blood pressure inside the vessels of the spleen is observed.
2. **Chronic infections:** In chronic infections like tuberculosis, typhoid, cytomegalovirus infection, and malaria spleen may enlarge.
3. **Glandular fever:** It is an infection caused by the Epstein-Barr virus.
4. **Haemolytic anaemia:** In hemolytic anemia, life span of red blood cells decrease considerably. Excessive destruction of red blood cells in spleen may lead to splenomegaly.
4. **Hodgkin's disease:** It is a type of cancer of the lymphatic system.
5. **Leukaemia:** A type of cancer of the bone marrow that affects the production of white blood cells.
6. **Lymphoma:** It is type of cancer of the lymph nodes of the lymphatic system.

Thymus Gland Disorders

Thymus gland may get enlarged due to diseases such as Addison's disease and thyrotoxicosis (enlargement of thyroid gland), mainly due to autoimmune disorder. Thymus gland also may affected due to myasthenia gravis (MG) and in hypogammaglobulinemia (very low gamma globulin values).

> **Objective:** To understand and explain the central theme of competency based medical and paramedical education (CBME): Horizontal and vertical integration of subjects.

BAQ: Show horizontal integration of physiology, and biochemistry with the following anatomical change: Enlargement of spleen and liver (hepatosplenomegaly).

Ans:

Horizontal Integration with Physiology

Affected intrahepatic circulation of bile pigments and bile salts.

Horizontal integration with Biochemistry

Increase in serum bilirubin, bile salts, and hepatic enzymes such as SGPT and SGOT (severe hepatic jaundice).

BIBLIOGRAPHY

1. "Anatomy of the Human Body". 42nd Edition. Henry Gray, Editor-in-chief: Susan Standring, Elsevier (2020).
2. Ross & Wilson Anatomy and Physiology in Health and Illness, 13th Edition, by Allison Wynn Grant, Anne Waugh, and Kathleen JW. Wilson (2018).

MULTIPLE CHOICE QUESTIONS (MCQs)

Select the correct option.

1. The lymphatic system is a part of:

(A) Circulatory system (B) The nervous system
(C) Immune system (D) Both (A) and (C)

2. The following one statement is not correct:

(A) The cardiovascular system is a closed system
(B) The lymphatic system is a closed system.
(C) Lymph is formed from blood fluid
(D) The lymphatic system is not a closed system

3. The cisterna chyli receives lymph from:

(A) The right lumber trunk
(B) The left lumbar trunks
(C) The abdominal wall
(D) All of the above

4. The following one statement is not correct:

(A) The lymph nodes monitor the lymph
(B) The lymph nodes filter the lymph
(C) The lymph nodes cannot produce and store lymphocytes
(D) The lymph nodes produce and store dentritic cells

5. Lymphatic vessels:

(A) Work like veins (B) Work like arteries
(C) Contain valves (D) Both (A) and (C)

6. The lymphatic vessels empty the lymph into:

(A) The thoracic duct
(B) The right atrium of the heart
(C) The left atrium of the heart
(D) Both (A) and (C)

7. The red pulp of the spleen contains:

(A) Red blood cells and white blood cells
(B) Lymphocytes
(C) Monocytes
(D) Both (A) and (C)

8. White pulp of spleen consists of:

(A) Red blood cells and white blood cells
(B) Lymphocytes and monocytes
(C) Platelets
(D) Both (A) and (C)

9. These cells are matured in the thymus gland:

(A) B lymphocytes
(B) T lymphocytes
(C) Macrophages
(D) Red blood cells

10. The following one statement is not correct:

(A) The tonsils are part of the immune system.
(B) The tonsils play an important role to protect the body from infectious diseases
(C) The tonsils trap bacteria and viruses that may enter body through the nose
(D) The tonsils are part of the digestive system

11. The heme released from destructed red blood cells in spleen is metabolized to:

(A) Porphyrin (B) Bilirubin
(C) Glycocholic acid (D) Taurocholic acid

12. The Payer's patches are small masses of:

(A) Connective tissue (B) Fibrous tissue
(C) Lymphatic tissue (D) Neurons

13. Generalized lymphadenopathy may be caused due to:

(A) Microbial infections (B) Malignancies
(C) Autoimmune diseases (D) All of the above

14. Hodgkin's disease is:

(A) Cancer of small intestine
(B) Cancer of lymphatic system
(C) Cancer of bones
(D) Cancer of pancreas

ANSWERS

1. D	2. B	3. D	4. C	5. D	6. A	7. A
8. B	9. B	10. D	11. B	12. C	13. D	14. B

MATCH THE COLUMNS

I	II
1. Speen	(A) Immune cells
2. Red pulp of spleen	(B) T cells
3. White pulp of spleen	(C) Largest lymphatic organ
4. Macrophages	(D) Bilirubin
5. Thymus gland	(E) Venous sinus
6. Payer's patches	(F) Accumulation of lymph
7. Very old RBCs	(G) Enlarged lymph nodes
8. Lymphedema	(H) Lymphoma
9. Lymphadenopathy	(I) Lymphatic tissue
10. Hodkin's disease	(J) Removal of old red blood cells

ANSWERS

1. C	2. E	3. A	4. J	5. B	6. I	7. D
8. F	9. G	10. H				

CHAPTER

11

Respiratory System

SAQ: Short answer question: Marks: 2
BAQ: Brief answer question: Marks: 4 or 5
LAQ: Long answer question: Marks: 9 or 10
MCQs: Multiple choice questions: Marks: 0.5 each
Match the columns: Marks: 0.5 each
Draw a labelled diagram: Marks: 5

Objective: To describe the basic components and functions of the respiratory system.

INTRODUCTION

BAQ: Briefly describe the respiratory system.

Ans: The respiratory system is a network of organs and tissues that help a person to breathe (Fig. 11.1). The main parts of the respiratory system are, nose, nasal cavity, pharynx, larynx, trachea, airways, lungs, blood vessels and blood circulation. The muscles that give strength to lungs are also part of the respiratory system. The respiratory system parts work together to move oxygen throughout the body and remove excretory gases like carbon dioxide formed during the metabolic activities of the cells. The exchange of oxygen and carbon dioxide in the body is called respiration, which is crucial for the life. Dysfunction of the respiratory system may take place due to infections of the respiratory system, cancerous growth and also due to trauma. Dysfunction of the respiratory system leads to hypoxia; means deficiency in the amount of oxygen reaching the tissues.

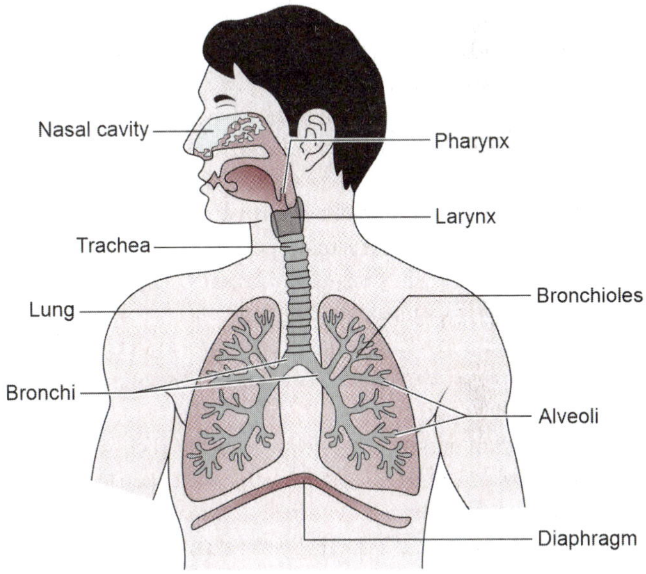

Fig. 11.1: Respiratory system

SAQ: Enumerate the functions of the respiratory system.

Ans: The following are the various functions of the respiratory system:

1. Facilitation of breathing.
2. Exchange of oxygen and carbon dioxide. From the air, oxygen is taken in the blood by inspiration and waste product carbon dioxide is expelled out in the expired air.
3. Protection from dust and microbes that may enter the body by means mucus production, function of cilia, and cough reflux mechanism.
3. Sound production by larynx
4. Facilitation of the sense of smell, through the specific nerves in the nose.

Objective: To identify the basic components of the respiratory system.

PARTS OF THE RESPIRATORY SYSTEM (Fig. 11.1)

SAQ: Enumerate the parts of the respiratory system.

Ans: The following are various parts of the respiratory system:

1. Nose and nasal cavity
2. Sinuses
3. Mouth
4. Pharynx (throat)
5. Larynx (voice box)

6. Trachea (windpipe)
7. Diaphragm
8. Lungs
9. Bronchial tubes/bronchi
10. Bronchioles
11. Air sacs (alveoli)
12. Blood capillaries

BAQ: Draw a labelled diagram of respiratory system.

Ans: Refer to Fig. 11.1.

Objectives: To describe the basic anatomical structure and related functions of various parts of the respiratory system. To describe the blood supply and innervation to the respiratory system. To describe the clinical conditions related to respiratory disorders.

NOSE (Refer to Chapter 7, Page 180)

LAQ: Describe the nose under the following heads: (1) Introduction, (2) applied anatomy, (3) functions and (4) the effects of nasal dysfunction.

Ans:

1. **Introduction:** The nose is an organ of the respiratory system that helps an individual to breathe and to smell.
2. **Nose anatomy**: The nose has two holes called nostrils (*see* Fig. 7.71). The internal nose is divided into the left and right nasal cavities by the nasal septum (*see* Fig. 7.72). The septum is made of very thin pieces of bone. Each nostril is connected with nasal cavity. Each nasal cavity contains a roof, floor, medial wall, and lateral wall. Each nasal cavity has the following three regions: (1) Nasal vestibule, (2) respiratory region, and (3) olfactory region (*see* Fig. 7.74). Three sections, the medial crus, the middle crus, and the lateral crus contribute to the outer shape of the nasal tip (*see* Fig. 7.73).
   The internal nose consists of a region known as the vestibule (*see* Fig. 7.74), which is supported by the cartilage of the nose. Vestibule is a skin-lined part, which contain small course hair and lined with tissue that contains small, course hairs (*see* Fig. 7.75). These hairs are useful to filter dust, sand, and other particles and to keep these from entering the lungs.
   Nose also contains the mucosa-lined region known as the nasal cavity proper (*see* Fig. 7.76). The nasal cavity proper is a large, air-filled space. It is present above and behind the nose and at the middle of the face.
   The cavity of the nose is lined with mucous membranes that have smell receptors connected to the olfactory nerve (*see* Fig. 7.76). The smell receptors are sensitive to various types of smell sensations.
3. **Functions:** The nose brings warm humidified air into the lungs. It facilitates filtering out particles in inspired air. It also serves to provide first-line immunologic defence by bringing inspired air in contact with mucous-coated membranes that contain immunoglobulins. Inspired air comes in contact with the olfactory nerves of nose and provides the sense of smell, which is associated with the taste sensation.
4. **Nasal dysfunction** leads to nasal congestion, sinus infections, postnasal drainage, headache, facial pressure and headache.

SAQ: What are sinuses and their functions as parts of the respiratory system?

Ans: The sinuses are hollow areas between the bones in head that regulate the temperature and humidity of the inhaled air (Refer Fig. 7.77).

Pharynx (Fig. 11.2)

LAQ: Describe the pharynx under the following heads: (1) Introduction, (2) applied anatomy with functions related to each part.

Ans:

1. **The pharynx** is a muscular tubular part that connects the oral and nasal cavity to the larynx and esophagus (Fig. 11.2). It extends from the base of the skull to the level of the sixth cervical vertebra.
2. **Applied anatomy and functions:** The pharynx is comprised of following three parts: (A) Nasopharynx, (B) oropharynx (Fig. 11.2) and, (C) hypopharynx (laryngopharynx).
   A. **Nasopharynx** (Fig. 11.2): The nasopharynx is lined with respiratory epithelium; ciliated pseudostrati-

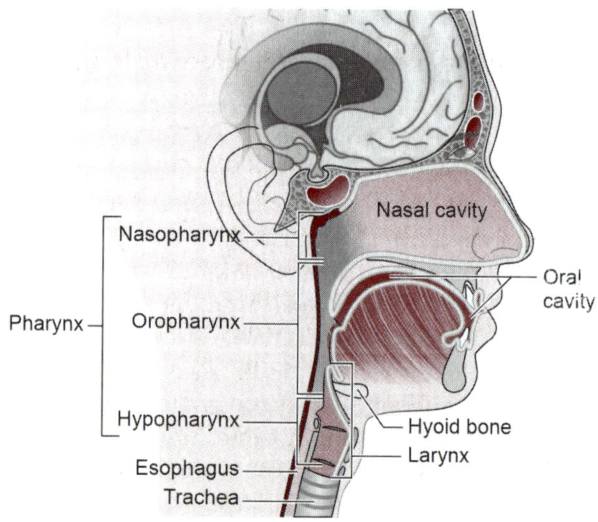

Fig. 11.2: Anatomy of pharynx

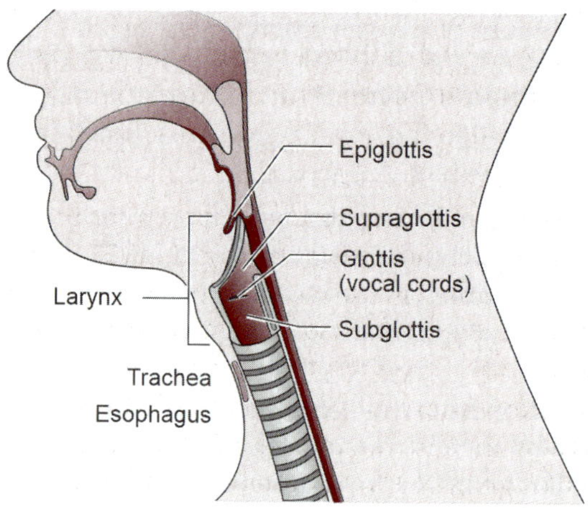

Fig. 11.3: Anatomy of larynx

fied columnar epithelium with mucous secreting goblet cells. The goblet cells trap dust particles and pathogens from the inspired air. The nasopharynx controls inspired air, which then gets propagated into the larynx.

The posterosuperior nasopharynx contains the adenoids and tonsils. The tonsils enlarge during 3–8 years of age and later on regress to reach the adult size. The adenoids and tonsils are important components of immune system and these protect the body from invading pathogens in the upper respiratory tract.

B. The oropharynx is the middle part of the pharynx, located between the soft palate and the superior border of the epiglottis. The four important parts contained within the oropharynx are, the base of the tongue, the palatine tonsils, tonsillar pillars, the soft palate, and the pharyngeal wall. Waldeyer's ring (the ring of lymphoid tissue) in the nasopharynx and oropharynx is formed by the paired palatine tonsils, the adenoid tonsils and lingual tonsil (Fig. 11.4).

The oropharynx is lined with a stratified squamous epithelium for extra protection from abrasion and exposures related to air and food. It joins the oral cavity and nasopharynx with the larynx and hypopharynx. The oropharynx is involved in the voluntary and involuntary phases of swallowing.

C. The hypopharynx (laryngopharynx) is placed between the superior border of the epiglottis and inferior border of the cricoid cartilage (C6). It remains continuous inferiorly with the esophagus. The laryngopharynx contains the middle and inferior pharyngeal constrictors (Fig. 11.5). Both food and air pass through the laryngopharynx.

The hypopharynx (laryngopharynx) is lined with squamous epithelium. When food and liquid are swallowed, these pass through the throat to the stomach. The hypopharynx action keeps food around the larynx and into the esophagus and food does not pass into the larynx.

BAQ: Draw a labelled diagram of pharynx.

Ans: Refer to Fig. 11.2.

BAQ: What are the general reasons for the blockage of the Eustachian tube?

Ans: The reasons for the general blockage of the Eustachian tube are as follows:

1. Due to microbial infections of the upper respiratory tract, the adenoid tonsils may get infected, become enlarged and can obstruct the opening of the Eustachian tube, which is located close to the adenoid tonsils in the nasopharynx (*see* Fig. 7.58).
2. Chronic infections of adenoid tonsils lead to chronic obstruction of the Eustachian tube, which prevents the equalising of pressure in the middle ear with the atmosphere and normal drainage of fluid. This may lead to chronic otitis media, means infection of the middle ear (*see* page 179).

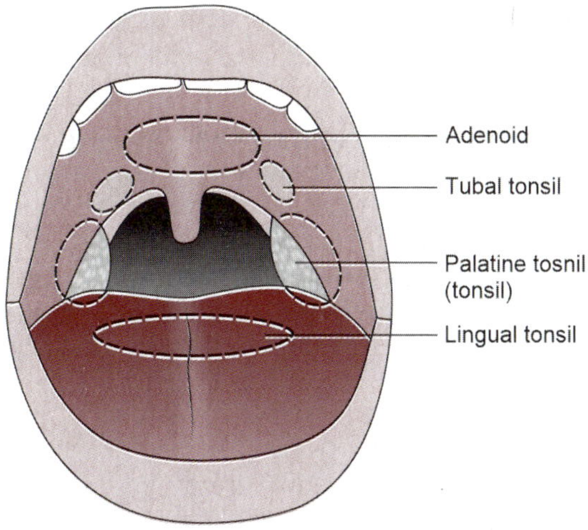

Fig. 11.4: Waldeyer's ring (the ring of lymphoid tissue)

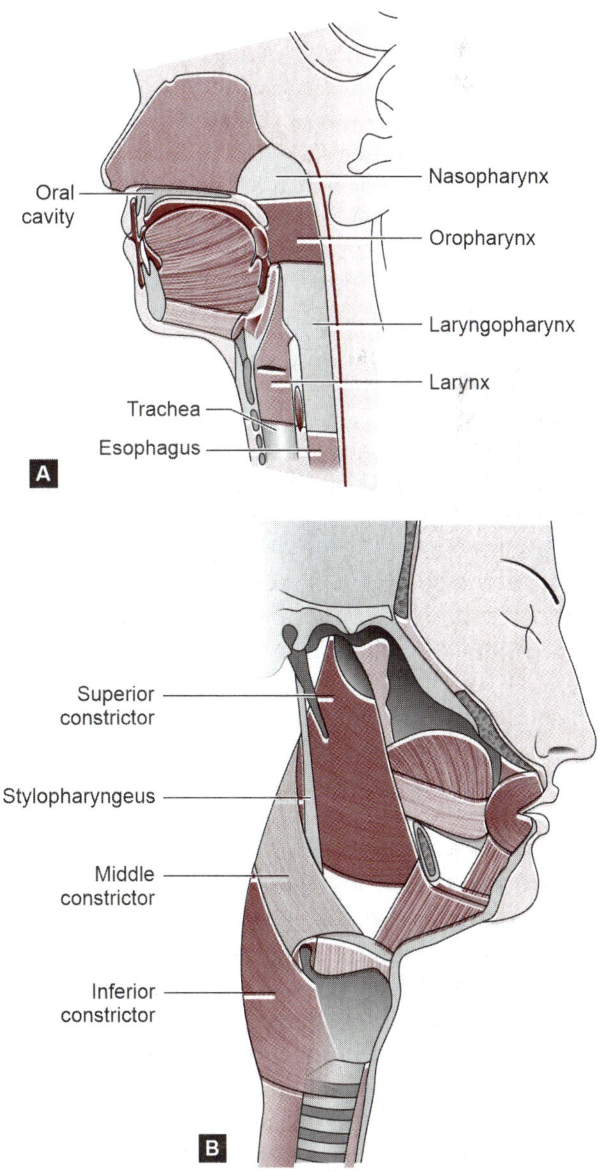

Figs 11.5A and B: Laryngopharynx (hypopharynx)

Uvula (Figs 11.6 A and B)

BAQ: Write a note on the uvula.

Ans: The uvula is a conical projection on the back edge of the middle of the soft palate (Fig. 11.6). It is composed of connective tissue. It contains serous glands, which produce saliva.

During swallowing, food is prevented from entering the nasal cavity as the soft palate and the uvula move together to close off the nasopharynx. Saliva produced by the uvula keep the throat very well lubricated. Uvula plays important role in the ability to speak. Enlarged uvula may contribute to heavy breathing (snoring) during sleep.

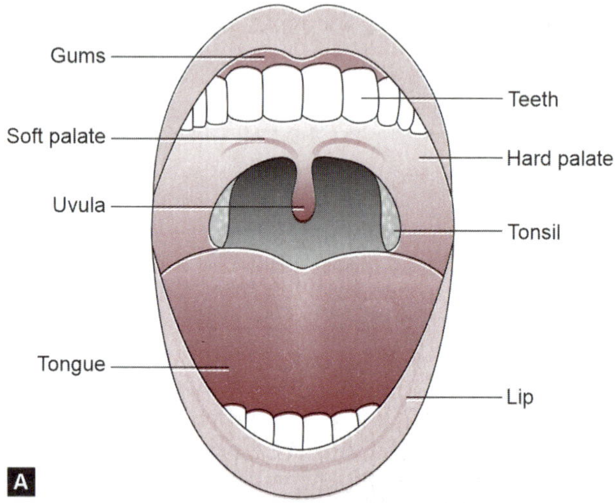

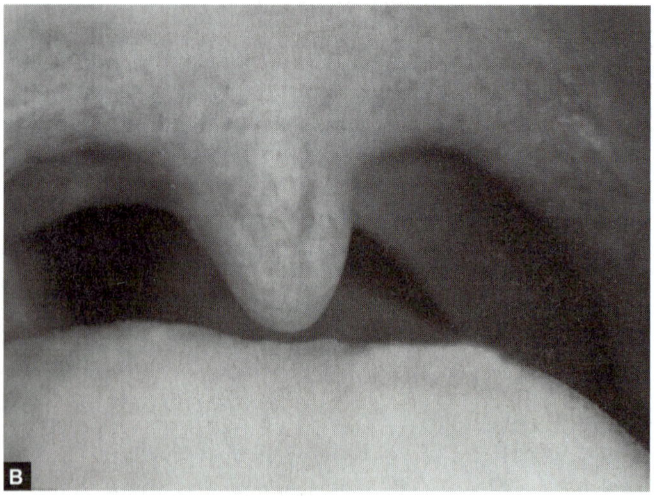

Figs 11.6A and B: Uvula

BAQ: Write role of the inferior pharyngeal constrictor muscle in the swallowing process.

Ans: The inferior pharyngeal constrictor muscle (skeletal muscle) splits into following two parts: (1) The thyropharyngeus and (2) the cricopharyngeus. Usually, during swallowing, the thyropharyngeus contracts and the cricopharyngeus relaxes. This action allows the bolus of food to pass into the oesophagus, prevents rise in the intra-pharyngeal pressure. If the coordinated relaxation of the cricopharyngeus fails to occur, the intra-pharyngeal pressure increases and pharyngeal mucosa forms a midline diverticulum (pouch) (Fig. 11.7) in the area between the thyropharyngeus and cricopharyngeus. Food may accumulate there, leading to difficulty in swallowing.

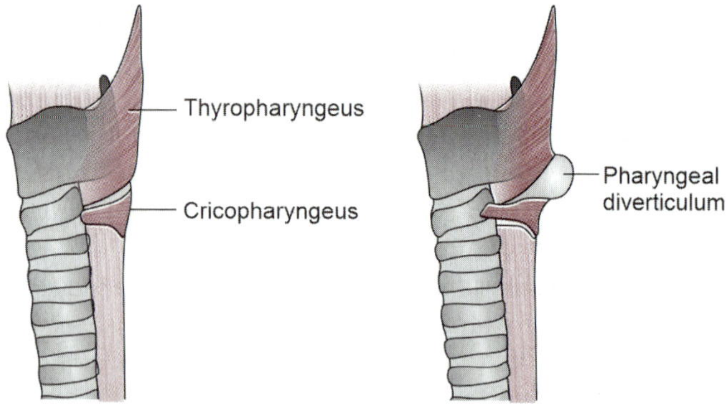

Fig. 11.7: Inferior pharyngeal constrictor muscle parts

Larynx

LAQ: Describe the larynx under the following heads: (1) Introduction, (2) anatomy and functions, (3) blood supply of larynx and (4) nerve supply of larynx.

Ans:

1. **The larynx (voice box)** is an organ located in the anterior neck. It is a component of the respiratory tract, and plays important in phonation, the cough reflex, and protection of the lower respiratory tract. Phonation is the process by which the vocal cord (Fig. 11.8), produces certain sounds through specific vibrations.

Anatomical Structure of the Larynx and Functions (Fig. 11.9)

2. **Anatomical structure and functions of larynx:** The larynx is formed of a cartilaginous skeleton. It is held together by ligaments and membranes. The larynx is composed of the following main parts: Three large unpaired cartilages: Cricoid, thyroid, and epiglottis. Three pairs of smaller cartilages: Arytenoids, corniculate, cuneiform. In addition to that it contains, epiglottis and intrinsic muscles. The laryngeal muscles play very important role in the movement of the components of the larynx for phonation and breathing. The internal cavity of the larynx can be divided into the following three sections:
   1. Supraglottis: It extends from the inferior surface of the epiglottis to the vestibular folds.
   2. Glottis: It contains vocal cords.
   3. Subglottis: It extends from inferior border of the glottis to the inferior border of the cricoid cartilage.

The interior surface of the larynx is lined by pseudostratified ciliated columnar epithelium. The true vocal cords are lined by a stratified squamous epithelium.

The portion of the cavity of the larynx above the vocal folds is the laryngeal vestibule, which provides protection to the larynx.

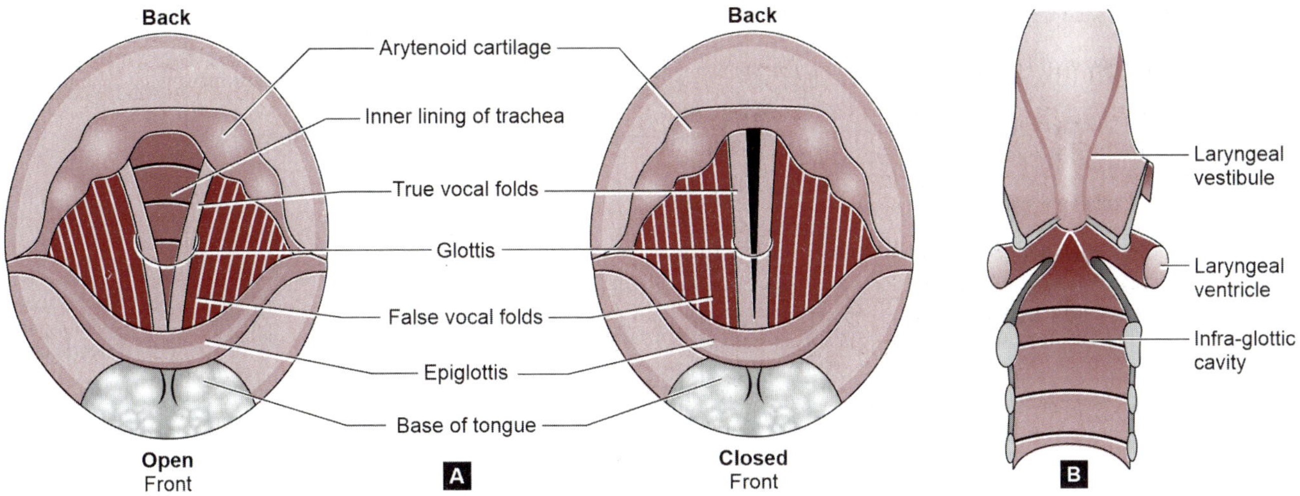

Figs 11.8A and B: (A) True vocal cord, made up of left and right muscle tissues; (B) laryngeal vestibule

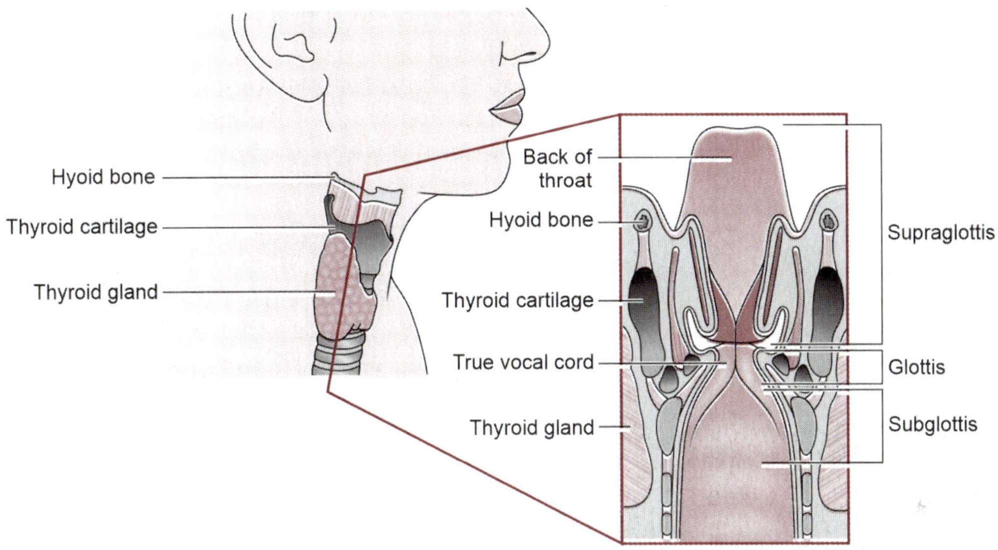

Fig. 11.9: Anatomy of larynx

The ventricular folds, located just above the vocal cords are false vocal cords. The false vocal cords divide the laryngeal vestibule. They function to protect the airway and do not play any role in phonation process.

Blood Supply of Larynx (Fig. 11.10)

3. **Blood supply of larynx:** The superior and inferior laryngeal arteries supply arterial blood to the larynx. Blood supply to the larynx is obtained from the external carotid and subclavian arteries. The external carotid gives rise to the superior thyroid artery, which bifurcates, forming the superior laryngeal artery.

The superior and inferior laryngeal veins carry venous blood.

The venous blood circulation of the larynx is through the inferior, middle, and superior thyroid veins. The middle and superior thyroid veins empty into the internal jugular vein.

Nerve Connections of Larynx (Fig. 11.11)

4. **Nerve connections of the larynx:** The larynx receives both motor and sensory nerve branches of the vagus nerve. The recurrent laryngeal nerve (RLN) branches off the vagus nerve and it supplies innervation to all of the deeply situated (intrinsic) muscles of the larynx, except for the cricothyroid muscles.

Superior laryngeal nerve provides sensory nerves to the upper part of larynx, and the external branch provides motor nerves to the cricothyroid muscle.

BAQ: Write a note on cough reflux?

Ans: Irritations due to foreign materials in the larynx trigger impulses. These impulses travel through the internal laryngeal nerve to the vagus nerve and then to the medulla of the brain and then cough reflux occurs.

Pulmonary cough receptors in the epithelium of the respiratory tract are sensitive to both mechanical and chemical stimuli. The bronchi and trachea are sensitive to small amounts of irritating foreign matter, that initiate the cough reflex, which plays important role in the removal of foreign material from the respiratory tract, before it reaches the lungs.

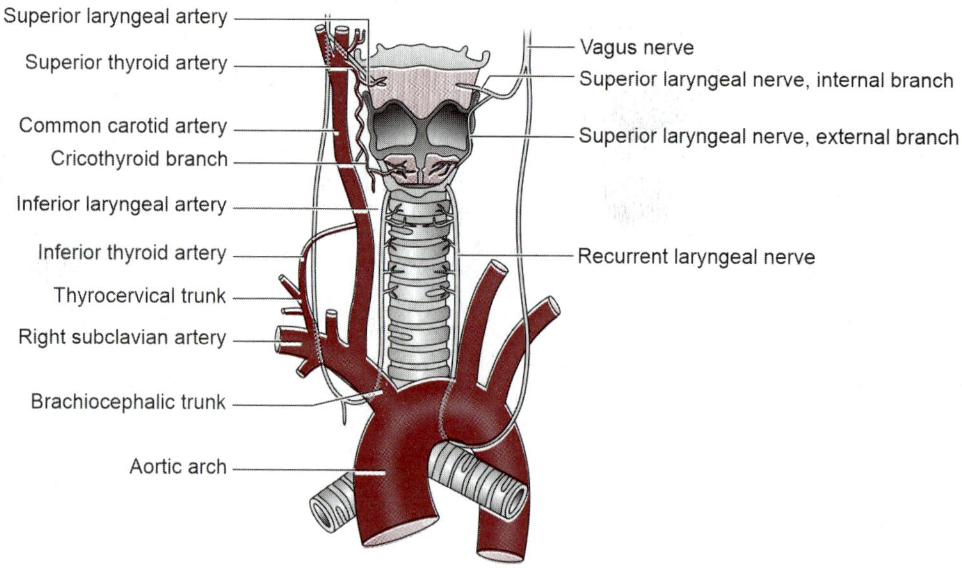

Fig. 11.10A: Arterial blood supply of the larynx

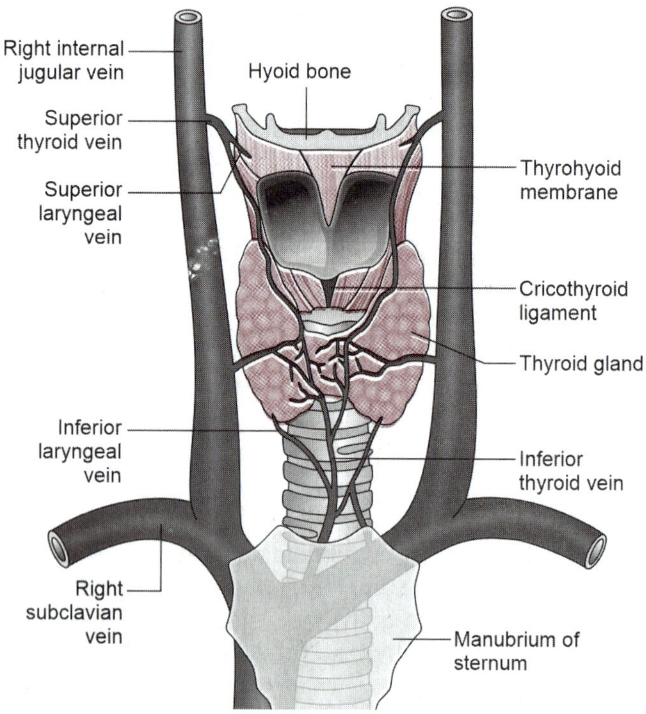

Fig. 11.10B: Venous drainage of the larynx

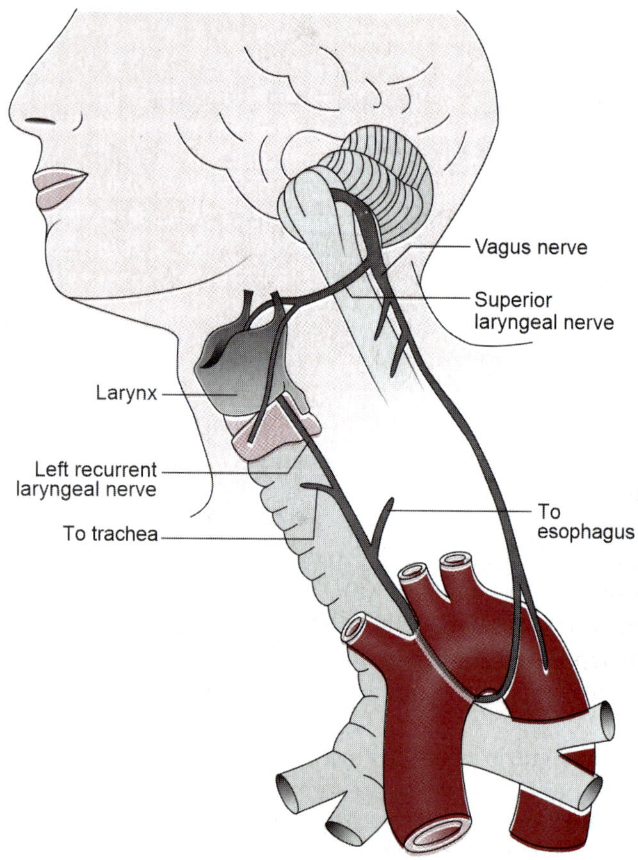

Fig. 11.11: Nerve supply of the larynx

SAQ: What is recurrent laryngeal nerve (RLN) palsy?

Ans: The vocal cords are responsible for the production of speech. Their movement is controlled by the intrinsic muscles of the larynx, mostly innervated by the recurrent laryngeal nerve (RLN). The RLN is susceptible to damage leading to RLN palsy, which result in voice changes or hoarseness. Various causes of RLN palsy include viral infections, nerve damage during surgery, thyroid cancer and certain other types of cancers.

Trachea (Windpipe)

BAQ: Write a note on the trachea.

Ans: The trachea is a tube-like structure. It is average, 3.9–4.3 inches long and 0.6–0.8 inch in diameter (Fig. 11.12A). The trachea begins just under the larynx and runs down behind the sternum bone (breastbone). The trachea then divides into two smaller tubes called bronchi. Each bronchus connects the lungs (Fig. 11.1).

The trachea transports air into the lungs and out of lungs during breathing process.

BAQ: Draw a labelled diagram of trachea.

Ans: Refer to Fig. 11.12B.

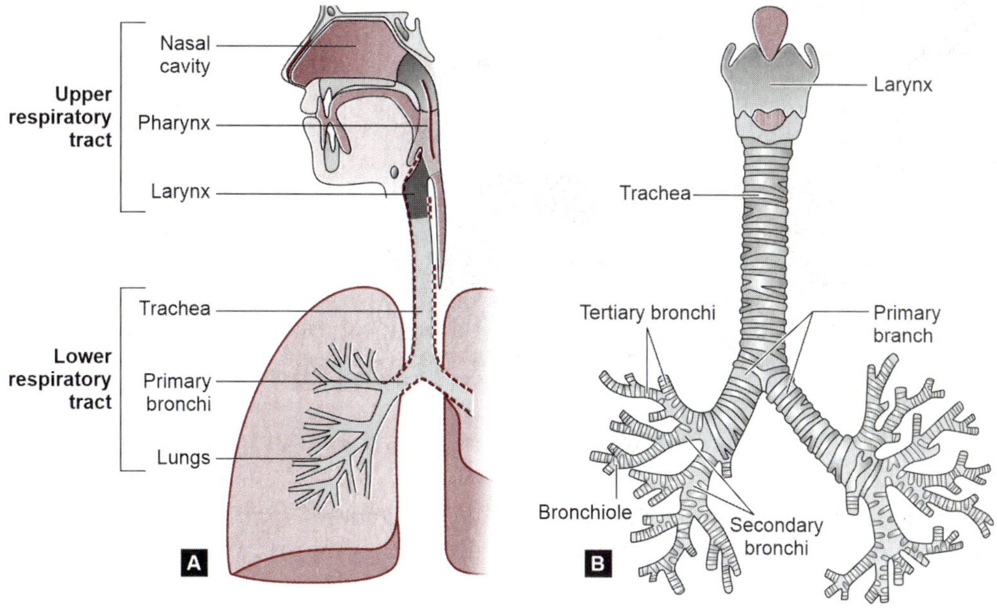

Figs 11.12A and B: Trachea and its position in the respiratory tract

> **Objective:** To describe the basic components and functions of the lungs to describe the blood supply and innervation to the lungs.

LUNGS (Fig. 11.13)

LAQ: Describe the lungs under the following heads: (1) Introduction, (2) applied anatomy and related functions, (3) blood supply and (4) nerve supply.

Ans: 1. **Introduction:** The lungs are a pair of spongy organs located on either side of the chest (thorax). These are the major organs of the respiratory system. A lung is divided into lobes. The left lung has two lobes. The right lung is comparatively larger than left lung and it has three lobes. The lungs are made up of pseudostratified ciliated columnar epithelium. The connective tissue contains cells and extracellular matter. Collagen and elastic fibers of lung tissue play important role in the mechanical activities of the lungs. The lungs are separated by the mediastinum, which contains the trachea, esophagus, many lymph nodes and the heart (Fig. 11.14).

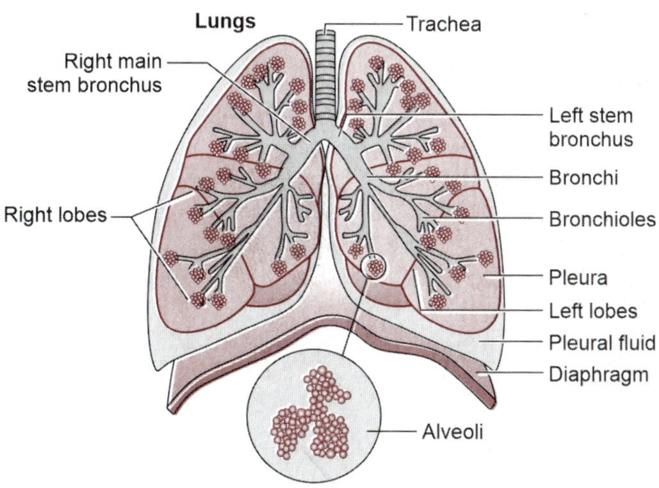

Fig. 11.13: Anatomical features of the lungs

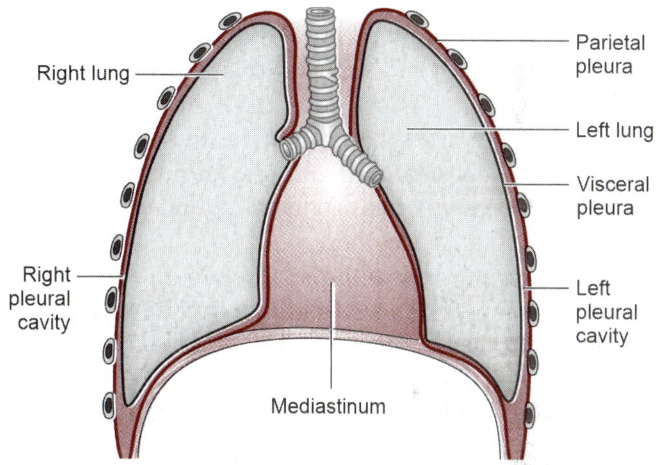

Fig. 11.14: Mediastinum region of the lungs

Parts of the Lungs (Fig. 11.13)

2. **Applied anatomy and related functions:** The following are the various parts of the lungs and their respective functions:
   A. *Bronchial tubes:* These are tubes at the bottom of windpipe that connect into each lung (Fig. 11.13).
   B. *Muscles and bones:* These help to move the inspired air into the lungs and expired air out of the lungs. The diaphragm is a muscle that helps lungs to pull air in and push it out and ribs are the bones that surround and protect the lungs and the heart (Fig. 11.13).
   C. *Tracheobronchial tree:* It is a branching structure of tubes of an ever-decreasing diameter that start at the larynx and end in the alveoli. It can broadly be divided into conduction and respiratory zones.
   Conduction zone: It is composed of the trachea, bronchi, bronchioles and terminal bronchioles. Their function is to optimise gas delivery to the functional portion of the lung. The walls of the conduction zone parts contain cilia to remove

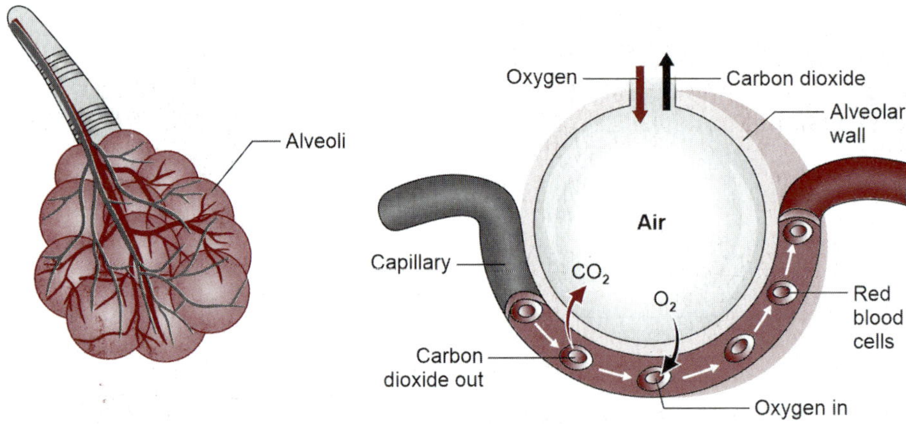

Fig. 11.15: Blood capillaries in the alveoli and gas exchange

particulates from the inspired gas and cartilages to ensure that they do not collapse during expiration process.

Respiratory zone: The respiratory zone is an extension of the tracheobronchial tree at the level of the terminal bronchioles. It is composed of respiratory bronchioles, alveolar ducts and alveoli, and it is the location of gas transfer within the lung.

D. *Bronchioles:* These are small branches of the bronchial tubes that lead to the alveoli (Fig. 11.14).

E. *Alveoli:* These are tiny air sacs in the lungs where the exchange of oxygen and carbon dioxide takes place (Fig. 11.15).

3. **Blood supply of the lungs:** The blood capillaries in the alveoli walls are responsible to move oxygen in the body and carbon dioxide out of the body (Fig. 11.15).
Pulmonary blood circulation (Fig. 11.16): The lungs have blood supply by bronchial circulation and by pulmonary circulation. The bronchial circulation supplies oxygenated blood to the airways of the lungs, by means of the bronchial arteries, which leave the aorta. The pulmonary circulation carries deoxygenated blood from the heart to the lungs and from the lung returns the oxygenated blood to the heart, which supplies it to the rest of the body.
4. **Pulmonary nerve supply** (Fig. 11.17): The vagus nerve connects the lungs through a small nerve plexus. The nerves of the pulmonary plexuses are important component of sympathetic, parasympathetic and visceral afferent fibres.

BAQ: What is pleura and its functions?

Ans: The pleura (Fig. 11.14) is a thin sac that surrounds each lung lobe and separates lungs from the chest wall. It is a serous membrane that form a membranous pleural sac of two layers. The outer layer is called the parietal pleura, which is attached to the chest wall. The inner layer is called the visceral pleura, which covers the lungs, blood vessels, nerves, and bronchi. Pleural fluid is present between the space in pleura membrane. Normal average quantity of pleural fluid is about 10–15 ml.

Function: Pleural fluid lubricates the space between the pleura and allow the pleura to glide smoothly during exhalation and inhalation.

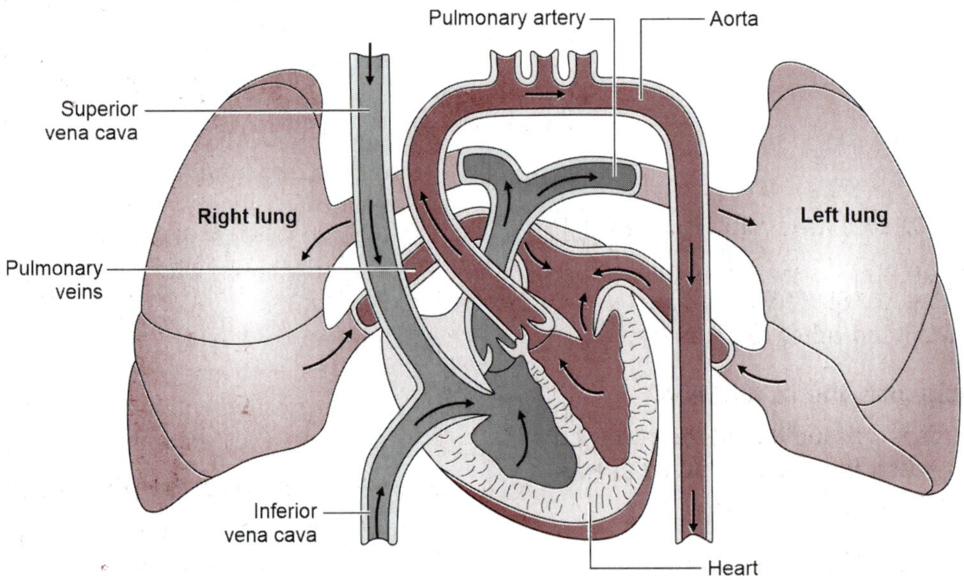

Fig. 11.16: Pulmonary blood circulation

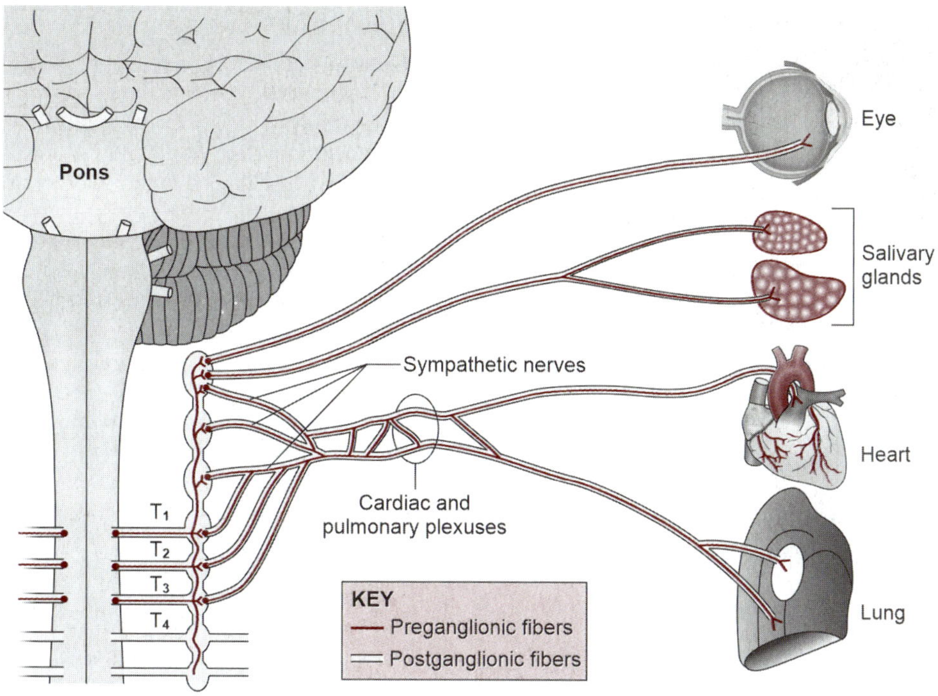

Fig. 11.17: Pulmonary nerve supply

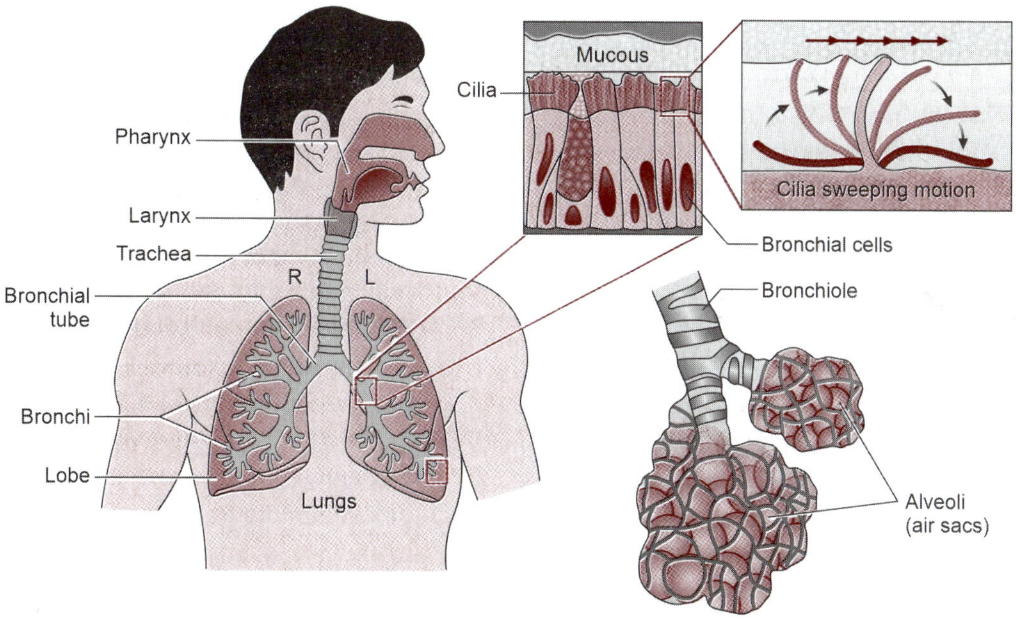

Fig. 11.18: Cilia in lungs and their sweeping motion

SAQ: What are cilia and their functions in the lungs?

Ans: Cilia are tiny hairs on the surface of the cells of the bronchial wall (Fig. 11.18). These move in a wave-like motion to filter dust and other irritants out of airways.

SAQ: What is epiglottis and its function.

Ans: The epiglottis is a tissue flap at the entrance to the trachea. It closes when food is swallowed to keep food and liquids out of airway (Fig. 11.19).

BAQ: Draw a labelled diagram of lungs.

Ans: Refer to Fig. 11.13.

Objectives: To define respiration and describe the physiology of respiration. To describe the exchange of gases in the lungs. To describe the role of respiratory system in the acid–base balance. To describe the transport of gases between the lungs and the cells.

PHYSIOLOGY OF RESPIRATION

LAQ: Write a note on the physiology of respiration.

Ans: The main function of the respiratory system is the respiration process. Respiration is the introduction of oxygen in lungs by inspiration from the external

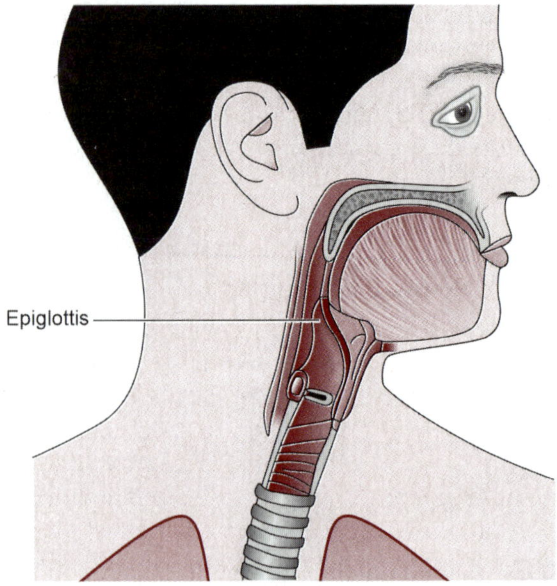

Fig. 11.19: Epiglottis

environment to the cells within the lung tissues and blood, and the removal of carbon dioxide produced in cellular metabolic activities, out of the body by expiration. The cells of the body need oxygen for the metabolic activities to produce energy in the form of ATPs, to remain alive. Similarly, it is also necessary to remove carbon dioxide to maintain acid–base balance and normal pH of the blood (Figs 7.38–7.42).

During inhalation process, the diaphragm moves downward toward the abdomen and the rib muscles pull the ribs upward. In this process the chest cavity increases and external air pushes through the nose or mouth into the lungs.

In exhalation process, the diaphragm moves upward and the chest wall muscles relax. In this process the chest cavity become smaller and push air out of the respiratory system through the nose or mouth.

About average 400 millions of alveoli are present per lung. With each inhalation, air fills a large portion of the alveoli. When the gases of the inspired air come in contact with the alveolar membrane of the lung, the exchange of gases takes place in accordance with the usual physical laws of diffusion. It is illustrated as follows: (The gas pressures in the blood are usually expressed as gas tensions.)

1. Oxygen tension in alveolar air: 107 mm Hg
2. Oxygen tension in venous blood: 40 mm Hg

   A pressure difference of 67 mm Hg serves to drive oxygen from alveoli of the lung into the blood.

   At the same time, when carbon dioxide passes into the alveoli.
3. CO_2 tension in alveolar air: 36 mm Hg
4. CO_2 tension in venous blood: 46 mm Hg

The difference of 10 mm Hg is sufficient to drive CO_2 from the blood into the lungs.

The carbon dioxide then passes out of the body in expired air.

> ***Note:***
> 1. Networks of neurons in the hindbrain (the pons and medulla) are responsible for breathing, which is an automatic and rhythmic act.
> 2. Respiratory system has ability to adjust breathing patterns according to changes in the internal as well as the external environment.
> 3. The pH of peripheral blood, measured as the pH of plasma in contact with red cells is normally within the range 7.36–7.42. Arterial blood (pH 7.40) is more alkaline than venous blood (pH 7.37).
> 4. On a mixed diet the metabolic processes cause an overall production of acids. The body contains buffering mechanisms. After intermediate buffering in the cells, final compensation for any change in the hydrogen ion concentration of the extracellular fluid is performed by lungs and kidneys.
> 5. The carbon dioxide formed in the metabolic reactions exists in blood in three main fractions (1) as small amount of carbonic acid (carbon dioxide dissolved in water), (2) the carbamino bound fraction transported in combination with protein (mainly hemoglobin) and (3) that carried as bicarbonate in combination with the cations, sodium and potassium.
> 6. It is estimated that in 24 hours the lungs remove equivalent of 20–40 liters of IN acid as carbonic acid from the circulated venous blood, with the help of the enzyme carbonic anhydrase which converts carbonic acid into carbon dioxide and water.

Diffusion of Gases in the Lungs

When the gases of the inspired air come in contact with the alveolar membrane of the lung, it is assumed that the exchange of gases takes place in accordance with the usual physical laws of diffusion. It is illustrated as follows: (The gas pressures in the blood are usually expressed as gas tensions).

1. Oxygen tension in alveolar air: 107 mm Hg
2. Oxygen tension in venous blood: 40 mm Hg

   A pressure difference of 67 mm Hg serves to drive oxygen from alveoli of the lung into the blood.
3. CO_2 tension in alveolar air: 36 mm Hg
4. CO_2 tension in venous blood: 46 mm Hg

The difference of 10 mm Hg is sufficient to drive CO_2 from the blood into the lungs. CO_2 and water vapors are expelled in expired air. After this exchange of gases has occurred, the blood becomes arterial (in the chemical sense).

At the normal pH of blood (7.40), a ratio of 20:1 must exist between the bicarbonate and carbonic acid fractions. Any change in 'H' ion activity will be met by an adjustment in the reaction. As long as this ratio is maintained the blood pH will be normal. This is maintained mainly by the following buffering system in blood

1. Carbonic acid-bicarbonate
2. Dihydrogen phosphate-monohydrogen phosphate
3. Protein proteinate
4. Hemoglobin in the red blood cells also plays important role in maintaining of the acid–base balance.

Objective: To describe the general infections of the respiratory tract.

RESPIRATORY TRACT INFECTIONS (RTIs)

SAQ: Write a note on respiratory tract infections (RTIs).

Ans: Respiratory tract infections (RTIs) are a number of infectious diseases, that involve the respiratory tract. RTIs are infections of the nose, sinuses, throat, airways and lungs. These are usually caused by viruses, bacteria and fungi. Respiratory tract infections can be further classified as upper respiratory tract infections (URTIs) or lower respiratory tract infections (LRTIs).

Upper Respiratory Tract Infections

BAQ: Write a note on upper respiratory tract infections (URIS).

Ans: The upper respiratory tract is generally considered to be the airway above the glottis or vocal cords. This includes the nose, sinuses, pharynx, and larynx. Typical infections of the upper respiratory tract include tonsillitis, pharyngitis, laryngitis, sinusitis, and otitis media. Symptoms of URIs can include cough, nasal congestion, headache, sore throat, runny nose, low grade fever, sneezing and increased facial pressure.

A throat infection (pharyngitis) can be mainly a viral or a bacterial infection leading to inflammation of the tissues of the throat that causes redness, pain and swelling of the walls or structures of the throat. Infective agents of the throat most often enter through the mouth or nose. Symptoms of throat infection most commonly include pain in the throat. The infection may also affect other structures within the throat, in particular the tonsils with swollen lymph nodes in the neck. Symptoms can range from mild to severe and may be accompanied by flu like symptoms such as fever, cough, congestion, and body ache.

Viral infections of throat comprise about 40–80% of all infectious cases and can be caused by many different types of viruses such as corona viruses, respiratory syncytial virus, parainfluenza virus, etc.

Different types of bacteria may infect the throat. The most common is Group A streptococcus and others include *Streptococcus pneumoniae*, *Corynebacterium diphtheriae*, etc. Fungi such as Aspergillus sp. also infects upper respiratory tract.

Lower Respiratory Tract Infections

BAQ: Write a note on lower respiratory tract infections (LRTIs).

Ans: The lower respiratory tract consists of the trachea (wind pipe), bronchial tubes, the bronchioles, and the lungs. Lower respiratory tract infections are generally more serious than upper respiratory infections. LRTIs are the leading cause of death among all infectious diseases. The more common LRTIs are bronchitis, pneumonia and tuberculosis. Influenza virus affects both the upper and lower respiratory tracts, however, more dangerous viruses such as SARS CoV1, Middle East Respiratory Syndrome (MERS) Virus and SARS CoV2, tend to bind to receptors deep in the lungs and cause life-threatening pneumonia.

Tuberculosis (TB)

BAQ: Write a note on tuberculosis.

Ans: Tuberculosis (TB) is caused by the bacteria, *Mycobacterium tuberculosis*. Although, *Mycobacterium tuberculosis*, can infect any part of the body, it mainly affects lungs. Most TB infections do not show symptoms. These type of TB infections are known as latent tuberculosis. However, latent infections may progress to active disease. The following are typical symptoms of active TB: Chronic cough, fever, chest pain, thick and sticky sputum, weight loss and night sweats. Tuberculosis spreads from one person suffering from active TB to another person by their actions such as coughing, sneezing, spitting, etc. The air around an active TB patient may carry air droplet with TB organisms. Number of drug-resistant cases are on increase in India.

Obstructive Lung Diseases

SAQ: What are obstructive lung diseases?

Ans: The obstructive lung diseases cause airway obstruction. In obstructive lung diseases bronchioles and bronchi of lungs become narrow due to inflammation and presence of excessive mucus, leading to difficulty in exhalation. The following are various types of obstructive lung diseases: Asthma, bronchiectasis, bronchitis, chronic obstructive pulmonary disease (COPD) and cystic fibrosis.

Asthma (Fig. 11.20)

BAQ: Write a note on asthma.

Ans: Asthma is an obstructive lung disease. In asthma, the airways become inflamed and produce excess mucus and the muscles around the airways become narrow (Fig. 11.20). Asthma is usually triggered by breathing in substances such as dust or pollen grains that produce an allergic reaction in certain persons. It may be triggered by other substances such as an upper respiratory tract infection, cold air, exercise or smoke. Asthma leads to recurring episodes of breathlessness, chest tightness, wheezing, and coughing, particularly at night or in the early morning.

Chronic Obstructive Pulmonary Disease (COPD) (Fig. 11.21)

BAQ: Write a note on chronic obstructive pulmonary disease (COPD).

Ans: Chronic obstructive pulmonary disease (COPD) is caused by long-term exposure to cigarette smoke,

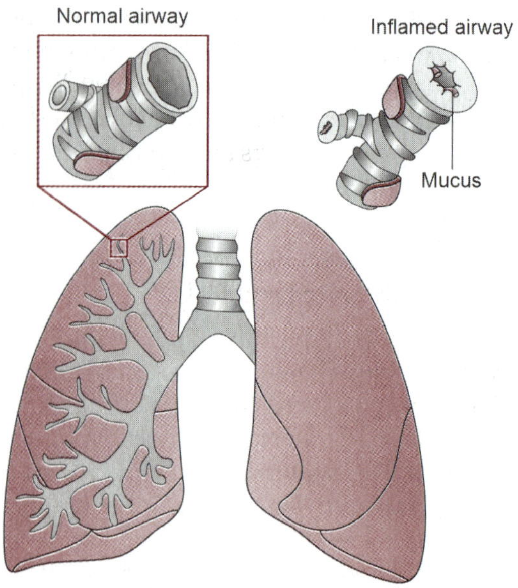

Fig. 11.20: Narrow air way in asthma (RHS)

polluted air particulate matter, and toxic gases (Fig. 11.20). Chronic bronchitis and emphysema are the two most common conditions that lead to COPD. Chronic bronchitis is inflammation of the lining of the bronchial tubes. Emphysema is a clinical condition in which the air spaces in bronchioles and alveoli of the lungs get significantly increased and subsequently get severely damaged. COPD is characterized by cough and excessive mucus production. In chronic obstructive pulmonary disease (COPD), the flow of air into and out of the lungs is impaired (Fig. 11.21).

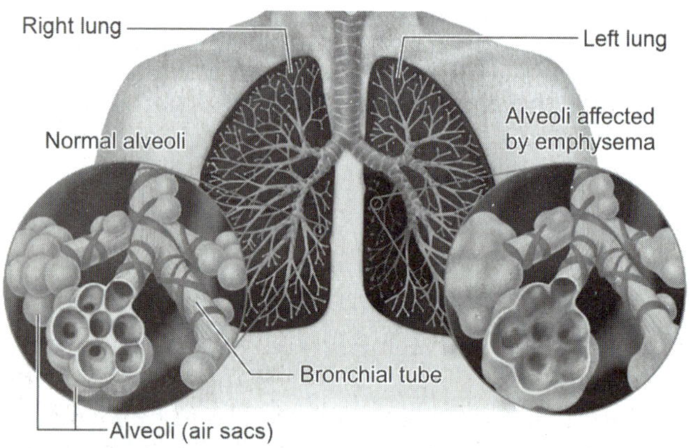

Fig. 11.21: Affected alveoli in chronic obstructive pulmonary disease (COPD)

Bronchitis (Fig. 11.22)

SAQ: Write a note on bronchitis.

Ans: Bronchitis is an inflammation of the bronchial tubes, due to bacterial, viral, fungal infections, or due to allergic reactions. It causes cough, that often brings up mucus. It can also cause shortness of breath, wheezing, fever, and chest tightness. There are two main types of bronchitis, acute bronchitis and chronic bronchitis. Acute bronchitis is characterized by sudden attack of persistent cough, with or without sputum production. It usually resolves spontaneously in over 1–3 weeks. The underlying cause may be a viral infection. Chronic bronchitis is a type of chronic obstructive pulmonary disease (COPD). It is characterised with the productive cough (with mucous). Chronic bronchitis causes long-term respiratory symptoms and airflow limitations.

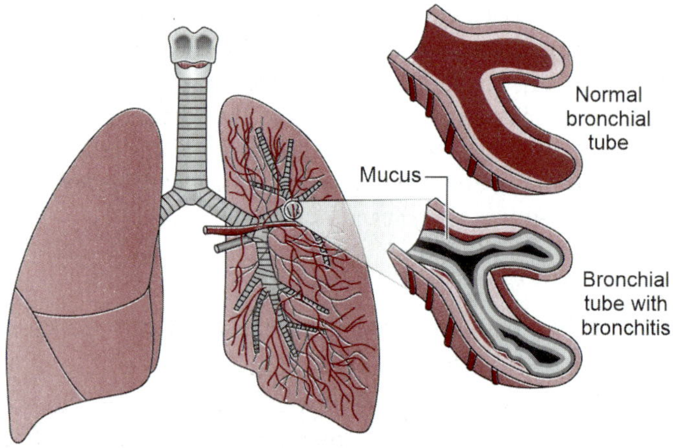

Fig. 11.22: Bronchial tube in bronchitis

Bronchiolitis (Fig. 11.23)

BAQ: Write a note on bronchiolitis.

Ans: Bronchiolitis is caused due to the infection of the bronchioles. Bronchiolitis is mainly an infection caused by respiratory viruses. It is a common lung infection observed in young children and infants. It causes inflammation and congestion in bronchioles (the small airways) of the lung (Fig. 11.22). The peak time of bronchiolitis is mainly observed during the months of winter season.

Bronchiectasis (Fig. 11.24)

BAQ: Write a note on bronchiectasis.

Ans: In bronchiectasis disease there is permanent enlargement of parts of the airways of the lung (Fig. 11.23). It may result from prolonged infectious state caused by pneumonia, tuberculosis, immune system disorders, and genetic disorder like cystic fibrosis.

Bronchiectasis is a chronic condition in which the bronchi become damaged and abnormally widened from recurring infection and related inflammation. Common symptoms of bronchiectasis are chronic cough that produces mucus, breathlessness, wheezing and fatigue.

BAQ: What is the difference between COPD and bronchiectasis?

Ans: The following is the difference between COPD and Bronchiectasis: Bronchiectasis is caused by consistent inflammation caused by irritants or infection in the lungs. However, most COPD conditions result from smoking, air pollution and allergies. Bronchiectasis may be irreversible in adults, while COPD severity may be reduced by appropriate treatment.

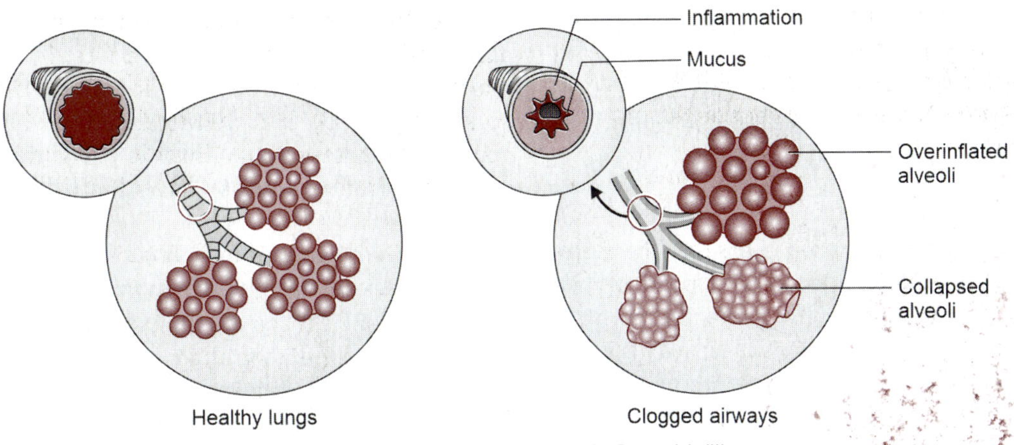

Fig. 11.23: Clogged air ways in Bronchiolitis

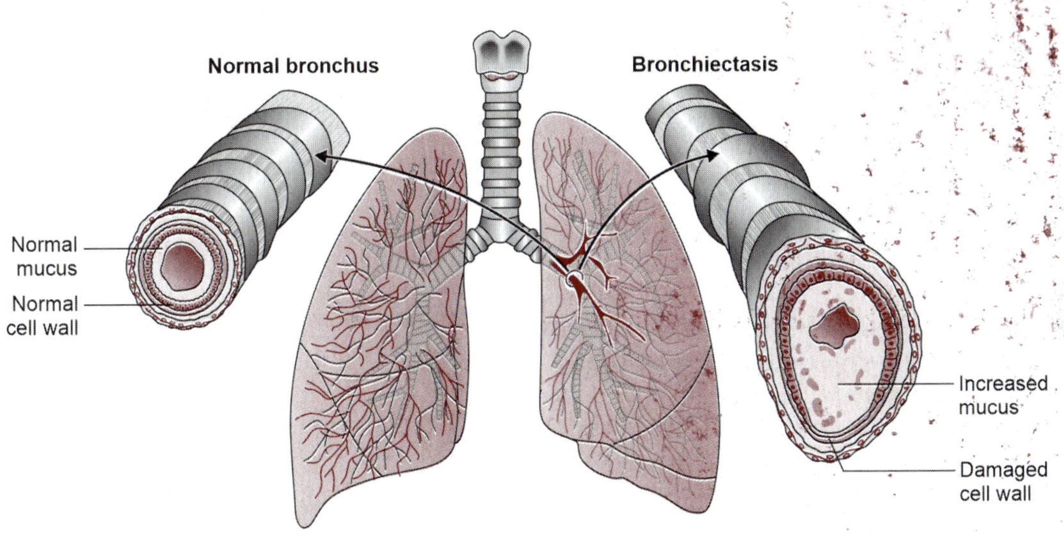

Fig. 11.24: Increased air ways in bronchiectasis

COVID-19

The COVID-19 is coronavirus disease caused by severe acute respiratory syndrome coronavirus 2 (SARS-CoV-2). The 2019 **Novel coronavirus (SARS-CoV-2)** affected about 216 countries in the world.

The virus spreads from one person to another person through small droplets formed while coughing or sneezing by a patient. It spreads when persons are close to each other and also when a person touches a surface with the virus, and then his face.

The time between when a person is exposed to the virus and when symptoms first appear is typically 5 to 6 days. It may range from 2 to 14 days. Hence, a person who might have been in contact with a confirmed case is instructed to self-isolate for 14 days.

Coronaviruses infected host respiratory cells. The cell damage triggers the production of inflammatory mediators, which increase nasal secretion and cause local inflammation and swelling. These responses in turn stimulate sneezing, obstruct the airway, and raise the temperature of the mucosa and body.

Increase in large amount of immune response may lead to **Cytokine storm**, which leads to large amount of fluid accumulates in the lung tissue. Lung alveoli are not able to exchange the gases in normal proportion, oxygen in inspired air and carbon dioxide in expired air and that leads to increase in CO_2 in blood and decrease in blood oxygen, leading to "acute respiratory distress syndrome" (ARDS), which is the reason to patients have breathing difficulty and chest pain.

Pneumonia

Pneumonia is an infection of the lungs that can cause mild to severe illness in people of all ages. It is the leading cause of death due to infection in children younger than 5 years of age worldwide. The following categories are at high risk for pneumonia: Immunocompromised individuals, children, older adults, and individuals with underlying health problems, such as diabetes mellitus, cancer, AIDs, etc.

Pneumonia can be caused by bacteria, viruses, or fungi. Bacterial pneumonia is the most common type in adults. Pneumonia causes inflammation in alveoli. When alveoli get filled with fluid or pus there is difficulty in breathing.

Signs and symptoms: The signs and symptoms of pneumonia may include, productive cough, which may produce greenish, yellow or even bloody mucus, rapid and shallow breathing, chest pain that gets worse when patient breathe deeply or cough, fever, sweating and shaking chills, loss of appetite, low energy, and fatigue.

The signs and symptoms of pneumonia vary from mild to severe, depending on factors such as the type of infection, patient's age and overall health. Mild signs and symptoms often are similar to those of a cold or flu, but they last longer.

Cystic Fibrosis (CF)

Cystic fibrosis (CF) is an inherited disorder. The cells of the persons suffering from cystic fibrosis produce thick and sticky mucus. Instead of acting as a lubricant, the thick mucus secretions tend to plug the air way passages of lungs and the ducts of the organs such as pancreas, small intestine, liver and kidneys.

Patients suffering from long-term CF suffer from difficulty in breathing and coughing up mucus as a result of frequent lung infections. Other signs and symptoms observed in CF are frequent sinus infections, fatty stool, infertility in most males and poor growth. A supportive therapy is suggested to manage the CF patients.

Objective: To understand and explain the central theme of competency based medical and paramedical education (CBME): Horizontal and vertical integration of subjects.

BAQ: Show horizontal integration of physiology, and biochemistry with the following anatomical change: Inflammation of lung tissue and alveoli.

Ans:

Horizontal Integration with Physiology

Decreased rate of carbon dioxide expiration and low circulation of blood oxygen.

Horizontal Integration with Biochemistry

Significant decrease in blood pH, leading to respiratory acidosis.

BAQ: Show vertical integration of a patient suffering from severe pneumonia with respiratory acidosis with microbiology and pharmacology.

Ans:

Vertical Integration with Microbiology

Study of the microorganism that caused pneumonia.

Vertical Integration with Pharmacology

Study of appropriate drugs to treat lung infection and to clear the air way passage.

BAQ: Show horizontal integration of physiology, and biochemistry with the following anatomical change: Inflammation of alveoli (asthama).

Ans:

Horizontal Integration with Physiology

Difficulty in breathing procedure.

Horizontal Integration with Biochemistry

Difficulty in the normal rate of exchange of carbon dioxide and oxygen gases at the alveoli.

BIBLIOGRAPHY

1. Medical Biochemistry, 1st Edition (2023). Godkar PB, Godkar DP, CBS Publishers, New Delhi, India.
2. Text book of Medical Laboratory Technology, 4th Edition, (2024). Godkar PB, Godkar DP, Bhalani Publishing House, Mumbai, India.
3. Anatomy of the Human Body. 42nd Edition. Henry Gray, Editor-in-chief: Susan Standring, Elsevier (2020).
4. Ross and Wilson Anatomy and Physiology in Health and Illness, 13th Edition, by Allison Wynn Grant, Anne Waugh, and Kathleen J. W. Wilson (2018).
5. Schaum's outline of theory and problems of Human anatomy and Physiology, 2nd Edition (1997), Tata MaGraw-Hill Publishing Company Limited, New Delhi, India.

MULTIPLE CHOICE QUESTIONS (MCQs)

Select the correct option.

1. Each nasal cavity has the following main three regions:

(A) Nasal vestibule (B) Respiratory region
(C) Olfactory region (D) All of the above

2. The outer shape of the nasal tip does not have the following section(s):

(A) Medial crus (B) Middle crus
(C) Nasal vestibule (D) Lateral crus

3. The following one statement is not correct.

(A) The cavity of the nose is lined with mucous membranes.
(B) The mucous membrane does not contain smell receptors.
(C) The smell receptors are connected to the olfactory nerve.
(D) The smell receptors are sensitive to various types of smell sensations.

4. Nasal dysfunction leads to:

(A) Nasal congestion
(B) Sinus infections
(C) Postnasal drainage
(D) All of the above

5. Contraction of this combination of muscles causes inspiration:

(A) Internal–external intercostals
(B) External intercostal–diaphragm
(C) Diaphragm–abdominal complex
(D) Diaphragm–external intercostal

6. These cells in the alveolar air wall are responsible to remove foreign particles in inspired air:

(A) Alveolar macrophage cells
(B) Kupffer cells
(C) Surfactant cells
(D) Both (B) and (C)

7. **Increase in blood carbon dioxide leads to:**
   (A) Metabolic acidosis (B) Respiratory acidosis
   (C) Metabolic alkalosis (D) None of these
8. **After inspiration carbon dioxide is transported in blood as:**
   (A) Carbonic acid (B) Bicarbonate
   (C) Carboxyhemoglobin (D) Both (A) and (B)
9. **Adenoids and tonsils are present in:**
   (A) Nasopharynx (B) Oropharynx
   (C) Hypopharynx (D) Both (A) and (B)
10. **The following one statement regarding the larynx is not correct:**
    (A) The larynx is formed of a cartilaginous skeleton.
    (B) It is held together by ligaments and membranes.
    (C) The larynx is composed of the following main parts: Two large unpaired cartilages.
    (D) It contains, epiglottis and intrinsic muscles.
11. **The following one statement regarding the lungs is not correct:**
    (A) These are the major organs of the respiratory system.
    (B) A lung is divided into lobes.
    (C) The left lung has three lobes.
    (D) The right lung has three lobes.
12. **The respiratory zone of lungs is composed of:**
    (A) Bronchioles
    (B) Alveolar ducts
    (C) Alveoli
    (D) All of the above
13. **During inspiration:**
    (A) Oxygen tension in alveolar air is 107 mm Hg
    (B) Oxygen tension in venous blood 40 mm Hg
    (C) Oxygen tension in venous blood 140 mm Hg
    (D) Both (A) and (B)
14. **This is not a part of the lower respiratory tract:**
    (A) Larynx (B) Trachea
    (C) Bronchial tubes (D) Lungs
15. **This part of lungs is located between two pleural sacs and is the central compartment of the thoracic cavity:**
    (A) Hilum (B) Mediastinum
    (C) Thoracic cage (D) Pleura
16. **The following statement about carbon dioxide during inspiration is *not* correct:**
    (A) CO_2 tension in alveolar air is 36 mm Hg
    (B) CO_2 tension in venous blood air is 46 mm Hg
    (C) Oxygen tension in venous blood air is 135 mm Hg
    (D) Oxygen tension in alveolar blood air is 107 mm Hg
17. **In this part of the respiratory system, gaseous exchange takes place in the:**
    (A) Bronchi (B) Alveoli
    (C) Trachea (D) All of the avove
18. **This statement is correct about the involuntary breathing?**
    (A) It is controlled by the neurons, located in the medulla and pons
    (B) It is controlled by the bronchioles
    (C) It is controlled by the pulmonary arterioles
    (D) It is controlled by the alveolar-capillary network
19. **This part of the lungs performs the filtering of inspired air and keeping the dirt away from the lungs?**
    (A) Macrophages in the lungs (B) Cilia
    (C) Bronchioles (D) All of the above
20. **Which one of the following statements is false about the trachea?**
    (A) It has 3.9–4.3 inches diameter
    (B) It splits into the right and left lungs
    (C) It is also called windpipe
    (D) The trachea divides into two smaller tubes
21. **Which following statement is not correct regarding larynx?**
    (A) It does not contain the vocal cords
    (B) It prevents the invading pathogens into the trachea
    (C) It connects the pharynx to the trachea
    (D) All of the above
22. **Asthama may get triggered by:**
    (A) An upper respiratory tract infection
    (B) Cold air
    (C) Smoke
    (D) All of the above

ANSWERS

1. D 2. C 3. B 4. D 5. B 6. A 7. B
8. D 9. D 10. C 11. C 12. D 13. D 14. A
15. B 16. C 17. B 18. A 19. B 20. A 21. A
22. D

MATCH THE COLUMNS

I	II
1. Pharyngitis	A. Infection of alveoli
2. Nasal cavity	B. Inflammation of bronchial tubes
3. Pneumonia	C. Role in speaking
4. Nasal vestibule	D. Upper respiratory infection
5. Bronchiolitis	E. Permanent widening of airways
6. Uvula	F. Keeps food particles away from airways
7. Bronchiectasis	G. Infection of bronchioles
8. Epiglottis	H. Filters dust particles
9. Pons and medulla	I. Olfactory region
10. Bronchitis	J. Breathing action

ANSWERS

1. D 2. I 3. A 4. H 5. G 6. C 7. E
8. F 9. J 10. B

CHAPTER

12

Digestive System

SAQ: Short answer question: Marks: 2
BAQ: Brief answer question: Marks: 4 or 5
LAQ: Long answer question: Marks: 9 or 10
MCQs: Multiple choice questions: Marks: 0.5 each
Match the columns: Marks: 0.5 each
Draw a labelled diagram: Marks: 5

Objectives: To identify and describe the basic components and functions of the digestive system.

INTRODUCTION

BAQ: Write a brief note on the digestive system.

Ans: The digestive system consists of the gastrointestinal tract (GI) and the accessory organs of digestion (Fig. 12.1). The digestive system includes: (1) A tubular gastro-intestinal tract and (2) accessory digestive organs.

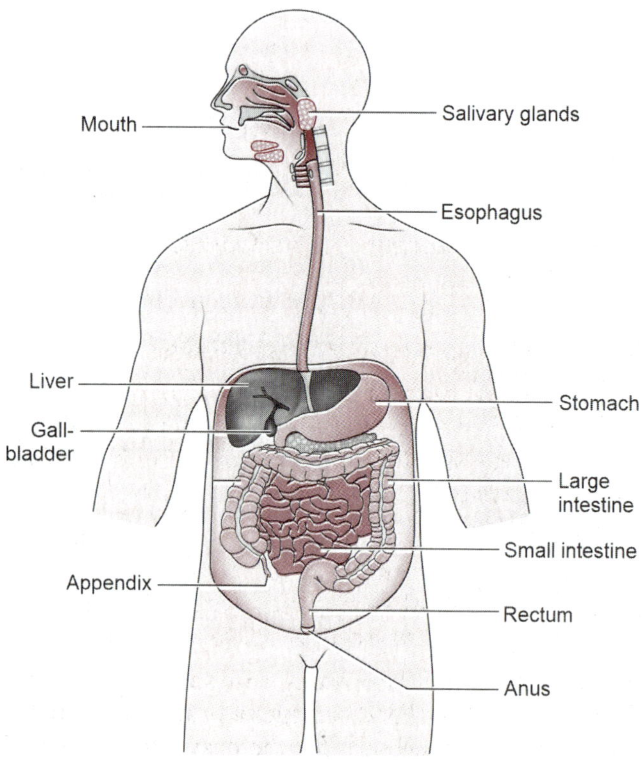

Fig. 12.1: Digestive system

The tubular gastrointestinal tract includes, the mouth, pharynx, esophagus, stomach, small intestine, large intestine, and anus. Accessory digestive organs are, the salivary glands, liver, gallbladder, and pancreas, which play very important role in digestion of food.

Upper GI organs are esophagus and stomach and lower GI organs are small intestine and large intestine.

The walls of the alimentary tract are formed of the following layers of tissues:

1. **Serosa (adventitia):** It is the outermost covering.
2. **Muscle layer:** It is mainly made up of smooth muscles. Tunica muscularis muscle provides the digestive tube the ability to remain motile during the food passage.
3. **Submucosa:** It is made up of loose areolar connective tissue. Blood vessels, lymph vessels, and nerves are present in this layer.
4. **Mucosa:** It is the lining of gastrointestinal tract.

The function of digestive system is to break food into very small components, which can be absorbed and assimilated into the body in useful form for the body cells, to derive energy for cellular metabolism and for growth purposes and repairing mechanisms.

In general, the passage of foods in gastrointestinal tract (GI) is a process comprised of: (1) Ingestions of food, (2) mastication (chewing) of food, (3) swallowing (deglutition) of food, (4) forward movement of food by peristalsis action of GI muscles, (5) digestion of food (6) absorption of food and (7) defecation of mainly waste materials.

SAQ: What is viscera and gut?

Ans: Viscera means abdominal organs, which perform digestion procedure and gut means GI tract.

SAQ: What is peritoneum and its function?

Ans: Abdominal organs are covered by a membrane called the peritoneum (Fig. 12.2). It supports the viscera, and provides pathways for blood vessels and lymph to pass to and the viscera.

SAQ: What are intraperitoneal organs?

Ans: Intraperitoneal organs are completely wrapped by visceral peritoneum. These organs are, the stomach, spleen, liver, superior part of the duodenum, jejunum, ileum, transverse colon, sigmoid colon and superior part of the rectum.

SAQ: Define digestion.

Ans: Digestion is the breakdown of large complex food components into very small components so that they can be absorbed in the gastrointestinal tract and then into the blood circulation and become available for the body cells for their metabolic reactions.

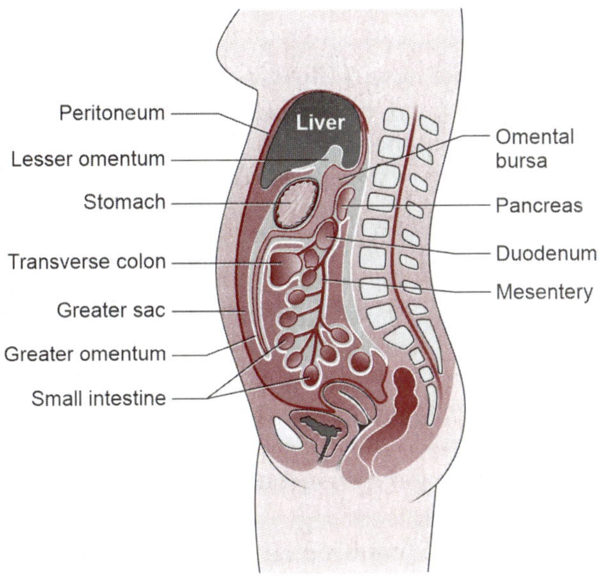

Fig. 12.2: Peritoneum covering the digestive system

> **Objectives:** To describe the anatomical structure and functions of various parts of the digestive system. To describe the various components of the mouth, teeth, oral cavity, pharynx and esophagus as parts of digestive system. To describe the various disorders related to the mouth, teeth, oral cavity, pharynx and esophagus.

MOUTH

SAQ: What are the components of the mouth and their general function?

Ans: The teeth, hard palate, soft palate, tongue and salivary glands are important components of the mouth. These mouth components play important role in the first step of digestion and ingestion of food in the gastrointestinal tract. Chewing (mastication) is the first step in the process of digestion (Fig. 12.3).

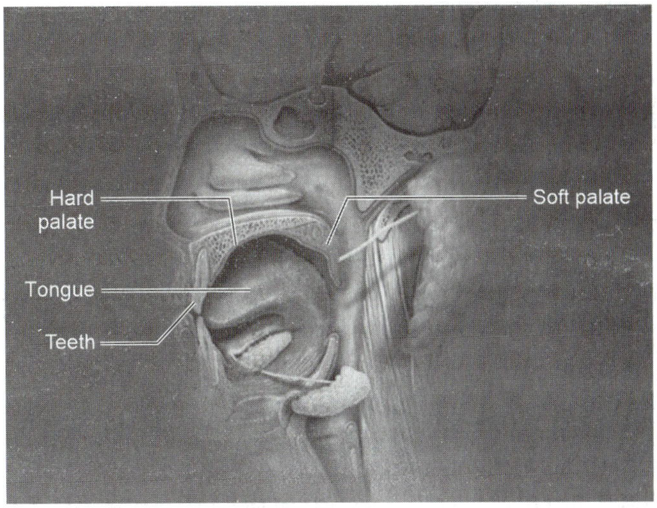

Fig. 12.3: Anatomical feature of the oral cavity

SAQ: Explain the role of the jawbones in the process of chewing.

Ans: The teeth grind food into small fragments due to the movement of the jaw. The jawbone (mandible) is the only bone in the head that moves, and the points where the temporal bones connect to the jawbone also are the only two movable joints in the head (Fig. 12.4).

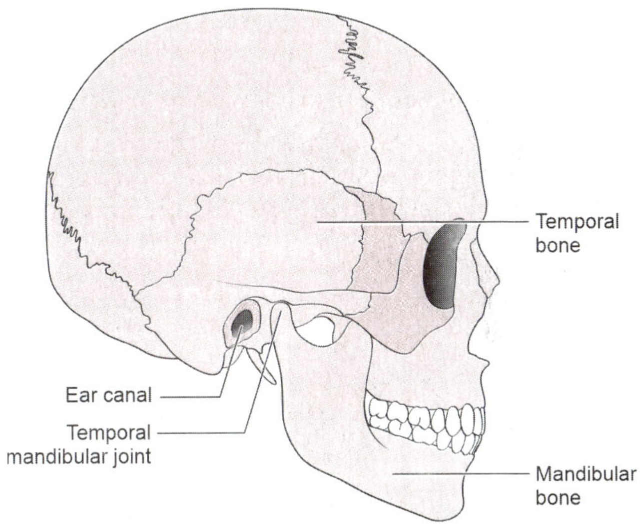

Fig. 12.4: Jawbones bones that facilitate chewing

SALIVARY GLANDS (Fig. 12.5A)

BAQ: Write a note on the salivary glands.

Ans: Salivary glands are present in the mouth (Fig. 12.5A). The following are three pairs of salivary glands: Parotid, sublingual, and submandibular (the submaxillary gland). These salivary glands secret saliva.

Saliva: It contains about 98% water, mucus and substances such as, mucus, electrolytes, white blood cells, antimicrobial antibodies (IgA), lysozymes, epithelial cells and enzymes (amylase and lipase).

Saliva functions: The mucus in saliva performs lubricating function. Food becomes wet and that initiates bolus formation necessary for the easy swallowing of food. Saliva plays important role in the sense of taste.

It also protects drying of the oral mucosa. Dry oral mucosa initiates microbial growth. Dry mouth also leads to bad breath. The saliva protects mouth cavity against microorganisms by means of antibodies and lysozymes. It clears food particles from teeth and reduces risk of formation of tooth cavities.

Saliva contains the following enzymes: Amylase (ptyalin) and lipase. Partial digestion of food takes place in the mouth due to these salivary enzymes. Salivary amylase acts on food starches to form simple sugars such as maltose and dextrins. Salivary lipase acts on food fats and fatty acids and glycerol are formed. Complete digestion of remaining food takes place in stomach and small intestine.

BAQ: Draw a neat and labelled diagram of the salivary glands.

Ans: Refer to Fig. 12.5A.

MUMPS

SAQ: Write a note on mumps.

Ans: Mumps is a viral disease caused by the mumps virus; which infect salivary glands. Inflammation of salivary glands takes place in mumps (Fig. 12.5B). Initial symptoms include difficulty in swallowing of food, headache, high fever, muscle pain, loss of appetite, and muscle pain. The treatment on mumps is supportive by using appropriate drugs to reduce high fever and pain and intake of plenty of fluids.

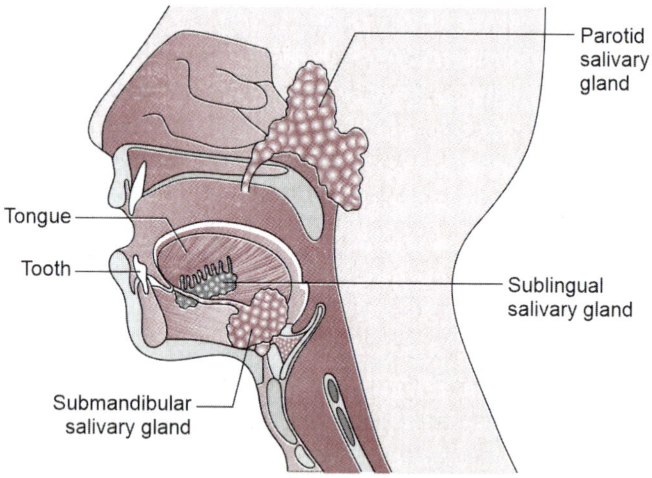

Fig. 12.5A: Salivary glands

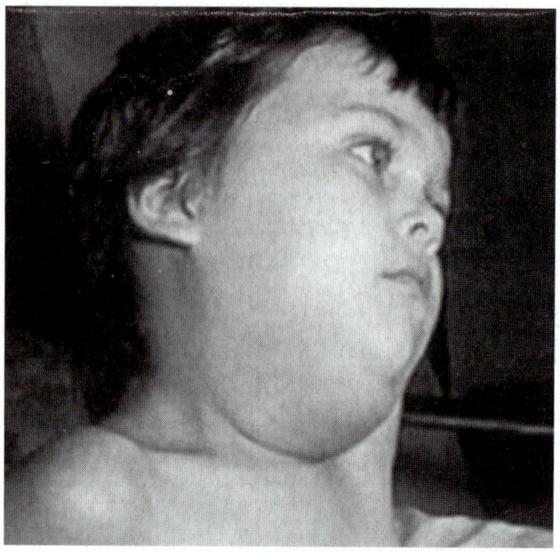

Fig. 12.5B: Swelling of throat due to mumps

TONGUE

BAQ: Write a note on the tongue.

Ans: Ref. Chapter 7, page 183.

SAQ. Write on the functions of the tongue as a part of the digestive system.

Ans: The tongue is useful to convert the chewed food into a small mass known as a bolus, which moves smoothly into the oropharynx. By involuntary action, the bolus passes through the pharynx and as the epiglottis closes off the trachea, the bolus is passed down the esophagus, and peristaltic waves move the bolus into the stomach (Fig. 12.6).

TEETH

SAQ: Write a brief note on the teeth and their functions.

Ans: Teeth are part of the digestive system. Teeth are the hardest component in the body. The function of teeth is to mechanically break down food by cutting and crushing actions so that food could be converted into bolus form, which is easy for swallowing and later on for digestion in the stomach and the intestine. With the lips and tongue, teeth play important role to form speech-words by controlling airflow out of the mouth.

Primary teeth or baby teeth start to appear around six months of age. The first set of primary teeth in the case of a normal baby contains 20 teeth by the age of three years. The baby teeth start to fall out during the years six to seven and adult teeth begin to grow. The adult teeth erupt by about 13 years of age, except wisdom teeth. A normal adult mouth contain 32 teeth. Wisdom teeth are the third and final set of molars that most adults get mainly in the early twenties.

BAQ: Describe the various types of teeth and their positions in the skull bones.

Ans: The following are four types of teeth: (1) Incisors, (2) canines, (3) premolars, and (4) molars. Each type of tooth performs a specific function. The incisors are used to cut the food. The canines are used to tear the food and the molars and premolars used to crush the food. The roots of teeth are embedded in the upper jaw (in the maxilla) and in the lower jaw (in the mandible), and these are covered by gums (Fig. 12.7).

SAQ: Write a brief note on primary (baby) teeth.

Ans: The primary teeth or baby teeth mainly start to appear around six months of age. The first set of primary teeth baby contains 20 teeth. These contain four second molars, four first molars, four cuspids (canine teeth), four

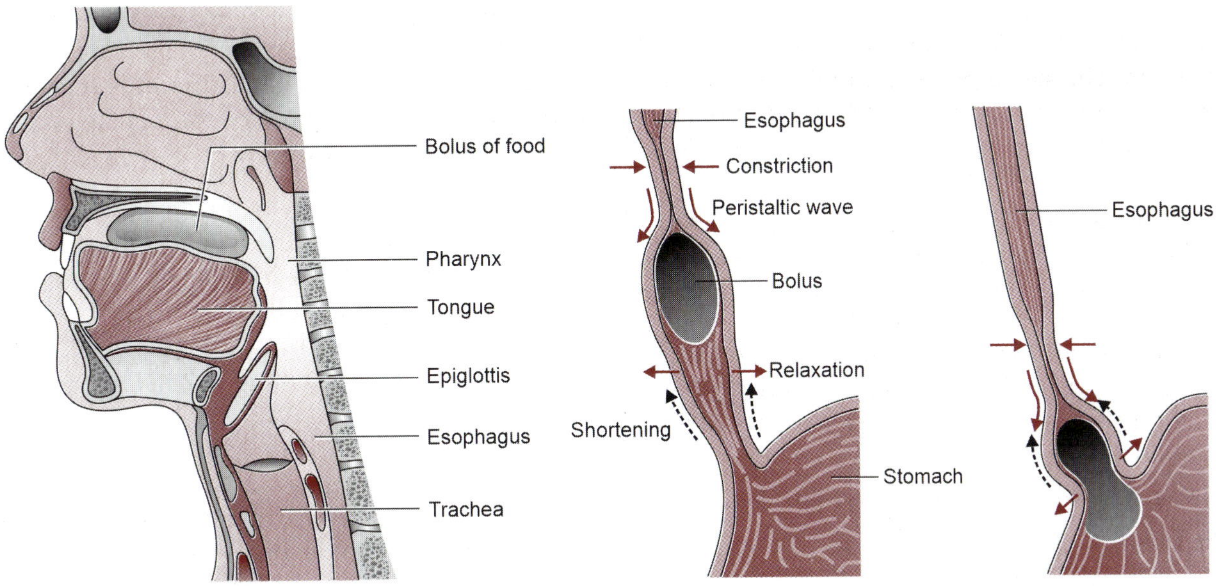

Fig. 12.6: Passage of bolus through esophagus

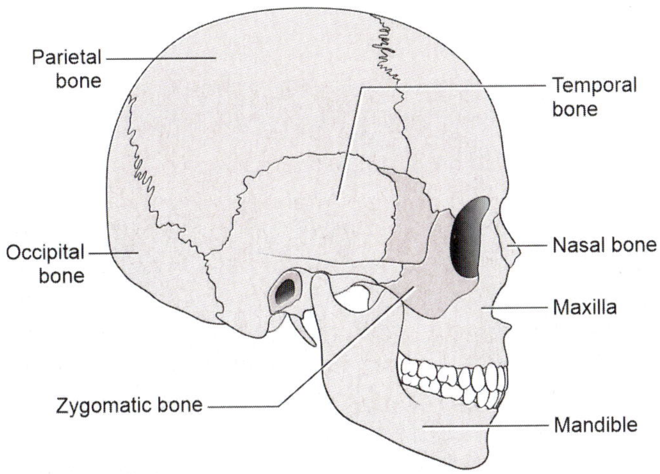

Fig. 12.7: Teeth position in the specific bones

lateral incisors and four central incisors. The baby teeth start to fall out during the years six to seven and adult teeth begin to grow. The adult teeth erupt by about 13 years of age, except wisdom teeth.

BAQ: Describe the important parts of tooth.

Ans: The following are important parts of the tooth (Fig. 12.8):

1. **Crown:** It is the top part of the tooth. The shape of the crown enables different functions. For example, incisors are sharp and are used for cutting food, while the molars have a flat surface for grinding the food (Fig. 12.8).
2. **Enamel:** It is the hardest, white outer part of the tooth. Enamel is mainly made up of calcium phosphate (Fig. 12.8).
3. **Dentin:** It is a layer underlying the enamel. It is a hard tissue, which contains microscopic tubes. If the enamel is damaged, heat or cold materials can enter the tooth through and cause irritation of nerves leading to pain (Fig. 12.8).
4. **Pulp:** It is the softer living inner structure of teeth. Blood vessels and nerves pass through the pulp of the teeth (Fig. 12.8).
5. **Cementum:** It is a layer of connective tissue that binds the roots of the teeth firmly to the gums and jawbone (Fig. 12.8).
6. **Periodontal ligament:** It is a tissue, which helps to hold the teeth tightly against the jaw (Fig. 12.9).
7. **Root:** It descends below the gum line and placed into the upper or lower jawbones. The toot anchors the tooth in the mouth. Different types of teeth have different number of roots. For example, incisors, canines and premolars have one root each, whereas, molars have two or three roots (Fig. 12.8).

> ***Note:*** Gumline is a line, where the gum and tooth meet (Fig. 12.10).

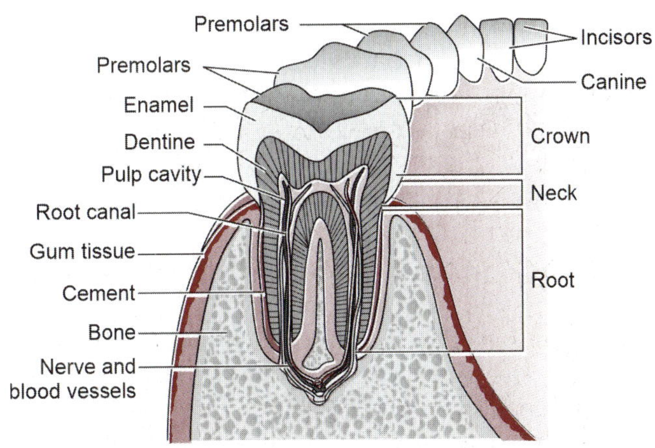

Fig. 12.8: Anatomical features of the tooth

BAQ: Draw a labelled diagram of anatomical features of a tooth.

Ans: Refer to Fig. 12.8.

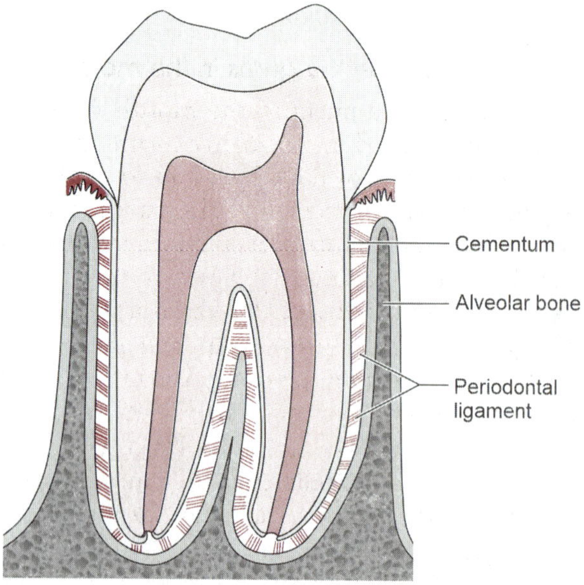

Fig. 12.9: Periodontal ligament

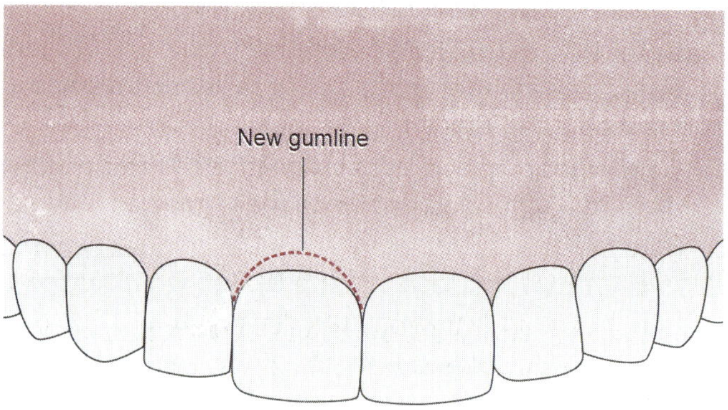

Fig. 12.10: Gum line

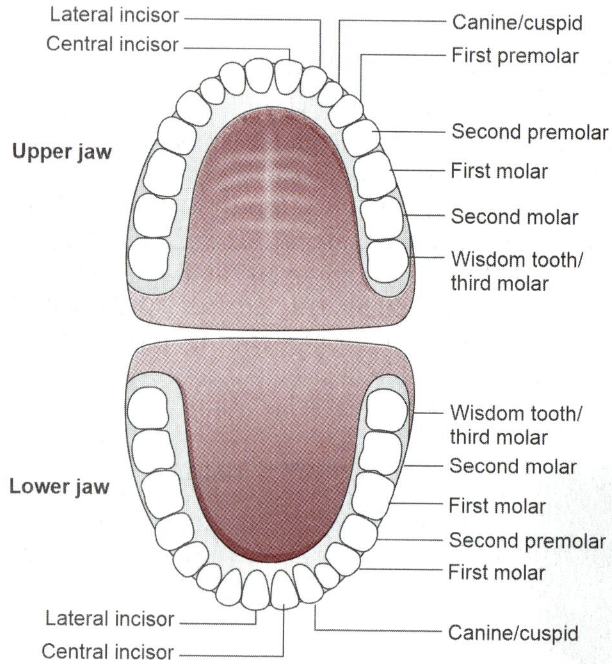

Fig. 12.11: Various types of teeth

Adult Teeth

BAQ: Write a note on the adult teeth.

Ans: A normal adult mouth has 32 teeth. These erupt by about 13 years of age, except wisdom teeth. Wisdom teeth are the third and final set of molars that most persons get mainly in the early twenties. The following are the various types of adult teeth (Fig. 12.11):

- Incisors: These are total eight teeth. Incisors are middlemost four teeth on the upper and lower jaws.
- Canines: These are four pointed teeth just outside the incisors.
- Premolars: These are eight teeth between the canines and molars.
- Molars: These are eight flat teeth in the rear of the mouth.
- Wisdom teeth: These are total four molars. These teeth erupt in the very back of the mouth, just behind the second molars (Fig. 12.11).

TEETH DISEASES

SAQ: What is the main reason of tooth decay?

Ans: Tooth decay (Fig. 12.12) takes place when bacteria in mouth act on the sugars that remain in the mouth after eating food to produce lactic acid. The lactic acid attacks the enamel. Tooth decay leads to formation of cavities (dental caries) (Fig. 12.13).

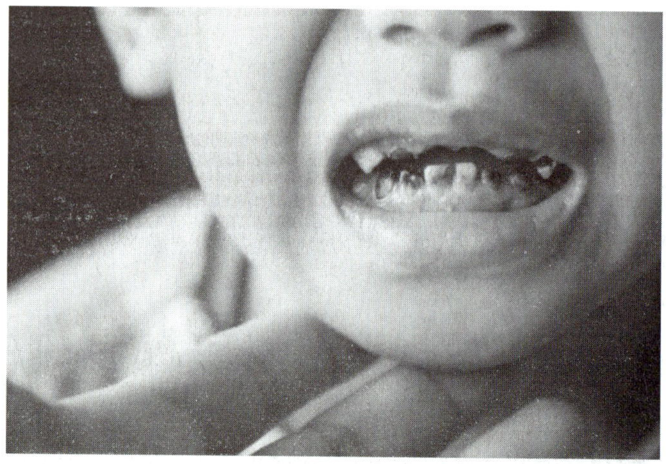
Fig. 12.12: Teeth decay

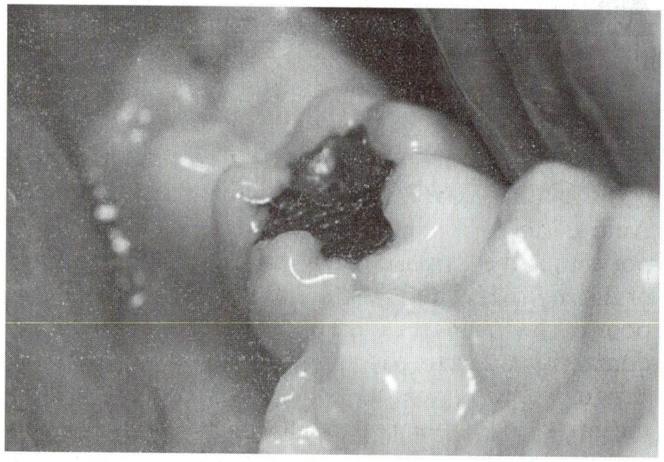
Fig. 12.13: Dental cavity

Dental Plaques

SAQ: What are dental plaques?

Ans: Dental plaque is a sticky film that form on tooth from time to time. Dental plaque contains bacteria, food particles and saliva. The bacteria present in the plaque act on the leftover sugary food particles and in the related chemical reactions lactic acid forms. The lactic acid act on teeth to form dental cavities. Regular tooth brushing and flossing usually get rid of dental plaques. If plaque accumulates, it hardens into tartar formation. The dental plaque can also lead to gingivitis, bad breath and eventually tooth loss (Fig. 12.14).

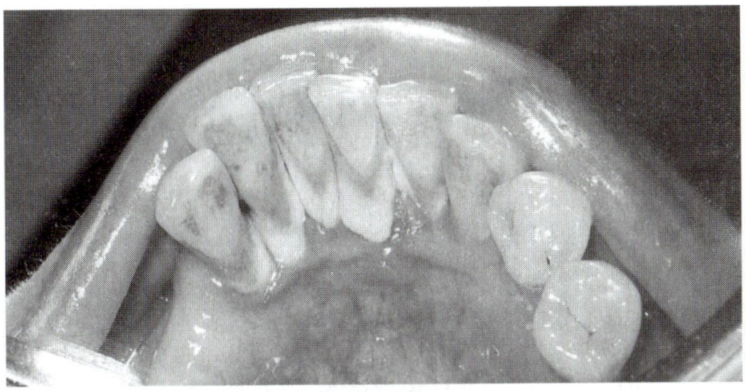

Fig. 12.14: Dental plaques

Peridontitis

SAQ: What is periodontium and periodontitis?

Ans: The periodontium is a specialized tissue. It surrounds and supports a tooth, and make it stable in the maxillary and mandibular bones (Figs 12.7 and 12.9). Periodontitis means inflammation of the periodontium structures of the teeth due to poor oral hygiene (Fig. 12.15).

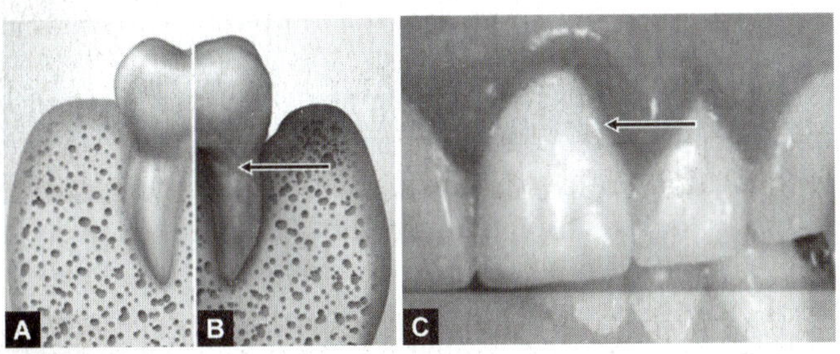

Figs 12.15A–C: (A) Normal tooth; (B) peridontitis; (C) gingivitis

Gingivitis

SAQ: What is gingivitis?

Ans: Gingivitis means inflammation of the surface portion of the gums, around and between the crowns of the teeth (Fig. 12.16). The main cause of gingivitis is poor care of teeth and gums, that lead to formation of dental plaques. The bacteria in the dental plaque act on the gums that surrounds the teeth and cause swelling of the gums. Tooth sensitivity increases, when tooth enamel gets damaged and dentin and nerves are exposed to hot or cold foods.

GUMS (GINGIVA) (Fig.12.16)

BAQ: Write a note on the gums in the mouth.

Ans: Gums are the parts in the mouth from which the teeth protrude (Fig. 12.16). The gum is made up of connective tissue of the upper and lower jaws that surrounds the base of the teeth. The gum is also called gingiva. Normal gums are pink in colour and these keep the teeth tightly anchored by covering the root of the tooth. Normal gums do not bleed by normal brushing.

The gums are able to resist the friction of food passing over them. Normal gums provide an effective protection to the of periodontal part of tooth (Fig. 12.16).

Increased in redness of gums together with swelling and tendency to bleed, indicate an inflammation of gums due to the accumulation of bacterial plaques.

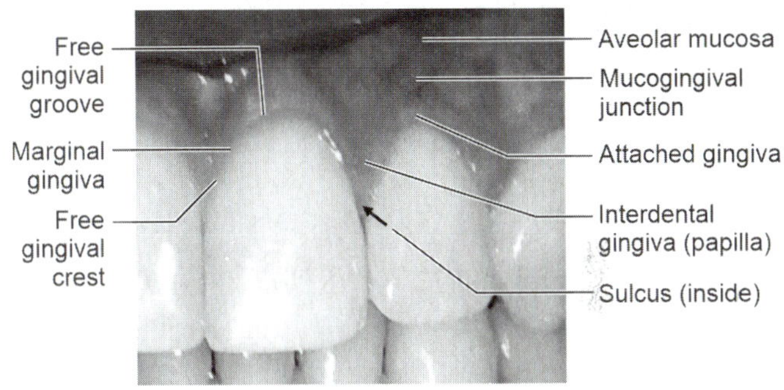

Fig. 12.16: Gum (gingiva)

BAQ: Draw a labelled diagram of anatomical features of the gum of mouth.

Ans: Refer to Fig. 12.17.

Gum Structure (Fig. 12.17)

BAQ: Write a note on the applied anatomy of tooth gum.

Ans: Anatomically, the gums are divided into following parts: (1) Marginal gingiva, (2) attached gingiva and, (3) interdental gingiva.

1. **Marginal gingiva** (Fig. 12.17): The marginal gingiva is the edge of the gums which surrounds the teeth. The marginal gingiva are stabilized by the gingival fibers, which do not have bony support.
2. **Attached gingiva** (Fig. 12.17): The attached gingiva are connected with the marginal gum. This part of the gum is firm and tightly bound to the underlying periosteum (dense layer of vascular connective tissue) of alveolar bone (Fig. 12.18).
3. **Interdental gum** (Fig. 12.17): The interdental gum is present between the teeth. These parts are resistant to the food-chewing pressures and are covered in the keratin.

The maxillary frenulum is a fold of the mucous membrane that connects the upper lip at the midline of the maxilla (Fig. 12.17).

The buccal frenum is a web of connective tissue formed bilaterally in the vestibule of the maxillary and mandibular arches (Fig. 12.17).

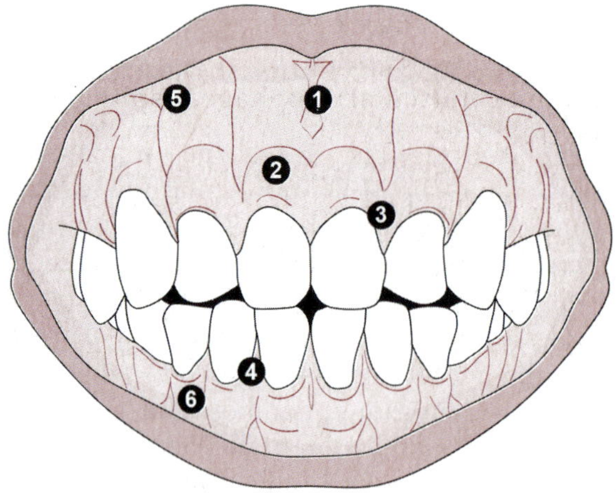

Fig. 12.17: Anatomical features of the gum: (1) Maxillary labial frenum, (2) attached gingiva, (3) marginal gingiva, (4) interdental gingiva and (5) alveolar mucosa, (6) interdental gingiva.

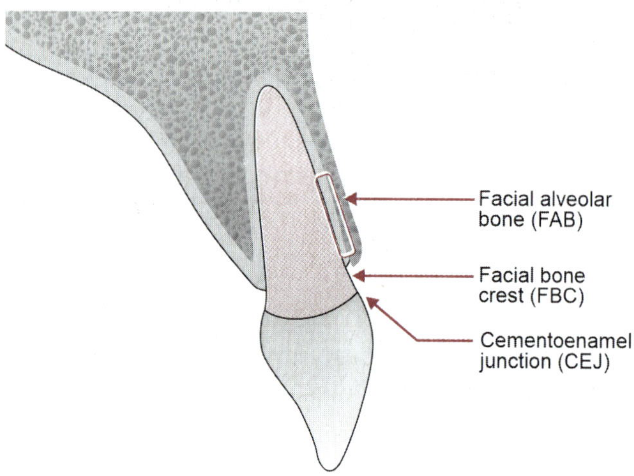

Fig. 12.18: Gum bound to facial alveolar bone

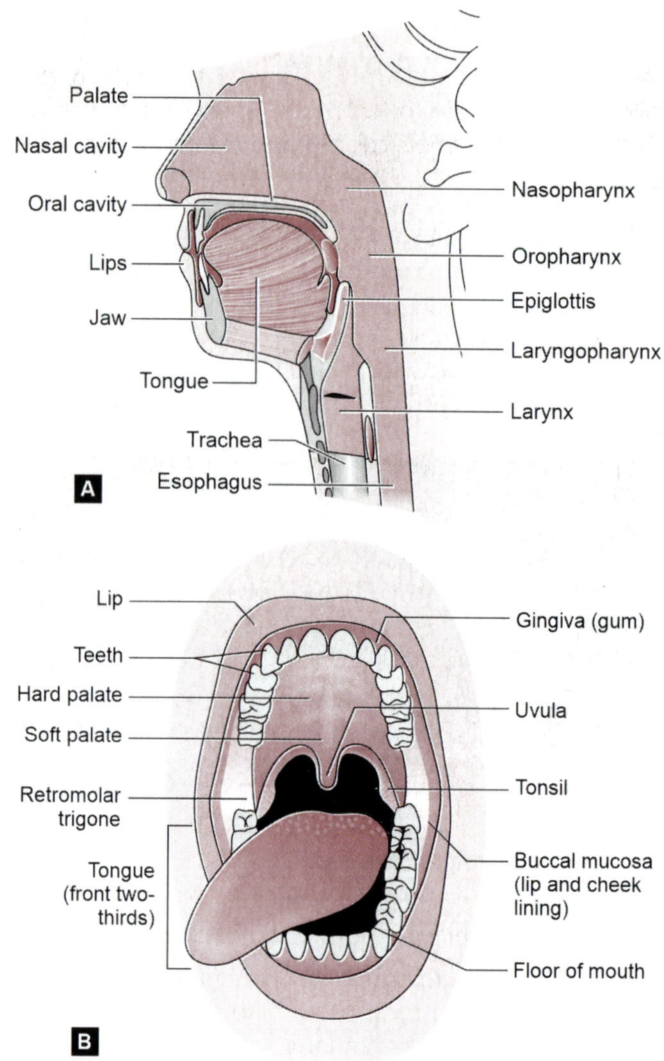

Figs 12.19A and B: Position of the palate in the mouth cavity

The alveolar mucosa is a thin and soft mucous membrane. It is present above the marginal gingiva and the attached gingiva, and continues across the floor of the mouth and lips (Fig. 12.17).

SAQ: Describe the location, structure and functions of the palate.

Ans:

Location: The palate is the roof of the mouth (Fig. 12.19). The palate separates the oral cavity from the nasal cavity.

Structure: The palate is divided into the following two parts: (1) The anterior bony hard palate and (2) the posterior fleshy soft palate.

Functions: The function of the hard palate is to separate the oral cavity from the nasal and sinus cavities. It facilitates proper articulation, breathing, chewing and phonation.

The soft palate plays important role in blocking food and other substances from entering the nasal passages during swallowing. It is also an important in the formation of specific sounds in the speech production.

BAQ: Write a note on mouth ulcers.

Ans: A mouth ulcer occurs on the mucous membrane of the oral cavity. These are very common and occur in association with specific incidences, drug side-effects and mainly related to specific clinical conditions. Usually, serious type of underlying cause is not present. However, a non-healing mouth ulcer may be a sign of oral cancer.

The mouth ulcers may cause pain and discomfort. The mouth ulcers often alter the choice of food of the affected person. Spicy and acidic foods and beverages tend to aggravate the mouth ulcers.

The following are the most common causes of oral ulcers:

1. **Oral sores caused by local trauma:** These may be caused from sharp edges of braces, dentures, and biting on any specific oral surface.
2. **Mouth sores caused by various other common reasons:** Mouth infections caused by bacteria, fungi or viruses, vitamin B complex deficiencies, specific chemicals in the food products and emotional stress.

ESOPHAGUS (Fig. 12.20)

LAQ: Describe the esophagus with respect to the following heads: (1) Introduction, (2) applied anatomy (3) functions (4) blood supply and (5) nerve supply.

Ans:

1. **Introduction:** The esophagus (the food pipe or gullet) is a fibromuscular tube. In adults, the length of esophagus is average 25 centimeters and the diameter is about 2 centimeters. It passes behind the trachea and heart, through the diaphragm, and connects the uppermost part of the stomach (Fig. 12.19).
2. **Applied anatomy:** The wall of the esophagus from the inner side to the outer side consists of the following components:
   a. *Mucosa:* It is made up of a stratified squamous epithelium formed of about three layers of squamous cells. It has two muscular rings called sphincters in its wall. One sphincter is present at the top and another sphincter is present at the bottom part of the esophagus (Fig. 12.20). The upper sphincter consists of skeletal muscle. However, it is not under voluntary control. The action of swallowing triggers the opening of the upper esophageal sphincter. The lower sphincter helps to prevent reflux of acidic contents from the stomach.
   b. The submucosa made up of connective tissue, and
   c. Muscle fiber layers between fibrous tissue layers, and
   d. An outer layer of connective tissue.
3. **Functions:** When bolus of food is swallowed, the esophagus receives food (Fig. 12.6). The epiglottis prevents food getting into windpipe. Peristalsis action in the esophagus (means a series of muscular contractions within the esophagus), introduces the food into the stomach.
   The upper muscular esophageal sphincter also protects against the reflux of food into the airways of lungs and prevent entry of air into the digestive tract (Fig. 12.20). Similarly, the muscular lower esophageal sphincter relaxes to allow the entry of food in the stomach. The lower esophageal sphincter then contracts and prevents the acidic contents of the stomach from flowing back into the esophagus (Fig. 12.21).
4. **Blood supply:** The upper parts of the esophagus receive blood from the inferior thyroid artery, partly from the bronchial arteries and branches directly from the thoracic aorta. The lower parts of the esophagus receive blood from the left gastric artery and the left inferior phrenic artery.
   The upper and middle parts of the esophagus drain into the azygos and hemiazygos veins, and blood from the lower part of the esophagus drains into the left gastric vein. All these veins drain into the superior vena cava, with the exception of the left gastric vein, which is a branch of the portal vein.
5. **Nerve supply:** The smooth muscle of the esophagus is innervated by the involuntary nerves, i.e. sympathetic nerves via the sympathetic trunk and parasympathetic nerves via the vagus nerve. The voluntary nerves innervate the striated muscles of the esophagus. These connects the vagus nerve.

SAQ: What is the difference between the pharynx and the esophagus.

Ans: The pharynx connects the oral and nasal cavities to the esophagus and trachea. It serves the digestive system as a passage of foods, as well as, respiratory system, as

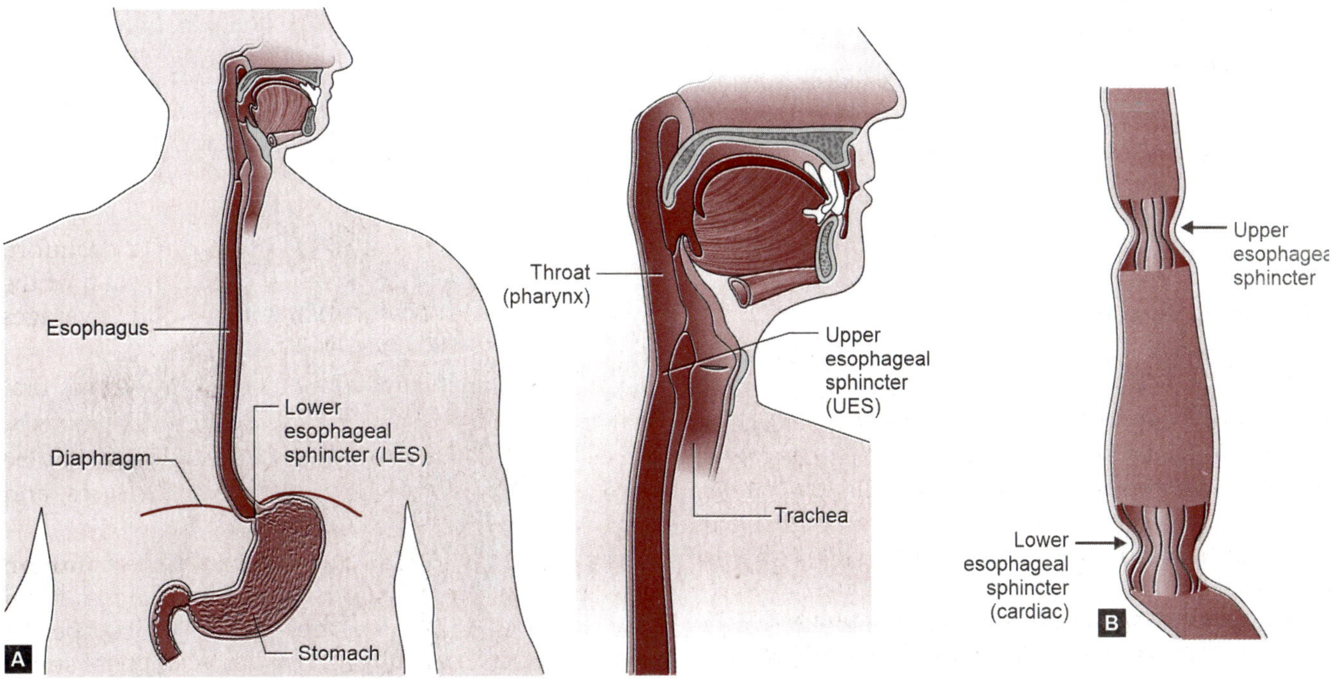

Figs 12.20A and B: (A) Esophagus; (B) esophageal sphincters

a passage of air. The esophagus connects the pharynx to the stomach.

SAQ: Describe the process of deglutition.

Ans: Deglutition (Figs 12.19–12.21) means the process of swallowing. It is a complex neuromuscular mechanism that uses both skeletal muscle in the form of tongue and smooth muscles of the pharynx and esophagus. The autonomic nervous system (ANS) coordinates this process in the pharyngeal and esophageal phases.

Deglutition takes place in the following three phases: (1) Oral phase, (2) pharyngeal phase and (3) esophageal phase. Each phase is controlled by a different neurological mechanism.

1. **Oral phase:** It includes food chewing, formation of food bolus and entry of bolus in the esophagus. The oral phase is voluntary and it is mainly controlled by the medial temporal lobes and limbic system of the cerebral cortex. The motor cortex and other cortical areas also play important role in this phase.
2. **Pharyngeal phase:** The pharyngeal swallow is involuntary and pharyngeal sensory receptors get stimulates by the passage of the bolus. The passage of the bolus is coordinated by the swallowing center on the medulla oblongata and pons. The reflex is initiated by the touch receptors in the pharynx as a bolus of food is pushed to the back of the mouth by the tongue and stimulation by palatal reflux.

   The bolus moves down by pharyngeal peristalsis towards the esophagus. It takes place by the sequential contraction of the superior, middle and inferior pharyngeal constrictor muscles.
3. **Esophageal phase:** This phase of swallowing is also involuntary. The upper esophageal sphincter relaxes to allow food to pass. Various striated constrictor muscles of the pharynx as well as peristalsis and relaxation of the lower esophageal sphincter sequentially push the bolus of food through the esophagus into the stomach.

As the bolus passes down the esophagus, the action of elevated uvula, hyoid bone and larynx and closing of nasal cavity takes place. The lower esophageal sphincter then relaxes and food enters the stomach.

BAQ: Write a note on dysphagia.

Ans: Dysphagia means difficulty in swallowing. The various symptoms of dysphagia are: Pain while swallowing, inability to swallow, drooling, coughing while eating, heart burn, etc. Dysphagia may be caused due to affected nervous system in the following clinical conditions: Stroke, head injury, dementia, mouth cancer, oesophageal cancer, gastroesophageal reflux disease (GERD), etc.

Barium meal swallow test and endoscopic examination could be useful to find out the cause of dysphagia, related to food pipe disorders.

Gastroesophageal Reflux Disease (GERD)

BAQ: Write a note on gastroesophageal reflux disease (GERD).

Ans: Gastroesophageal reflux disease (GERD) is a chronic disorder that occurs due to a weak lower esophageal sphincter (LES) or inability of the lower esophageal sphincter to close completely, when food enters the stomach (Fig. 12.21).

In GERD stomach hydrochloric acid or bile flows into the food pipe and irritates and damages the internal lining and causes further damage to the lower esophageal sphincter. The following are the specific symptoms of GERD: Dysphagia, regurgitation, heartburn, chest pain, hoarseness, chronic cough, and acid reflux-induced laryngitis, etc. The cause of GERD could be diagnosed by endoscopic examination of the food pipe and the stomach.

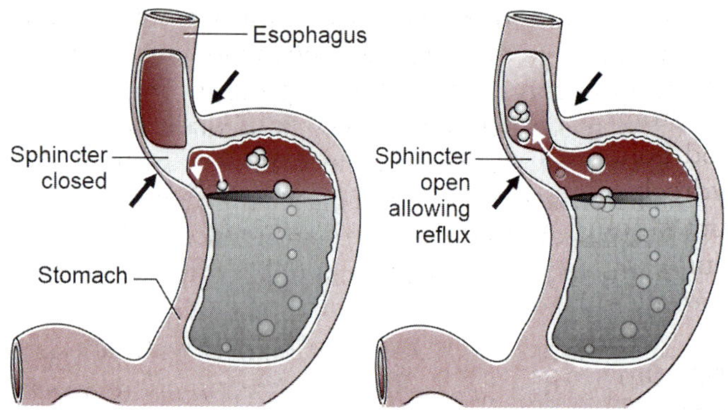

Fig. 12.21: Weak lower esophageal sphincter leading to GERD

Objectives: To describe the anatomical features and functions of the stomach, small intestine and large intestine. To describe the various disorders related to the stomach, small intestine and large intestine. To describe the blood supply and innervation of the gastrointestinal system.

STOMACH (Fig.12.22)

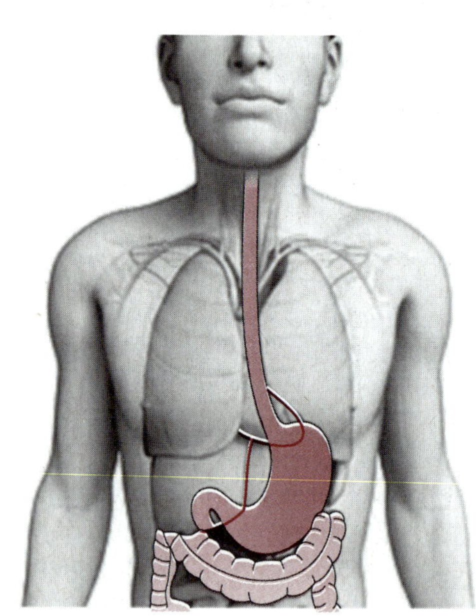

Fig.12.22: Stomach

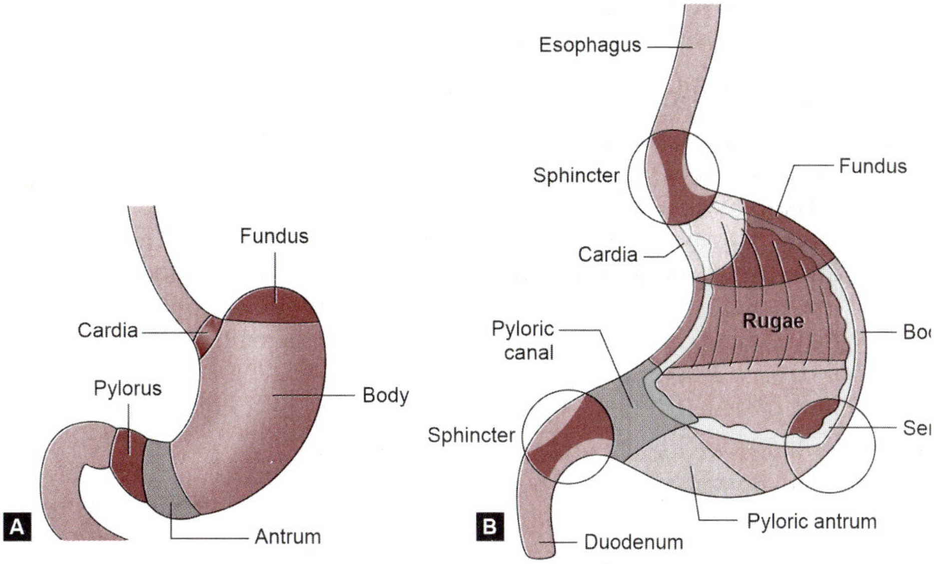

Figs 12.23A and B: Sections of the stomach

Introduction

The stomach is a muscular hollow organ. It receives food bolus from esophagus. The stomach cells secret hydrochloric acid and enzymes. Food bolus gets mixed with stomach acid and enzymes, which break down complex food into simple form, which then passes to intestine for further processing.

BAQ: Draw a labelled diagram of the parts of the stomach.

Ans: Refer to Fig. 12.23A.

Position and the Sections of the Stomach (Figs 12.23 A and B)

BAQ: Write a note on the position and the sections of the stomach.

Ans: The stomach lies just below the diaphragm in the upper part of the abdominal cavity. It is situated primarily to the left of the midline under a specific portion of the liver. The main parts of the stomach are as follow:

1. **Cardia** (Figs 12.23A and B): It is the opening of the esophagus into the stomach.
2. **Fundus** (Figs 12.23A and B): The fundus is the enlarged portion of the left side of stomach and it is seen above the cardiac orifice.
3. **Body** (Figs 12.23A and B): The body of stomach or corpus, is the central part of the stomach.
4. **Pyloric antrum** (Fig. 12.23B): The pyloric antrum is the lower portion of stomach above the duodenum. The opening between the stomach and the small intestine is the pylorus.
5. **Pyloric sphincter** regulates the passage of food in the form of chyme into the duodenum (Fig. 12.23B).

Anatomical Features of the Body of the Stomach and their Functions (Fig. 12.24)

BAQ: Write a note on the anatomical parts of the body of the stomach and their functions.

Ans: The body of the stomach is composed of the following three layers of muscles: (1) The innermost longitudinal layer of the stomach muscle, (2) the middle circular layer, and (3) the inner oblique layer of gastric folds called rugae (Fig. 12.24).

The innermost longitudinal layer of stomach helps in peristalsis action of stomach.

The middle circular layer aids in digestion by grinding the food together with digestive juices.

The inner oblique layer, the rugae, are folds in the stomach lining made up of epithelial tissue. Function of the gastric rugae is to allow the stomach to expand after the intake of foods and liquids. Expansion of stomach result in formation of greater surface area useful in absorption of partially digested nutrients. The rugae also facilitates increases in volume of the stomach to hold large amount of food. In addition to the circular and longitudinal muscle layers of the tunica muscularis,

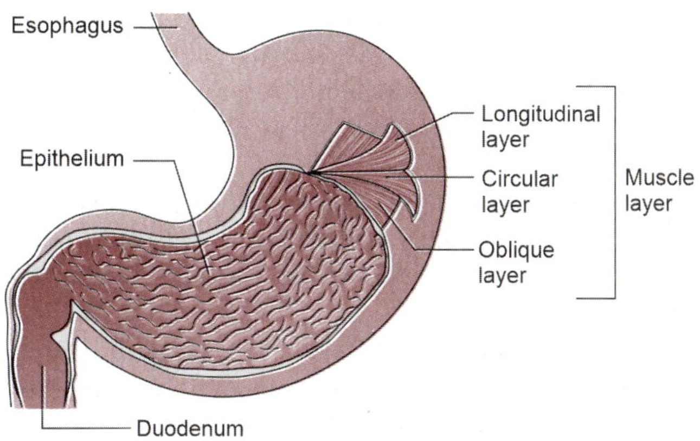

Fig. 12.24: Anatomical features of the stomach

the stomach also contains an oblique layer. These muscle layers facilitate churning movements in the stomach for the formation of chyme.

Gastric rugae facilitate stretching of the stomach and the tunica mucosa contains gastric gland. The gastric glands contain various types of secretary cells. The secretory cells contain chief cells and parietal cells that secret gastric juice containing digestive enzymes and hydrochloric acid, which are useful in the digestion of food in the stomach.

Ligaments and Omentum (Fatty Tissue) that Support the Stomach (Fig. 12.25)

SAQ: Write a note on the ligaments and omentum (fatty tissue) that support the stomach.

Ans: The stomach is suspended from the abdominal wall by the lesser omentum. The greater omentum attaches the stomach to the transverse colon, spleen and diaphragm. The omentum is made up of adipose tissue (Fig. 12.25).

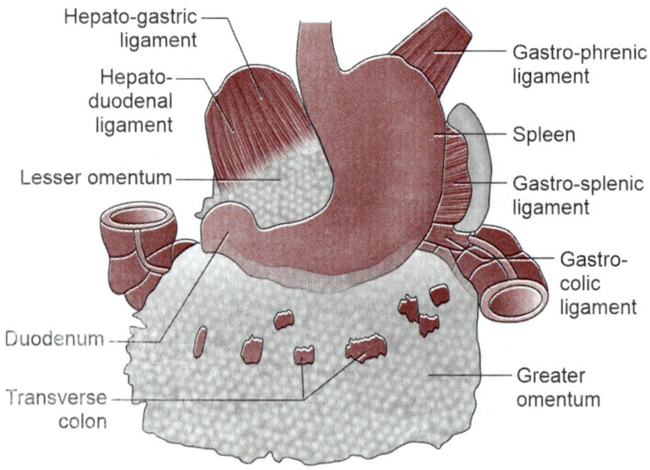

Fig. 12.25: Ligaments and omentum (fatty tissue) that support the stomach

Passage of Food and Digestion in the Stomach

BAQ: Write a note on the passage of food and digestion in the Stomach

Ans: The stomach secretes gastric juice. Average 1.5 liters of gastric juice is produced per day. Gastric juice is a mixture of water, hydrochloric acid, pepsinogen, mucin and electrolytes. pH of gastric juice is 1.5–3. The Gastric juice initiates digestion of food bolus arriving in the stomach and converts it to a semiliquid form called chyme.

The physiologic stimulation of acid secretion has been divided into the following three interrelated phases: (1) Cephalic phase, (2) gastric phase, and (3) intestinal phase.

1. **Cephalic (cerebral) phase:** It is triggered by the thought, sight, or smell, of food, which initiates the digestive process with the salivary and gastric secretions mediated through the autonomic nervous system.
2. **Gastric phase:** When food enters the stomach in the form of a bolus, it is churned by the stomach muscles by muscular contractions. The stomach chief cells release pepsin enzyme, which plays important role in the digestion of proteins in the food bolus. Hydrochloric acid secreted by parietal cells destroy bacteria and provides the acidic medium for conversion of inactive enzyme pepsinogen to pepsin. Pepsin acts on food proteins to form amino acids and small protein fragments called peptides. Further digestion of peptides takes place in the small intestine. In the stomach of infants and children renin enzyme is present. It helps in the partial digestion of milk proteins.

During stomach digestion the food bolus gets converted into chyme, which is partially digested form of food. In the stomach, the food remains in the stomach for about 40 minutes to two hours. Partial absorption of certain small molecules takes place in blood through stomach lining. This includes water, amino acids, caffeine, and certain medicines such as aspirin, etc.

Intestinal phase of gastric secretion: The presence of acidic chyme into the duodenum secretes secretin hormone, which inhibits gastric secretion. Presence of chyme in the duodenum initiates secretions of the enzymes of small intestine.

Control of Secretion of Enzymes and Motility of Bolus in the Stomach

SAQ: How control of secretion of enzymes and motility of bolus takes place in the stomach?

Ans: The movement and the flow of various food molecules and secretion of enzymes into the stomach and intestine are controlled by both the autonomic nervous system and controlled by the various digestive hormones of the digestive system.

BAQ: Enumerate the functions of the stomach.

Ans: The following are the important functions of the stomach:

1. The stomach acts as a reservoir for storage of food for initial digestion process with the secretion of gastric juice. Due to the reservoir capacity of the stomach, its volume increases significantly, while internal pressure does not increase significantly.
2. Secretion of gastrin hormone by neuroendocrine G-cells of the stomach. Gastrin stimulates parietal cells of stomach to secrete hydrochloric acid (HCl) and the chief cells to secret the inactive pepsinogen. Hydrochloric acid and pepsinogen are very important digestive components.
3. HCl protects against invading pathogens and provides suitable acidic pH for conversion of inactive pepsinogen to active pepsin.
4. Action of active pepsin on proteins in food and formation of intermediate digestive products, peptones and proteoses.

5. Important role of stomach in the mixing of stomach contents and initiation in the gastrointestinal motility.
6. The stomach also plays an important motility role as a pump, which is anatomically provided by the distal two thirds of the corpus, the antrum and the pylorus.

BAQ: Describe the various phases of gastric acid secretion.

Ans: The physiologic stimulation of acid secretion has been divided into the following three interrelated phases: (1) Cephalic phase, (2) gastric phase, and (3) intestinal phase.

1. Cephalic phase of gastric secretion: It is initiated by the sense of thought, sight, smell, taste, and swallowing of food. This stimulation occurs from the centres in the brain through the vagus nerve.
2. The gastric phase of gastric secretion is mediated by the by the release of gastrin hormone. The gastrin acts on the parietal cells to secret hydrochloric acid. The chief are stimulated mainly by the cholinergic activity from the vagus nerve and acidic pH in the stomach.
3. Intestinal phase of gastric secretion: The presence of acidic chyme into the duodenum secretes secretin hormone, which inhibits gastric secretion.

BAQ: What are the chief constituents of gastric secretion and their respective functions?

Ans: The chief constituents of gastric secretion are: (1) Hydrochloric acid, secreted by the parietal cells, (2) pepsinogen, secreted by the chief cells, (3) renin, (4) intrinsic factor, and (5) mucus.

The gastric secretion is produced in response to psychic factors (i.e. sight, taste, smell, etc.), by the action of gastrin hormone secreted by the gastric mucosa when food is present in the stomach. Insulin stimulates the vagus nerve by creating hypoglycemia, which increases the output of both acid and pepsin.

The various functions of gastric juice components are as follows:

1. HCl protects against invading pathogens and provides suitable acidic pH for conversion of inactive pepsinogen to active pepsin.
2. Pepsinogen is activated to pepsin by gastric acid, which also provides the acid medium for the enzyme action on food proteins. The proteins present in food are partially broken down into peptones and proteoses.
3. Renin clots milk by converting milk protein caseinogen to casein.
4. The intrinsic factor (IF) is a glycoprotein produced by the parietal cells of the stomach. Intrinsic factor plays an important role in the transportation and absorption of vitamin B_{12} by the terminal ileum.
5. The intestinal mucus protects the stomach epithelium from bacteria by promoting their clearance and separating from the epithelial cells, plays important role in the inhibition of inflammation and infection.

SAQ: Describe the clinical condition hyperchlorhydria.

Ans: Hyperchlorhydria term is used when the maximum free acid exceeds 50 mEq/liter. After the initial fall from a high fasting acidity, there may be a fairly rapid rise to concentrations exceeding 100 mEq/L. These findings are seen occasionally in gastric ulcers and are most characteristic of duodenal ulcers. Blood, together with hyperchlorhydria, is suggestive of gastric ulcer and may also be found occasionally in gastric carcinoma. In pyloric stenosis (obstruction to the entry of chyle in the intestine), the volume of residual and resting contents may be very high with the presence of starch. A small percentage of cases of cancer of the stomach are found to have hyperchlorhydria.

SAQ: Describe the clinical conditions achlorhydria and achylia gastrica.

Ans: Achlorhydria term is used when there is no secretion of hydrochloric acid. The enzyme pepsin may be present. When free acid and the enzyme both are absent, the term achylia gastrica is used. Achlorhydria is associated with persons belonging to older age groups, tuberculosis of the stomach, Addison's disease, ulcerative colitis, later stage of malignancy, and in pernicious anemia.

SAQ: What are gastrointestinal hormones? Name three gastrointestinal hormones.

Ans: Gastrointestinal hormones are polypeptides produced by mucosal endocrine cells of the stomach and small intestine. They are involved primarily in the regulation of the stomach, small intestine, pancreas, liver, and biliary tract. The major gastrointestinal hormones are gastrin, secretin, and cholecystokinin (pancreozymin).

SAQ: Write three functions of gastrin.

Ans: The following are the functions of gastrin:

1. It is the most effective activator of gastric acid secretion.
2. It causes chief cells to secrete pepsinogen, the zymogen (inactive) form of the digestive enzyme pepsin. It also stimulates intrinsic factor release from gastric mucosa.
3. It stimulates secretin release.

SAQ: What is Zollinger-Ellison syndrome?

Ans: Gastrin-producing pancreatic tumors cause Zollinger-Ellison syndrome. It is characterized by high levels of gastrin and elevated gastric acid secretion, leading to gastrointestinal ulcers.

SAQ: What is autoimmune gastritis.

Ans: In autoimmune gastritis, the immune system attacks the parietal cells leading to hypochlorhydria. This results in an elevated gastrin level in an attempt to compensate for increased pH in the stomach. Eventually, all the parietal cells are lost, and achlorhydria results leading to a loss of negative feedback on gastrin secretion.

Stomach Ulcers (Gastric Ulcers)

SAQ: What are stomach (gastric) ulcers?

Ans: A stomach (gastric) ulcer is an open sore in the stomach lining, due to excessive acid secretion. The most common causes of gastric ulcers are infection by *Helicobacter pylori* bacteria and also by long-term use of nonsteroidal anti-inflammatory drugs (NSAIDs) (Fig. 12.26). A chronic pain the middle of the stomach may indicate presence of gastric ulcers. The following are the typical symptoms: Pain in the stomach, heart burn, acid reflux, bloating, nausea, vomiting, etc. The gastric ulcers could be managed by the appropriate treatment and use of anti-acid drugs.

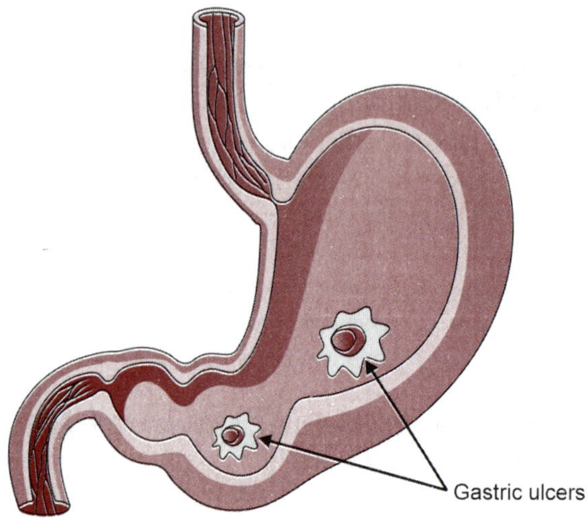

Fig. 12.26: Gastric ulcers

Nerve Supply of the Gastrointestinal Tract (Fig. 12.27)

BAQ: Write a note on the nerve supply of gastrointestinal tract.

Ans: The gastrointestinal tract is innervated by intrinsic (internal) neurons of the enteric nervous system (ENS) and by the axons of extrinsic (outside) sympathetic, parasympathetic, and visceral afferent neurons.

The gastrointestinal (GI) tract is responsible for the digestion and absorption of food components. GI utilizes digestive system organs to achieve processes of digestion and absorption. The digestive system organs involved in digestion and absorption are, mouth, esophagus, stomach, small and large intestine, liver, biliary tract, pancreas, and various glands that work together through a complex mechanisms. The following three distinct centers of control are used by the GI tract of the body: 1) Muscular control 2) hormonal control and 3) Neural control

These three processes work together to obtain four major actions required for a proper functioning of GI tract: Motility of food, digestion of food, secretion of hormones and enzymes and absorption of end products of food digestion.

Blood and Lymph Circulation of the Gastrointestinal Tract (Figs 12.28 and 12.29)

BAQ: Write a note on the blood and lymph circulation of the gastrointestinal tract.

Ans: The following are the major arteries that supply the gastrointestinal tract: (1) The celiac artery (2) superior mesenteric artery and (3) inferior mesenteric arteries.

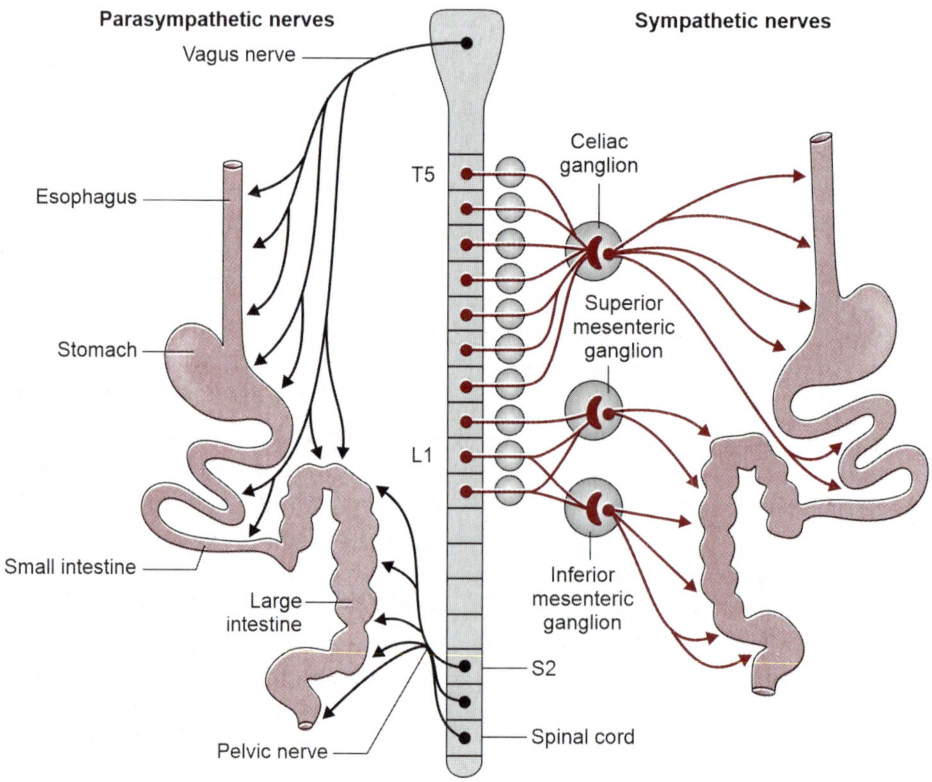

Fig. 12.27: Autonomic nerves of gastrointestinal tract

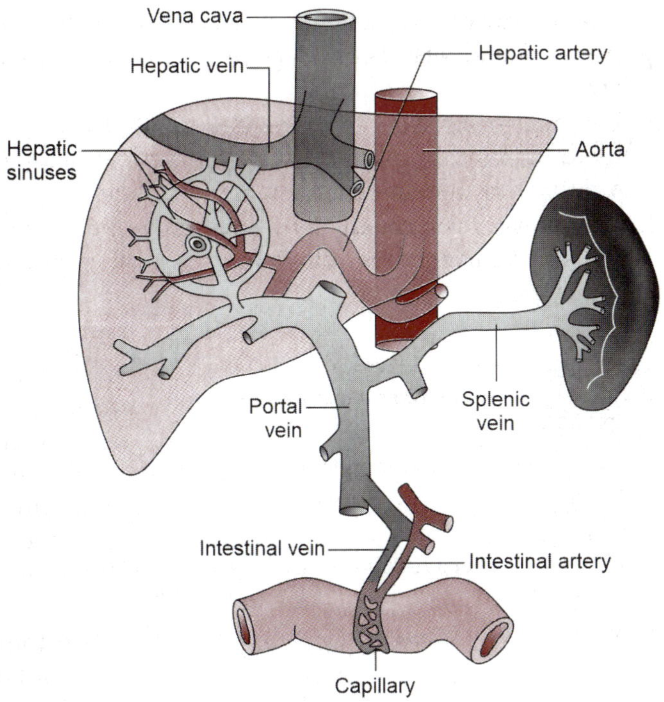

Fig. 12.28: Blood circulation of liver, spleen and the gastrointestinal tract

The celiac artery supplies the stomach and the duodenum, the superior mesenteric supplies the rest of the small intestine and proximal portion of the colon, while the inferior mesenteric artery supplies the distal portion of the colon (Fig. 12.29).

The splenic vein drains the stomach, the superior mesenteric vein drains the upper small intestine, and the inferior mesenteric vein drains the distal portions of the colon. These three veins drain into the portal vein, which passes to the liver. From liver venous flow is delivered back to the heart (Fig. 12.30).

The lymph vessels draining the gastrointestinal tract run in association with blood vessels and enter various lymph nodes. The efferent lymphatic vessels from the lymph nodes empty in the systemic circulation via the thoracic duct (Fig.12.31).

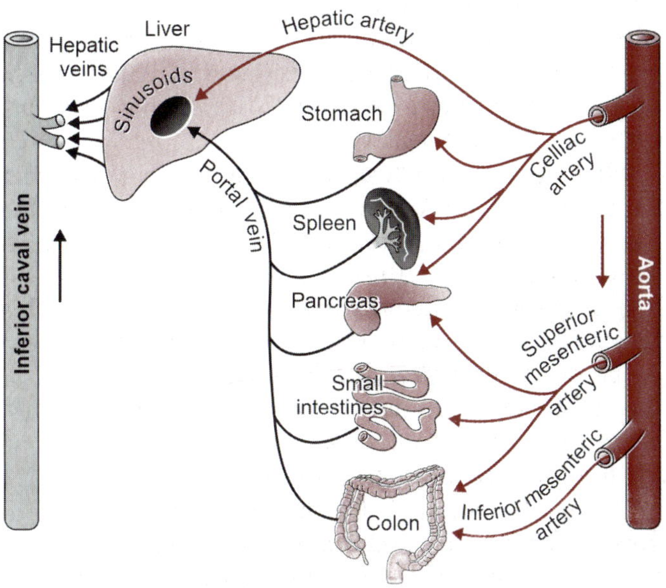

Fig. 12.29: Arterial and venous supply of gastrointestinal tract

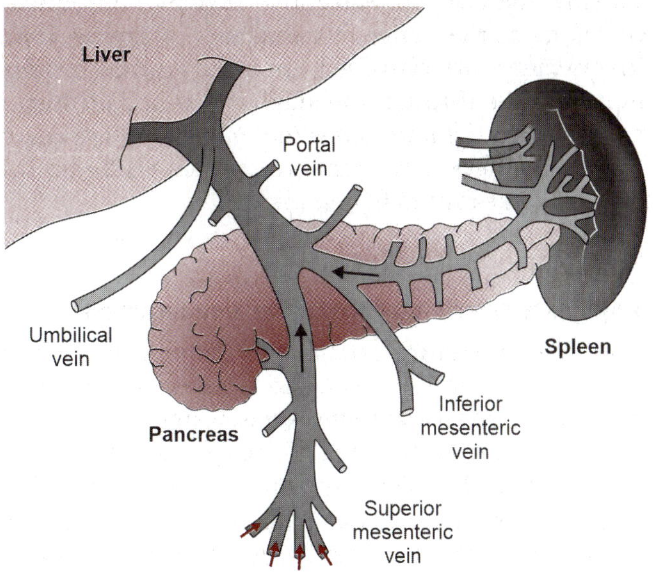

Fig. 12.30: Venous circulation of the gastrointestinal tract

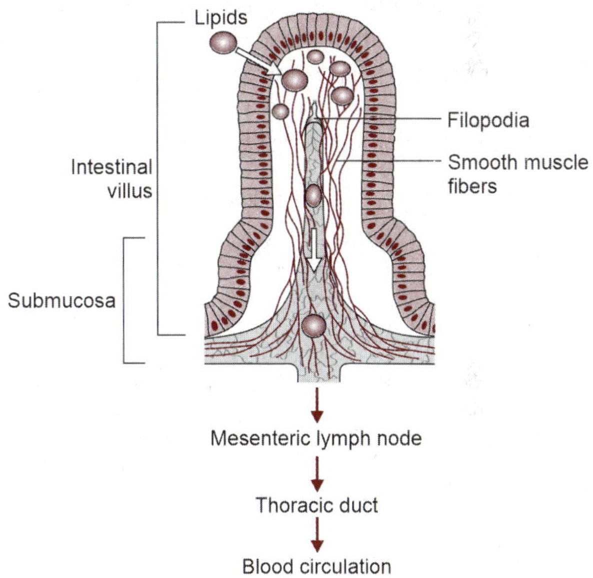

Fig. 12.31: Lymph circulation of the gastrointestinal tract

SMALL INTESTINE

BAQ: Write a note on the small intestine.

Ans: The small intestine is about 22 feet muscular tubular structure. It is made up of three segments, the duodenum, jejunum, and ileum. It plays very important role in the completion of digestion of food using enzymes released by the pancreas and bile from the liver and also enzymes released by the intestinal cells. Digested food gets mixed and moves forward to large intestine by peristalsis action.

The duodenum is the first segment of the small intestine. It is mainly responsible for the continuous digestion of chyme. The jejunum and ileum parts in the intestine are mainly responsible for the absorption of nutrients into the bloodstream.

The contents of the small intestine are semi-solid initially and at the end of passage through end in digested liquid form. Water, bile, enzymes and mucus contribute to the change in consistency of chyme. Once the nutrients are absorbed, the leftover-food residue liquid passes through the small intestine and then it moves on to the large intestine. Normally passage of food in the form of chyme through the small intestine takes average four to five hours.

Duodenum (Fig.12.32)

BAQ: Write a note on the duodenum segments.

Ans: The duodenum connects to the pylorus part of stomach. It is initial C-shaped segment of the small intestine. It connects with the jejunum and ileum distally. The duodenum is about 8 to 10 inches long. Duodenum is made up of the following four segments (Fig. 12.32):

1. **First segment** (the duodenal bulb): It is connected to the lower part of the liver through the hepatoduodenal ligament, which contains the portal vein, the hepatic artery, and common bile duct.
2. **Second or descending segment:** It is just above the inferior vena cava and right kidney.
3. **Third segment:** It passes from right to left in front of the aorta and inferior vena cava.
4. **Fourth segment:** It connects the jejunum.

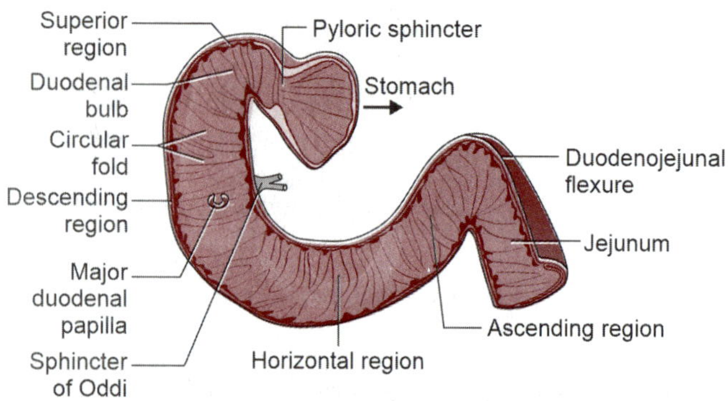

Fig. 12.32: Various segments of the duodenum

BAQ: Draw a labelled diagram of the various segments of the duodenum.

Ans: Refer to Fig. 12.32.

Tunics (Layers) of Duodenum (Fig. 12.33)

BAQ: Write a note on the tunics (layers) of the duodenum.

Ans: The wall of the duodenum is made up of the following four layers of tissues (from innermost to the outermost layer): (1) The mucosa layer, (2) the submucosa layer, (3) the muscularis layer and, (4) the serosa layer.

1. The mucosal layer lines the inner surface of the duodenum. It is made of simple columnar cells with microvilli and numerous mucous glands. Nutrients from the digested fluid are absorbed through microvilli, and pass into the blood capillaries and lymphatics and made available to cells of the body.
2. The submucosal layer is mostly a layer of connective tissue. Blood vessels and nerves pass through this layer.
3. The muscularis layer contains the smooth muscle of the duodenum. It plays an important role in mixing and forward peristaltic movement of chyme.
4. The serosal layer is made up of squamous epithelium. It acts as a barrier for the duodenum from other organs of the body.

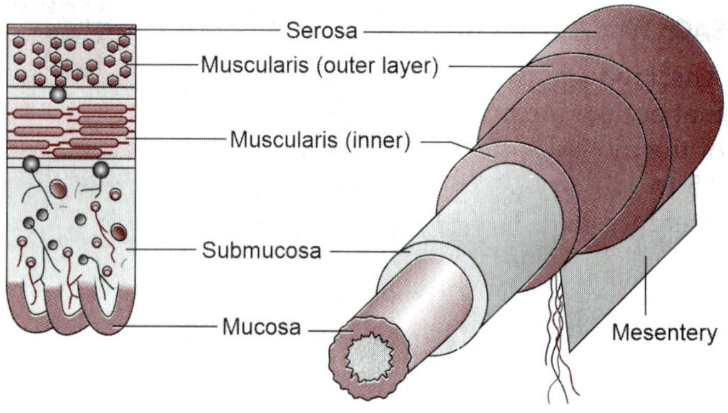

Fig. 12.33: Tunics (layers) of the duodenum

BAQ: Draw a neat labelled figure of the tunics of the duodenum.

Ans: Refer to Fig. 12.33.

Digestive Functions of the Duodenum

BAQ: Describe the digestive functions of the duodenum.

Ans: The duodenum receives chyme from the stomach through pyloric sphincter, which is a controlled valve between the stomach and the duodenum (Fig. 12.32). Inside the duodenum digestion of chyme takes place by the action of digestive enzymes and intestinal juices secreted by the intestinal wall as well as the digestive fluids received from the liver, gallbladder, and pancreas. These secretions are received into the duodenum by the major and minor papilla in the second part of the duodenum. The duodenal papilla is surrounded by a semicircular fold and the sphincter of Oddi muscle (Fig. 12.32), which prevents reflux of duodenal secretions into the bile and pancreatic ducts.

The duodenum has the ability to regulate its environment with hormones that are released from the duodenal epithelium. These hormones are secretin and cholecystokinin. Secretin is released, when the pH of the duodenum decreases towards alkaline level. This hormone acts to neutralize the pH of the duodenum by stimulating water and bicarbonate secretion into the duodenum. This aids in the digestion process since pancreatic amylase and lipase enzymes require alkaline pH to function at the optimum alkaline level.

The cholecystokinin is released in the presence of food containing fats and protein inside the duodenum. It acts to inhibit gastric emptying and also to stimulate contraction of the gallbladder which delivers bile acids in the duodenum required for fat digestion. At the same time relaxation of the sphincter of Oddi takes place to allow delivery of bile into the duodenum.

SAQ: What are the functions of the muscularis muscles of the duodenum?

Ans: The muscles in the muscularis layer of the duodenum contain the circular and longitudinal muscles. The coordination of contraction of these muscles leads to peristalsis to occur throughout the gastrointestinal tract.

SAQ: What is hypertrophic pyloric stenosis?

Ans: Hypertrophic pyloric stenosis is a clinical condition that occurs due to increased mass of the smooth muscle of the pyloric sphincter. This condition occurs in about 0.5 to 1% of infants. Child keeps on vomiting shortly after feeding (Fig. 12.34).

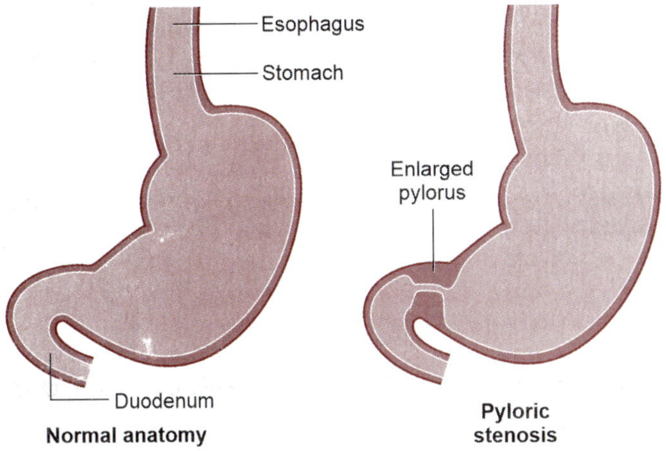

Fig. 12.34: Pyloric stenosis compared to normal anatomy of duodenum

SAQ: What is duodenal atresia?

Ans: Duodenal atresia is a congenital intestinal obstruction that can cause child vomiting within the first 24–38 hours of neonatal life, following the first oral feeding. Duodenal atresia occurs due to complete closure of the lumen of the duodenum (Fig. 12.35).

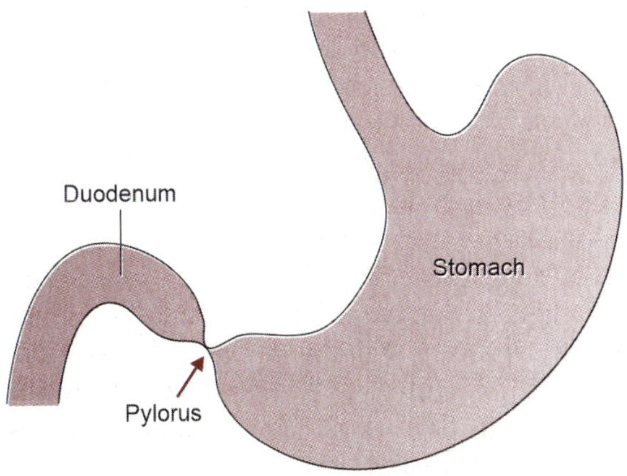

Fig. 12.35: Duodenal atresia

SAQ: Write a brief note on duodenal ulcer.

Ans: Duodenal ulcer is a type of peptic ulcer that occurs due to the damage in the mucosal surface of the duodenum, leading to ulceration. The ulceration may extend beyond the superficial layer of the duodenum. Duodenal ulcer is most commonly observed in patients who are infected with *Helicobacter pylori* bacterial infection and may have gastric ulcers (Fig. 12.36).

Duodenal ulcer also may be observed in persons on long-term use of nonsteroidal anti-inflammatory drugs (NSAIDs). A chronic pain in the upper part of the abdomen may indicate presence of stomach ulcers. The following are the typical symptoms: Pain in the abdomen, heart burn, bloating, nausea, vomiting, etc. The gastric ulcers could be managed by the appropriate treatment and use of anti-acid drugs.

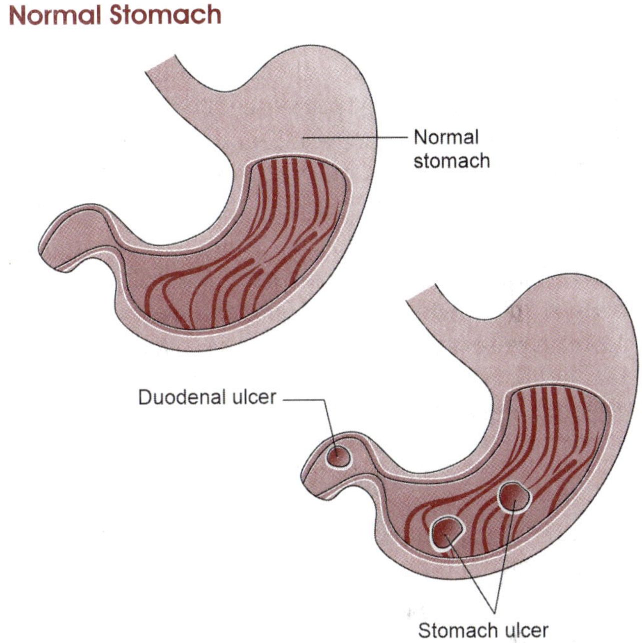

Fig. 12.36: Duodenal ulcer

SAQ: What is gastritis?

Ans: Gastritis means inflammation of the mucosa (lining) of stomach. Excessive intake of alcohol, spicy food, stress, prolonged use of anti-inflammatory drugs and bacterial infection like *Helicobacter pylori* may lead to gastritis.

Jejunum

BAQ: Describe the jejunum on the basis of the following heads: (1) Introduction and (2) applied anatomical features with respective functions.

Ans:

1. **Introduction:** The jejunum is the second part of the small intestine (Fig. 12.37). It lies between the duodenum and the ileum. Average length of the jejunum is about 8 feet. Lining of jejunum is specialised for the absorption of small nutrient molecules which have been previously digested by enzymes in the duodenum. Absorption of digested food takes place by enterocytes, which are simple columnar epithelial cells which line the inner surface of the jejunum.

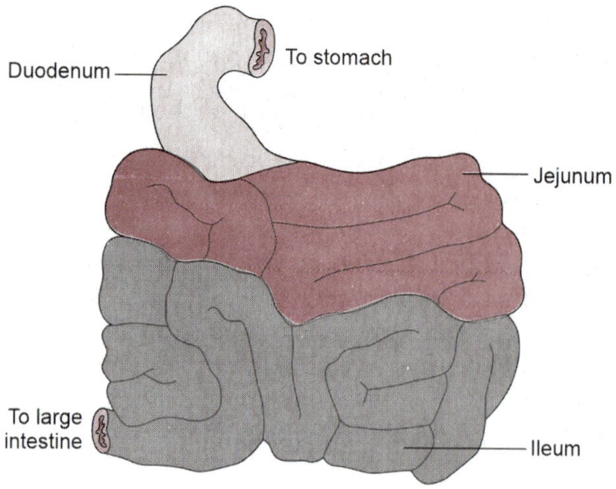

Fig.12.37: Duodenum, jejunum and ileum parts of the small intestine

2. **Applied anatomical features with respective functions:** The interior surface of the jejunum is covered by finger–like projections of mucosa, called villi (Fig. 12.38). The villi increase the surface area of jejunum to absorb nutrients from ingested food. The villi in the jejunum are longer than that in the duodenum or ileum. The pH in the jejunum is usually slightly alkaline, between 7 and 8. The villi have epithelial cells which line microvilli (Fig. 12.38). Microvilli are microscopic cellular membrane projections that increase the surface area for diffusion of digested food micromolecules. The absorbed micronutrients pass from the enterocytes into the enterohepatic circulation and enter the liver through the hepatic portal vein (Fig. 12.39).

SAQ: What is mesentery and its functions?

Ans: The jejunum and the ileum are suspended by a fold of membrane called mesentery (refer to Fig. 1.28). It gives the bowel mobility within the abdomen. It also contains circular and longitudinal smooth muscle which helps to move food through the intestinal passage by peristalsis.

Ileum (Fig. 12.37)

BAQ: Write a note on the ileum.

Ans: Ileum is the last part of the small intestine. It is about 11 feet long. It connects to the cecum, the first part of the large intestine. The main function of the ileum is to absorb products of digestion which are not absorbed by the jejunum including vitamin B_{12} and bile acids.

The wall of ileum has villi on its surface. Thus, the ileum has large surface area for the absorption of end-products of digested food. The villi contain large numbers of capillaries that take the amino acids and glucose produced by digestion to the hepatic portal vein and the liver (Fig. 12.38). Lacteals (small lymph vessels) present in villi absorb fatty acids and glycerol, the products of fat digestion (Fig. 12.38). Layers of circular and longitudinal smooth muscles enable the digested food and water to be pushed along the ileum by peristalsis.

LARGE INTESTINE (Fig. 12.40)

BAQ: Write a note on the large intestine.

Ans: The large intestine is average 5–6 feet long, tube-like organ. It is connected to the small intestine at one

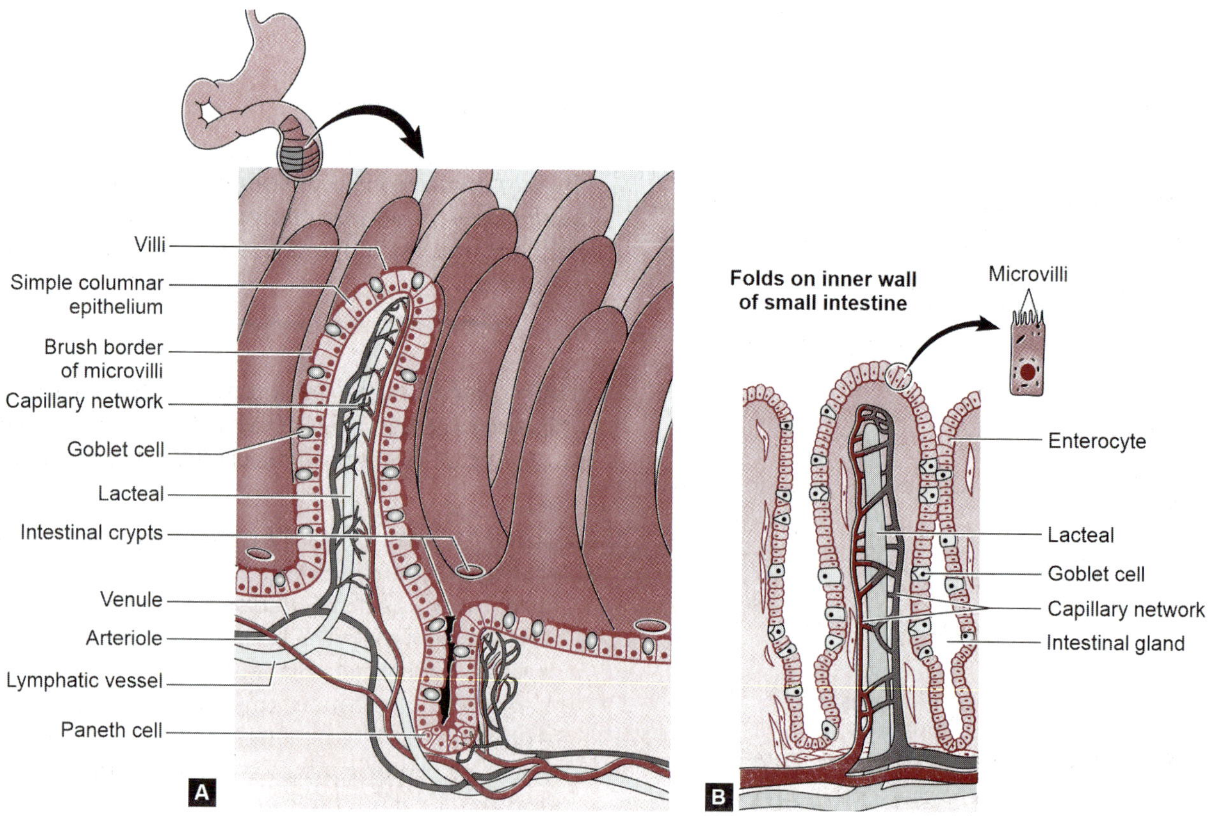

Figs 12.38A and B: (A) Anatomy of villi; (B) villi and microvilli

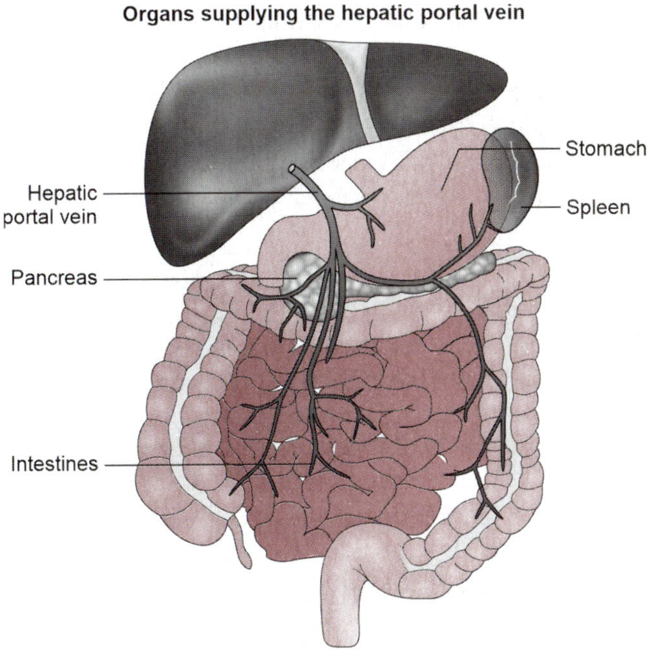

Fig. 12.39: Absorbed food passage to liver

end and the anus at the other end. The large intestine has following four parts: Cecum, colon, rectum, and anal canal. Digested food moves from ileum to the cecum and then into the colon, where water and some nutrients and electrolytes are absorbed and remaining waste products passed out through anus as stool or feces.

Stool is passed through the colon by means of peristalsis. Normally, it takes about average 10–35 hours for stool to pass through the colon. When stool passes through the colon, water is absorbed. Stool is stored in the sigmoid (S-shaped) colon until a "mass movement" empties it into the rectum once or twice a day.

Cecum (Fig. 12.40)

SAQ: Write a brief note on the cecum.

Ans: The cecum is the beginning of the large intestine. It is located on the right side of the body. The cecum receives chyme from the ileum, and passes it to the ascending colon of the large intestine. It is separated from the ileum by the ileocecal valve (ICV) known as Bauhin's valve (Fig. 12.41). The ileocecal valve is a sphincter muscle valve that separates the small intestine and the large intestine. The function of ICV is to control the reflux of colonic contents into the ileum. About two liters of fluid enters the colon through the ileocecal valve per day.

Colon (Fig. 12.40)

BAQ: Describe the colon on the basis of the following heads: (1) Introduction and (2) applied anatomical features with respective functions.

Ans: The average length of the colon is about 5 feet. It has the following four parts: (1) Ascending colon, (2) the transverse colon, (3) descending colon and (4) the sigmoid colon.

Ascending colon: It is the part of the colon situated between the cecum and the transverse colon. The function of the ascending colon is to absorb part of water and remaining nutrients from the indigestible material and then solidifying it to form stool. (Figs 12.40 and 12.41).

Transverse colon: It is the longest and most movable part of the colon. The transverse colon absorbs water and salts (Figs 12.40 and 12.41).

Descending colon: It is the part of the large intestine from the splenic flexure to the beginning of the sigmoid colon (Figs 12.40 and 12.41). The function of the descending

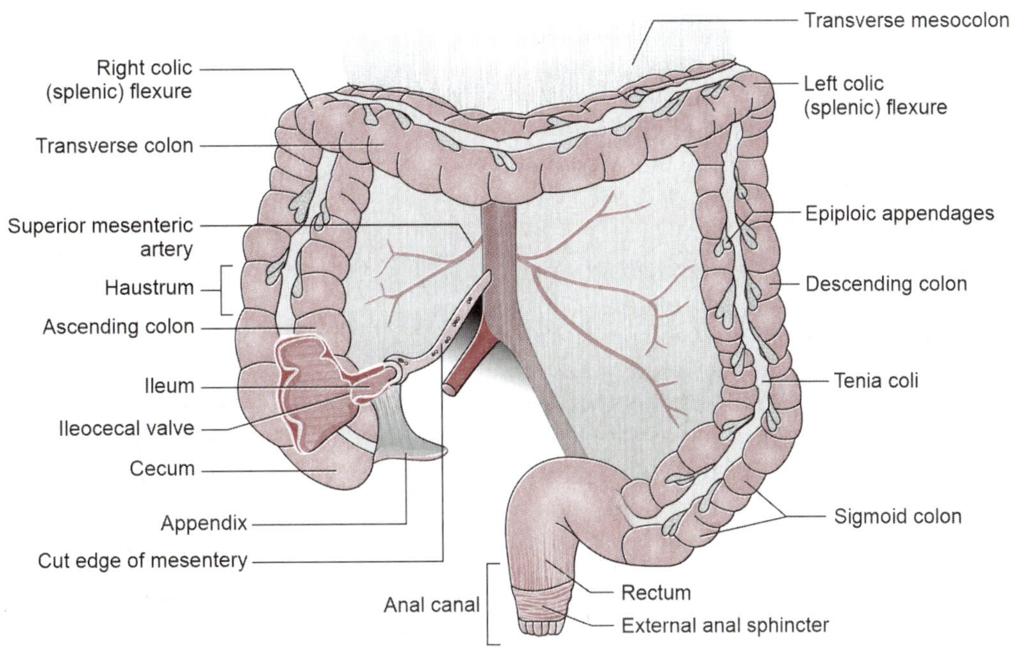

Fig. 12.40: Large intestine

Digestive System 12

colon is to store remaining material from digested food that later on passes into the rectum.

Sigmoid colon: It is the S-shaped last part of the large intestine, which leads into the rectum. The function of sigmoid colon is to store fecal wastes until they pass out of the body (Fig. 12.41).

SAQ: What is the flexure of a colon?

Ans: A "flexure" is a specific part where the colon bends. The colon has two flexures: One on the right side and one on the left. The splenic flexure is near the spleen. It is also called the left colic flexure, since it is on the left side of the body (Fig. 12.41).

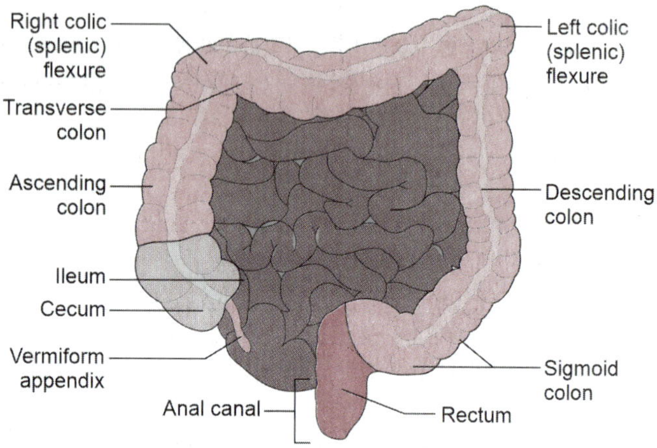

Fig. 12.41: Flexures of the colon

Rectum (Fig. 12.41)

BAQ: Write a note on the rectum.

Ans: The rectum is a tubular organ that is connected to the colon by the sigmoid colon (Fig. 12.41). The average length of the rectum is about 5 inches. The end of rectum connects to anus in a specific structure called an ampulla (Fig. 12.42).

The rectum is a temporary storage site for feces. The rectum receives fecal material from the descending colon, which is transmitted by peristalsis. The rectal walls expand due to the materials filling it from within, leading to stimulate stretch receptors located in the nervous system of the rectal walls, which create the desire to pass feces, a process called defecation.

An internal and external anal sphincter, and resting contraction of the puborectalis muscle (Fig. 12.43) prevent leakage of feces. As the rectum becomes more distended, the sphincters relax and a reflex expulsion of the contents of the rectum occurs. Expulsion occurs through contractions of the muscles of the rectum.

The urge to voluntarily defecate occurs after the rectal pressure increases significantly. In voluntary defecation, abdominal muscle contraction, and relaxation of the puborectalis muscle also necessary (Fig. 12.44). This action of puborectalis muscle leads to arrange the angle between the rectum and anus straighter, which facilitate defecation.

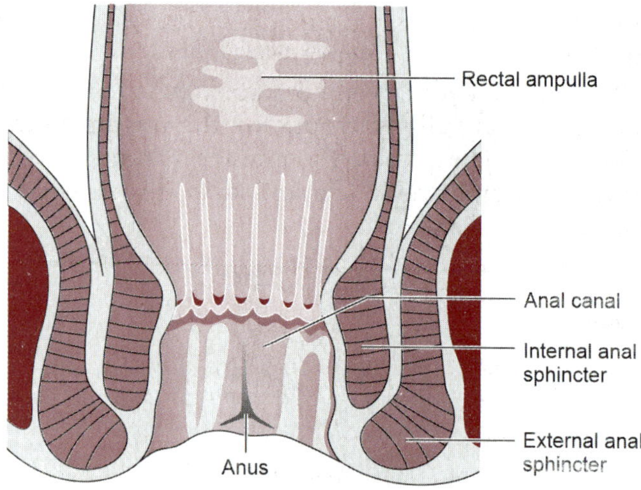

Fig. 12.42: Anatomical features of the anal canal

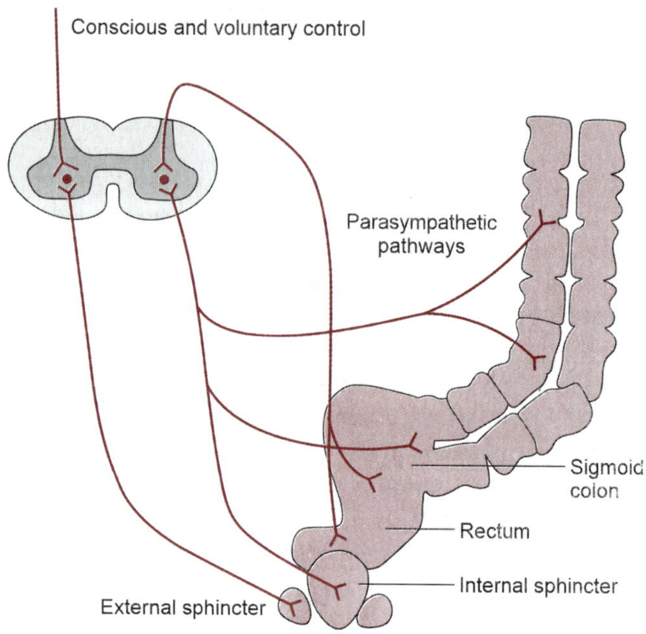

Fig. 12.43: Neuronal control on contraction of rectum

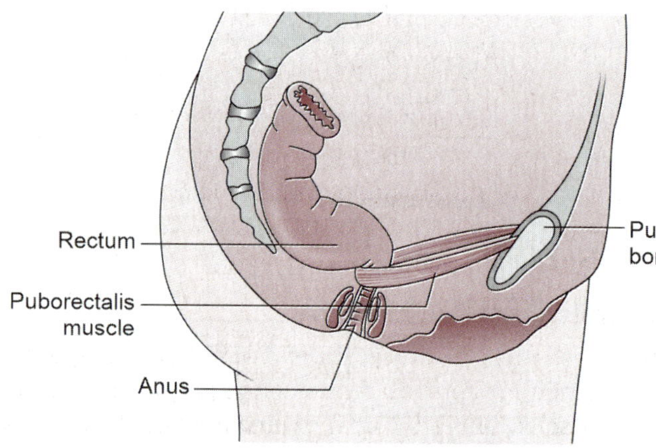

Fig. 12.44: Puborectalis muscle

Blood Supply of the Rectum (Fig. 12.45)

BAQ: Write a note on the blood supply of the rectum.

Ans: Blood to the upper two-thirds part of rectum is supplied by the superior rectal artery. The lower one-third portion of rectum is supplied by the middle and inferior rectal arteries (Fig. 12.45).

The superior rectal vein, or superior hemorrhoidal vein, connects veins surrounding the rectum to the inferior mesenteric vein. The inferior mesenteric vein brings blood from the large intestines to the splenic vein (Fig. 12.46).

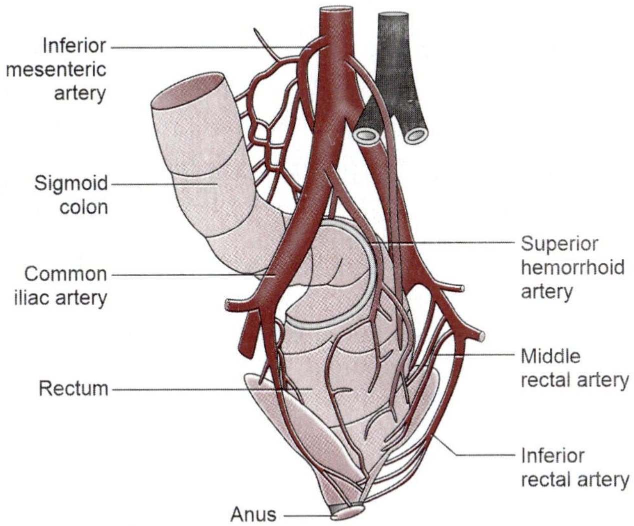

Fig. 12.45: Blood supply to rectum

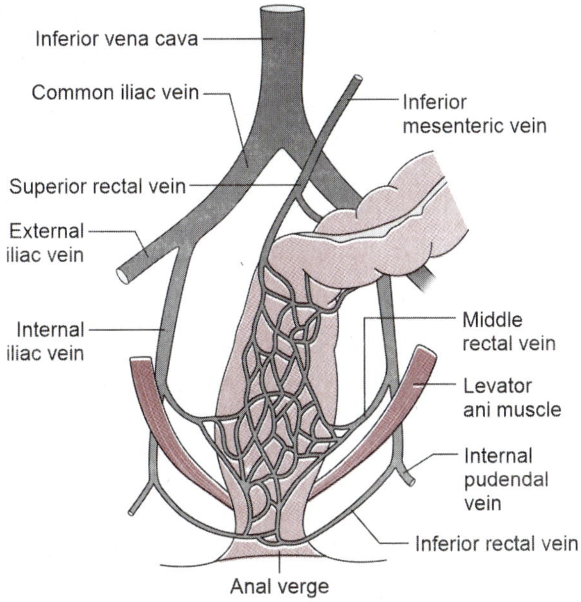

Fig.12.46: Venous drainage of rectum

Anus (Fig. 12.47)

BAQ: Write a note on the anus.

Ans: Anus is the opening at the end of the intestinal tract. It is a 2-inch long canal. Anus consisting of the pelvic floor muscles, internal and external anal sphincters (Fig. 12.47). These are important in control of defecation process. The pelvic floor muscle makes an angle between the rectum and the anus so that stool is prevented from expelling out. The internal sphincter remains tight till significant pressure builds by stool quantity. This action prevents involuntary defecation, mainly during sleeping conditions and travelling. External sphincter holds the stool until person with an urge for defecation reaches a toilet.

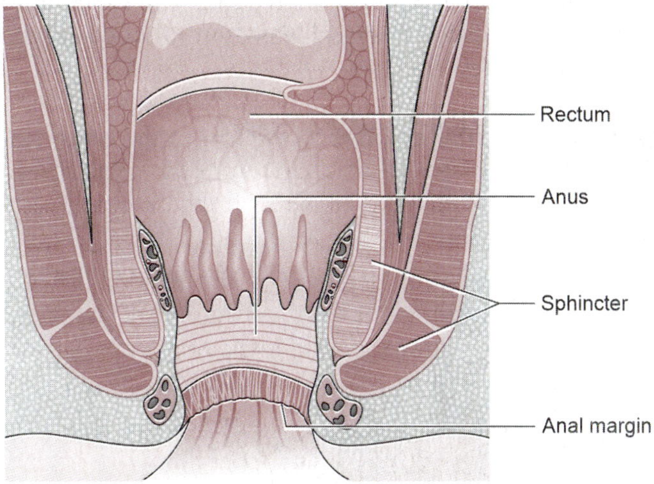

Fig. 12.47: Anatomical features of the anus

BAQ: Describe the tunics of the large intestine and their respective functions.

Ans: There are four layers of the large intestine. These layers from the internal lumen to outwards are: (1) The mucosa, (2) the submucosa, (3) the muscular layer, and (4) the serosa.

1. Mucosa is the inner lining of the large intestine. It is made up of a thin layer of epithelial cells. The mucosa does not have villi. It contains large number of goblet cells. Mucus secreted by the mucosa helps for the movement of the undigested food. Mucosa absorbs water and remaining nutrients in the remaining undigested food.
2. Submucosa is a fibrous connective tissue layer. It surrounds the mucosa. The submucosa contains major branches of blood and lymph vessels that supply the large intestine.
3. The muscular layer is made up of the following two layers of smooth muscles: The inner circular layer and the outer longitudinal layer. These layers contribute to the motility of the large intestine.
4. The serosa consists of a continuous sheet of squamous epithelial cells, the mesothelium, and it is separated from the underlying longitudinal muscle layer by a thin layer of loose connective tissue.

The serous layer provides a partition between the internal organs and the abdominal cavity. The serosa layer secretes a lubricating fluid. It provides lubrication to reduce friction with the abdominal cavity layer. The connective tissue layer provides blood vessels and nerves. It facilitates the sliding motion between the opposite surfaces.

BAQ: Draw a neat and labelled figure of anatomical features of the anus.

Ans: Refer to Fig. 12.47.

Hemorrhoids (Piles) (Fig. 12.48)

SAQ: What are hemorrhoids?

Ans: Hemorrhoids (piles) are swollen, enlarged veins that form inside and outside the rectum and anus. These could be painful and may cause rectal bleeding.

SAQ: What are the reasons for the formation of hemorrhoids?

Ans: Constipation leads to formation of hard stool. Prolonged straining to pass hard stool increase intra-abdominal pressure, leading to obstruction of the venous return and results in the swelling of the rectal venous plexus (hemorrhoidal plexus).

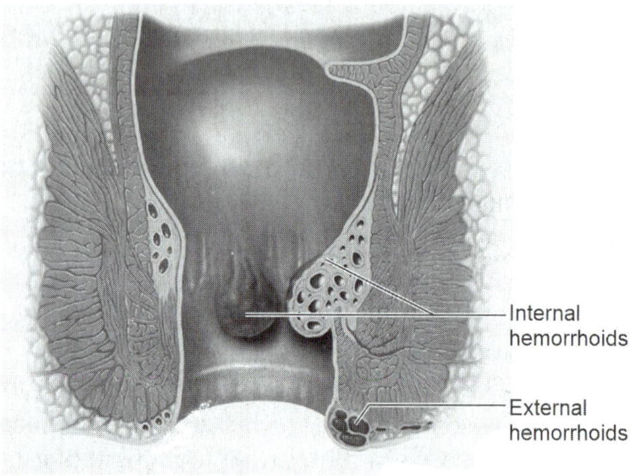

Fig. 12.48: Hemorrhoids (piles)

Anal Fistula (Fig. 12.49)

SAQ: What is anal fistula?

Ans: Anal fistula is an infected tunnel between the skin and the anus. These are caused due to an infection near anus that spreads to the skin. Symptoms of anal fistula include swelling of the affected part, pain, swelling and discharge of pus and blood.

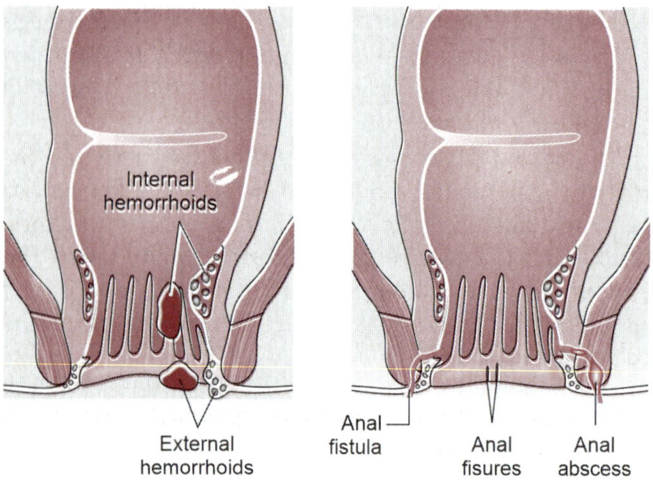

Fig. 12.49: Anal fistula, fissures and abscess

Anal Fissures (Fig. 12.49)

SAQ: What are anal fissures?

Ans: Anal fissures are cracks in the lining of anal opening. These occur due to frequent passages of very hard or watery stools. The crack in the anal lining exposes the underlying muscles that control the passage of stool through the anus (Fig. 12.49).

Appendix (Fig. 12.50)

SAQ: What is an appendix?

Ans: The appendix is a finger-like tubular part connected to the cecum (Fig. 12.50). The appendix is usually located in the lower right quadrant of the abdomen. The average length of appendix is about 3.5 inch and average diameter is about 0.24 inches. During the early years of development, the appendix has been observed to function as a lymphoid organ and exhibit protective functions against invading microorganisms.

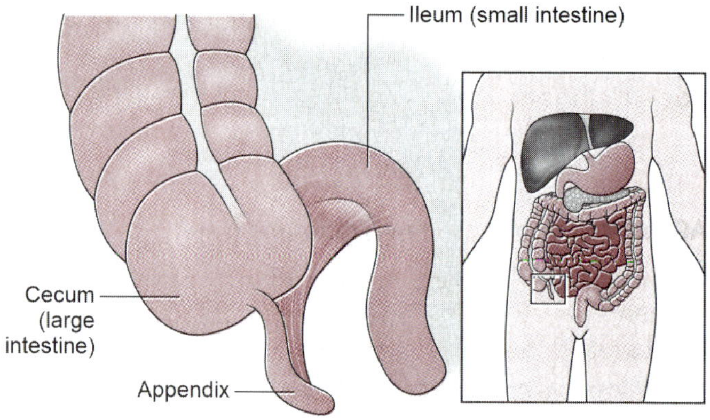

Fig. 12.50: Appendix

SAQ: What is appendicitis?

Ans: Appendicitis is an inflammation of the appendix. Appendicitis is caused, mostly due to blockage of the appendix by the entry of fecal particles inside appendix. This leads to microbial infection and rapid multiplication of microorganisms takes place. Due to the spread of infection, the appendix becomes inflamed, swollen and fill with pus. Appendicitis causes pain mostly in lower right abdomen.

The standard treatment on appendicitis is surgical removal of appendix, since, antibiotic treatment may not be effective. This procedure is known as appendicectomy.

SAQ: What are the symptoms of diarrhea?

Ans: The following are the symptoms of diarrhea: Loose watery stools, bloating, cramps in the stomach, loss of appetite, nausea, fatigue, and fever if infection is severe.

SAQ: What is the difference between diarrhea and dysentery?

Ans: Diarrhea is a clinical condition that involves the frequent passing of loose or watery stools, mainly due to microbial, or parasitic infections. The presence of blood in the stool of a person suffering from diarrhea is a sign of dysentery.

Objectives: To describe the anatomical features and functions of the liver, gallbladder and pancreas as the accessory parts of the digestive system. To describe the various disorders related to the liver, gallbladder and pancreas as the accessory parts of the digestive system. To describe the blood supply to the liver, gallbladder and pancreas.

LIVER (Fig. 12.51)

BAQ: Write a brief note on liver.

Ans: Liver is the largest organ in the human body. It weighs 1.2–1.5 kg in adult. It is located in the right upper quadrant of the abdomen and is attached beneath the diaphragm by its ligaments. It is divided into four lobes, left, right, quadrate and caudate. These are supplied by the left and right branches of the portal vein and the hepatic artery. The biliary drainage is into the left and right hepatic ducts. A thin connective-tissue capsule covers the entire liver surface (Fig. 12.52).

The liver is of vital importance in intermediary metabolisms, in the detoxification and in the elimination of toxic substances.

Ligaments of the Liver (Fig. 12.53)

BAQ: Write a note on liver ligaments.

Ans: A ligament means a tough band of tissue. The ligaments of liver attach the liver to the surrounding structures. These are formed by a double layer of peritoneum. The following are ligaments of liver:

1. The falciform ligament attaches the anterior surface of the liver to the anterior abdominal wall.
2. The coronary ligament attaches the superior surface of the liver to the inferior surface of the diaphragm.
3. The left triangular ligament attaches the left lobe of the liver to the diaphragm.
4. The lesser omentum attaches the liver to the lesser curvature of the stomach and first part of the duodenum.

BAQ: Draw a neat and labeled figure of liver ligaments.
Ans: Refer to Fig. 12.53.

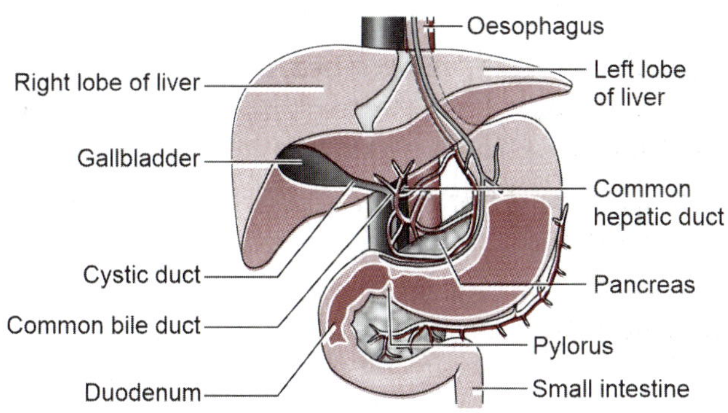

Fig. 12.51: Anatomy of liver

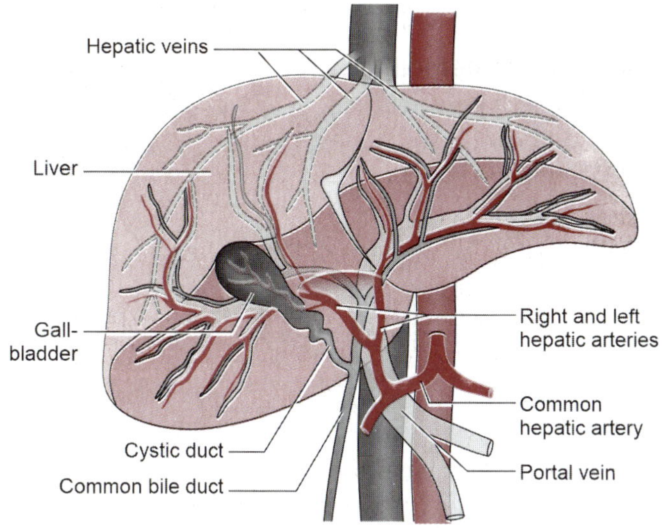

Fig. 12.52: Blood circulation of liver

Liver Anatomy (Fig. 12.54)

LAQ: Write a note on the liver with respect to the following points: (1) Applied anatomical features, (3) blood supply, (3) bile circulation (4) functions of various anatomical components and (5) innervation of liver.

Ans:

1. The liver is made up of various types of cells. The majority of cells in the liver (nearly two-thirds of liver mass) are hepatocytes. The remaining cell types are Kupffer cells, stellate (fat storing) cells, endothelial cells, blood vessels, cells of bile ducts and supporting structures.

   #### Microscopic Anatomy of Liver (Fig. 12.54)

   The liver is composed of a large number of functional units or lobules. A lobule is a polyhedral prism of tissue demarcated by connective tissue septa and by the vascular and biliary vessels.

2. **Blood supply:** Each lobule consists of row of hepatocytes (liver cells) radiating from the central vein. The hepatocytes are supplied with arterial blood through a hepatic arteriole and arterial sinusoids, and with blood from the portal vein through a portal venule and venous sinusoids. The central vein is in the center of the lobule (Fig. 12.54A).

   The circulating system of the liver is characterized by a dual blood supply. The portal vein carries blood from the capillary bed of the alimentary tract, which is rich in nutrients absorbed from the gastrointestinal tract. Hepatic artery (a branch of the celiac trunk) carries well-oxygenated blood to the liver (Fig. 12.54B). About 20% of the blood flow is oxygen-rich blood from the hepatic artery, and 80% blood is nutrition-rich from the portal vein. The venous drainage from the liver is through the right and left hepatic veins, which enter into inferior vena cava near the right atrium. In addition, numerous lymphatic channels are also seen in the liver.

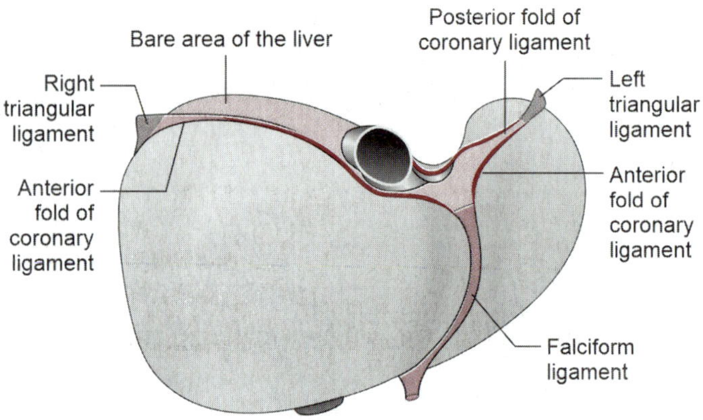

Fig. 12.53: Liver ligaments

The portal triad consists of bile ducts that accompany the hepatic artery and portal vein (Fig. 12.54B). Bile flows from the hepatocytes into the bile canaliculi and ductules, to the larger intrahepatic bile ducts, and finally to the left and right hepatic bile ducts. These emerge from the liver and form a common bile duct.

3. **Bile circulation:** The bile canaliculi run between the rows of hepatocytes. These collect the bile made by the hepatocytes. These bile canaliculi drain into terminal bile ducts, by way of larger interlobular bile ducts, into the main hepatic duct which drains into the gall-bladder (Fig. 12.55).
4. **Functions of various anatomical components:**
   A. The venous sinusoids are lined with phagocytic cells called Kupffer cells which remove bacteria (of intestinal origin) and other foreign bodies from the blood before it enters the systemic circulation. Kupffer cells form about 20% of the hepatic cell mass.

   Kupffer cells represent the largest group of fixed macrophages in the body.

   B. The hepatocytes demonstrate pinocytotic (ingestion of liquid droplets) and endocytotic activity (internalization of substances) with active and passive uptake of nutrients. Hepatocytes perform various functions in maintaining homeostasis and health. These functions include, synthesis of albumin, coagulation factors, carrier proteins, hormonal and growth factors, production of bile and its constituents (bile salts, cholesterol, lecithin,

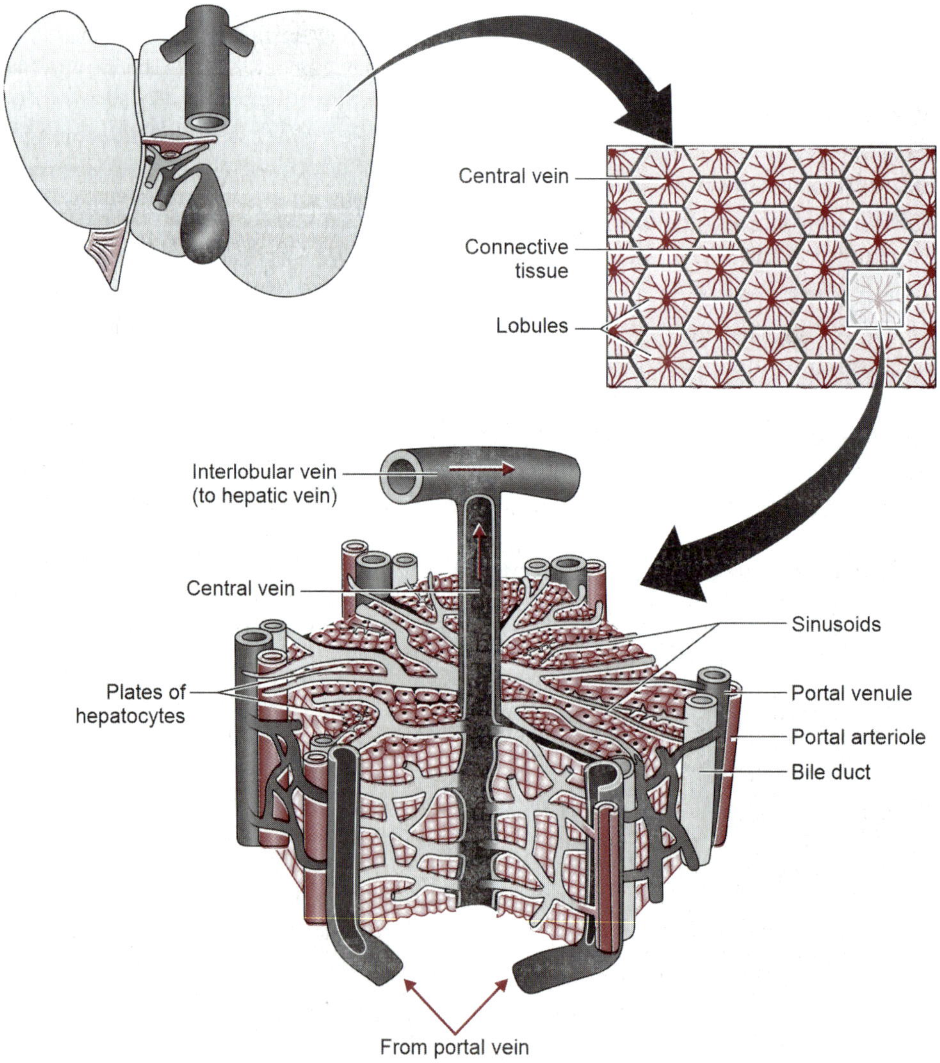

Fig. 12.54A: Microscopic anatomy of liver–I

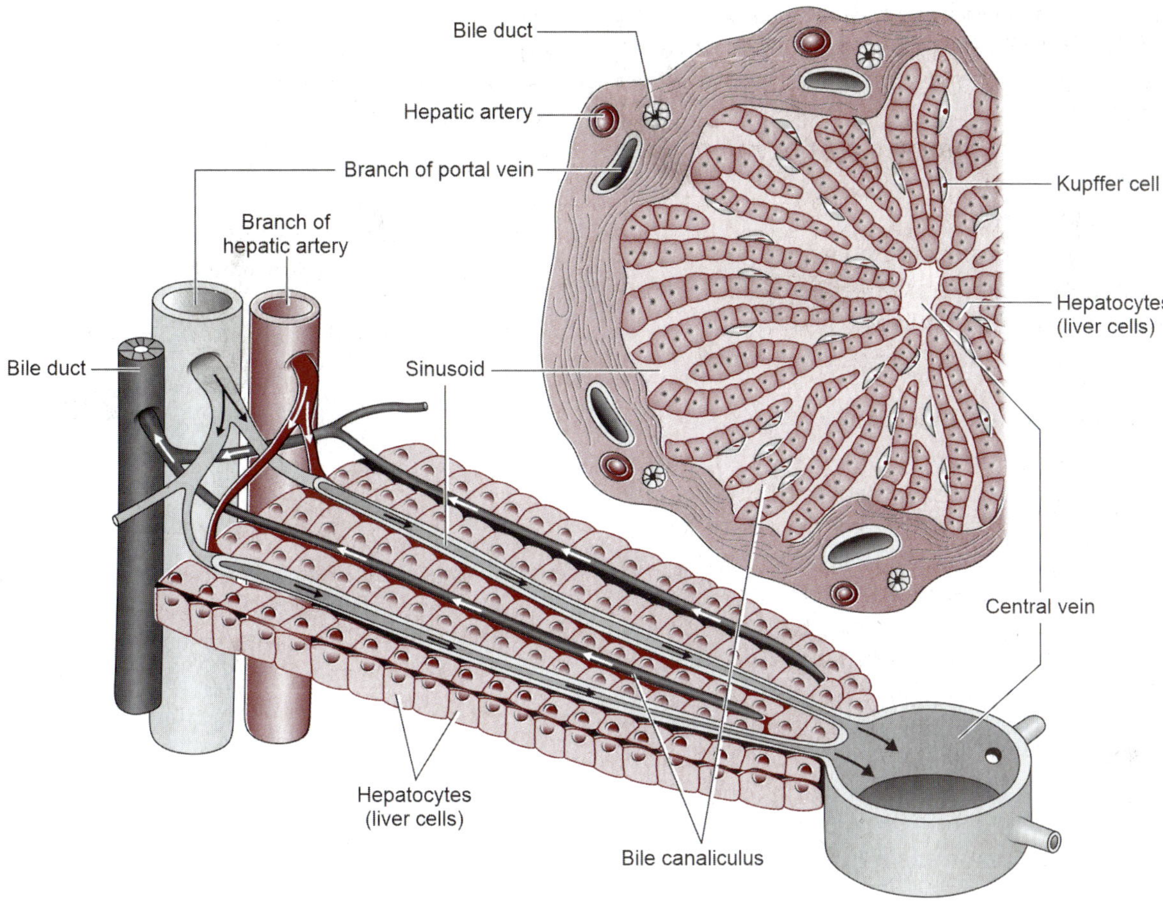

Fig. 12.54B: Microscopic anatomy of liver–II

phospholipids etc.), metabolism of glucose, glycogen, cholesterol, fatty acids, amino acids, lipoproteins, drugs, bilirubin etc.

5. **Innervation of the liver:** It is provided by hepatic nerve plexus, which enters the liver at the porta hepatis. Parasympathetic innervation is derived from the preganglionic fibers of the vagus and sympathetic innervation is derived from preganglionic fibers.

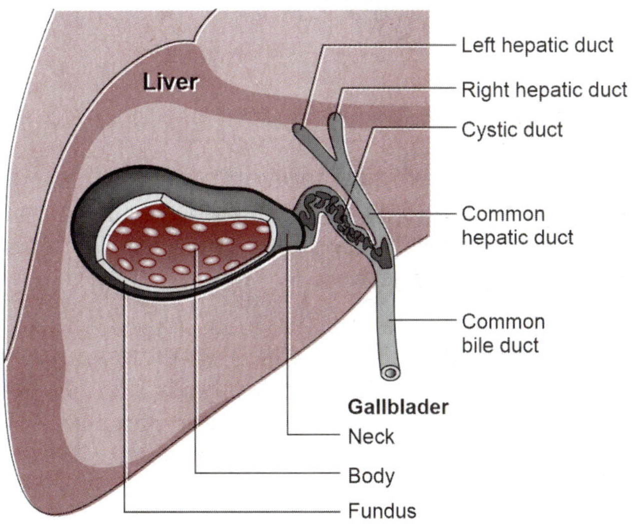

Fig. 12.55: Bile storage in the gallbladder

LIVER FUNCTIONS

BAQ: Enumerate various functions of the liver.

Ans:

1. **Excretory functions**
   a. Bile formation and excretion of bile into the intestine.
   b. Excretion of bilirubin.
   c. Secretion of bile salts, water-soluble bilirubin and cholesterol through bile; which are produced from the liver parenchymal cells.
   d. Excretion of substances like heavy metals and alkaline phosphatase enzyme; withdrawn from the blood by hepatic blood circulation.
2. **Metabolic functions:** Liver is the main center of metabolic reactions of carbohydrate, protein and lipids.
3. **Protective functions and detoxication**
   a. Kupffer cells remove foreign bodies from blood (phagocytosis).
   b. Detoxication by conjugation, methylation, oxidation and reduction reactions.
   c. Removal of ammonia from blood, particularly that absorbed from the intestine by way of the portal vein.
4. **Hematologic functions** (Hematopoiesis and coagulation):
   a. Blood formation in the embryo.

b. Production of blood coagulation factors (I to XIII, PK, HMWK, etc.) fibrinogen, prothrombin and heparin, which play important role in blood coagulation.
c. Destruction of erythrocytes (at the end of their respective life span.
5. **Circulatory functions**
a. Transfer of blood from portal to systemic circulation.
b. Activity of its reticuloendothelial system (Kupffer cells) in immune mechanisms.
c. Blood storage (regulation of blood volume).

SAQ: Write a note on the bile.

Ans: The bile is secreted by the liver cells. It mainly contains; water, mineral salts, cholesterol, bile salts, bile pigments, and mucus. Bile salts play important role in the digestion of fats in the small intestine. The yellow colour of the bile is due to bilirubin, which is an excretory substance formed from the degenerated red blood cells. Through the biliary capillaries (biliary tree) the bile circulates in the liver cells and by the common hepatic duct and cystic duct; it is stored in the gallbladder (Figs 12.56 and 12.57). When food reaches the duodenum, enterocrinin hormone secretes from the intestinal wall. It stimulates the gallbladder to secrete bile through the common bile duct in the duodenum (Fig. 12.57).

BAQ: Describe the gallbladder on the basis of the following heads: (1) Introduction and (2) applied anatomical features with respective functions.

Ans:

1. **Introduction:** The gallbladder is located in the upper right side of the abdomen under the liver (Figs 12.52, 12.55, 12.56). The primary function of gallbladder is to store and secrete bile, which is necessary to digest fats in the small intestine and also excretion of bilirubin. The gall bladder stores about 30–50 ml of bile.
2. Applied anatomical features with respective functions: The gallbladder is divided into the following three sections: (1) fundus, (2) body and (3) neck.
   1. **Fundus:** It is a large rounded base of gall bladder. It stores the bile.
   2. **Body:** It is the part of the gallbladder that taper into the neck.
   3. **Neck:** At this part, the gallbladder continues to taper and become narrow as it joins the cystic duct, which joins the common bile duct and the biliary tree. The neck of the gallbladder has a folded area of tissues called "Hartmann Pouch."

The wall of the gallbladder is made up of the following four layers:

1. **Inner mucosa:** It is made up of thin layer of epithelium. It lines the inside part of the gallbladder.
2. **Lamina propria:** It is a layer of loose connective tissue and part of the inner mucosa.
3. **Tunica muscularis:** It is a layer of smooth muscle tissue that enables the gallbladder to contract to release bile into the bile duct.
4. **Serosa:** It is the outer fibrous connective tissue layer, that surrounds the tunica muscularis. The serosa contains blood vessels and lymphatics.

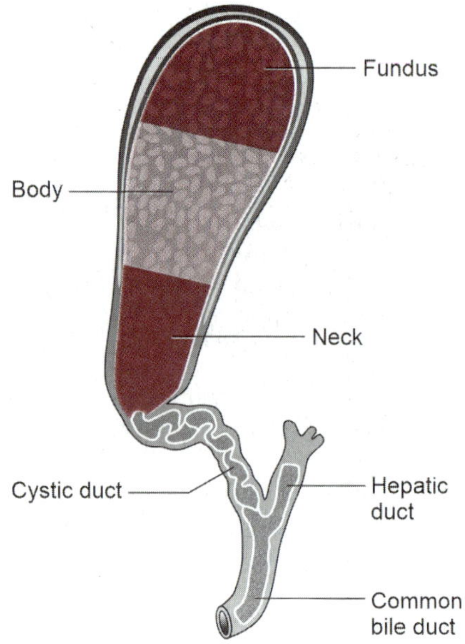

Fig. 12.56: Gallbladder

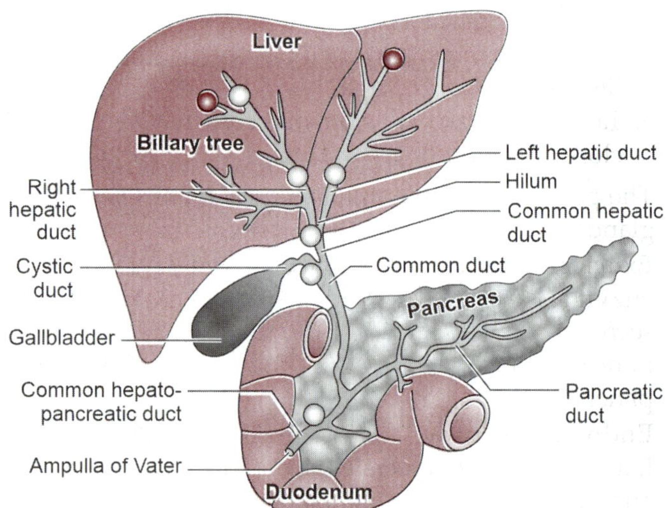

Fig. 12.57: Gallbladder connections

PANCREAS (Figs 12.57 and 12.58)

LAQ: Describe the pancreas with respect to the following points: (1) Introduction and (2) applied anatomical features with respective functions, (3) blood supply and (4) innervation.

Ans:

1. **Introduction:** The pancreas is an elongated and tapered organ behind the stomach (Fig. 12.58). With the exception of the tail of the pancreas, it is placed outside the peritoneum (retroperitoneal) organ. Tail of the pancreas is inside the peritoneum (intraperitoneal). It is located deep within the upper abdomen in the epigastrium and left hypochondrium

regions. The average size of pancreas in adults is about 4.7–5.9 inches long. It is lobulated, and salmon-coloured in appearance.

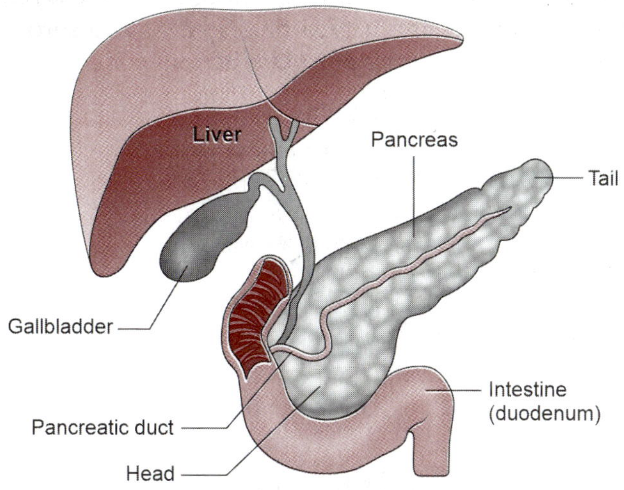

Fig. 12.58: Pancreas

2. **Anatomical features with the respective functions:** The pancreas can be divided into the following main three parts (Fig. 12.58):
   1. *Head:* It is the widest part of the pancreas. It lies within the C-shaped curve of the duodenum. Head of pancreas is connected to duodenum by connective tissue.
   2. *Body:* It is centrally located part of the pancreas. It lies behind the stomach.
   3. Tail: It is the left end of the pancreas that lies within close proximity to the spleen.

The pancreas is made up of the following two types of glands:

1. **Exocrine glands:** These glands secrete digestive enzymes, amylase and lipase. These enzymes are secreted into a network of ducts that join the main pancreatic duct, which runs the full length of the pancreas.
2. **Endocrine glands:** These consists of the islets of Langerhans, which secretes hormones such as insulin and glucagon into the bloodstream.

Exocrine Part of the Pancreas

The exocrine part of the pancreas is a lobulated, serous gland which produces digestive enzyme precursors. It is composed of approximately one million clusters of cells, known as acinar cells, which are connected by short intercalated ducts (Figs 12.59 and 12.60).

The intercalated ducts unite and pass secretions into a network of intralobular collecting ducts, which in turn drain into the main pancreatic duct.

The pancreatic duct runs the full length of the pancreas and unites with the common bile duct and form the hepatopancreatic ampulla of Vater (Fig.12.57), which opens into the duodenum through the major duodenal papilla.

The passage of secretions from liver and pancreas into the duodenum are controlled by the sphincter of Oddi (Fig. 12.60B). It surrounds the ampulla of Vater, acting as a valve.

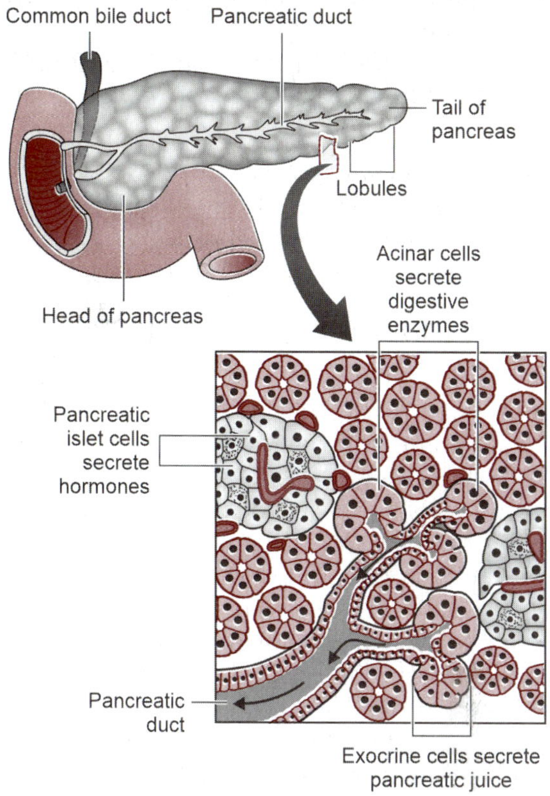

Fig. 12.59: Anatomy of pancreatic lobule

Endocrine Part of Pancreas (Figs 12.59 and 12.60)

The tissues of pancreas contain clusters of cells called islets of Langerhans (Figs 12.59 and 12.60). These cells are distributed throughout the pancreas. Pancreatic islets contain alpha cells, beta cells, and delta cells. Alpha cells secrete glucagon hormone. Beta cells secrete insulin hormone. Insulin and glucagon play very important role in the management of glucose molecules for the body cells. Delta cells secrete somatostatin hormone, which controls the secretions of insulin and glucagon. Gamma cells produce pancreatic polypeptide (PP) hormone, which regulates both the endocrine and exocrine pancreatic secretions.

Islets are composed of about 3,000 secretory cells, which contain small arterioles and venules that facilitate passage of the hormones secreted by the cells to enter the systemic circulation.

Enterochromaffin cells are also scattered throughout the islets. These cells play crucial role in regulation of gastrointestinal motility and secretion by secreting serotonin hormone.

Blood Supply of Pancreas (Fig. 12.61)

3. **Blood supply:** The pancreas is supplied with blood by splenic artery. Following branches of splenic artery extend to the body and to the tail of the gland: The dorsal pancreatic artery, inferior pancreatic artery, greater pancreatic artery, artery to tail of pancreas, and pancreatic branches (Fig. 12.61).

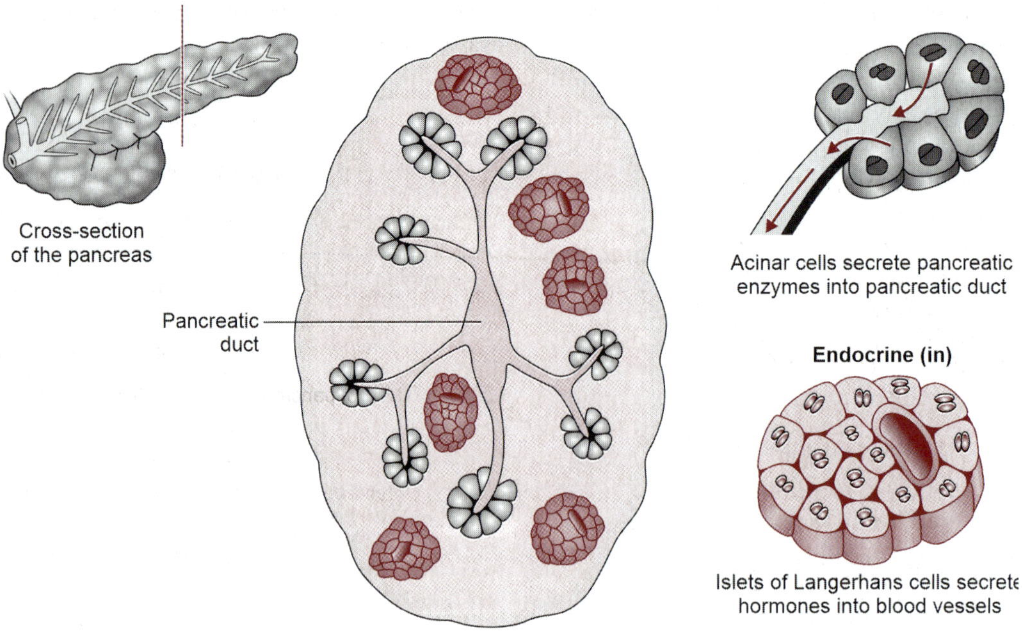

Fig. 12.60A: Cross section of the pancreas

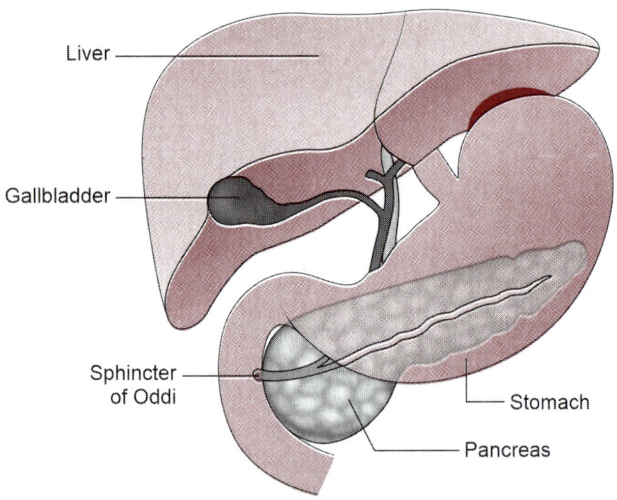

Fig. 12.60B: Sphincter of oddi

The venous drainage of the pancreas head part is into the superior mesenteric branches of the hepatic portal vein. The rest of the pancreas blood drainage is via the splenic vein (Fig. 12.61).

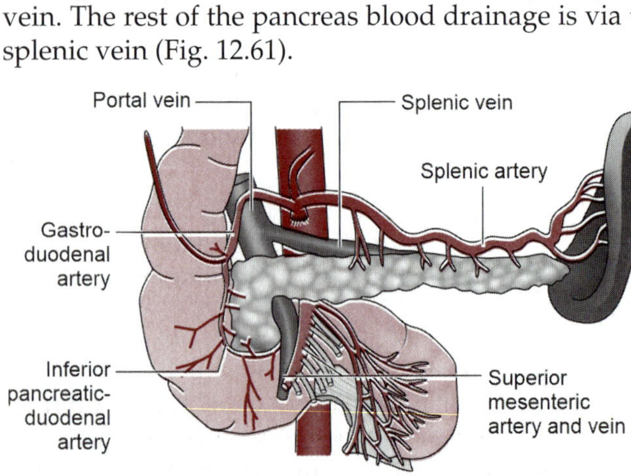

Fig. 12.61: Blood supply of pancreas

4. **Innervation of the pancreas:** The pancreas receives involuntary innervation via the autonomic nervous system. The parasympathetic innervation of pancreas originates from the vagus nerve (CN X). The sympathetic innervation of pancreas originates from the greater and lesser splanchnic nerves (T5–T12).

Lymphatic Drainage of Pancreas (Fig. 12.62)

SAQ: Write a note on the lymphatic drainage of the pancreas.

Ans: The pancreas drains into lymphatic vessels that travel alongside its arteries, and has a rich lymphatic supply. The lymphatic vessels of the body and tail drain into splenic lymph nodes, and eventually into lymph nodes that lie in front of the aorta (Fig. 12.62).

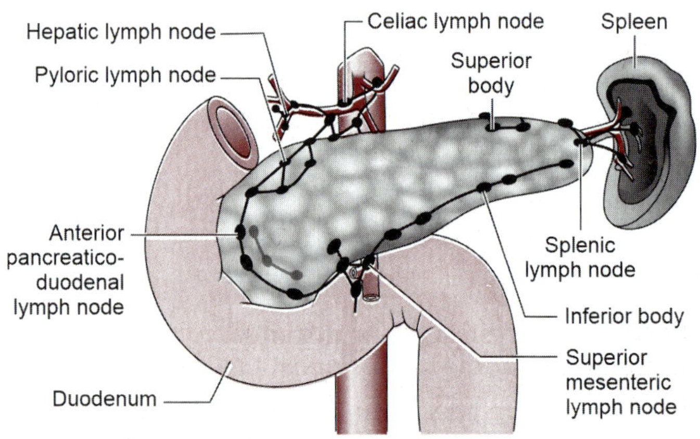

Fig.12.62: Pancreatic lymph drainage

BAQ: Enumerate the functions of the pancreas.

Ans: The various functions of the pancreas are as follows:

1. The pancreas secretes digestive enzymes such as amylase, trypsin and lipase, which break down carbohydrates, protein and fats in the duodenum, respectively into simplified forms respectively. These simplified food products are processed further and

absorbed in the duodenum, jejunum and ileum during chyme passage through the small intestine.
2. The main hormones secreted by the endocrine gland in the pancreas are insulin, glucagon and somatostatin. These hormones regulate the level of blood glucose and somatostatin hormone controls the release of insulin and glucagon.

Objective: To describe the anatomical structure and functions of peritoneum and related disorders.

PERITONEUM (Fig. 12.63)

BAQ: Write a note on the peritoneum.

Ans: The peritoneum is a membrane that lines the abdominal cavity and covers the abdominal organs. The peritoneum consists of following two layers: (1) The parietal peritoneum and (2) the visceral peritoneum. Both types are made up of simple squamous epithelial cells called mesothelium (Fig. 12.63).

1. **Parietal peritoneum:** The parietal peritoneum lines the internal surface of the abdominal wall.
2. **Visceral peritoneum:** The visceral peritoneum turns inside out to cover the majority of the abdominal viscera.

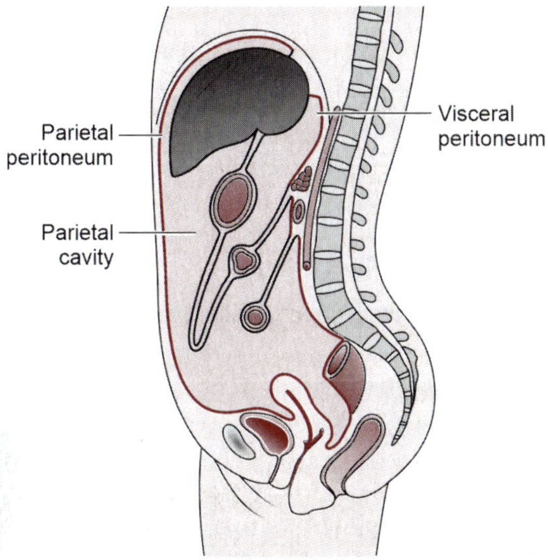

Fig. 12.63: Peritoneum

Functions of the Peritoneum

Peritoneum protects the abdominopelvic organs. It connects abdominal organs with each other and maintain the position of organs by suspending them with ligaments. Peritoneum provides pathways for nerves, blood vessels and lymph to viscera and away from viscera. Peritoneum also prevents friction of the various internal organs.

Peritoneal Cavity (Fig. 12.63)

SAQ: What is peritoneal cavity?

Ans: The peritoneal cavity is a potential space between the parietal and visceral peritoneum. It normally contains only a small amount of lubricating fluid called peritoneal fluid (Fig. 12.64).

Peritoneal Fluid (Fig. 12.64)

BAQ: Write a note on the peritoneal fluid.

Ans: The peritoneal fluid is present in the peritoneal cavity, which is a space between the wall of the abdomen and the organs inside the abdomen. It is a serous (serum like) fluid produced by passage of fluids from blood vessels across the peritoneal membrane.

The primary function of peritoneal fluid is to reduce the friction between the abdominal organs when they move during digestion procedure.

The peritoneal cavity normally contains approximately 50–75 ml of peritoneal fluid. An increased volume of peritoneal fluid is called ascites (Fig. 12.64). It is observed when pressure builds up in the veins of liver, which blocks blood flow in the liver. Various reasons for the ascites are, cirrhosis of liver, heart failure, kidney failure, development of cancer, or due to an infection.

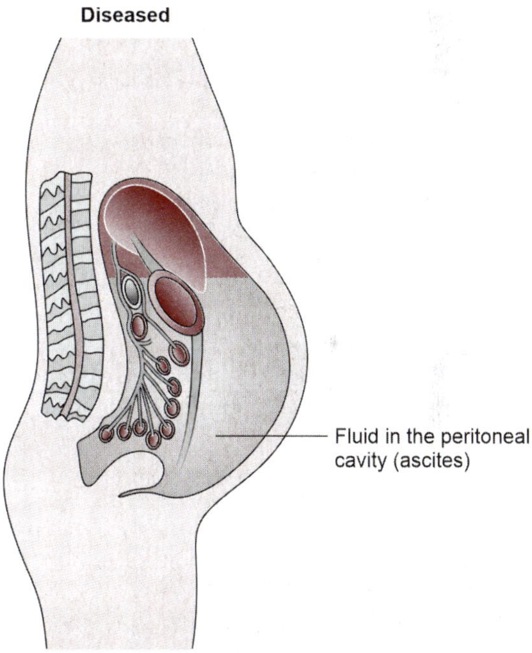

Fig. 12.64: Increased peritoneal fluid (ascites)

HERNIA (Figs 12.65–12.68)

SAQ: Write a brief note on hernia.

Ans: A hernia occurs when an internal organ pushes through a weak spot in muscle or tissue. A hernia mainly involves the stomach or the intestine. Symptoms of a hernia include a lump in the affected area of the body and related pain. The following are the most common types of hernia: (1) Inguinal hernia (inner groin), (2) incisional hernia (resulting from an incision), (3) femoral hernia (outer groin), (4) umbilical hernia (belly button), and (5) hiatal hernia (upper stomach).

Although hernias may not be life-threatening, surgery may be required to prevent future complications.

Inguinal Hernia (Fig. 12.65)

BAQ: Write a note on inguinal hernia.

Ans: Inguinal hernia is the most common type of hernia. In this type of hernia, the intestine pushes through a weak spot in the lower abdominal wall, in the inguinal canal in groin (Fig. 12.65).

Inguinal hernias are more common in men, since, the testicles descend through the inguinal canal after birth. When the inguinal canal does not close properly, a weakened area remains, through which intestine may push through (Fig. 12.65). When the intestinal part gets trapped in the abdominal wall, it may obstruct the bowel, leading to severe pain and other symptoms such as, nausea, vomiting, and the inability to have a normal bowel movement. When surrounding muscle clamps around the protruding tissue, the blood supply to the small intestine may stop. This is called strangulation of the small intestine. It may lead to intestinal perforation, shock, or gangrene and it is a life-threatening condition.

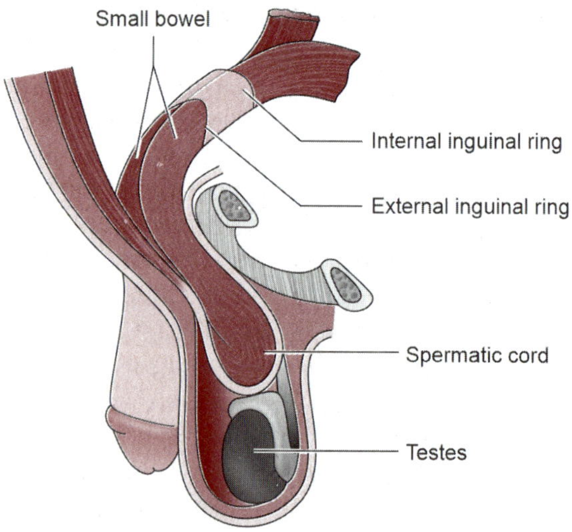

Fig. 12.65: Inguinal hernia

Hiatal Hernia (Fig. 12.66)

BAQ: Write a note on hiatal hernia.

Ans: A hiatal hernia occurs when part of the stomach protrudes up through the diaphragm into the chest cavity.

This type of hernia is most common in elderly persons with age above 50 years. A child also may have hiatal hernia; caused by a congenital birth defect.

Hiatal hernia leads to gastroesophageal reflux disease (GERD). In GERD, the stomach contents containing hydrochloric acid leak backward into the esophagus. Reflux of gastric acid may damage the pharynx, esophagus, or the respiratory tract.

Umbilical Hernia (Fig. 12.67)

BAQ: Write a note on hiatal hernia.

Ans: An umbilical hernia occurs when part of intestine bulges through the opening in abdominal muscles near navel (small lump at the middle of stomach) (Fig. 12.67). Umbilical hernia is the most common in infants, however, it can also be seen among obese adults. Umbilical hernias are common and harmless; and it may go away on its own; when the abdominal wall muscles get stronger.

Ventral (Incisional) Hernia (Fig. 12.68)

BAQ: Write a note on ventral (incisional) hernia.

Ans: A ventral (incisional) hernia occurs when tissue bulges through an opening in the muscles of the abdomen (Fig. 12.68). Common features observed in ventral hernia are pregnancy, obesity and strenuous activities.

Ventral hernias may also occur at the site of a surgical incision. This is called an incisional hernia and it results from scarring or weakness caused due to surgery of the abdominal muscles (Fig. 12.68). A strangulated ventral hernia is an emergency and require surgery.

Femoral Hernia (Fig. 12.69)

BAQ: Write a note on femoral hernia.

Ans: In femoral hernia, a portion of tissue pushes through the wall of the femoral canal. A femoral hernia appears as a bulge near the groin or thigh. Although, femoral hernias can occur in both males and females; due to the increased width of the female pelvis, it is more common among female. Femoral hernias are also more common in adults than in children.

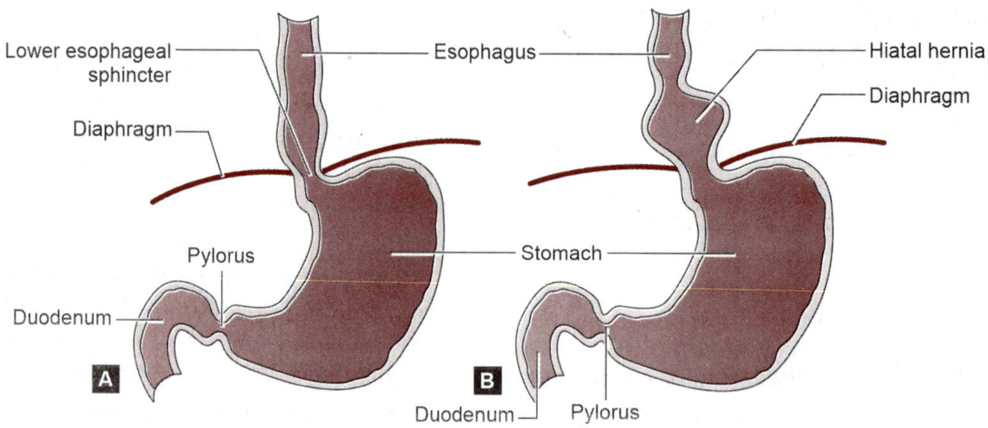

Figs 12.66A and B: (A) Normal stomach; (B) hiatal hernia

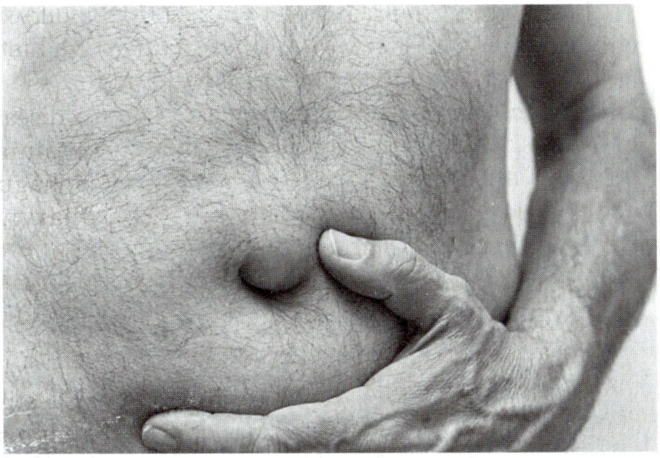

Fig. 12.67: Umbilical hernia

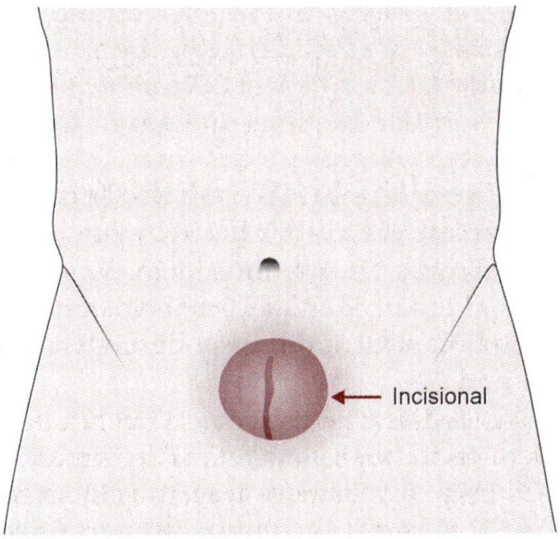

Fig. 12.68: Incisional hernia

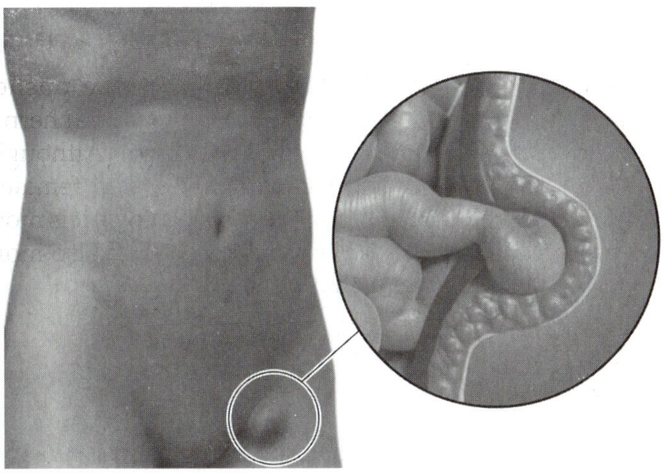

Fig. 12.69: Femoral hernia

Objective: To describe the physiology of digestion and absorption.

PHYSIOLOGY OF DIGESTION

LAQ: Write a note on the physiology of digestion.

Ans: Digestion is the process of breaking down of complex food components in gastrointestinal tract into microparticles; which are suitable for the absorption into the bloodstream. The food contains mainly carbohydrates, proteins, fats, minerals, vitamins and water. The macronutrients are broken down into micromolecules; that get absorbed in GI and enter the bloodstream. Digested micromolecules are used by body cells for their various activities. The digestion is comprised of mechanical digestion and chemical digestion.

Mechanical digestion takes place in mouth by mastication process. Teeth break down food substances into smaller particles. Chemical digestion is further degradation of mechanically broken food particles by the digestive enzymes, secreted by salivary glands in the mouth; in the stomach and in the small intestine.

Salivary amylase (ptyalin) acts on starch to form maltose and maltotriose. The lingual lipase hydrolyses the ester bonds in triglycerides to form diacylglycerols and monoacylglycerols. This partially digested food present in bolus form is swallowed into the esophagus and the bolus passes to the stomach by peristalsis actions. Food digestion does nor take place in the esophagus.

Mechanical digestion of the bolus also takes place in the stomach by the peristaltic contractions of the smooth muscle. The antrum part of the stomach functions to grind the bolus by forceful peristaltic contractions. The size of food particles reduces further by the grinding of bolus by the antrum. Food particles smaller than 2 mm in diameter pass through the contracted pylorus into the duodenum. The rest of the bolus is pushed back for further mechanical and chemical digestion.

When bolus arrives in the stomach, pyloric glands present in the lines of stomach secrete gastrin hormone. Gastrin stimulates parietal cells of stomach to secret hydrochloric acid.

Mucous cells present in the stomach secrete a bicarbonate-rich mucous on the surface of the gastric mucosa to protect it from the acidic contents of the stomach.

Functions of hydrochloric acid are as follows:

Hydrochloric Acid

1. Maintain pH about 1.5–3.0, to prevent growth of microorganisms in the food.
2. Denatures proteins for further enzymatic actions and
3. Activate the inactive pepsinogen to active pepsin form.

Pepsin converts proteins into the following simplified forms, peptones and proteoses.

Parietal cells in the stomach also secrete intrinsic factor, a substance necessary for the absorption of vitamin B_{12} in the ileum.

Digestion of carbohydrates does not take place in the stomach. Bolus is converted to chyme in the stomach.

The chyme passes through the pylorus by peristalsis into the duodenum. It is controlled by the nervous and hormonal control. In the small intestine, mechanical digestion of chyme takes place to some extent.

When chyle arrives in small intestine, cholecystokinin (CCK) and secretin hormones are released from the neuroendocrine cells of the upper small intestine. CCK and secretin stimulate gall bladder to secret bile in the small intestine and also stimulate pancreas to secret pancreatic juice in the small intestine. Pancreatic juice contains digestive enzymes such as amylase, trypsinogen, chymotrypsinogen, procarboxypeptidase, and proelastase. These enzymes function optimally at pH from 6 to 7 due to presence of bicarbonate in the pancreatic juice.

Pancreatic amylase acts on starch and glycogen to form maltose and trisaccharides.

Pancreatic lipase along with a colipase, acts on emulsified triglycerides in lipids to form monoglycerides, diacylglycerols and glycerol. Bile secreted by gall bladder is necessary to emulsify the lipids.

Duodenal enzyme enterokinase converts, inactive, trypsinogen into active form, trypsin. Trypsin converts chymotrypsinogen, procarboxypeptidase, and proelastase to their active forms.

Trypsin, chymotrypsin, and elastase are all endopeptidases that hydrolyze proteins and various digested forms of proteins into peptones, proteases and dipeptides.

The duodenum also contains digestive enzymes such as disaccharidases and dipeptidase. The disaccharidases are maltase, lactase, and sucrase. Maltase acts on maltose to produce two glucose molecules. Lactase acts on lactose to produce glucose and galactose. Sucrase acts on sucrose to produce glucose and fructose.

Dipeptidase acts on dipeptides to produce two amino acid molecules.

End products of digestion are mainly, monosaccharides, fatty acids, glycerol, amino acids and vitamins (already present in the food).

PHYSIOLOGY OF ABSORBTION OF DIGESTED FOOD

LAQ: Write a note on the absorption of digested food.

Ans: The absorption of most of the digested food takes place in the jejunum. The end products of carbohydrate digestion are glucose, fructose and galactose. Glucose and galactose are absorbed in blood by active transport system. Other monosaccharides are absorbed by diffusion. Fructose and sugar alcohols are absorbed down their concentration gradient. After a high intake of fructose, some may remain in the intestinal lumen leading to bacterial fermentation.

The end products of fat digestion are, 2-monoacyl glycerols, 1-monoacyl glycerols and free fatty acids. In the presence of bile salts, emulsification of these end products along with cholesterol and phospholipids takes place in the formation of micelles. Since micelles are soluble, they allow the products of lipid digestion and fat-soluble vitamins to be transported through the aqueous environment of the intestinal lumen.

Within the intestinal epithelium, 1-monoacylglycerols are hydrolysed to fatty acids and glycerol and 2-monoacylglycerols are re-cycled to triglycerides. Glycerol and free fatty acids along with other products form chylomicrons and enter the bloodstream via thoracic duct. Short- and medium-chain fatty acids are mainly absorbed into hepatic portal vein.

The end-products of protein digestion are free amino acids and small peptides. Free amino acids are absorbed across the intestinal mucosa by active transport. Dipeptides and tripeptides enter the brush border of the intestinal mucosal cells, where they are hydrolysed to free amino acids. The amino acids are then transported into the hepatic portal vein.

Vitamins and minerals are released from food during digestion. The fat-soluble vitamins are absorbed in the lipid micelles formed in the lipid digestion. Water-soluble vitamins are absorbed either by active transport or by diffusion. Absorption of calcium requires vitamin D. Iron absorption requires vitamin C. Calcium and inorganic phosphorus are absorbed in a controlled manner by the influence of parathyroid hormones. Most mineral salts are absorbed in blood by simple diffusion.

Iron is absorbed in the duodenum. Vitamin B_{12} and bile salts are absorbed in the terminal ileum and Water is absorbed by passive diffusion throughout the small intestine and also in the colon.

The absorbed food micronutrients are then transported through the blood vessels to different organs of the body. The body cells use them for various cellular activities. The food that remains undigested and unabsorbed passes into the large intestine.

Objective: To describe the effects of ageing on the gastro-intestinal tract.

EFFECTS OF AGEING ON THE GASTROINTESTINAL (GI) SYSTEM

Due to the advancing age, the elderly may suffer from the following various changes in the anatomical features of the gastrointestinal tract and related clinical conditions:

1. Decrease in the muscle mass of the tongue and decrease in the salivation. Similarly, the number of taste buds may decrease Eating difficulties may arise due to the loss of teeth and use of dentures.
2. Decrease in the strength of esophageal contractions and in the tension in the upper esophageal sphincter. The passage of food through the esophagus may be affected in some older adults.
3. The capacity of the stomach lining to resist damage decreases. It may increase the risk of peptic ulcers in those individuals who use nonsteroid anti-inflammatory drugs and aspirin. The elasticity of the stomach decreases and the capacity to accommodate more food also decreases. The rate at which the stomach empties food into the small intestine also decreases. In some elderly individuals, acid secretion

may decrease, leading to poor absorption of vitamin B_{12} and the tendency of overgrowth of intestinal bacteria.

4. Some elderly individuals may suffer from decrease in the level of lactase in the brush border of small intestine. These individuals may suffer from lactose intolerance and may need to avoid milk and other dairy products.
5. Bacterial overgrowth becomes more common in elderly and it can lead to bloating, pain and weight loss. Bacterial overgrowth may also lead to decreased in the absorption of iron, calcium, vitamin A, vitamin D and vitamin B_{12}.
6. The normal rate of peristalsis decreases, leading to increase in the tendency of constipation.
7. Pelvic floor may become weak in older women, which may contribute to fecal incontinence.
8. Normal mass of liver and pancreas decreases. Decrease in the mass of liver may lead to overall decrease in various types of metabolic reactions. Decrease in the mass of pancreas may lead to decrease in the exocrine functions.

Objective: To describe the general diseases of the gastrointestinal tract.

GENERAL DISEASES OF THE GATROINTESTINAL TRACT

LAQ: Write a note on the diseases of the gastro-intestinal tract.

Ans: Gastrointestinal diseases affect any specific part of the gastrointestinal tract. The affected part may be from the oesophagus to the rectum. The gastrointestinal diseases also include diseases of liver, gallbladder and pancreas. The following common symptoms give indication of gastrointestinal diseases: Constipation, nausea, vomiting, mouth inflammation, excessive gas formation, diarrhea and gastrointestinal bleeding.

The following are two main categories of gastro-intestinal (GI) diseases: (1) Functional gastrointestinal diseases and (2) structural gastrointestinal diseases.

Functional Gastrointestinal (GI) Diseases

The functional gastrointestinal disorders are common GI disorders. These are characterized by persistent and recurring GI symptoms such as constipation, diarrhea, vomiting, etc. These may occur due to abnormal functioning of the GI tract. The functional gastrointestinal disorders are not caused by GI structural abnormality. These GI disorders are related to gut and brain interactions. It is a group of disorders classified by any combination of the following observations: Visceral hypersensitivity, altered mucosal function, motility disturbance, altered central nervous system (CNS) processing, and altered immune function.

Endoscopy examination, X-ray examination, CT scan or blood tests may not be useful in the detection of a specific functional gastrointestinal disease. The following are some examples of functional GI disorders: Irritable bowel syndrome (IBS), functional vomiting, functional indigestion, discomfort in the upper abdominal area, functional abdominal pain, functional diarrhea, and functional constipation.

Structural Gastrointestinal Diseases

Structural GI disorder occur when a specific gastro-intestinal organ appears abnormal and does not work normally. Structural disorders could be easy to identify by medical examination. Common examples of structural GI disorders are Crohn's disease, presence of hemorrhoids, presence of intestinal polyps, ulcerative colitis, colorectal cancer and anal fistulas.

Lactose Intolerance

SAQ: Write a note on lactose intolerance.

Ans: Lactose intolerance is usually caused by a deficiency of lactase in the small intestine, which is required for lactose digestion. Undigested lactose passes in the colon. Bacteria in the colon ferment lactose, leading to formation of gases that cause various abdominal symptoms. The unabsorbed sugars and fermentation products raise the osmotic pressure of the colon, causing an increased flow of water into the bowels leading to diarrhea. Symptoms of lactose tolerance include abdominal cramps and bloating.

Constipation

SAQ: Write a note on constipation.

Ans: Constipation is defined as having dry and hard bowel movements or passing stool less than three times a week. Constipation may occur due to functional or structural disorders of gastrointestinal tract.

Various other factors that lead to constipation are, stress, pregnancy, uncontrolled diabetes mellitus, thyroid diseases, irregular eating habits, over use of laxatives and older age. Constipation also occurs due to inadequate intake of fibers in foods.

Irritable Bowel Syndrome (IBS)

SAQ: Write a note on irritable bowel syndrome (IBS).

Ans: Irritable bowel syndrome (IBS) is a common functional disorder that affects the large intestine. Symptoms of IBS include abdominal pain, abdominal cramps, excessive gas formation in the intestine, constipation or diarrhea or both. IBS is a chronic condition that needs long term treatment.

Ulcerative Colitis (Fig. 12.70)

SAQ: Write a note on ulcerative colitis.

Ans: Ulcerative colitis is an autoimmune inflammatory bowel disease. Ulcerative colitis affects the innermost lining of the colon and the rectum. Patients with ulcerative colitis are at increased risk of developing colon cancer. Symptoms of ulcerative colitis include abdominal cramps, pain, and rectal bleeding, leading to dysentery.

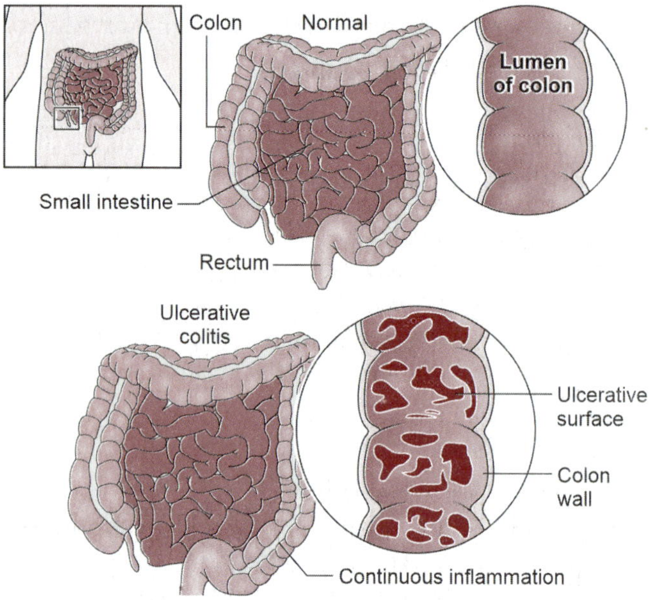

Fig. 12.70: Colon in ulcerative colitis

Colon Polyps (Fig. 12.71)

SAQ: Write a note on colon polyps.

Ans: Colon polyps are small clump of cells that form on the lining of the colon. Most colon polyps are harmless. However, some colon polyps may develop into colon cancer. Cancer development takes place when cells grow out of control, forming abnormal cells, leading to formation of tumor (mass of tissue).

Common symptoms of colon cancer include changes in bowel movements, prolonged abdominal discomfort, changes in stool consistency, and blood in the stool.

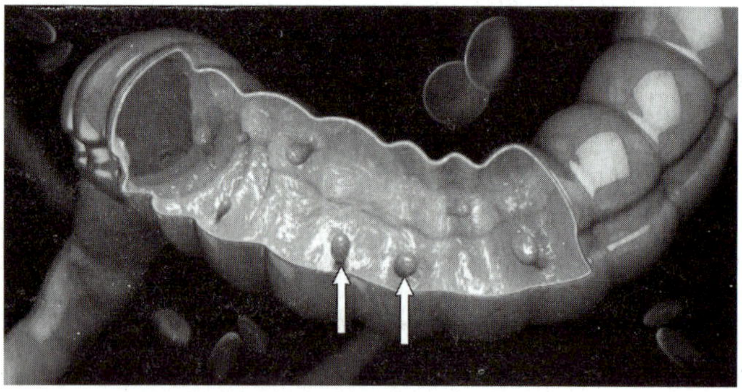

Fig. 12.71: Colon polyps

Perianal Abscess

SAQ: Write a note on perianal abscesses.

Ans: Perianal abscess is a structural disease. It can occur when the tiny anal gland inside the anus becomes blocked. Bacteria present in these glands causes an infection, leading to pus and abscess formation. Sexually transmitted diseases that can cause perianal abscess and affect the anus include AIDS, gonorrhea, chlamydia, and herpes.

Diverticular Disease (Fig. 12.72)

SAQ: Write a note on diverticulosis.

Ans: Diverticulosis occurs when small, bulging pouches known as diverticula develop in the gastrointestinal tract. The diverticula usually occur in the sigmoid colon, which is a high pressure region in the large intestine. Diverticulitis means inflammation of the diverticula, due to bacterial infection. Obstruction to passage of stool, and bleeding may be observed in diverticulitis.

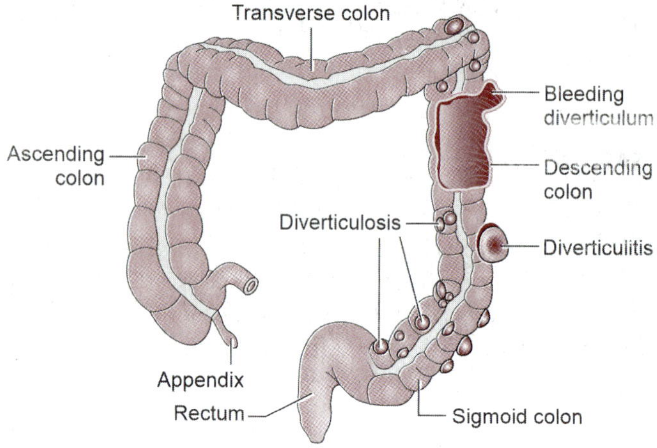

Fig. 12.72: Diverticulosis

Gallstones (Fig. 12.73)

SAQ: Write a note on gallstones.

Ans: Gallstones are solid small pieces of varying sizes formed from bile in the gallbladder. The presence of gallstones in the gall bladder in small number may not cause symptoms. However, a gallstone may lodge in a bile duct and causes a blockage of the bile flow. It may lead to severe pain in the upper right portion of abdomen, nausea and vomiting. Obstruction of main bile duct may lead to obstructive jaundice. The gallstones form due to presence of high concentration of cholesterol and bile pigments and low concentration of bile salts. The gallstones or gallbladder is removed by surgical procedures to treat the patient.

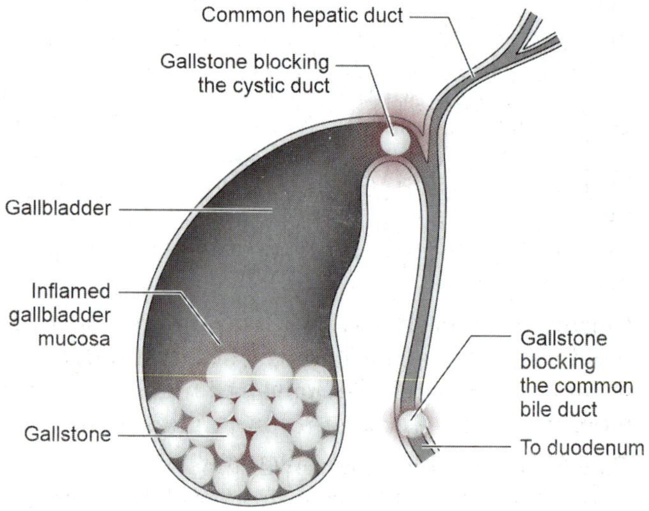

Fig. 12.73: Gallstones

Celiac Disease

SAQ: Write a note on celiac disease.

Ans: Celiac disease is caused due to an immune reaction to gluten, a protein present in wheat, barley and rye. The related autoimmune reaction lead to inflammation of intestinal lining. Celiac disease causes poor absorption of digestion products. Common celiac disease symptoms are bloating and fatigue. Malnutrition caused by celiac disease may lead to anemia and osteoporosis. The celiac disease can be diagnosed by clinical laboratory tests. The patients are advised to have diet free from glutein containing foods.

Gastrointestinal Infections

SAQ: Write a note on gastrointestinal infections.

Ans: Gastrointestinal infections are caused by bacterial, viral, fungal or parasitic infections. These infections cause gastroenteritis, means an inflammation of the gastrointestinal tract; which may involve both the stomach and the small intestine. Symptoms of general gastrointestinal infections include vomiting, diarrhea, and abdominal pain.

Inflammation caused by GI infection leads to a loss of the normal surface area of GI; which is associated with decrease in food digestion and absorption procedures, leading to malnutrition and related weight loss.

Diarrhea

BAQ: Write a note on diarrhea.

Ans: Diarrhea is a condition that involves the frequent passing of loose or watery stools. It can have many causes, which may be infectious or non-infectious. Diarrhea is defined by the World Health Organization (WHO) as having three or more loose or liquid stools per day, or as having more stools than is normal for that individual. Diarrhea can be acute or chronic.

Acute Diarrhea

Acute diarrhea (short-term diarrhea) is defined as an abnormally frequent discharge of semisolid or fluid fecal matter from the bowel, lasting less than 14 days. Acute diarrhea (short-term diarrhea) is a very common cause of death especially among young children and babies. It usually appears rapidly and may last from between 5 and 10 days.

Causes of acute diarrhea: It is usually caused by an infection leading to gastroenteritis. This may be caused by food or water contaminated with bacteria, viruses and parasites.

Chronic diarrhea (long-term diarrhea): Chronic diarrhea is defined as passing of loose and watery stools, for three or more times within 24 hours and which may last for more than four weeks.

Causes of chronic diarrhea: Chronic diarrhea may be caused by an infection, inflammatory bowel syndrome (IBS), Crohn's disease, or by an allergy.

Chronic diarrhea is the second cause of death among children. People with diarrhea often have fever and (or) abdominal cramps.

Jaundice (Figs 12.74–12.76)

SAQ: Write a note on jaundice.

Ans: Jaundice is a clinical condition in which bilirubin in blood increases above 2 mg%. Increased bilirubin imparts yellow colour to the skin, sclera of eyes and mucous membranes. Increased water-soluble bilirubin also imparts yellow colour to urine.

Jaundice is caused due following three reasons: (1) Due to increased break-down of red blood cells as seen in hemolytic anemia, (2) due to viral, bacterial and parasite infections of liver or drug reactions and (3) due to obstruction to the flow of bile to intestine, due to gall-stones or narrowing of common bile duct.

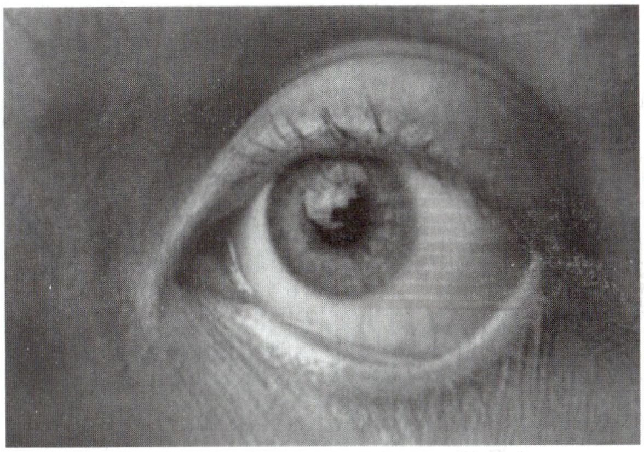

Fig. 12.74: Yellow colour of sclera in jaundice

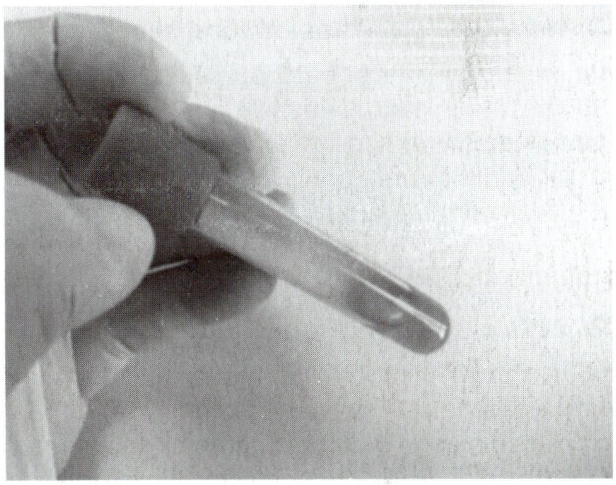

Fig. 12.75: Yellow colour of serum in jaundice

Cirrhosis of Liver (Fig. 12.77)

Cirrhosis of liver may be caused by long-term high intake of alcohol. It also can be of non-alcoholic type. Cirrhosis of liver is mainly associated with irreversible chronic injury of the hepatic parenchyma and include extensive fibrosis with regenerative nodules. Loss of functioning hepatocellular mass may lead to edema, jaundice, fibrosis, and coagulopathy. Distorted vasculature of liver tissue leads to portal hyper tension, splenomegaly and acites.

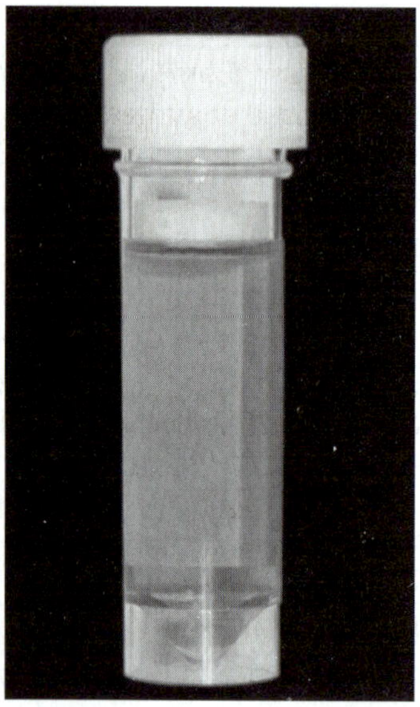

Fig. 12.76: Yellow colour of urine in jaundice

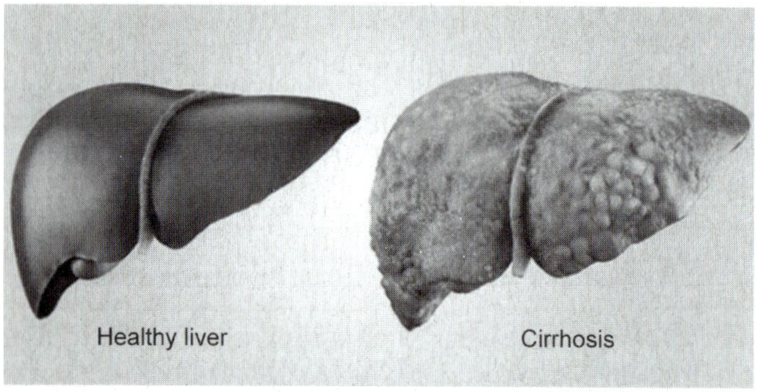

Fig. 12.77: Normal liver (LHS). cirrhosis of liver (RHS)

Autoimmune Hepatitis

SAQ: Write a note on autoimmune hepatitis.

Ans: Autoimmune hepatitis occurs when specific antibodies are created against the liver cells. It is a chronic disorder characterized by progressive hepatocellular necrosis and inflammation leading to fibrosis, cirrhosis and ultimately liver failure.

Chronic Hepatitis

SAQ: Write a note on chronic hepatitis.

Ans: In chronic hepatitis a series of liver disorders of varying causes and severity continue for at least six months and lead to hepatic inflammation and necrosis. Severe forms of chronic hepatitis ultimately lead to cirrhosis of liver. Chronic hepatitis includes various categories such as chronic viral hepatitis, drug-induced chronic hepatitis and autoimmune chronic hepatitis.

Alcoholic Liver Disease

SAQ: Write a note on alcoholic liver disease.

Ans: Excessive alcohol ingestion may lead to liver injury in three major forms such as fatty liver, alcoholic hepatitis and cirrhosis. Nutritional, social, immunologic and host factors are responsible in the development of pathogenic process. Chronic hepatitis B and C infection are important risk factor in the progression of alcoholic liver disease. Fatty liver is the initial most common histologic response to excessive alcohol ingestion. It could be reversed by appropriate medical advise and treatment.

DISEASES OF PANCREAS

Acute Pancreatitis (Fig. 12.78)

Ans: Acute pancreatitis is inflammation of pancreas. It is characterized by sudden severe upper abdominal pain. The pain may be severe and last several days. Other symptoms of acute pancreatitis include fever, nausea, vomiting, bloating, and diarrhea. Various causes of pancreatitis include trauma, infections, chronic alcohol consumption, increased gall stones in liver, and high blood lipid levels, etc.

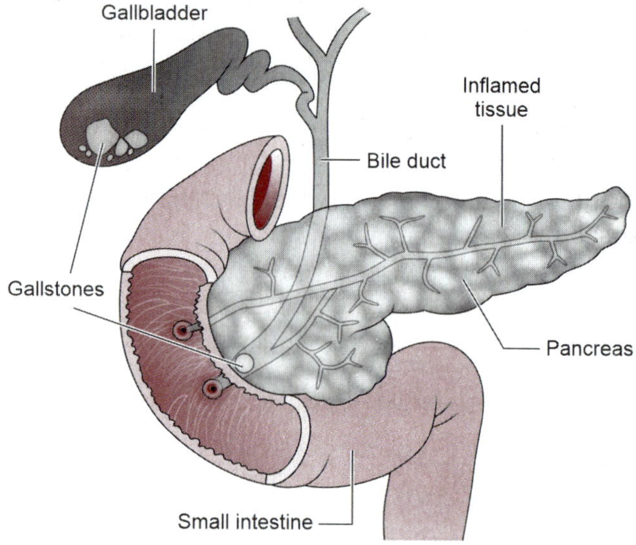

Fig. 12.78: Pancreatitis

Chronic Pancreatitis

SAQ: Write a note on chronic pancreatitis.

Ans: Chronic pancreatitis is inflammation of the pancreas, which gets worse over time. Chronic pancreatitis is a progressive disorder; which is associated with the destruction of the pancreas. Symptoms of chronic pancreatitis include deep epigastric pain, vomiting, abdominal pain, weight loss, steatorrhea and high levels of blood glucose. The most common cause of chronic pancreatitis is chronic alcohol consumption, cystic fibrosis and hereditary disorders of the pancreas.

Diabetes Mellitus

BAQ: Write a note on diabetes mellitus.

Ans: Diabetes mellitus is caused; when beta cells of the pancreas are unable to secret sufficient insulin, as seen in type-1 diabetes mellitus or body cells are unable to use insulin, as seen in type-2 diabetes mellitus. Insulin hormone is necessary for the body cells to use glucose to derive energy in the form of ATP molecules. In the case of a person suffering from uncontrolled diabetes, the following symptoms are observed: High blood glucose levels (hyperglycemia), passing of glucose in urine, (glycosuria), increased frequency of urination (polyurea), weight loss and immuno-compromised state.

Type-1 diabetes mellitus occurs due to destruction of beta cells of the pancreas due to genetic reasons, autoimmune disorder or due to attack by viruses (mumps virus). Type-1 diabetic person require appropriate insulin therapy.

The main reason of type-2 diabetes mellitus is obesity caused due to the life-style changes made by an individual. Excessive fats in the adipose tissue cause resistance to the functions of the insulin hormone (insulin resistance). Appropriate treatment to get rid of obesity and initial oral drug treatment could control type 2 diabetes mellitus.

Objective: To understand and explain the central theme of competency based medical and paramedical education (CBME): Horizontal and vertical integration of subjects.

BAQ: Show horizontal integration of physiology, biochemistry and nutrition with the following anatomical change: Damage of the lower sphincter of esophagus.

Ans:

Horizontal Integration with Physiology

Failure of the lower esophageal sphincter to prevent the acidic contents of the stomach from flowing back into the esophagus (GERD).

Horizontal Integration with Biochemistry

Secretion of inflammatory markers such as prostaglandins and C-reactive proteins due to action of hydrochloric acid on the mucosa of the esophagus, leading to inflammation of internal layers of the esophagus.

Horizontal Integration with Nutrition

Suggested diet should contain low spices and restriction on alcohol intake to prevent irritation of the inflammatory part of esophagus.

BAQ: Show horizontal integration of physiology and biochemistry with the following anatomical change: Destruction of chief cells of the stomach.

Ans:

Horizontal integration with Physiology

Digestion of proteins is affected.

Horizontal integration with Biochemistry

No secretion of pepsinogen.

BAQ: Show horizontal integration of physiology, biochemistry and nutrition with the following anatomical change: Ulcers in the duodenum.

Ans:

Horizontal Integration with Physiology

Presence of highly acidic chyle in the duodenum.

Horizontal Integration with Biochemistry

Inhibition of maximum activities of amylase, trypsin, chymotrypsin and lipase enzymes at strong acidic pH, in the duodenum.

Horizontal Integration with Nutrition

Suggested diet should contain low spices and restriction on alcohol intake.

BAQ: Show horizontal integration of physiology, biochemistry and nutrition with the following anatomical change: Inflammation of liver (hepatic jaundice).

Ans:

Horizontal Integration with Physiology

Obstruction to the intrahepatic bile circulation.

Horizontal Integration with Biochemistry

Increase in bile pigments and bile salts in blood and urine.

Horizontal Integration with Nutrition

Suggested diet should contain normal amount of carbohydrates, low fats and moderate amount of protein.

BIBLIOGRAPHY

1. Medical Biochemistry, 1st Edition (2023). Godkar PB, Godkar DP, CBS Publishers, New Delhi, India.
2. Text book of Medical Laboratory Technology, 4th Edition, (2024). Godkar PB, Godkar DP, Bhalani Publishing House, Mumbai, India.
3. Anatomy of the Human Body. 42nd Edition. Henry Gray, Editor-in-chief: Susan Standring, Elsevier (2020).
4. Ross & Wilson Anatomy and Physiology in Health and Illness, 13th Edition, by Allison Wynn Grant, Anne Waugh, and Kathleen J. W. Wilson (2018).
5. Schaum's outline of theory and problems of Human anatomy and Physiology, 2nd Edition (1997), Tata MaGraw-Hill Publishing Company Limited, New Delhi, India.

MULTIPLE CHOICE QUESTIONS (MCQs)

Select the correct option.

1. **The outermost covering of the walls of the alimentary tract is:**
   (A) Serosa (B) Muscle layer
   (C) Submucosa (D) Mucosa
2. **The abdominal organs are covered by:**
   (A) Submucosa (B) Mucosa
   (C) Peritoneum (D) Both (A) and (C)
3. **This one is not an intraperitoneal organ:**
   (A) Duodenum (B) Jejunum
   (C) Ileum (kidney) (D) None of these
4. **Saliva does not contain the following component:**
   (A) Pepsin (B) Amylase (ptyalin)
   (C) Lipase (D) Mucus

5. **Primary teeth or baby teeth start to appear around:**
   (A) Six months of age (B) Three months of age
   (C) Tenth months of age (D) First year of age
6. **One of the following statements is not correct:**
   (A) The canines are used to tear the food.
   (B) The canines are used to crush the food.
   (C) The molars are used to crush the food.
   (D) The premolars are used to crush the food.
7. **The following one statement is not correct:**
   (A) The crown is the top part of the tooth.
   (B) The enamel is the hardest, white outer part of the tooth.
   (C) The enamel is mainly made up of sodium phosphate.
   (D) The dentin is a layer underlying the enamel.
8. **Only the following one statement is correct:**
   (A) The incisors have two roots
   (B) The canines have two to three roots
   (C) The premolars have two to three roots
   (D) The molars have two or three roots
9. **Dental caries are due to the attack of this acid on enamel:**
   (A) Lactic acid
   (B) Acetic acid
   (C) Butyric acid
   (D) Hydrochloric acid
10. **Dental plaque contains:**
    (A) Bacteria (B) Food particles
    (C) Saliva (D) All of the above
11. **Only the following one statement is not correct:**
    (A) The mucosa of esophagus is made up of a stratified squamous epithelium.
    (B) The mucosa is formed of about two layers of squamous cells.
    (C) The mucosa has two muscular rings called sphincters in its wall.
    (D) One sphincter is present at the top and another sphincter is present at the bottom.
12. **The following one statement is not correct:**
    (A) Gastroesophageal reflux disease (GERD) is a chronic disorder.
    (B) GERD occurs due to a weak upper esophageal sphincter (LES).
    (C) GERD occurs due to inability of the lower esophageal sphincter to close completely, when food enters the stomach.
    (D) In GERD, stomach hydrochloric acid or bile flows into the food pipe.
13. **This is the enlarged portion on the left side part of stomach:**
    (A) Cardia (B) Fundus
    (C) Body (D) Pyloric antrum
14. **The functions of the gastric rugae is:**
    (A) To allow the stomach to contract after the intake of foods and liquids.
    (B) To form greater surface area useful in absorption of partially digested nutrients.
    (C) To create more space to hold large amount of food in the stomach.
    (D) Both (B) and (C)
15. **The average amount of gastric acid produced per day is:**
    (A) 1.5 liters (B) 5–6 liters
    (C) 0.5–0.8 liters (D) 3–4 liters
16. **The main constituents of gastric juice are:**
    (A) Water (B) Hydrochloric acid
    (C) Pepsinogen (D) All of the above
17. **pH of gastric juice is:**
    (A) 2.0–4.0 (B) 5.0–6.0
    (C) 3.0–5.0 (D) 1.5–3.0
18. **In the gastric phase of the stomach:**
    (A) Secretion of gastric juice takes place
    (B) Partial digestion of food takes place
    (C) Inhibition of gastric secretions takes place
    (D) Complete digestion of food proteins takes place
19. **In the intestinal phase of the stomach:**
    (A) Secretion of gastric juice takes place
    (B) Partial digestion of food takes place
    (C) Inhibition of gastric secretions take place
    (D) Complete digestion of food proteins takes place
20. **The following one statement is correct about the stomach:**
    (A) The secretion of gastrin hormone by the chief cells.
    (B) Gastrin stimulates parietal cells of the stomach to secrete hydrochloric acid (HCl).
    (C) Gastrin inactivates the chief cells.
    (D) Pepsinogen is active digestive component.
21. **The intrinsic factor (IF):**
    (A) Is a glycoprotein produced by the parietal cells of the stomach.
    (B) Plays an important role in the transportation and absorption of vitamin B_{12} by the terminal ileum.
    (C) Is an inactive form of pepsin.
    (D) Both (A) and (B)
22. **The following one is not a major gastrointestinal hormone:**
    (A) Gastrin (B) Secretin
    (C) Cholecystokinin (D) Cholecystokinine
23. **The duodenal epithelium secretes these hormones:**
    (A) Secretin
    (B) Cholecystokinin
    (C) Renin
    (D) Both (A) and (B)

24. Duodenal ulcer is most commonly observed in patients who are infected with:

(A) *Helicobacter pylori* (B) *Escherichia coli*
(C) *Proteus vulgaris* (D) *Vibrio cholerae*

25. The average length of the jejunum is about:

(A) 12 feet (B) 4 feet
(C) 8 feet (D) 16 feet

26. The pH in the jejunum is usually about:

(A) 1.5–3 (B) 4.0–6.0
(C) 5–7 (D) 7–8

27. Lacteals (small lymph vessels) present in villi of ileum absorb:

(A) Fatty acids and glycerol
(B) Amino acids
(C) Glucose
(D) Lactose

28. The following is not a part of large intestine:

(A) Cecum (B) Colon
(C) Ileum (D) Rectum

29. One of the following statements is not correct:

(A) The rectum is a tubular organ that is connected to the colon by the sigmoid colon.
(B) The average length of the rectum is about 5 feet.
(C) The end of rectum connects to anus.
(D) At the end of the rectum a specific structure called ampulla is present.

30. One of the following statements is not correct:

(A) The appendix is a finger-like tubular part connected to the cecum.
(B) The appendix is usually located in the lower right quadrant of the abdomen.
(C) The average length of appendix is about 3.5 inch
(D) The average diameter of appendix is about 2.4 inches

31. Infectious diarrhea is caused due to gastrointestinal infection caused by:

(A) Bacteria (B) Parasites
(C) Viruses (D) All of the above

32. One of the following statements is correct:

(A) The liver is the smallest organ in the human body.
(B) The liver weighs 2.2 to 3.5 kg in adult.
(C) The liver is located in the right upper quadrant of the abdomen.
(D) The liver is divided into two lobes, left and right.

33. The majority of cells in the liver are:

(A) Hepatocytes (B) Kupffer cells
(C) Stellate cells (D) Endothelial cells

34. These are phagocytic cells in the liver:

(A) Hepatocytes (B) Kupffer cells
(C) Stellate cells (D) Both (B) and (C)

35. Hepatocytes perform the following various functions:

(A) Synthesis of albumin
(B) Synthesis of coagulation factors
(C) Synthesis of bile
(D) All of the above

36. One of the following statements is not correct:

(A) The gallbladder is located in the upper right side of the abdomen.
(B) The primary function of gallbladder is to store and secrete bile.
(C) Bile is necessary to digest proteuns in the small intestine
(D) One of the function of the gallbladder is excretion of bilirubin.

37. One of the following statements is not correct:

(A) The pancreas is an elongated and tapered organ behind the stomach.
(B) The tail of the pancreas is inside the peritoneum (intraperitoneal).
(C) The tail of pancreas is located deep within the upper abdomen.
(D) The average size of pancreas in adults is about 4.7–5.9 centimeter long.

38. This enzyme is secreted by the exocrine glands of the pancreas:

(A) Pepsin (B) Ptylin
(C) Sucrase (D) Amylase

39. These hormones are secreted by the endocrine glands of the pancreas:

(A) Corticosteroids
(B) Insulin
(C) Glucagon
(D) Both (B) and (C)

40. The exocrine part of the pancreas is composed of:

(A) Acinar cells
(B) Kupffer cells
(C) Stellate cells
(D) Both (B) and (C)

41. The delta cells of the pancreas secrete:

(A) Insulin
(B) Somatostatin
(C) Insulin
(D) Glucagon

42. Inguinal hernia occurs when:

(A) Part of the stomach protrudes up through the diaphragm into the chest cavity.
(B) The intestine pushes through a weak spot in the lower abdominal wall.
(C) Part of intestine bulges through the opening in abdominal muscles near navel.
(D) The tissue bulges through an opening in the muscles of the abdomen.

43. A hiatal hernia occurs when:

(A) Part of the stomach protrudes up through the diaphragm into the chest cavity.

(B) The intestine pushes through a weak spot in the lower abdominal wall.

(C) Part of intestine bulges through the opening in abdominal muscles near navel.

(D) The tissue bulges through an opening in the muscles of the abdomen.

44. An umbilical hernia occurs when:

(A) Part of the stomach protrudes up through the diaphragm into the chest cavity.

(B) The intestine pushes through a weak spot in the lower abdominal wall.

(C) Part of intestine bulges through the opening in abdominal muscles near navel.

(D) The tissue bulges through an opening in the muscles of the abdomen.

45. One of the following statements is not correct regarding absorption of digested food products:

(A) Water-soluble vitamins are absorbed either by active transport or by diffusion.

(B) Absorption of calcium requires vitamin A.

(C) Iron absorption requires vitamin C.

(D) Calcium and inorganic phosphorus are absorbed in a controlled manner by the influence of parathyroid hormones.

46. One of the following statements is not correct:

(A) Pancreatic amylase acts on starch to form maltose and trisaccharides.

(B) Pancreatic amylase acts on glycogen to form maltose and trisaccharides.

(C) Pancreatic lipase along with a colipase, acts on emulsified triglycerides.

(D) Bile pigments secreted by gall bladder in bile is necessary to emulsify the lipids.

47. One of the following is not a disaccharidase:

(A) Dipeptidase (B) Maltase
(C) Lactase (D) Sucrase

48. One of the following statements is not correct:

(A) Maltase acts on maltose to produce two glucose molecules.

(B) Lactase acts on lactose to produce glucose and galactose.

(C) Sucrase acts on sucrose to produce two glucose molecules.

(D) Pancreatic amylase acts on starch to form maltose and trisaccharides.

ANSWERS

1. A	2. C	3. D	4. A	5. A	6. B	7. C
8. D	9. A	10. D	11. B	12. B	13. B	14. D
15. A	16. D	17. D	18. B	19. C	20. B	21. D
22. D	23. D	24. A	25. C	26. D	27. A	28. A
29. B	30. D	31. D	32. C	33. A	34. B	35. D
36. C	37. D	38. D	39. D	40. A	41. B	42. B
43. A	44. C	45. B	46. D	47. A	48. C	

MATCH THE COLUMNS

I	II
1. Enterokinase	A. Inflammation of salivary glands
2. Saliva	B. Converts proenzyme to pepsin
3. GERD	C. Salivary or pancreatic
4. Mumps	D. Inflammation of esophagus
5. HCl	E. Activates pancreas to secrete trypsin
6. Lactase	F. Stimulates secretion of HCl and pepsinogen
7. Amylase	G. Ptylin
8. Gastrin	H. Fat emulsification
9. Secretin	I. Responsible to produce two monosaccharides
10. Bile	J. Inhibits gastric phase

ANSWERS

1. E	2. G	3. D	4. A	5. B	6. I	7. C
8. F	9. J	10. H				

CHAPTER 13

Urinary System

SAQ: Short answer question: Marks: 2	**MCQs:** Multiple choice questions: Marks: 0.5 each
BAQ: Brief answer question: Marks: 4 or 5	**Match the columns:** Marks: 0.5 each
LAQ: Long answer question: Marks: 9 or 10	**Draw a labelled diagram:** Marks: 5

Objective: To identify the basic components of the urinary system.

INTRODUCTION (Figs 13.1 and 13.2)

SAQ: Write a note on the urinary system.

Ans: The urinary system (the renal system) consists of the following important parts: (1) Kidneys, (2) ureters, (3) bladder, and (4) urethra. The main function of the urinary system is to eliminate waste end-products of cellular activities from the body, by forming and excreting urine. Other important functions of kidneys are, regulation of blood volume, blood pressure, blood pH, blood levels of electrolytes and metabolic products.

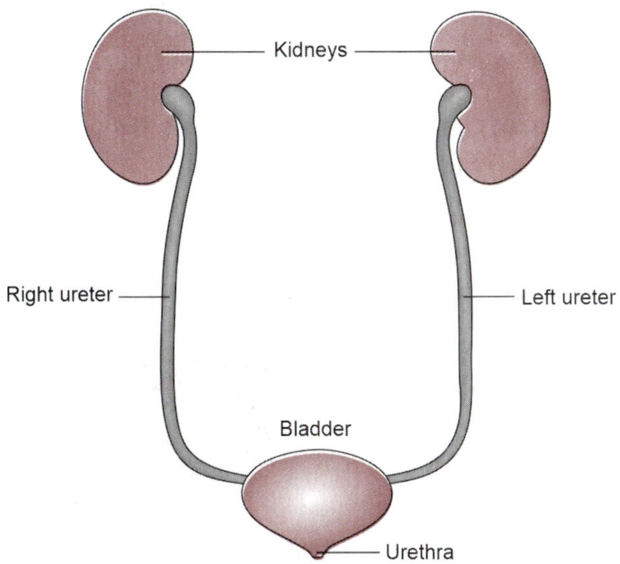

Fig. 13.1: Urinary system

BAQ: Draw a labelled diagram of the urinary system.

Ans: Refer to Fig. 13.1.

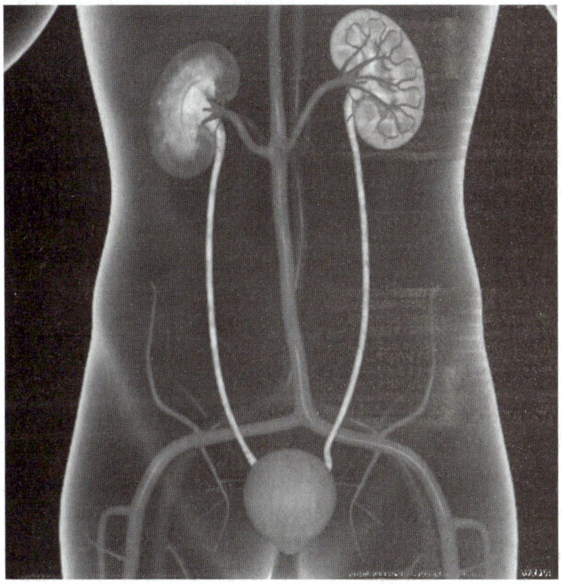

Fig. 13.2: Position of kidneys in the body

Objective: To describe the terms and anatomical features of the components of the urinary system.

KIDNEYS (Figs 13.1 and 13.2)

BAQ: Write a note on the kidneys.

Ans: The kidneys are a paired organ system located in the retroperitoneal space embedded in adipose and fibrous capsule (13.2). The kidneys extend from the level of the lower part of the 11th thoracic vertebra to the upper portion of the 3rd lumbar vertebra. Each kidney weighs about 150 g in an adult human.

The kidney parenchyma is divided into lobes that consist of an outer cortex, which covers a pyramidal medulla (Fig. 13.3). The cortex is composed mostly of glomeruli and the proximal and distal convoluted

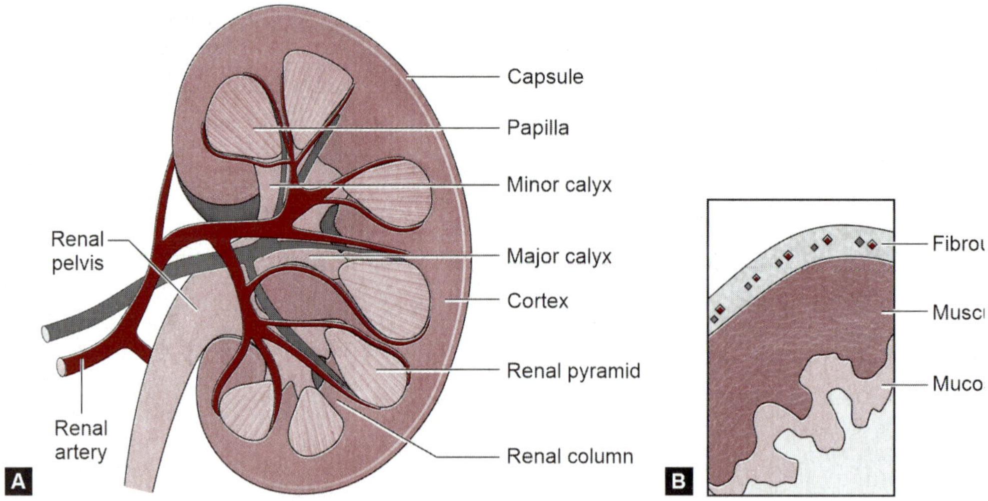

Figs 13.3A and B: (A) Kidney anatomy; (B) anatomy of ureter

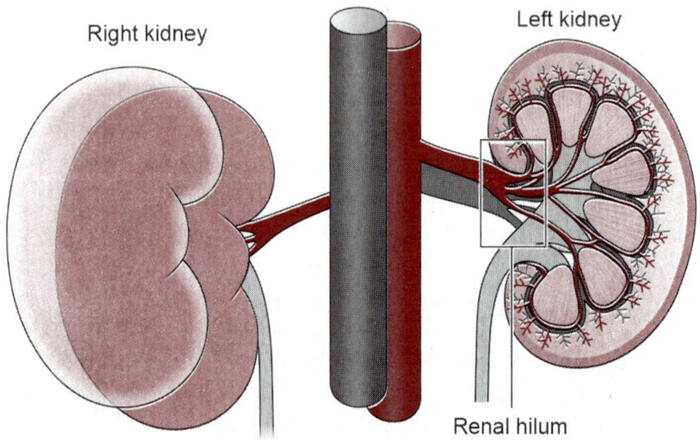

Fig. 13.3C: Renal hilum

tubules of nephrons, which are very important urine producing microscopic units of kidneys (Fig. 13.3). The medulla consists mostly of loops of Henle and collecting ducts (Figs 13.3, 13.10, 13.11 and 13.14).

The renal medulla is composed of a series of triangular renal pyramids. The apex of each pyramid is called a renal papilla. Each papilla projects into a minor calyx. Many minor calyces unit to form a major calyx. The major calyx joins to form the renal pelvis (Fig. 13.3).

The collecting ducts drain through the rounded apex of the pyramid into branches of the calyces. From the calyses, urine collects in the pelvis and flows through the ureteropelvic junction into the ureter (Fig. 13.3). The ureters carry urine from each kidney into the bladder. It is stored there until voided through the urethra.

The hilum is the concave part of kidney (Fig. 13.3C); where blood vessels and nerves enter and exit the kidney. It is also the point of exit for the ureters which passes urine into the urinary bladder.

Ureters (Fig. 13.1)

BAQ: Write a note on the ureters with respect to the following points: (1) Introduction, (2) description, (3) applied anatomy and (4) functions.

Ans:

1. **Introduction:** A ureter is a tube that carries urine from the kidney to the urinary bladder (Fig. 13.1).
2. **Description:** There are two ureters. These are attached to the kidneys. One ureter is attached to the left kidney and another ureter is attached to the right kidney. A ureter is about 25–30 cm long and about 3 mm diameter in a normal adult. The upper half of the ureter is located in the abdomen (abdominal ureter) and the lower half is located in the pelvic area (pelvic ureter). The ureters enter the bladder from its back surface. It passes about 1.5–2 cm before opening into the bladder. When urine accumulates in the bladder, pressure in the bladder rises; leading to constriction of ureters. This prevents back flow of urine into ureters.
3. **Anatomy of ureter**
   The wall of the ureter consists of the following three parts: (1) Outer covering of fibrous connective tissue, (2) middle layer of smooth muscle fibers and (3) inner mucosa made up of transitional epithelium.
4. **Functions of the ureters:** The smooth muscle layer of the ureter has property of peristalsis. Urine in small quantities is passed through ureters by peristalsis and gets collected into the bladder.

SAQ: What is vesicoureteral reflux?

Ans: Normally, urine flows from the kidneys in downward direction to the bladder. Vesicoureteral reflux (VUR) means back flow of urine from the bladder to the kidneys. Vesicoureteral reflux can be caused due to urinary tract infection.

Objective: To describe the anatomical features and functions of the urinary bladder.

Urinary Bladder (Figs 13.1 and 13.4)

BAQ: Write a note on the urinary bladder with respect to the following points: (1) Introduction, (2) description, (3) applied anatomy and (4) functions.

Ans:

1. **Introduction:** The urinary bladder is a hollow muscular organ. Urine formed by the kidneys is stored in the bladder; before it is excreted by urination. In men, the bladder is situated in front of the rectum and above the prostate gland. In women, the bladder is located in front of the vagina and below the uterus.
2. **Description:** The urinary bladder is present on the pelvic floor in the pelvic cavity. Urine enters the bladder through the ureters and exits through the urethra (Fig. 13.1). Normal bladder is capable of holding average 300–500 ml urine. The important property of the wall of the bladder is to relax and expand to store urine; and contract and become flat to empty urine through the urethra.
3. **Applied anatomy:**
   a. The wall of the urinary bladder is average 3–5 mm thick. The bladder has three openings. The two ureters enter the bladder at ureteric orifices. The bladder connects urethra at the trigone of the bladder. The trigone is a part of smooth muscle that forms the floor of the bladder above the urethra. It facilitates smooth flow of urine into and from the bladder.
   b. The ureteric openings have mucosal flaps in front of them. The flaps act as valves in preventing the backflow of urine into the ureters (vesicoureteral reflux). Between the two ureteric openings is a raised area of tissue called the interureteric crest. It makes the upper boundary of the trigone (Fig. 13.4C).
   c. The walls of the bladder have a series of ridges. These are thick mucosal folds known as rugae. Rugae are useful for the expansion of the bladder. The detrusor muscle is a smooth muscular layer of the bladder wall (Fig. 13.4C). It is arranged in circular, spiral, and longitudinal bundles. The detrusor muscle is able to change its length and able to contract for a long time whilst voiding. It remains relaxed, when urine is collected in the bladder.
4. **Functions:** The bladder has the following main functions: (1) The storage of urine and (2) controlling of urination by storage of average 400–500 ml of urine and then emptying urine, when the bladder is full.

Microanatomy of the Urinary Bladder (Fig. 13.5)

BAQ: Write a note on the microanatomy of the urinary bladder.

Ans: The bladder has an inner lining of transitional epithelium, three layers of muscle fibres, and an outer adventitia. The outside part of the bladder is protected by adventitia. The inner wall of the bladder is called urothelium. It is formed of three to six layers of cells. The cells may become more cuboidal or flatter depending on the bladder status, whether it is empty or full. A mucous membrane protects the cells beneath it from the nature of the urine. The epithelium lies on a thin basement

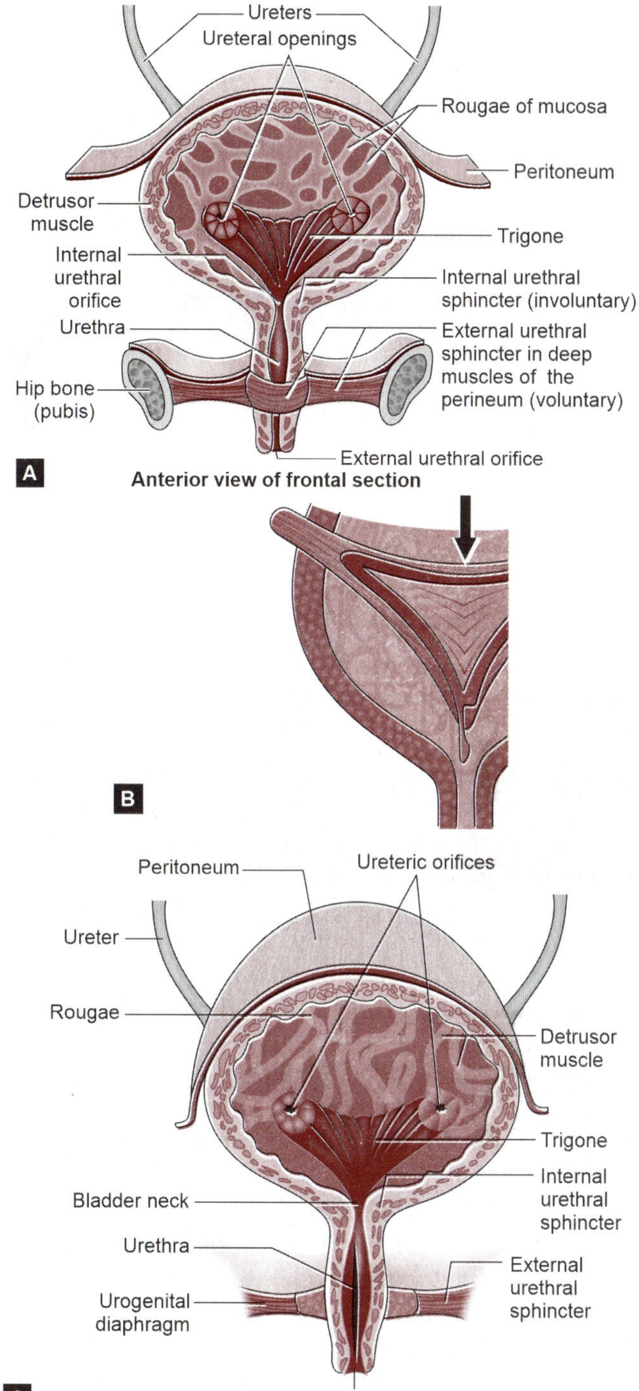

Figs 13.4A–C: Anatomical features of the urinary bladder

membrane, and a lamina propria. The mucosal lining also acts as a urothelial barrier against the microbial infections. These layers of muscles are surrounded by detrusor muscle.

Objective: To describe the anatomical structure and functions of male and female urethra.

Urethra (Figs 13.6A and B)

SAQ: Write a note on urethra.

Ans: The urethra is a fibromuscular tube that connects the neck of the bladder to the urethral opening on external genitals, from where urine passes out of the body. It is lined by stratified columnar epithelium, which

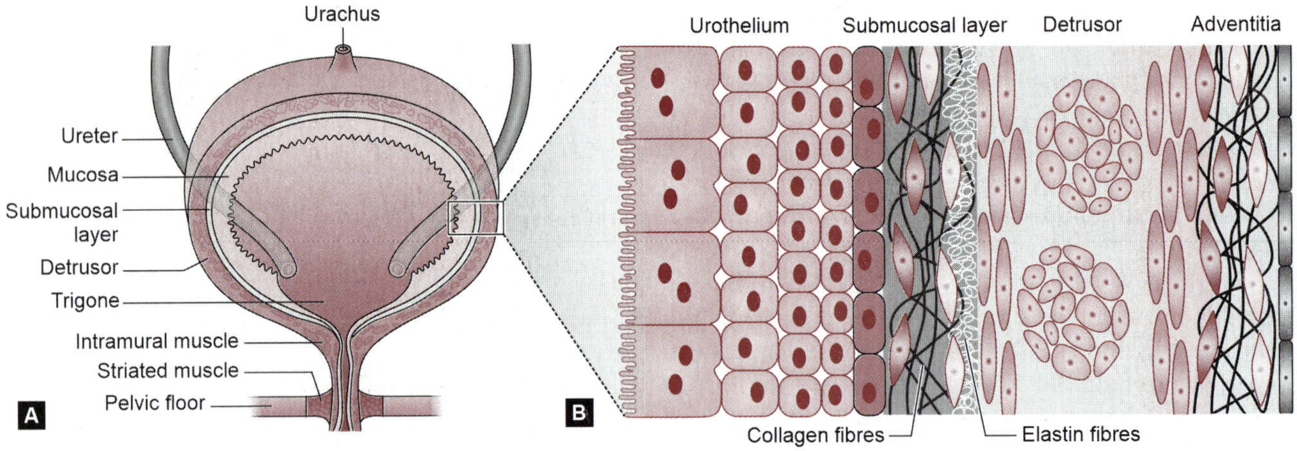

Figs 13.5A and B: Microanatomy of the urinary bladder

is protected from the acidic urine by mucus secreting glands.

Male Urethra

SAQ: Write a note on the anatomical feature of the male urethra.

Ans: The male urethra is average 15–20 cm long with 8–9 mm diameter. In addition to urine, the male urethra also transports semen. The male urethra can be divided anatomically into the following three parts (proximal to distal): (A) Prostate urethra, (B) membranous urethra and (C) penile urethra (Fig. 13.6).

a. The prostatic urethra acts as a continuation of the bladder neck and passes through the prostate gland. It receives the ejaculatory ducts (containing spermatozoa from the testes and seminal fluid from the seminal vesicle glands) and the prostatic ducts (containing alkaline fluid). Prostatic urethra is a wide part and able to dilate.

   The internal urethral sphincter is a muscle that constricts the internal urethral orifice. It is located at the junction of the urethra with the urinary bladder and is continuous with the detrusor muscle (Fig. 13.6B).
b. The membranous urethra passes through the pelvic floor and the deep perineal pouch. It is surrounded by the external urethral sphincter (Fig. 13.6B); which has voluntary control of micturition. It a narrow and least dilatable portion of the urethra.
c. Penile (bulbous) urethra passes through the bulb and corpus spongiosum of the penis, ending at the external urethral orifice (the meatus).

SAQ: What is urinary catheterisation?

Ans: Urinary catheterisation is the process, in which a tube is inserted through the urethra and into the bladder (Figs 13.7 and 13.8).

Urinary catheterisation is performed in situations where urine output needs to be monitored during operations related to kidneys. It is also performed when a patient is not able to pass urine, due to obstruction to the excretion of urine.

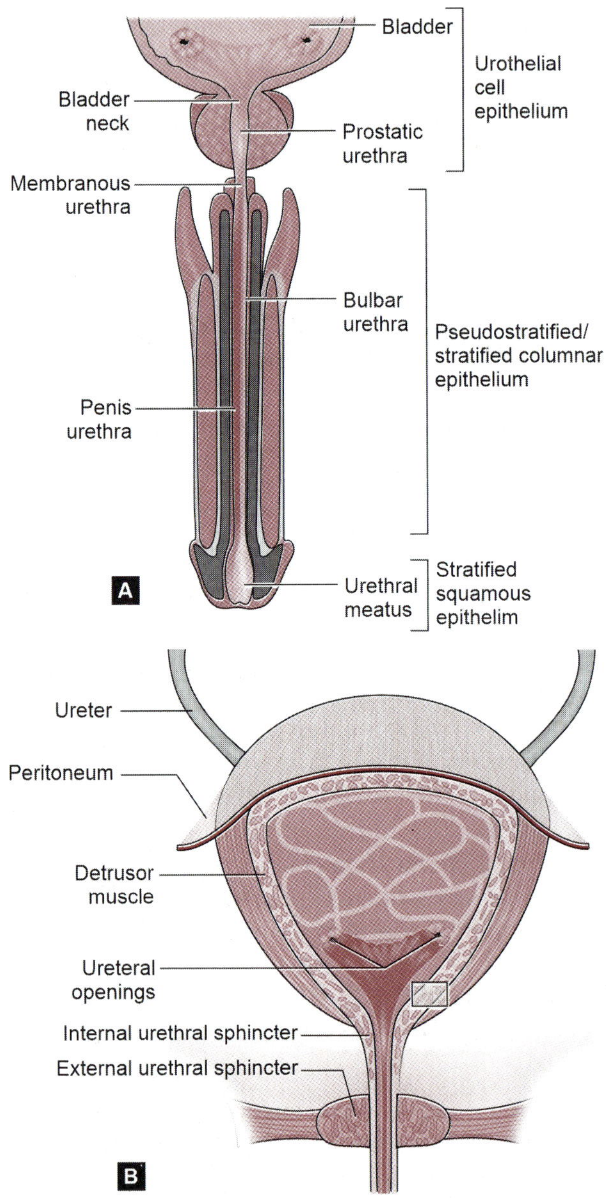

Figs 13.6A and B: Male urethra

Female Urethra (Figs 13.9A and B)

SAQ: Write a note on the description and anatomical feature of the female urethra.

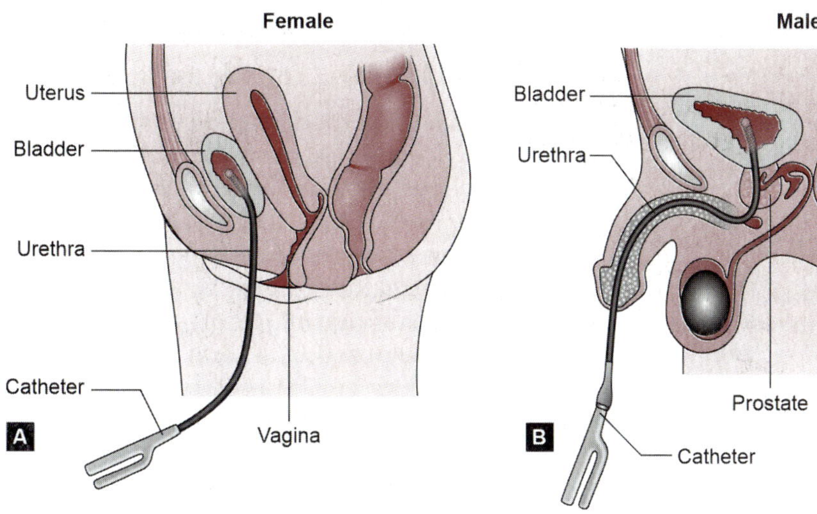

Figs 13.7A and B: Urinary catheterization

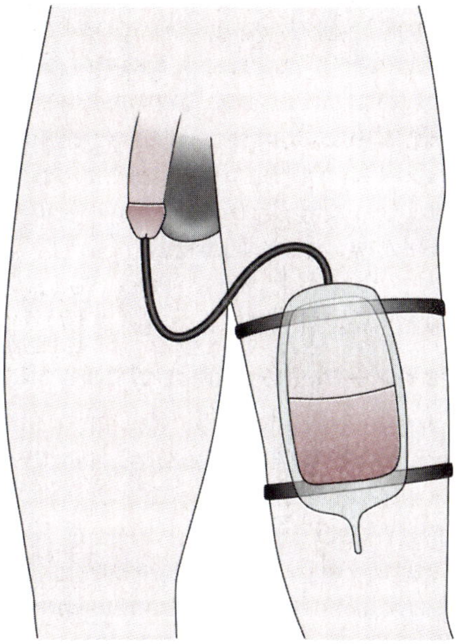

Fig. 13.8: Urine collected by urinary catheterization

Ans: Description: Female urethra is short compared to male urethra. It is average 4 cm in length. It begins at the neck of the bladder and opens directly onto the perineum, in the vestibule (an area between the labia minora) (Fig. 13.7A).

Within the vestibule, the urethral orifice is located anteriorly to the vaginal opening, and 2–3 cm posteriorly to the clitoris (refer Chapter 14, Fig. 14.15).

Anatomical features: The wall of the female urethra is made up of an outer muscular layer and an inner layer of mucosa, which remains continuous with the bladder. The muscular layer has inner smooth muscle, which is under autonomic nervous control and outer layer is made up of striated muscle, which is under voluntary control. The mucosa contains loose fibroelastic tissue. It contains nerves and blood vessels. Transitional epithelium forms the proximal part of mucosa layer and striated epithelium forms the distal part.

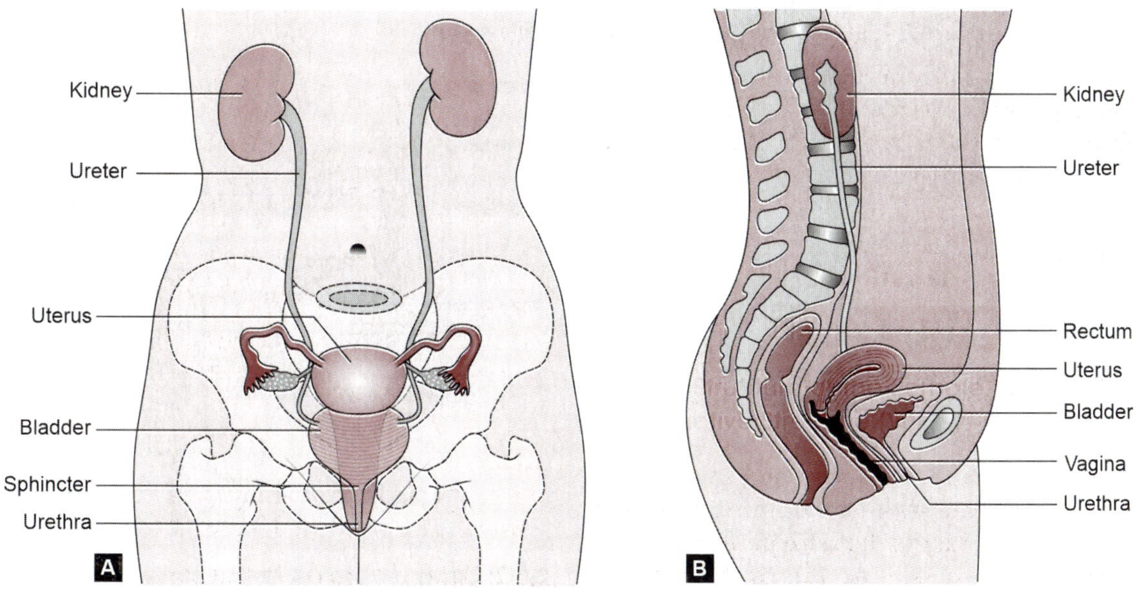

Figs 13.9A and B: Female urethra

SAQ: Why women are more susceptible to infections of the urinary tract?

Ans: Women are more susceptible to infections of the urinary tract; due to the short length of the urethra (Fig. 13.9).

> **Objectives:** To describe the functional microunits of the kidney. To describe blood supply and innervation of the functional microunits of the kidney. To describe the process of filtration. To describe the process of absorption and secretion by the tubules.

FUNCTIONAL MICROUNITS OF KIDNEY

Nephron (Fig. 13.10)

BAQ: Write a note on the nephron.

Ans: A nephron is the functional microunit of the kidney. More than one million nephrons are present in the kidneys. The nephron produces urine by excreting waste and excess metabolic substances in the blood and retains useful substances in the blood. It consists of the following parts:

1. **Bowman's capsule (glomerular capsule):** It is a part of the nephron that forms a cup-like sack which surrounds the glomerulus. Bowman's capsule encloses "Bowman's space"(Fig. 13.10). It is in contact with the proximal convoluted tubule of the nephron (Fig. 13.11).
2. **A glomerulus:** It is a network of blood capillaries (known as tuft), located at the beginning of a nephron in the kidney (Figs 13.10 and 13.11).
3. **A tubule:** It is made up of epithelial cells. It is continuous with the glomerular epithelial space and ultimately leads to collecting ducts that empty into the renal pelvis. The tubule is divided into proximal convoluted tubule, loop of Henle, distal convoluted tubule and excretory tubule or ducts (Fig. 13.11).

Anatomy of the Bowman's Capsule (Fig. 13.10)

BAQ: Write a note on the Bowman's capsule.

Ans: The Bowman's capsule is composed of inner visceral layer of simple squamous epithelial cells and outer parietal layer made up of simple squamous epithelial cells. The visceral layer lies just beneath the glomerular basement membrane and only allows fluid and small molecules like glucose and ions like sodium to pass through into the nephron. The basement membrane is composed of several dense layers. These layers are separated by translucent layers and contain bundles of microligaments.

Special types of cells called podocytes are present in the visceral layer of Bowman's capsule. These cells have the foot-like processes called pedicels. Podocytes play important role in the glomerular filtration process.

Red blood cells and large proteins, such as serum albumins, cannot pass through the glomerular basement membrane under normal circumstances. However, when the visceral layer and the basement membrane are damaged, these may be able to pass through and can cause blood and protein content to enter the urine. Presence of blood and protein in urine is a sign of diseased condition of the kidney.

Proximal Convoluted Tubule (Fig. 13.11)

BAQ: Write a note on the proximal convoluted tubule.

Ans: The proximal tubule is the first site of water reabsorption into the bloodstream, and the site where the majority of water and salt reabsorption takes place (Fig. 13.11). Water reabsorption in the proximal convoluted tubule occurs due to passive diffusion across the basolateral membrane. Water is also reabsorbed by active transport along with glucose, sodium, and potassium ions across the basolateral membrane.

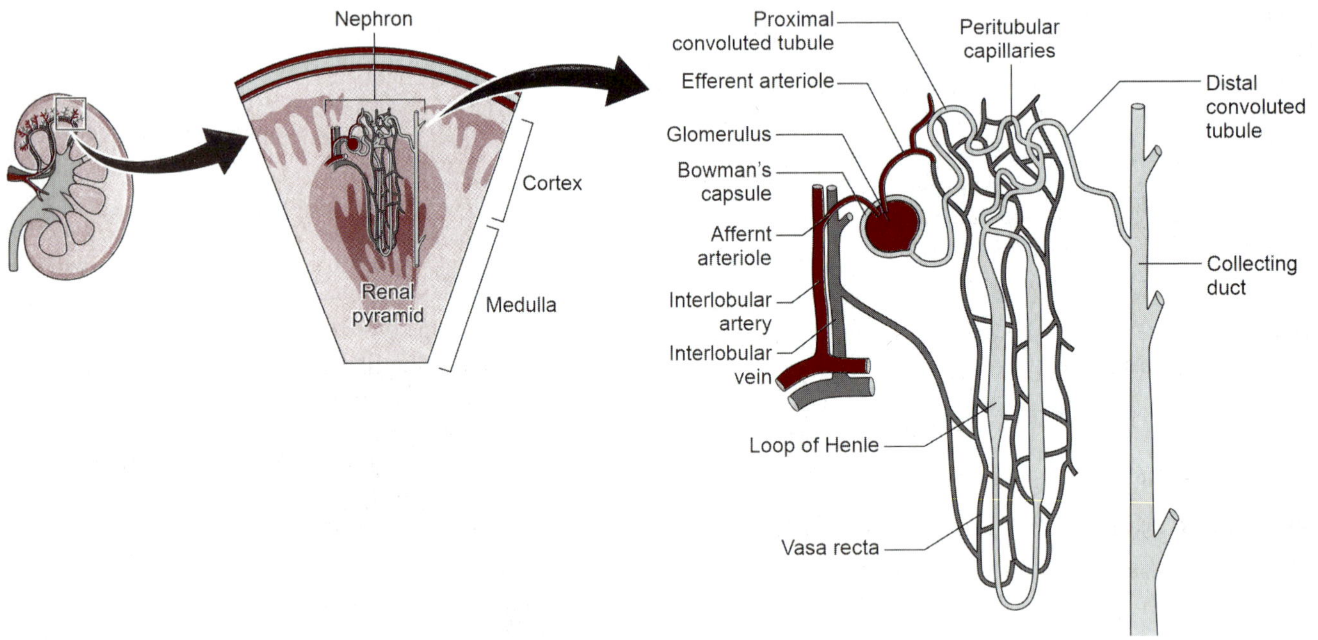

Fig. 13.10: Anatomy and functions of various parts of the nephron

Approximately, two-thirds of water in the nephron and 100% of the glucose in the nephron are reabsorbed in the proximal convoluted tubule.

Loop of Henle (Fig. 13.11)

BAQ: Write a note on the loop of Henle.

Ans: The loop of Henle is a U-shaped tube that consists of a descending limb and ascending limb (Fig. 13.11). It transfers fluid from the proximal to the distal tubule. The descending limb is highly permeable to water but completely impermeable to the ions; causing a large amount of water to be reabsorbed. In contrast, the ascending limb of Henle's loop is impermeable to water but highly permeable to ions.

Distal Convoluted Tubule and Collecting Duct (Fig. 13.6)

BAQ: Write a note on the distal convoluted tubule and the collecting duct.

Ans: The distal convoluted tubule and collecting duct is the final site of reabsorption in the nephron (Fig. 13.11). Unlike the other components of the nephron, its permeability to water is variable depending on the action of antidiuretic hormone (ADH).

Normally, distal convoluted tubule is impermeable to water and permeable to ions. However, ADH secreted from the pituitary gland (as a part of the homeostasis) acts on the distal convoluted tubule to increase the permeability of the tubule to water to increase water reabsorption.

The hormone aldosterone, (secreted by adrenal cortex gland) mediates sodium ion absorption by the distal tubule. Increase in the water and sodium ions in the blood leads to appropriate increase in blood volume and increase in the blood pressure.

The collecting duct is similar in function to the distal convoluted tubule and generally responds the same way to ADH stimuli. It is, however, different in terms of histology to distal convoluted tubule. The osmolarity of fluid through the distal tubule and collecting duct is highly variable depending on the hormone stimulus. After passage through the collecting duct, the fluid is brought into the ureter, where it leaves the kidney as urine.

BAQ: Draw a labelled diagram of the anatomical features of a nephron.

Ans: Refer to Fig. 13.11.

Nerve Supply of the Kidneys (Fig. 13.12)

BAQ: Write a note on the nerve supply of the kidneys.

Ans: Nerve supply of the kidneys consists of both afferent and efferent nerves. These nerves make up the renal plexus, and receive inputs from the celiac and aorticorenal plexuses and the splanchnic nerves.

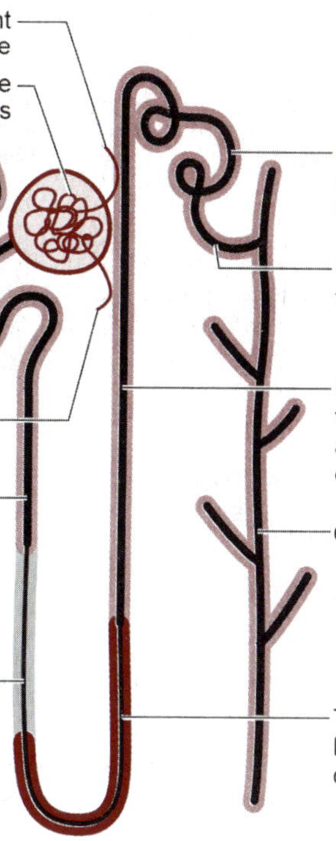

Fig. 13.11: Anatomy of the nephron

The kidney and nervous system communicate via the renal plexus. Inputs from the sympathetic nervous system trigger vasoconstriction in the kidney, leading to reduction in the renal blood flow. The kidney also receives inputs from the parasympathetic nervous system, by the way of the renal branches of the vagus nerve. Parasympathetic stimulus trigger vasodilation, leading to increase in the renal blood flow. Sensory input from the kidney travels to the T10–11 levels of the spinal cord. It is then sensed in the corresponding dermatome (that connect to specific nerves).

Blood Supply of the Kidneys (Fig. 13.13)

BAQ: Write a note on the blood supply of the kidneys.

Ans: The kidneys receive blood from the left and right renal arteries, which branch directly from the abdominal aorta (Fig. 13.13). The kidneys receive approximately 20–25% of cardiac output in an adult individual. Each renal artery branches into segmental arteries, dividing further into interlobar arteries, which penetrate the renal capsule and extend through the renal columns between the renal pyramids. The interlobar arteries then supply blood to the arcuate arteries that run through the boundary of the cortex and the medulla. Each arcuate artery supplies several interlobular arteries that feed into the afferent arterioles that supply the glomeruli.

Blood drains from the kidneys, ultimately into the inferior vena cava. After filtration takes place, the blood moves through a small network of small veins (venules) that converge into interlobular veins. Similar to the arteriole distribution, the veins follow the same pattern. The interlobular vein provide blood to the arcuate veins then back to the interlobar veins, which come to form the renal veins which exit the kidney.

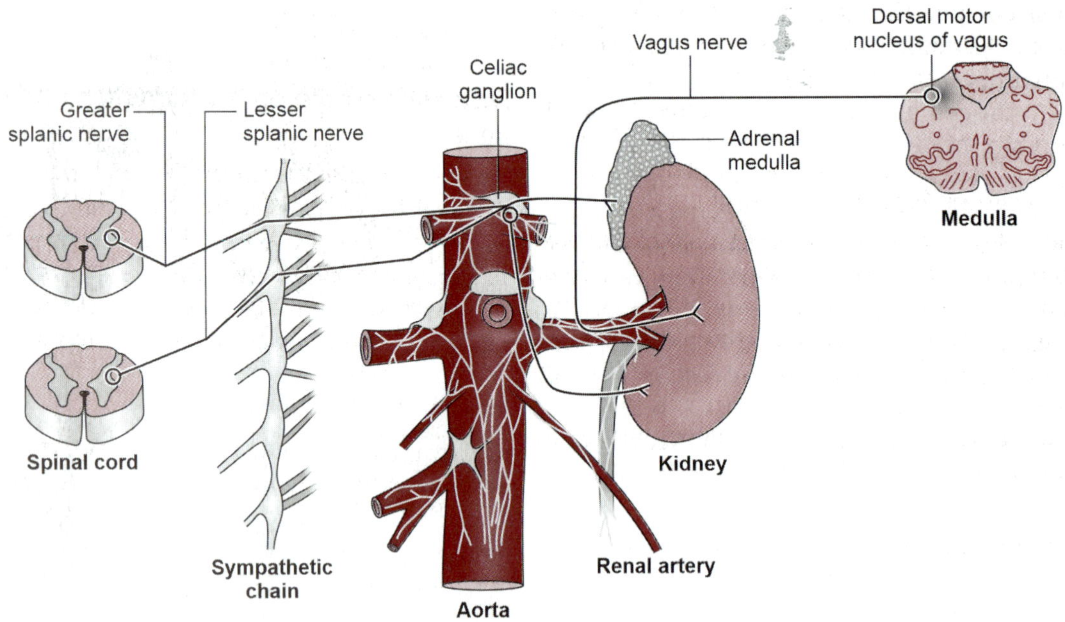

Fig. 13.12: Innervation of kidneys: Nerves pass from the spinal cord, sympathetic chain to the celiac ganglion and then connect to the adrenal medulla and kidney and then pass to the vagus nerve and the medulla

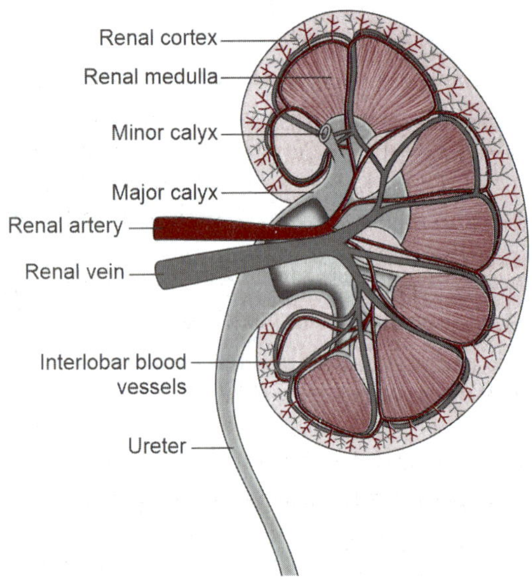

Fig. 13.13: Blood supply of the kidneys

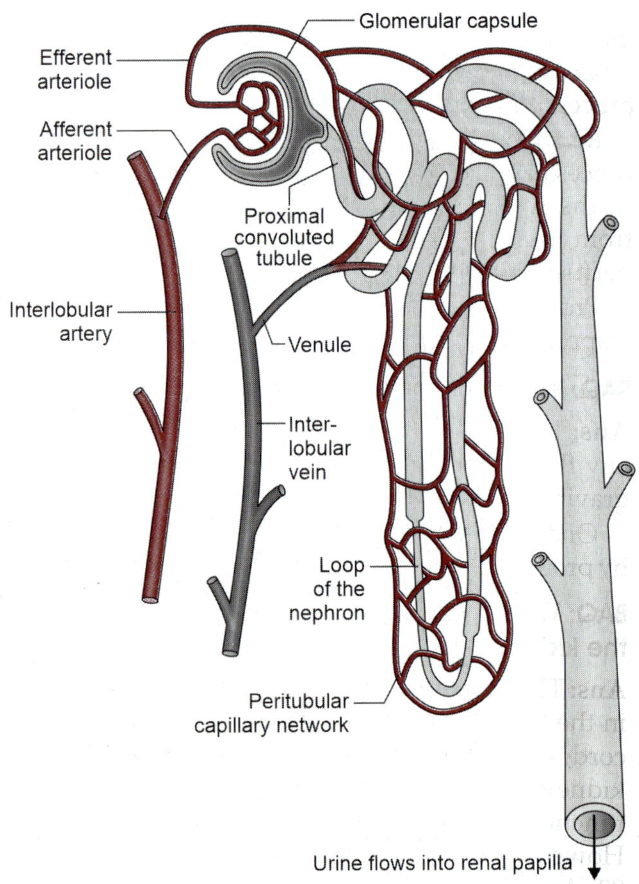

Fig. 13.14: Blood supply of the nephron

Blood Supply of the Nephron (Fig. 13.14)

BAQ: Write a note on the blood supply of the nephron.

Ans: The renal artery divides into posterior and anterior portions, and ultimately terminate in the afferent arterioles. Each afferent arteriole supply blood to a single glomerulus (Fig. 13.14). Efferent arterioles form capillary plexuses as well as elongated vessels around the loops of Henle (Fig. 13.14). It provides blood circulation necessary for the highly active tubular cells to reabsorb various essential substances in the urine.

The efferent vessel breaks up to form a second capillary network around the uriniferous tubules. These capillaries eventually reunite to form renal vein, which conveys the blood from the kidneys to the inferior vena cava (Fig. 13.14).

Objective: To enumerate and describe the functions of the kidneys.

KIDNEY FUNCTIONS

BAQ: Describe the functions of the kedneys.

Ans: The following are the functions of the kidneys:

1. **Excretory function:** This function serves to excrete of most of the undesirable end products of metabolism. These substances are urea, creatinine, uric acid, ammonia, hydrogen ions, etc. Certain ions in higher concentration, such as phosphates, sulphates, carbonates are also excreted in a controlled manner.
2. **Acidification of urine:** Initially, when glomerular filtrate is formed, its pH is about 7.4 (alkaline). However, pH of freshly voided normal urine is always acidic (average about pH 6.3). This is due to the continuous excretion of hydrogen ions (by the tubules) in urine. This is extremely important in maintaining the acid–base balance of the body.
3. **The endocrine functions of the kidneys:** Kidneys produce erythropoietin, renin, and prostaglandin. The functions of these compounds are as follows:

Erythropoietin: Both anemia and hypoxia are major stimuli for erythropoietin production. The target cells for erythropoietin activity are erythroid progenitor cells in the bone marrow. The maturation of erythroid progenitor cells by erythropoietin results in an increase in red blood cell mass.

Prostaglandins and thromboxanes: These play an important role in regulating the physiological action of other hormones on renal vascular tone and the tubular processing of salt and water.

Renin: It is produced within juxtaglomerular cells after processing and cleavage of prorenin, which is produced in the liver. The primary stimuli for renin released from juxtaglomerular cells include reduction of renal perfusion pressure and decrease in sodium ions.

Production of vitamin D_3: The kidneys are primarily responsible for the production of vitamin D_3.

SAQ: What are hydrostatic and oncolytic pressures?

Ans: Hydrostatic pressure is the pressure exerted by any fluid at resting or equilibrium at any point due to gravitational force.

Oncotic pressure is a form of osmotic pressure exerted by proteins either in the blood plasma or interstitial fluid.

BAQ: Write a note on the embryonic development of the kidneys.

Ans: The formation of the nephrogenic cord takes place in the fourth week of the fetus. Along the nephrogenic cord, the pronephros, mesonephros and metanephros kidney units also form. The metanephric kidneys act as functional excretory units by the 11th week of the fetus. However, nephrogenesis is not complete until the week 32. At this stage, multiple branching events form that include, about 1–3 million collecting tubules. Complex interactions between the following various embryonic tissues takes place: The mesonephric duct, ureteric bud, and metanephric blastema and finally, the appropriate development of the urinary tract takes place in the fetus.

Objective: To describe the role of the kidneys in the formation of urine.

PHYSIOLOGY OF KIDNEY

Formation and Excretion of Urine

LAQ: Write a note on the formation and excretion of urine.

Ans: The kidneys form urine which passes through the ureters to the bladder for excretion. The composition of urine reflects the activities of the nephrons in the maintenance of homeostasis. The following are the three phases in the formation of urine: (1) Simple filtration, (2) selective reabsorption and (3) secretion.

1. Simple Filtration

A large volume of blood approximately one liter per minute flows through the kidneys. In four or five minutes a volume of blood equal to the total blood volume passes through the renal circulation.

A net filtration pressure of about 15 mm Hg in the glomerulus; drives the filtrate through the glomerular membrane. The filtrate is called an ultrafilter because its composition is essentially the same as that of plasma. However, ultrafilter does not contain most of the proteins present in plasma having molecular weight greater than 15,000 and also the blood cells.

Each nephron produces 100 microliters of ultrafilter per day. Since each kidney contains about one million nephrons, about 170–200 liter of ultrafilter is produced per day and per minute about 125 ml of filtrate is formed. It is known as glomerular filtration rate (GFR), which is 125 ml/minute. Chemically, glomerular filtrate is an essentially protein-free extracellular fluid or a protein and cell free filtrate of whole blood.

2. Selective Reabsorption

The glomerular filtrate contains various substances such as high threshold substances (glucose, amino acids, bicarbonate, proteins, etc.) and low threshold substances (sodium, potassium, calcium, etc.). High threshold substances are reabsorbed almost completely by the tubule when their concentrations in the plasma are within the normal range but are not completely reabsorbed when their normal plasma levels (also called threshold levels) are exceeded. The high threshold substances such as glucose, amino acids and small amounts of proteins (that pass through the glomeruli) are completely reabsorbed in the first part of the proximal tubule (Fig. 13.15). Nearly 60–80% of ultrafilter is reabsorbed in the proximal part of the tubule. The other substances reabsorbed in the proximal part of the tubule are sodium, chloride, bicarbonate, calcium and phosphate ions. Aldosterone hormone secreted by the adrenal cortex act on distal part of tubules and regulate absorption of sodium ions and secretion of potassium ions. Similarly, parathyroid hormones secreted by parathyroid gland regulate absorption of calcium ions and excretion of inorganic phosphates. In the loop of Henle, chloride and sodium ions without water are reabsorbed, generating dilute urine. Water reabsorption in the distal tubules and collecting ducts is then regulated by antidiuretic hormone (ADH).

3. Secretion in the Distal Tubule

Some substances are actively transported (or actively excreted) into the tubular lumen. The substances secreted by the tubular epithelium are creatinine and potassium. Similarly, hydrogen and ammonium ions are also excreted and reabsorption of sodium and bicarbonate takes place in this region.

The hydrostatic pressure gradient across the glomerular capillary membrane provides the driving force for glomerular filtration of urine.

The oncotic pressure difference between the capillary lumen and Bowman's space opposes filtration. Since most proteins are not normally filtered, the oncotic pressure in the glomerular capillary progressively rises until filtration stops. This controls the amount of filtrate that could be obtained from a specific volume of plasma. The maintenance of glomerular filtration rate (GFR) is dependent on an adequate renal blood flow and adequate normal blood pressure.

Out of 170 liters of glomerular filtrate produced in a day, the tubules reabsorb about 168.5 liters of the filtrate. Average 1.5 liters of urine is excreted in 24 hours, which contains average, 25–30 g urea, 2–3 g creatinine, 1–1.5 g uric acid, 15 g sodium chloride, etc.

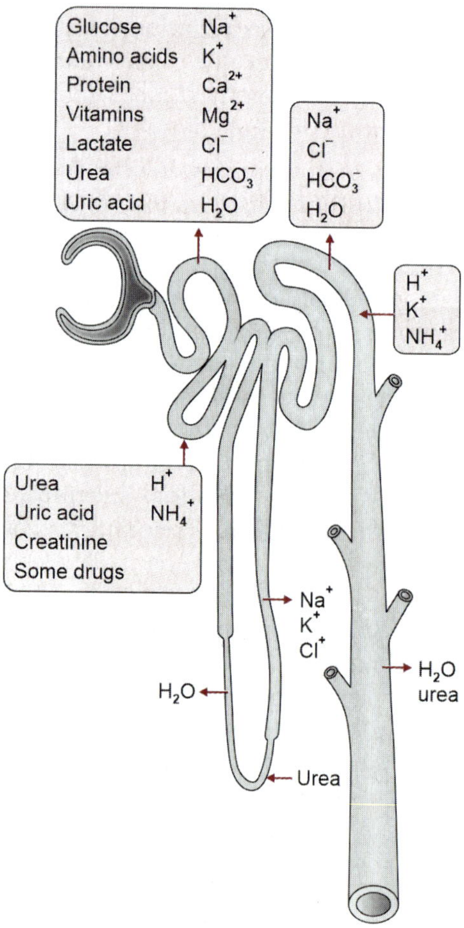

Fig. 13.15: Role of nephron in selective absorption and excretion of ions

SAQ: What is an juxtaglomerular apparatus (JGA)?

Ans: A group of specialized cells known as juxtaglomerular apparatus (JGA) are located around the afferent arteriole where it enters the renal corpuscle. The JGA secretes an enzyme called renin, due to a variety of specific stimuli (e.g. decrease in glomerular filtration). The renin plays very important role in the maintenance of homeostasis, by the appropriate regulation of blood pressure.

Objective: To describe the renin–angiotensin–aldosterone system (RAAS) and related functions.

RENIN–ANGIOTENSIN–ALDOSTERONE SYSTEM (RAAS) (Fig. 13.16)

BAQ: Write note on the renin–angiotensin–aldosterone system (RAAS).

Ans: The renin–angiotensin–aldosterone system (RAAS) is a hormone system that regulates blood pressure and fluid and electrolyte balance. The RAAS performs actions as follows (Fig. 13.16):

1. When renal blood flow is reduced, juxtaglomerular cells in the kidneys convert the precursor prorenin, present in the blood into renin and secrete it into blood circulation. Plasma renin then carries out the conversion of angiotensinogen (Alpha-2-globulin) released by the liver, to angiotensin I.
2. Angiotensin I is then converted to angiotensin II by the angiotensin-converting enzyme (ACE) found on the surface of vascular endothelial cells, mainly of the lungs.
3. Angiotensin II action decreases volume of blood vessels, leading to increase in the blood pressure. Angiotensin II also stimulates the secretion of the hormone aldosterone from the adrenal cortex. Aldosterone causes the renal tubules to increase the reabsorption of sodium and water into the blood, causing the secretion of potassium in urine, to maintain electrolyte balance. This increases the volume of extracellular fluid in the body, which also increases blood pressure.

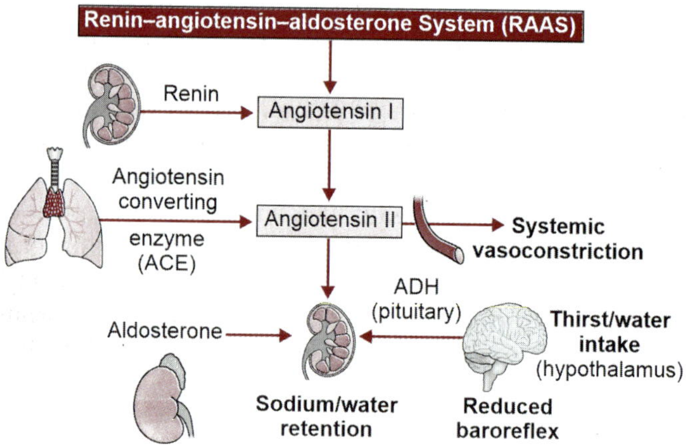

Fig. 13.16: Renin–angiotensin system

If the RAAS action is abnormally active (as in kidney and heart diseases), blood pressure will be very high. There are several types of drugs which includes ACE inhibitors, angiotensin receptor blockers (ARBs), and renin inhibitors that interrupt different steps in this system to improve blood pressure. These drugs are one of the primary ways to control high blood pressure, heart failure, kidney failure, and harmful effects of diabetes.

Objective: To describe the micturition process and associated factors.

Micturition (Figs 13.17 and 13.18)

LAQ: Write a note on micturition.

Ans: Micturition is the physiological process of urination. It involves nerve impulses and muscular responses. Urination means voiding of urine from the urinary bladder. The detrusor muscle in the bladder wall (Fig. 13.17) is the smooth or involuntary muscle. The main function of the detrusor muscle is to contract during urination to push the urine out of the bladder and into the urethra. The process of emptying the urine into the urethra is regulated by nervous signals from the autonomic and the somatic nervous system.

When the volume of urine in the bladder reaches about 250 ml, the stretch receptors in the bladder walls get stimulated and excite sensory parasympathetic nerve fibres. Parasympathetic nerves relay information to the lower part of the spine, which is relayed to following different sets of neurons.

Excited parasympathetic motor neurons act to contract the detrusor muscles in the bladder (Fig. 13.17). By detrusor muscle contraction; bladder pressure increases and the internal sphincter opens. At this time, somatic motor neurons supplying the external sphincter through the pudendal nerve are inhibited. Due to this action, the external sphincter opens and urine flows out, which is assisted by gravitational force.

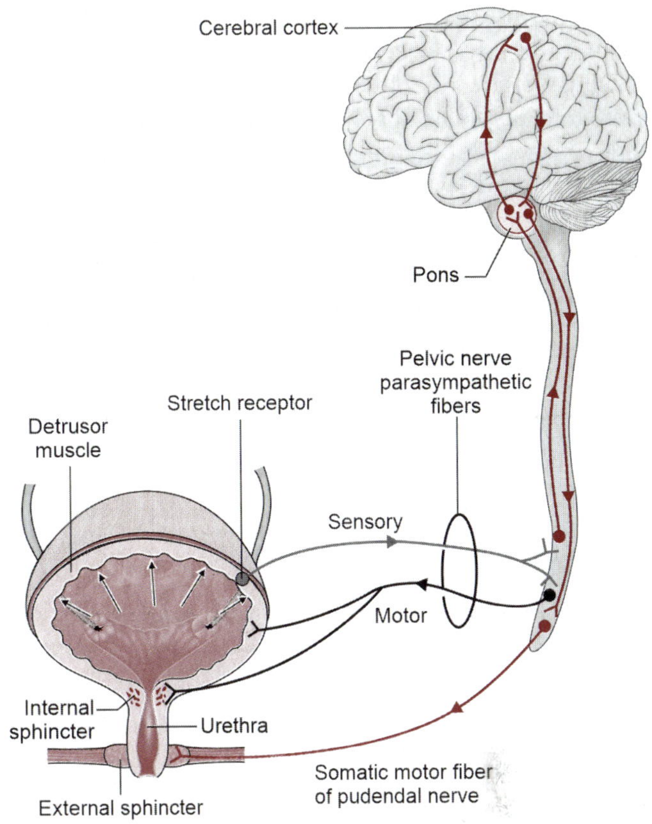

Fig. 13.17: Neuronal control on micturition

Control of Micturition

In healthy humans, micturition (urination) is under voluntary control. In infants, urination may occur as a reflex. They are not able to control bladder action

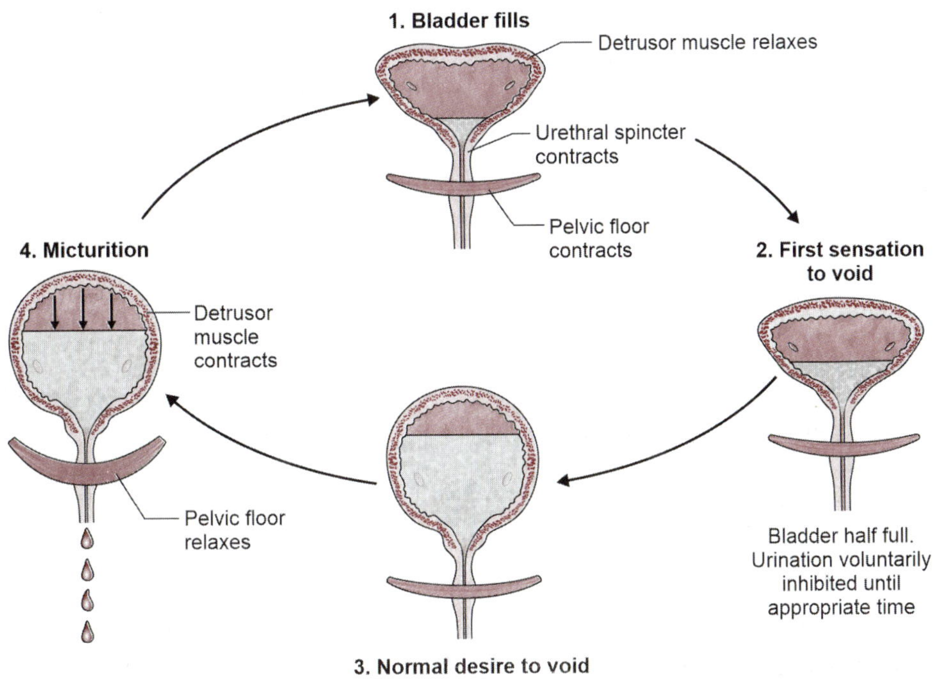

Fig. 13.18: Micturition process

related to micturition like older children and adults. That means, infants pass urine by reflex action, when urinary bladder is full. Only after the age of 2–3, a child could be trained to have bladder control and pass urine like older children and adults (toilet training). In the case of some elderly individuals, urination may occur as reflex, since the detrusor muscle function declines due to advancing age. Similarly, in individuals with neurological injury also urination may occur as reflex. With normal intake of water and other fluids, the average rate of urination is about 8–10 times in a day.

Older children and adults have considerable control over urination. They are able to decide, when and where to pass urine. They are also able to increase or decrease the rate of flow of urine. Similarly, they can stop and start urination at will.

Micturition-associated Factors

BAQ: What are the various factors associated with normal micturition?

Ans: The following are the various factors associated with normal micturition: (1) Normal nerve pathways to the urinary tract; (2) normal muscle tone in the detrusor muscles, sphincters and pelvic floor muscles; (3) absence of any obstruction to urine flow in the urinary tract; (4) Normal bladder capacity; (5) absence of inhibitors such as environmental or psychological factors. Loss of any one of these normal factors may lead to urgency to urinate.

BAQ: What are the various factors associated with micturition disorders?

Ans: The following are the various factors associated with micturition disorders:

1. Neurological disorders that lead to disorder in urination include Alzheimer's disease (AD), stroke and any other neurological clinical condition. In these diseases and disorders, the neuronal pathways to and from the spine and brain are injured or blocked.
2. Enlarged prostate, inflammation of urinary passage and renal stones may obstruct the flow of urine and may result in an increased frequency of urination with small amounts of urine and retention of urine.
3. Bladder tumours and pregnancy also reduce normal bladder capacity.
4. Environmental and psychological factors may also affect the ability of a person to pass urine.
5. Muscles at the bladder neck, around the urethra and in the pelvic floor may become weak in prolonged diabetes mellitus and due to aging. In such cases there is urge to pass urine with relatively small bladder pressure changes.
6. Certain drugs which act on nervous system and stress also may lead to urination with small pressure on bladder.

SAQ: What is the difference between micturition and urination?

Ans: Micturition is the physiological process of urination, which includes nerve impulses and muscular responses. Urination means voiding of urine from the urinary bladder.

Objective: To describe the role of the kidneys in the maintenance of acid–base balance.

BAQ: Write a note on the acidification of urine function of the kidneys.

Ans: When blood passes through the glomeruli of the nephron of kidney, glomerular filtrate forms. The pH of this initial filtrate is about 7.4 (alkaline). As this part of the filtrate passes to the proximal part of the tubules, and through distal part of the tubules, excess hydrogen ions from the blood are secreted in the filtrate (Fig. 13.19). The hydrogen ions and phosphate are formed from the following reactions:

1. CO_2 and H_2O formed in cellular metabolism are combined by the action of the enzyme, carbonic anhydrase to form carbonic acid (H_2CO_3). It dissociates to form H^+ ions and HCO_3^- ions.
2. H^+ ions are secreted by the tubules
3. HCO_3^- ions combine with reabsorbed sodium ions to form sodium bicarbonate ($NaHCO_3$), which are reabsorbed in the blood.
4. Excess phosphate and sodium ions in the filtrate combine and acidic sodium hydrogen phosphate compound forms. As a result; the pH of the filtrate in the urine form now becomes about 6.3 (acidic).

Hence, pH of freshly voided normal urine is always acidic. This is mainly due to the continuous excretion of hydrogen ions by the tubules in urine. This is extremely important for the maintenance of the acid–base balance of the body.

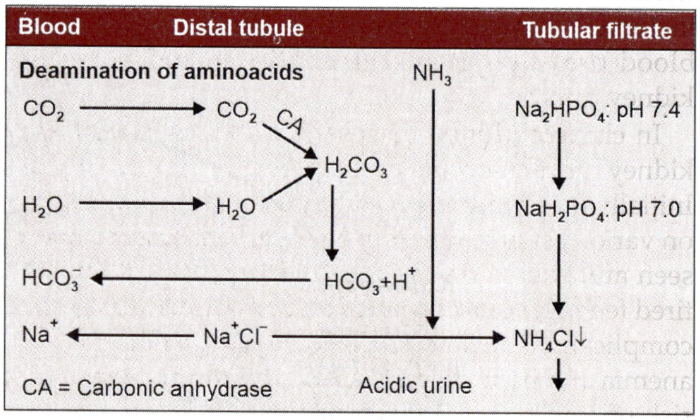

Fig. 13.19: Acidification of urine by the kidneys

Objective: To describe the various diseases of the kidneys.

DISEASES OF THE KIDNEYS

BAQ: Write a note on kidney diseases.

Ans: Kidney disease is caused due to various clinical conditions leading to diminished blood supply, immunological injury of the glomeruli, infection to tubular cells, etc. The ultimate result of kidney disease is loss of nephrons. The loss of more than 90% of nephrons leads to failure of renal functions leading to acute renal failure (ARF). If patient survives the acute illness, normal renal function can be regained. Chronic renal failure (CRF) develops insidiously, often over many years and is irreversible. Chronic renal failure may lead eventually to end-stage renal disease.

Patients with renal disease may present with systemic abnormalities, such as hypertension, edema, anemia, loss of weight, pyrexia and oliguria (very low excretion of urine).

Acute Renal Failure (AFR)

BAQ: Write a note on acute renal failure.

Ans: Acute renal failure results from a variety of problems affecting the kidneys. Usually, it presents as a sudden deterioration of renal function. In ARF urine output falls below 400 ml/24 hr (oliguria), with elevated serum urea nitrogen and creatinine. There is reduced glomerular filtrate and tubular selective reabsorption and secretion due to variety of conditions not primarily associated with the kidneys. ARF results due to severe and prolonged shock caused due to (a) incompatible blood transfusion, (b) severe hemorrhage, (c) extensive burns, (d) severe dehydration and (e) acute intestinal obstruction.

Chronic Renal Failure (CRF)

BAQ: Write a note on chronic renal failure.

Ans: Chronic renal failure (CRF) is a progressive and irreversible destruction of kidney tissue. The major adverse effects of CRF are due to the significant loss of normal nephrons. The causes of chronic kidney disease include prolonged uncontrolled diabetes mellitus, high blood pressure, glomerulonephritis, and polycystic kidney disease.

In chronic kidney disease (CKD) a gradual loss of kidney function occurs over a period of months to years. Initially no symptoms may be observed, however, later on various symptoms may be observed. The symptoms seen are, edema on the face and legs, loss of appetite, tired feeling, vomiting, and loss of appetite. The general complications related to CKD are high blood pressure, anemia and bone disease. CKD patients have increased risk of cardiovascular complications, related frequent hospitalizations and increased risks of death.

Post-streptococcal Glomerulonephritis (PSGN)

BAQ: Write a note on post-streptococcal glomerulonephritis (PSGN).

Ans: Post-streptococcal glomerulonephritis (PSGN) is an acute glomerulonephritis. The damage to the glomerulus is caused by antigen–antibody (immune) complexes produced due throat infection caused by the bacteria, Group A streptococci. Local inflammatory reactions are caused, due to the deposition of these antigen–antibody complexes in the walls of the glomerular capillaries, glomerular capsule and mesangial cells.

Chronic Glomerulonephritis

BAQ: Write a note on chronic glomerulonephritis.

Ans: Chronic glomerulonephritis may develop with no previous history of kidney disease. It may develop due to acute poststreptococcal glomerulonephritis caused by bacteria, Group A streptococci or due to corona virus infection. The rate at which the disease progresses may vary considerably. There is progressive loss of renal function due to gradual loss of nephrons.

Acute Pyelonephritis

BAQ: Write a note on acute pyelonephritis.

Ans: Acute pyelonephritis is an acute microbial infection of the kidney pelvis and calyces and may spread to other parts of the kidneys. The infection may travel up to the urinary tract from bloodborne infection and source of infection may be elsewhere in the body, e.g. wound infections, boils, abscesses or it may be in the lower urinary tract, following surgical procedures. This is a common cause of renal failure.

Chronic Pyelonephritis

SAQ: Write a note on chronic pyelonephritis.

Ans: Repeated attacks of acute pyelonephritis may lead to chronic pyelonephritis with scar tissue formation. This may lead to concurrent hypertension and then to renal failure and uremia.

Diabetic Kidney

BAQ: Write a note on diabetic kidney.

Ans: In prolonged uncontrolled diabetes mellitus, person may suffer from hypercholesterolemia (high serum cholesterol), leading to renal ischemia (inadequate blood supply to kidney tissue). There may be progressive atrophy (decrease in size) of the tubules, blockages of the renal arteries due to lipid and dead cell deposits. Renal failure is one of the cause of death in uncontrolled diabetes mellitus.

Nephrotic Syndrome

BAQ: Write a note on nephrotic syndrome.

Ans: Nephrotic syndrome is a group of signs and symptoms resulting from significant loss of nephrons of the kidney. The signs and symptom are as follows:

a. Massive proteinuria and hypoalbuminemia
b. Hyperlipidemia
c. Generalized edema
d. Reduced renal blood flow
e. Stimulation of renin–angiotensin–aldosterone mechanism causing hypertension and increased

reabsorption of water leading to widespread edema and reduced plasma volume.

Nephrotic syndrome can be associated with a number of complications that can affect the kidneys of an individual. The following are some examples: Chronic infections, prolonged uncontrolled diabetes mellitus, prolonged uncontrolled hypertension, chronic glomerulonephritis, acute kidney failure, protein malnutrition, presence of autoimmune antibodies, etc.

Renal Condition Caused by Renal Calculi

BAQ: Write a note on renal calculi (kidney stones).

Ans: Stones may form in the kidneys and bladder. Usually low concentrations of uric acid, calcium phosphate, oxalic acid remain in solution form in the filtrate formed at the glomeruli. However, prolonged high concentrations of these constituents, may precipitate in the kidneys and form urinary calculi. The kidneys stone formation takes place mainly from high concentrations of calcium oxalate, calcium phosphate, and uric acid in the glomerulus filtrate. Most of these renal calculi originate in collecting tubules or in renal papillae. They pass into the pelvis of the kidney; where they may increase in size. Some become very large to pass through the ureter and may obstruct the flow of urine and others pass to the bladder and may obstruct the urethra. Patient may suffer from severe pain on lower back, nausea, vomiting and hematuria (presence of blood in urine). Specific medicines and lithotripsy techniques are used to remove kidney stones.

> **Objective:** To understand and explain the central theme of competency based medical and paramedical education (CBME): Horizontal and vertical integration of subjects.

BAQ: Show horizontal integration of Physiology, and Biochemistry with the following anatomical change: Glomerular damage (in renal disease).

Ans:

Horizontal Integration with Physiology

Decrease in the glomerular filtration rate (GFR), leakage of serum albumin in urine, increase in blood pressure.

Horizontal Integration with Biochemistry

Secretion of renin, activation of renin–angiotensin system, leading to increase in blood pressure.

BAQ: Show horizontal integration of physiology, biochemistry and nutrition with the following anatomical change: Blockage of ureters due to renal calculi (post-renal condition).

Ans:

Horizontal Integration with Physiology

Obstruction to the normal excretion of urine.

Horizontal Integration with Biochemistry

Increase in the blood circulation of excretory substances such as urea, creatinine and uric acid.

BIBLIOGRAPHY

1. Medical Biochemistry, 1st Edition (2023). Godkar PB, Godkar DP, CBS Publishers, New Delhi, India.
2. Text book of Medical Laboratory Technology, 4th Edition, (2024). Godkar PB, Godkar DP, Bhalani Publishing House, Mumbai, India.
3. Anatomy of the Human Body. 42nd Edition. Henry Gray, Editor-in-chief: Susan Standring, Elsevier (2020).
4. Ross and Wilson Anatomy and Physiology in Health and Illness, 13th Edition, by Allison Wynn Grant, Anne Waugh, and Kathleen J. W. Wilson (2018).
5. Schaum's outline of theory and problems of Human anatomy and Physiology, 2nd Edition (1997), Tata MaGraw-Hill Publishing Company Limited, New Delhi, India.

MULTIPLE CHOICE QUESTIONS (MCQs)

Select the correct options.

1. One of the following sentence is not correct:
(A) The bladder has an inner lining of transitional epithelium.
(B) The bladder has three layers of muscle fibres and an outer adventitia.
(C) The inner part of the bladder is protected by adventitia.
(D) The inner wall of the bladder is called urothelium.

2. The transport of urine through the ureter is by:
(A) Active transport (B) Passive transport
(C) Pressure of fluid (D) Peristalsis

3. The podocyte cells are found within:
(A) The Bowman's capsule
(B) The urinary bladder
(C) The urethra
(D) Both (B) and (C)

4. The transitional epithelium is predominantly present in:
(A) Urethra (B) Urinary bladder
(C) Glomerulus (D) Nephron

5. The following one statement is not correct:
(A) Female urethra is short compared to male urethra.
(B) Female urethra is average 4 cm in length.
(C) Female urethra begins at the neck of the bladder
(D) Female urethra opens directly onto the perineum

6. These substances are absorbed by the proximal part of the tubules:
(A) Water (B) Glucose
(C) Sodium (D) All of the above

7. ADH acts on:

(A) Proximal part of the tubule
(B) Loop of Henle
(C) Distal convoluted part of the tubule
(D) None of these

8. These are phases in formation of urine:

(A) Simple filtration (B) Selective reabsorption
(C) Secretion (D) Both (A) and (B)

9. Average glomerulus filtration rate (GFR) is:

(A) 75 ml (B) 125 ml
(C) 50 ml (D) 25 ml

10. Each nephron produces following amount of ultra-filter per day:

(A) 10 μl (B) 100 μl
(C) 1000 μl (D) 500 μl

11. Total ultra-filter produced per day is about:

(A) 1.0–2.0 liters (B) 5–10 liters
(C) 25–50 liters (D) 170–200 liters

12. Normal urinary excretion per day is about:

(A) 1.5–2.0 liters (B) 500–700 ml
(C) 5.0–10.0 liters (D) 300–500 ml

13. These all are essential substances, *except*:

(A) Urea (B) Glucose
(C) Amino acids (D) Proteins

14. These are all low threshold substances, *except*:

(A) Sodium (B) Potassium
(C) Calcium (D) Amino acids

15. Increase in all these substances in blood indicates renal diseae, *except*:

(A) Urea (B) Glucose
(C) Creatinine (D) Uric acid

16. Water reabsorption in distal tubules is regulated by:

(A) ADH
(B) FSH
(C) Parathyroid hormones
(D) All of the above

17. These hormones increase reabsorption of calcium ions and decrease reabsorption of phosphate ions at kidney level:

(A) Mineralocorticoids
(B) Parathyroid hormones
(C) Corticosteroids
(D) Androgens

18. pH of freshly voided urine (sample collected after 8–12 hours fasting) is:

(A) Acidic
(B) Basic
(C) Neutral
(D) Either (B) or (C)

19. A volume of blood equal to the total blood volume passes through the kidneys in

(A) 10–15 minutes (B) 2–4 hours
(C) 4–5 minutes (D) 4–5 hours

20. Anuria means

(A) Excretion of urine <500 ml
(B) Excretion of urine <50 ml
(C) Complete suppression of urine formation
(D) Excretion of urine 25–100 ml

21. Which of the following renal structure is not a component of the nephron?

(A) Loop of Henle
(B) Renal capsule
(C) Proximal convoluted tubule
(D) Collecting duct

22. The renal structure that drains urine directly into the ureter is the:

(A) Major calyx (B) Urethra
(C) Collecting duct (D) Renal pelvis

23. Activation of the renin–angiotensin system stimulates the secretion of:

(A) Antidiuretic hormone
(B) Aldosterone
(C) Atrial natriuretic peptide
(D) Cortisol

24. Increased levels of aldosterone stimulate the reabsorption the following molecules:

(A) Sodium and water (B) Potassium and sodium
(C) Glucose and sodium (D) Calcium and water

25. Hormone affected in the case of damage to posterior pituitary:

(A) Renin
(B) Antidiuretic hormone
(C) Erythropoietin
(D) Aldosterone

26. Which of the following hormones is produced and secreted by the juxtaglomerular apparatus in response to low blood pressure?

(A) Aldosterone
(B) Renin
(C) Antidiuretic hormone
(D) Natriuretic peptide

27. Main observation in routine examination in nephrotic syndrome is:

(A) Presence of red blood cells
(B) Polyuria
(C) Glycouria
(D) Massive proteinuria

28. The primary manifestation of acute renal failure is:

(A) Proteinuria (B) Oliguria
(C) Hematuria (D) Diuresis

29. Which of the following dietary nutrients must be restricted in individuals with advanced chronic renal failure?

(A) Lipids (B) Carbohydrates
(C) Protein (D) Vitamins

30. Which of the following complications associated with renal failure creates the greatest need for immediate dialysis?

(A) Very high serum urea and creatinine
(B) High serum potassium
(C) Hypertension
(D) Both (A) and (B)

31. Which of the following factors have a major influence on the development of renal calculi?

(A) Urine urea levels (B) Serum lactate levels
(C) Urine pH (D) Urine creatinine levels

32. Which one of the following microorganisms causes the vast majority of urinary tract infections (UTIs)?

(A) *Klebsiella aerogenes* (B) *Candida albicans*
(C) *Escherichia coli* (D) *Shigella flexneri*

33. This is an important cause of bacterial persistence resulting in recurring urinary tract infections includes

(A) Alkaline pH of urine
(B) Increased mucus secretion by the urinary tract
(C) Microbial resistance to antibiotics
(D) Acidic urine pH

34. Which of the following infections is most commonly associated with the development of acute post-streptococcal glomerulonephritis?

(A) Wound infections (B) Throat infections
(C) Endocarditis (D) Skin infections

35. What is the cause of the peripheral edema that often manifests with glomerulonephritis and nephrotic syndrome?

(A) Systemic inflammation
(B) Potassium retention
(C) Significant proteinuria
(D) Sodium retention

36. Renal calculi are formed from all of the following substances, *except*:

(A) Uric acid (B) Bilirubin
(C) Calcium oxalate (D) Struvite

37. Which of the following promotes sodium retention and potassium loss from the blood across the wall of the distal convoluted tubule?

(A) Renin (B) ADH
(C) Aldosterone (D) Angiotensin I

ANSWERS

1. C	2. C	3. A	4. B	5. A	6. D	7. C
8. D	9. B	10. B	11. D	12. A	13. A	14. D
15. B	16. A	17. B	18. A	19. C	20. C	21. B
22. D	23. B	24. A	25. B	26. B	27. D	28. B
29. C	30. D	31. C	32. C	33. C	34. B	35. C
36. B	37. C					

MATCH THE COLUMNS

I	II
1. Polyurea	A. Physiological event leading to excretion of urine
2. Cystisis	B. Secreted by juxtaglomerular cells of kidney
3. Micturition	C. Excretion of 24-hr urine >2,500 ml
4. Anuria	D. Secreted by zona glomerulosa of adrenal gland
5. Renin	E. Inflammation of bladder
6. Aldosterone	F. Urination during sleep
7. Oliguria	G. Complete suppression of excretion of urine
8. Nocturia	H. Basic functional unit of kidneys
9. Nephron	I. Stimulation of zona glomerulosa cells of the adrenal gland
10. Angiotensin II	J. Excretion of 24-hr urine <500 ml

ANSWERS

1. C	2. E	3. A	4. G	5. B	6. D	7. J
8. F	9. H	10. I				

CHAPTER 14

Reproductive System

SAQ: Short answer question: Marks: 2	**MCQs:** Multiple choice questions: Marks: 0.5 each
BAQ: Brief answer question: Marks: 4 or 5	**Match the columns:** Marks: 0.5 each
LAQ: Long answer question: Marks: 9 or 10	**Draw a labelled diagram:** Marks: 5

Objectives: To identify male and female sex organs. To differentiate between primary and secondary sex organs. To describe secondary sex characters.

INTRODUCTION (Fig. 14.1)

SAQ: Write a brief introduction on the reproductive system.

Ans: The reproductive system (the genital system) (Fig. 14.1), is made up of all the anatomical organs involved in sexual reproduction. The male reproductive system mainly includes: The penis, scrotum, testes, epididymis, vas deferens, prostate, and seminal vesicles. The main female reproductive system consists of: The vagina, the uterus, the bilateral Fallopian tubes and the ovaries. The outer sex organs are known as the external genitalia, which are visible at birth in both the sexes. The inner sex organs are known as the internal genitalia, which are present internally in both the sexes.

The following are the main functions of the male reproductive system: (1) To produce testosterone hormone, which is responsible to maintain the male reproductive functions, (2) to promote sperm synthesis and (3) transport of sperms into the female reproductive system for fertilization.

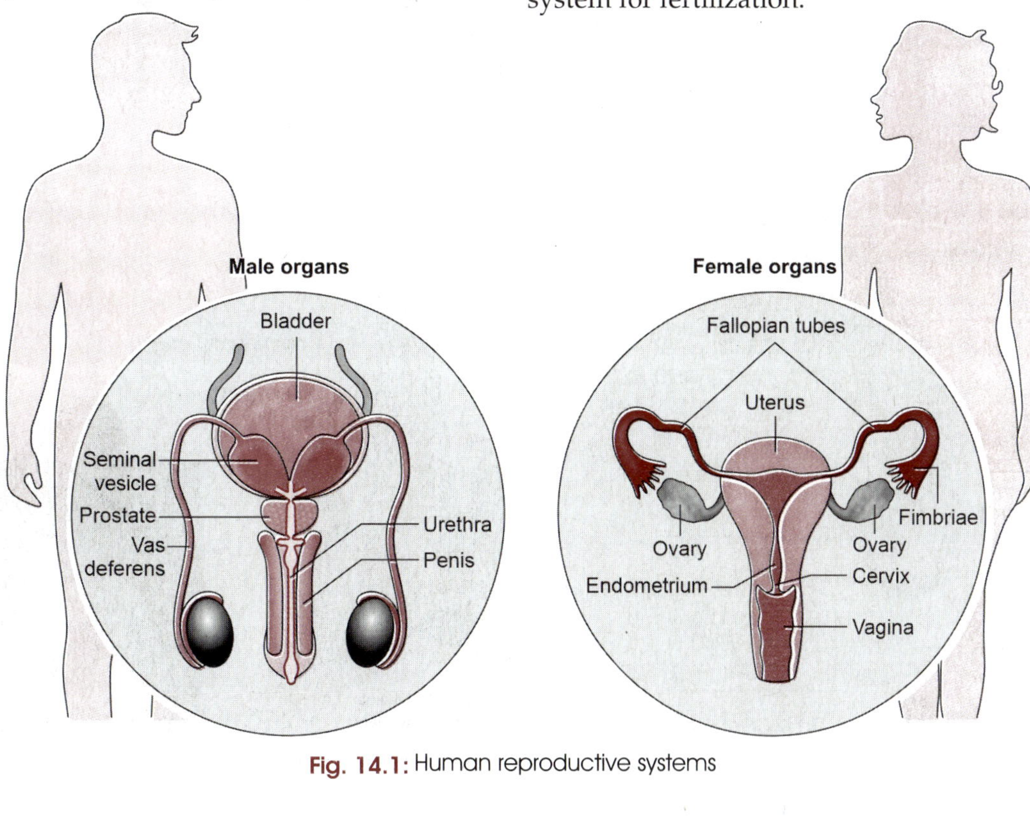

Fig. 14.1: Human reproductive systems

The following are the main functions of the female reproductive system: (1) To produce ova (gametes or eggs) (2) to regulate sex hormones and (3) maintenance of fertilized egg as it develops into mature fetus, set for delivery.

SAQ: What is the difference between primary and secondary sex organs?

Ans: The primary sex organs are the gonads, which are internal sex organs that produce gametes and hormones necessary for reproduction. The secondary sex organs develop after puberty. In the case of male, the testes are the primary sex organs, which produce sperms while, penis, epididymis, vas deferens, prostate, and seminal vesicles are the secondary sex organs.

In the case of female, the ovaries are primary sex organs, which produce ova, while, the cervix, the bilateral Fallopian tubes, the uterus, and breasts are the secondary sex organs.

SAQ: What are secondary sex characters?

Ans: Secondary sex characters develop during puberty. In the case of normal males the secondary sex characteristics include, hair pattern changes, hair become thick, Adam's apple becomes prominent, voice become deep, hair growth appears in the pubic area, under the arms and on the face, shoulders become broad, increase in the growth of skeletal muscles, increase in musculature and increase in height.

The secondary sexual characteristics in normal females are, development of breasts, lighter musculature, broadening of hips due to fat deposition, voice becomes relatively deep, hair growth appears in the pubic area and under the arms and increase in height.

Objectives: To describe anatomical features of the male sex organs and related functions. To describe the basic disorders of the male sex organs. To describe the composition of semen and the factors associated with male fertility. To describe the morphology of human spermatozoa.

MALE REPRODUCTIVE SYSTEM (Fig. 14.2)

SAQ: What are the components of male reproductive system?

Ans: The male reproductive system includes the penis, scrotum, testes, epididymis, vas deferens, prostate, and seminal vesicles (Fig. 14.2).

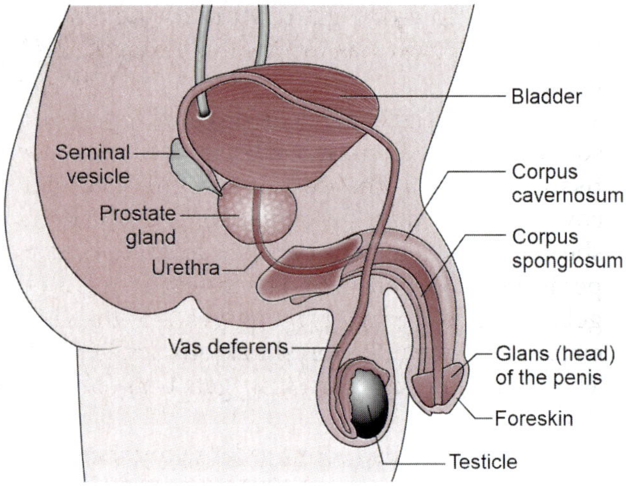

Fig. 14.2: Male reproductive system

Penis (Fig. 14.3)

BAQ: Write a note on the applied anatomy and related functions of the penis.

Ans: The penis is the male sex organ. It attains full size during puberty. The penis is the organ involved in sexual intercourse. The penis also acts as a tube for urine excretion.

The following are the main parts of the penis: The base, the shaft, the glans, and the foreskin. The tissues of the penis contain blood vessels, the dorsal nerve, connective tissue, and the erectile tissues, corpus cavernosum and corpus spongiosum.

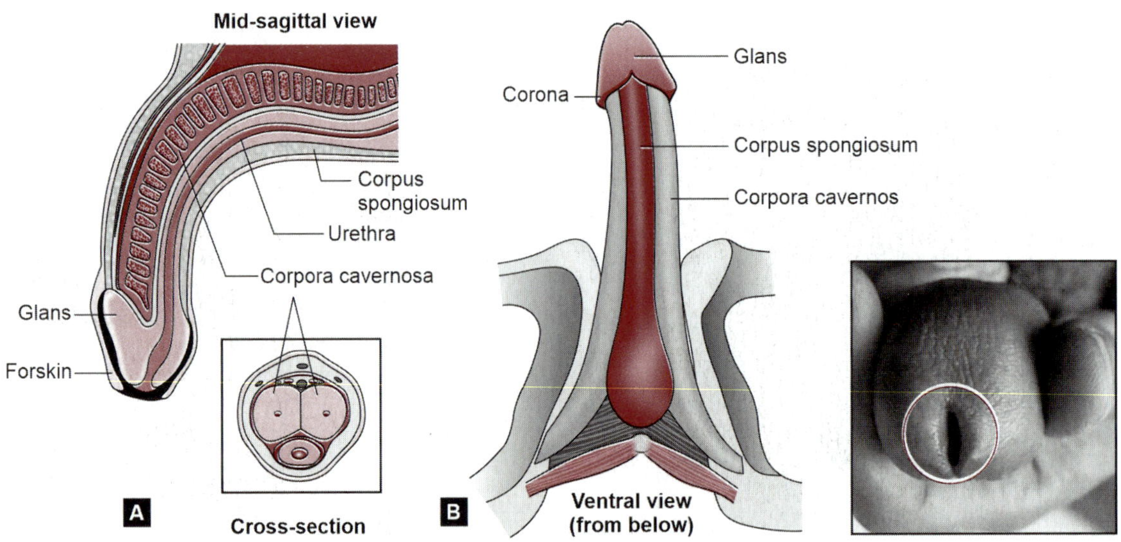

Figs 14.3A and B: (A) Anatomical feature of the penis; (B) meatus of penis

Anatomical Features

The description of the anatomical features of the penis is as follows (Fig. 14.3):

1. **Glans (head) of the penis:** It is the distal part of the penis. The proximal portion of the glans is termed the corona. The corona is a rounded projecting border that forms at the base of the glans (Fig. 14.3). The neck of the corona glans separates it from the body of the penis. The tip of the glans contains the opening to the urethra, known as the meatus (external urethral orifice).

   The human glans penis is covered by stratified squamous epithelium and a dense layer of connective tissue similar to the dermis of skin. The glans is covered by the foreskin (prepuce). The foreskin is the sheath of skin and at the birth it is fully attached to the penis (Figs 14.3 and 14.6). The foreskin separates and gets retracted during growing years of the child. In circumcised men, the foreskin is surgically removed. The mucosa on the glans then gets transformed into dry skin.

   The glans penis also contains large number of nerve endings. Hence, the glans is the most sensitive part of the penis. The large number of nerves contribute in the sensitivity of the glans, which is important for sexual stimulation and ejaculation.

   The glans penis plays important role in urination and in the ejaculation of the semen. The glans penis also plays a protective role for the female genitalia, during intercourse.
2. **Corpus cavernosum:** It is a smooth muscle in the penis. It exhibits a resting form and tone. On stimulation, the muscle cells of corpus cavernosum relax and cavernous spaces fill with blood; which results in an erection of the penis.
3. **Corpus spongiosum:** It is a column of sponge-like tissue that covers the front of the penis. It fills with blood during an erection of penis; keeping the urethra open.
4. The urethra passes through the corpus spongiosum. Urine passes out of the body, through the urethra.

Function: When a man becomes sexually aroused, nerves cause penis blood vessels to expand. An erection of penis takes place due to blood flow in the penis; leading to hardening the tissue in the corpus cavernosum. Penis erection is a complex process in which the brain, nerves, muscles and blood vessels play very important role.

Erectile Dysfunction

SAQ: Write a note on erectile dysfunction (impotence).

Ans: Erectile dysfunction (impotence) is the inability of a man to get and keep firm erection of penis for sex. Due to erectile dysfunction; penis of a man does not achieve sufficient hardness for effective intercourse. The various reasons of erectile dysfunction include psychological problems, poor health conditions, trauma and specific lifestyle factors.

Prolonged erectile dysfunction problem can cause stress, affect self-confidence and mainly contribute to the relationship problems. It is necessary for the patient to seek advise of an appropriate physician.

SAQ: Write a note on priapism.

Ans: Priapism is an abnormal erection of penis; that remains for several hours. Priapism may be caused due to inappropriate use of erectile dysfunction drugs, antidepressants, and blood thinner drugs.

Scrotum (Fig. 14.4)

SAQ: Write a note the scrotum.

Ans: The scrotum is a sac of skin; that contains the testicles (Fig. 14.4). The scrotum hangs from the body at the front of the pelvis, between the legs. It is below the penis and placed next to the upper thighs.

The cremaster muscle of scrotum surrounds the testicles and spermatic cords. The spermatic cord is

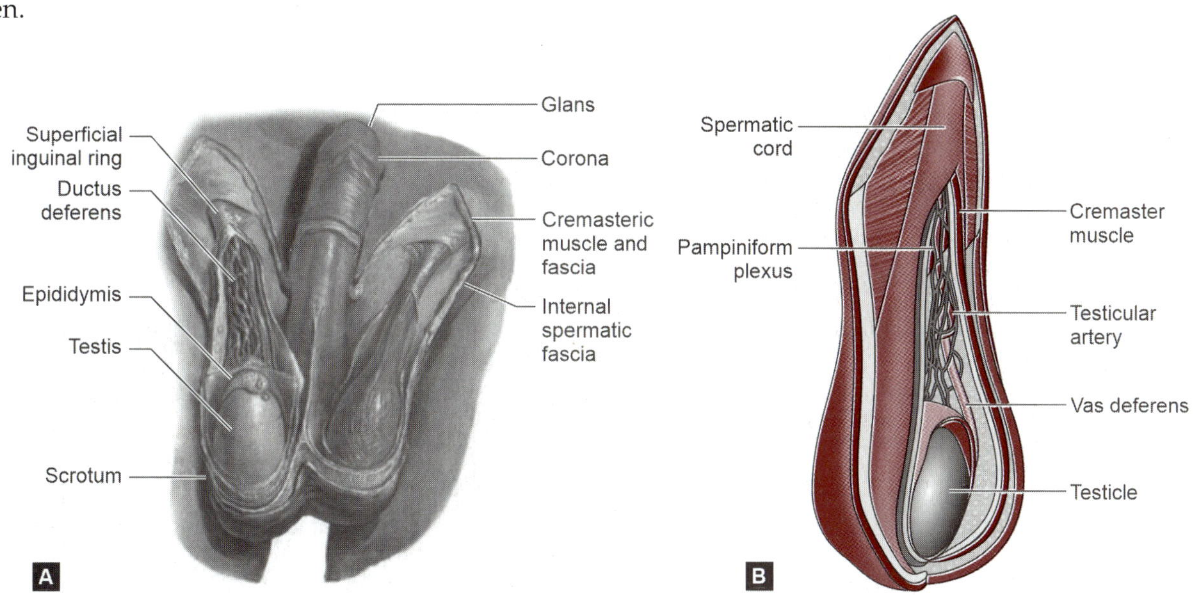

Figs 14.4A and B: Anatomy of the scrotum

composed of arteries, veins, lymphatics, nerves, and the excretory duct of the testis. Cremaster muscle facilitates the movement of the testicle toward and away from the body; which maintain the ideal temperature for sperm production.

Contents of scrotum are surrounded by the scrotal wall. This wall is lined with a smooth muscle. This muscle, along with the cremaster muscles, is used to expand or tighten the skin of the scrotum as it moves up and down.

Each side of the scrotum usually contains a testicle, epididymis, and spermatic cord (Fig. 14.4B).

Testis (Fig. 14.5)

LAQ: Write a note on the testis with respect to the following points: (1) Introduction (2) applied anatomy and (3) functions.

Ans:

1. **Introduction:** The testis are male gonads. These are contained in the scrotum. Each testis is an ovoid organ. The average length of testes is about 5 cm. Each testis lies in the scrotum on either side of a septum that divides the scrotal cavity into two halves (Fig. 14.4). The testis contains several looped tubules. These are known as the seminiferous tubules (Fig. 14.5). Seminiferous tubules are responsible for the production of the sperm cells by a process called spermatogenesis. Inside seminiferous lumen, the development and production of the spermatozoa takes place.
2. **Applied anatomy:** The following two types of cells are present in the testis: (1) Leydig cells and (2) Sertoli cells.

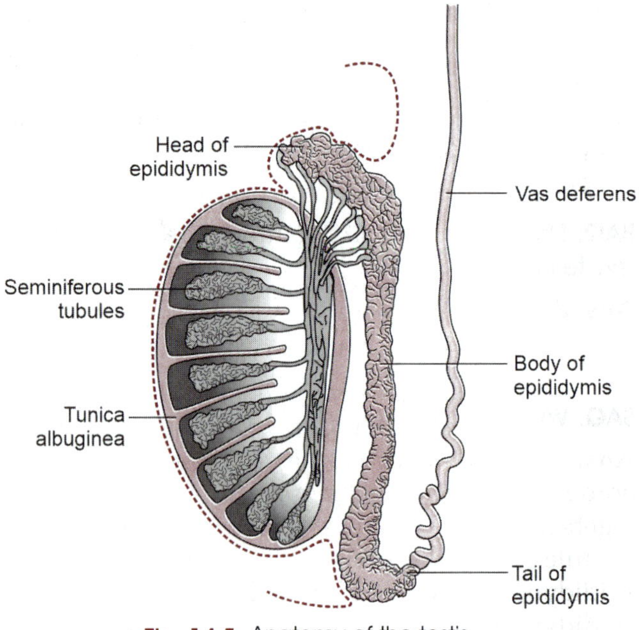

Fig. 14.5: Anatomy of the testis

Leydig Cells (Fig. 14.6)

These lye within the connective tissue that binds the convolutions of the seminiferous tubules together. The pituitary hormone, luteinizing hormone (LH), acts on the leydig cells to stimulate production of testosterone.

Sertoli Cells (Fig. 14.6)

Seminiferous tubules are lined by Sertoli cells. These are sensitive to stimulation by pituitary hormone, follicle stimulating hormone (FSH). Sertoli cells are responsible for the production of spermatozoa from germ cells. Spermatozoa are then regulated by FSH.

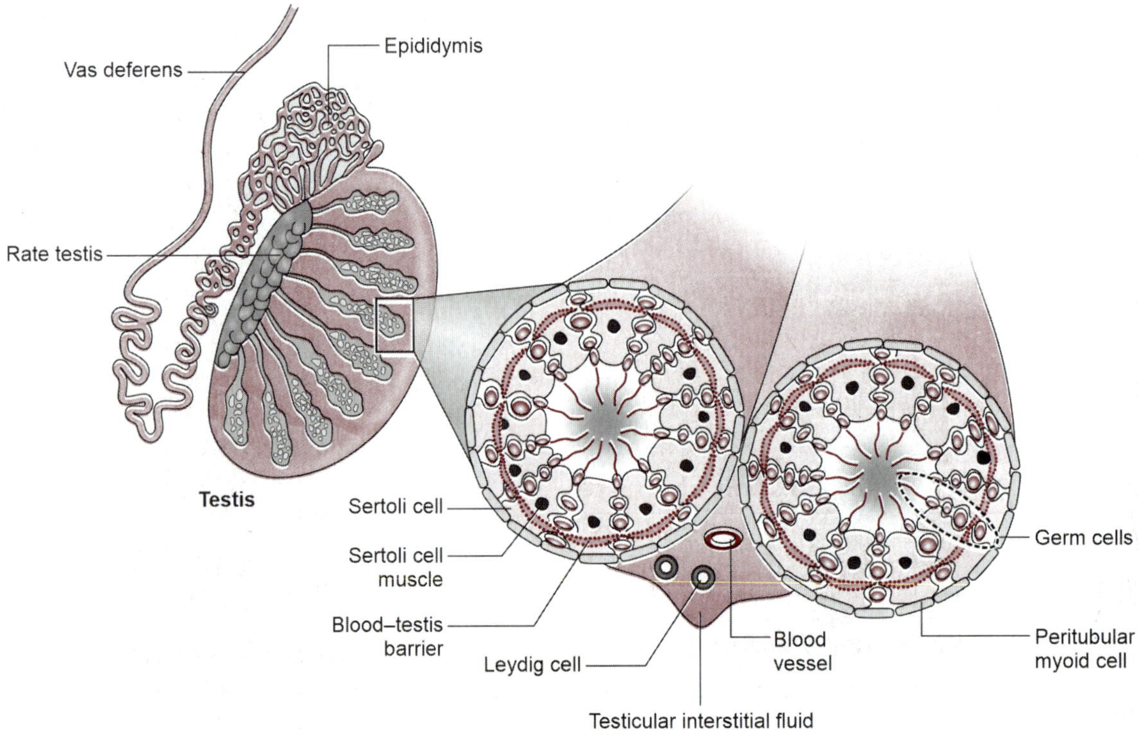

Fig. 14.6: Leydig cells and Sertoli cells

Sertoli cells also stimulate production of a hormone called inhibin, which provides a negative feedback mechanism; which controls the secretion of FSH.

3. **Functions:** The testis has two main functions, synthesis of testosterone hormone and production of spermatozoa.

BAQ: Draw a neat and labelled figure of anatomy of the testis.

Ans: Refer to the Fig. 14.5.

Epididymis (Fig. 14.5)

SAQ: Write a note on the epididymis.

Ans: The epididymis lies among the posterolateral border of each testis. It is made up of tubules packed together in loose connective tissue. The small efferent ductule in the upper end of a larger duct known as the epididymal duct. Within the tail of the epididymis, the epididymal duct increases its diameter and remains in the shape of a roll (convoluted) to form vas deferens. The main function of the epididymis is to store the sperms for maturation and transport these to the vas deferens.

Vas Deferens and Seminal Vesicle (Fig.14.7)

SAQ: Write a note on vas deference and seminal-vesicle.

Ans: The vas deferens passes up into the pelvis. Behind the bladder, the vas dilates to form a chamber known as ampulla. Each ampulla narrows and joins with the duct of the seminal vesicle. The seminal vesicles have a thick muscular coat which contracts strongly during ejaculation of semen. In ampulla of vas deferens and in the cauda (tail of) epididymis the mature sperms are stored. The vas deferens transports mature sperms to the urethra for ejaculation, during sexual intercourse.

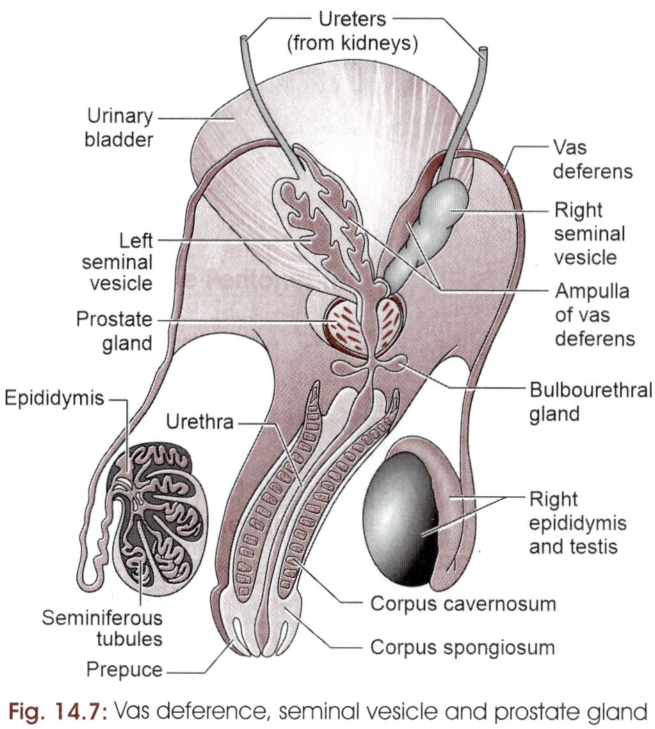

Fig. 14.7: Vas deference, seminal vesicle and prostate gland

Prostate Gland (Fig. 14.7)

SAQ: Write a note on the prostate gland.

Ans: The prostate gland is enclosed within a muscle coat which contracts during ejaculation process. The secretions of the prostate; which are expelled during ejaculation, enter the prostatic urethra. The function of the prostate gland is to form seminal fluid.

Bulbourehral Glands and Urethral Glands (Fig. 14.7)

SAQ: What are bulbourethral glands (Cowper's gland) and urethral glands?

Ans: The bulbourethral glands (Cowper's glands) are two small lobulated glands; which secrete mucus and these open into the urethra.

The urethral glands are small glands located in the mucosa of the anterior male urethra. The urethral glands also secrete mucus. Mucous plays important role as a lubricant during sexual intercourse.

MORPHOLOGY OF HUMAN SPERMATOZOA (Figs 14.8 and 14.9)

BAQ. Write a note on the morphology of spermatozoa.

Ans: The following description of the structure of a human sperm is by the use of a high resolution of electron microscopy:

Each normal human spermatozoan is made up of two main parts, a head and a tail.

Sperm head: It is flat and measures approximately 4.5 micrometer in length, 3 micrometer in width and 1.5 micrometer thick.

The head consists of the nucleus and the acrosome. The nucleus holds whole of the chromatin. The acrosome is made up of a collection of many enzymes that aid in penetration of the zona pellucida (the thick transparent membrane surrounding a mammalian ovum before implantation) by the sperm. Breakdown of the outer acrosomal membrane and release of these enzymes occurs in the female genital tract. This phenomenon is known as the acrosome reaction.

The connecting piece that joins head to the tail of spermatozoa; is a small area in a very short segment. This part contains the proximal centriole. Any defect in the proximal centriole leads to formation of immobile sperms; which may lead to infertility.

Sperm Tail

The tail of a sperm measures about 50 micrometer. It consists of three parts. The mid piece, the principal piece and the terminal segment. The whole length of the tail contains a central contractile unit known as the axoneme.

By means of the tail, the sperm moves. Due to its complexity, abnormalities of the sperm tail can often be a cause of poor sperm movement and therefore of reproductive failure.

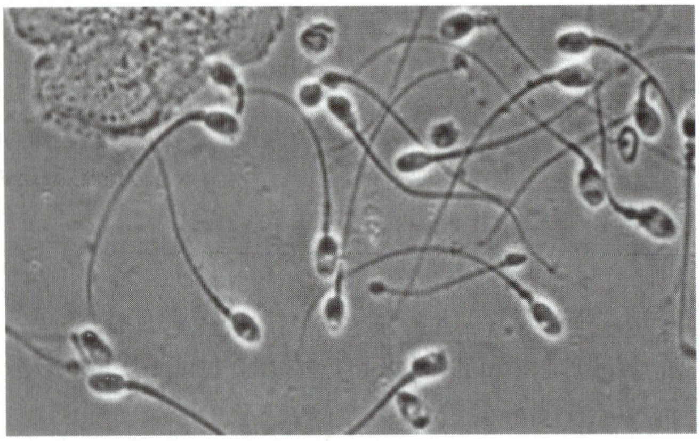

Fig. 14.8: Microscopic image of spermatozoa as seen under the higher power of a compound microscope

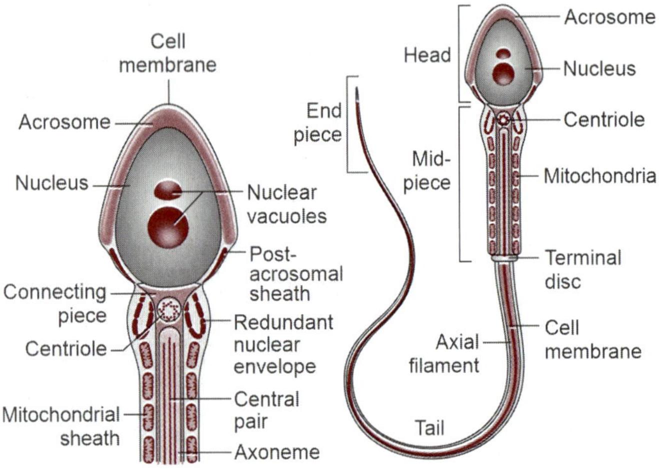

Fig. 14.9: Anatomy of spermatozoa

Objective: To describe blood supply and innervation of the male sex organs.

Blood Supply to Male Reproductive System (Fig. 14.11)

BAQ: Write a note on the blood supply to male reproductive system.

Ans: Two major blood vessels, the femoral artery and femoral vein pass through the pelvic bone and transport

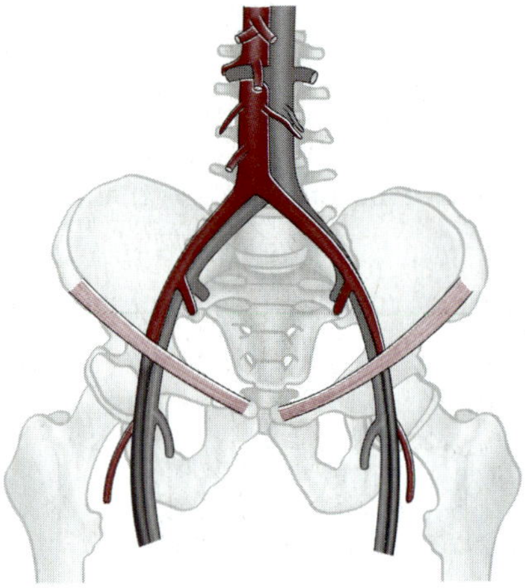

Fig. 14.10: Femoral artery and femoral vein blood transport to male reproductive system

blood to male reproductive system (Fig. 14.10). The femoral artery branches, external iliac artery and internal iliac artery supply arterial blood to the male reproductive parts.

The internal pudendal artery is the main vessel that supplies oxygenated blood to the penis, which is necessary for penis erection. Any problems with the blood flow to the penis can result in erectile dysfunction.

The deoxygenated blood is collected from the superficial inguinal ring, external and internal pudendal veins to testicular vein and from there the deoxygenated blood passes to the inferior vena cava (Fig. 14.12).

Nerve Supply of the Male Reproductive System (Fig. 14.13)

BAQ: Write a note on the nerve supply of the male reproductive system.

Ans: The organs of the male reproductive system receive visceral afferent and efferent nerve supply. A group of ganglia near the spinal cord, the celiac, aortic, caudal mesenteric, hypogastric, and pelvic ganglia connect to male reproductive system. The scrotum and external cremaster muscle also receive a somatic innervation (component of the peripheral nervous system).

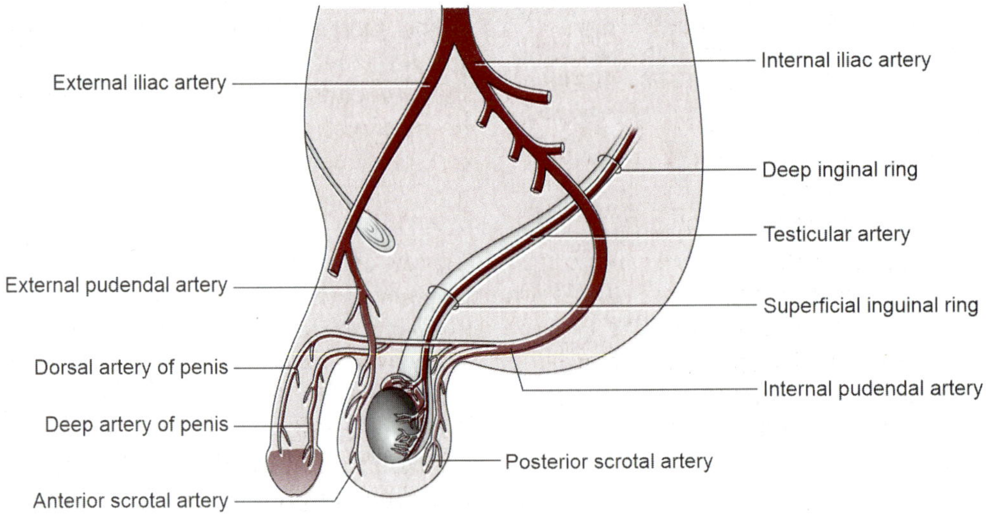

Fig. 14.11: Arterial blood transport to male reproductive system

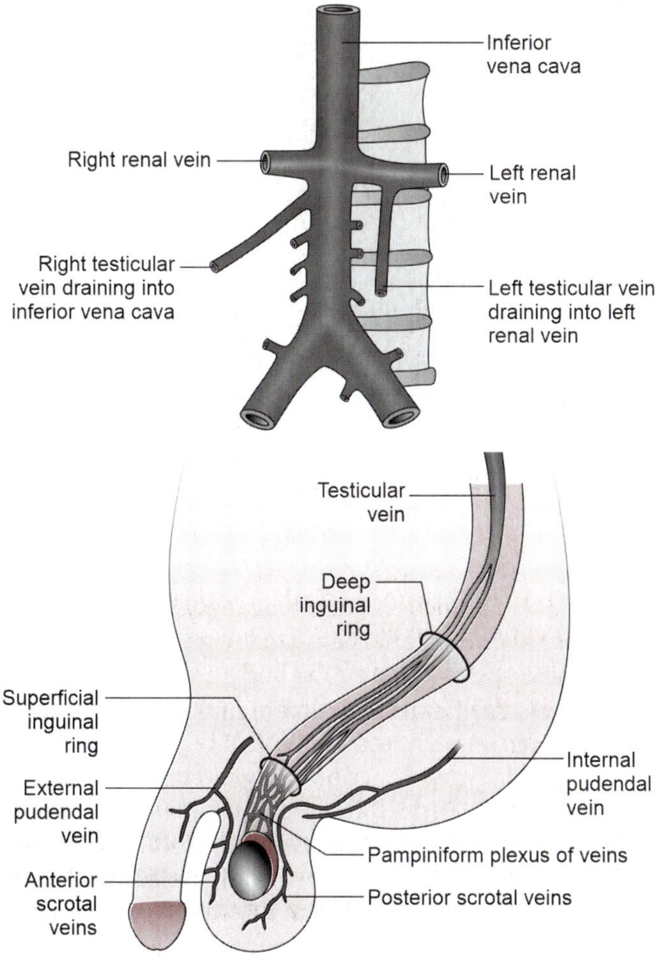

Fig. 14.12: Venous blood transport from male reproductive system

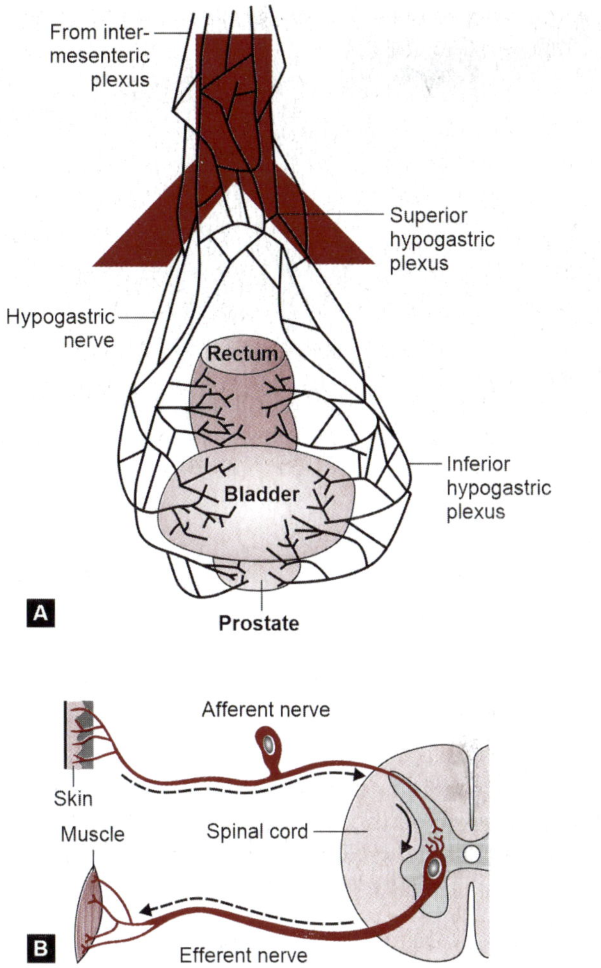

Figs 14.13A and B: Nerve supply of male reproductive system

Objective: To describe anatomical features of the female sex organs and related functions.

FEMALE REPRODUCTIVE SYSTEM (Fig. 14.14)

BAQ: Write a brief note on the female reproductive system.

Ans: The female reproductive anatomy includes external and internal structures. The main female reproductive system mainly consists of the vagina, the uterus, the bilateral Fallopian tubes and the ovaries (Fig. 14.14).

The ovaries are placed near the Fallopian tubes; located on either side of the uterus. The ovaries are responsible for the production of ova and also for the secretion of the sex hormones, estrogens and progesterone.

The Fallopian tubes arise from the uterus and extend towards the ovaries. After the intercourse and ejaculation of semen, sperms travel upwards from the uterine cavity (cavity of uterus) and Fallopian tubes provide the site for fertilization of oocyte. The fertilized egg is transported back along the Fallopian tubes to the uterine cavity. Endometrium of uterine cavity undergoes cyclical changes in preparation for implantation of fertilized egg and pregnancy.

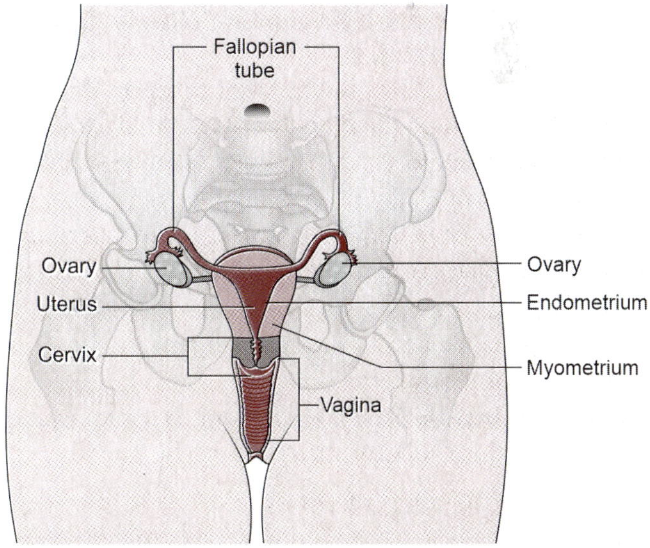

Fig. 14.14: Female reproductive system

External Structure of the Female Reproductive Structure (Vulva)

BAQ: Write a note on the external structure of the female reproductive system with respect to the applied anatomy and related functions.

Ans: Following are the main external structures of the female reproductive system (vulva): Mons pubis, labia majora, labia minora, pudendal cleft, Bartholin's glands and clitoris (Fig. 14.15).

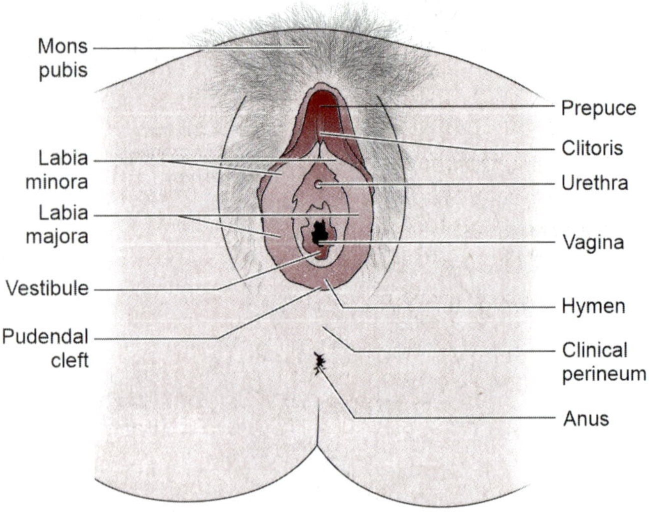

Fig. 14.15: External structure of female reproductive structure (vulva)

Mons Pubis (Fig. 14.15)

The mons pubis is a rounded mass of fatty tissue over the joint of the pubic bones. The function of mons pubis is to provide cushion during sexual intercourse. The mons pubis also contains sebaceous glands that secrete pheromones to induce sexual attraction.

Labia Majora (Fig. 14.15)

The labia majora (singular: Labium majus) are a pair of rounded folds of skin and adipose tissue. Their function is to cover and protect more delicate and sensitive; inner structures such as the labia minora, clitoris, urinary orifice, and vaginal orifice.

During puberty, hair growth takes place on the skin of the labia majora, which also contain sweat and oil-secreting glands.

Labia Minora (Fig. 14.15)

The labia minora are inner skin folds and lie inside the labia majora. These skin folds protect the opening of the urethra and the vagina.

Pudendal Cleft (Fig. 14.15)

It is the cleft between the labia majora. It contains and protects the more delicate structures of the vulva.

Bartholin's Glands (Fig. 14.16)

The Bartholin's glands are located on each side of vaginal opening. Their primary function is the production of a mucous secretion, which aids in vaginal lubrication.

Clitoris (Fig. 14.15)

The clitoris is a small and sensitive protrusion. It is covered by a fold of skin, called the prepuce. The clitoris is similar to the foreskin at the end of the penis. The clitoris is very sensitive to stimulation and can erect.

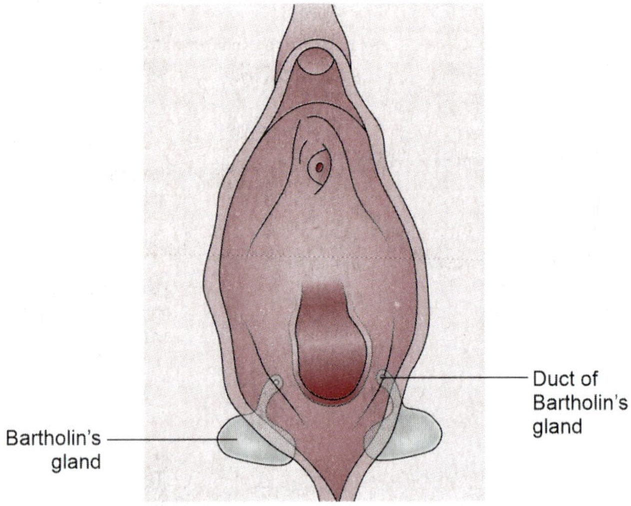

Fig. 14.16: Bartholin's gland

Functions of the External Female Reproductive Structures (the Genitals)

1. To enable sperm to enter the body and
2. To protect the internal genital organs from infectious organisms.

Internal Reproductive Organs (Fig. 14.17)

LAQ: Write a note on the internal structure of the female reproductive system with respect to the applied anatomy and related functions.

Ans: Following are the internal reproductive organs: Vagina, uterus, ovaries and the Fallopian tubes.

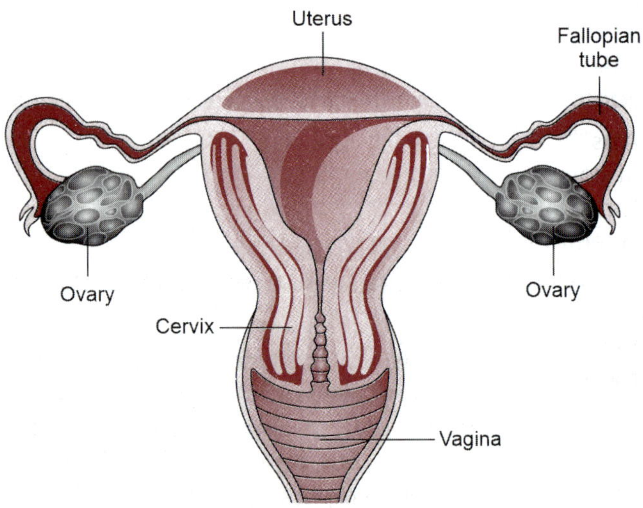

Fig. 14.17: Internal reproductive organs

VAGINA (Fig. 14.17)

The vagina is a muscular, elastic canal of female internal genital tract that joins the cervix to the outside of the body (Fig. 14.17).

The outer vaginal opening is normally covered partially by a thin layer of mucosal tissue called the hymen (Fig. 14.18). The vagina passage is used for sexual intercourse and also for delivering child following birth. Menstrual cycle blood flow (menses) also passes through the vagina.

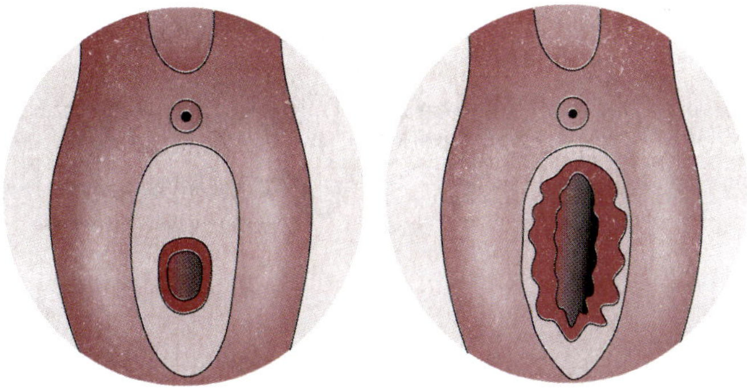

Fig. 14.18: Normal hymen and after defloration

To accommodate smooth penetration of the penis through vagina during sexual intercourse, vaginal moisture increases during sexual arousal. The Bartholin's glands are responsible for the supply of mucus for the lubrication of the entrance to the vagina during sexual excitement.

The space that exists between the opening of the cervix and the wider back wall of the vaginal canal makes up the vaginal fornix. It exists as anterior fornix and posterior fornix (Fig. 14.19).

The anterior fornix is the point, where the tip of the penis reaches, during sexual intercourse. The posterior fornix is an important part of the vagina. Due to pocket-like shape of the posterior fornix; ejaculated semen remains in there up to 20–30 minutes in liquid form. This facilitates the easy permeation of sperms through the cervical canal.

SAQ: What is the reason for the change of colour of vaginal discharge.

Ans: The vaginal discharge is most often a normal type of colourless discharge. However, due to bacterial or fungal infections; abnormal green, or yellow and foul smelling discharge may be produced.

Microanatomical Layers of the Vagina

BAQ: Write a note on the microanatomical layers of the vagina.

Ans: The vagina is composed of the following four histological layers (internal to external) (Fig. 14.20):

1. **Stratified squamous epithelium:** This layer provides protection and is lubricated by cervical mucus.
2. **Elastic lamina propria:** It is a dense connective tissue layer which projects papillae into the overlying epithelium.
3. **Muscularis (Fibromuscular layer):** It is comprised of following two layers of smooth muscle: An inner circular layer and an outer longitudinal layer.
4. **Adventitia:** It is a fibrous layer. It provides additional strength to the vagina and also binds it to surrounding structures.

Objectives: To describe blood supply and innervation of the female sex organs.

Blood Supply of the Vagina (Figs 14.21 and 14.22)

BAQ: Write a note on the blood supply of the vagina

Ans: Blood is supplied to the vagina is through the vaginal artery. It emerges from a branch of the internal iliac artery. Three groups of lymphatic vessels accompany these arteries. Two main veins drain blood from the vagina, which form a network, the vaginal venous plexus, on the sides of the vagina and connect with similar venous plexuses of the uterus, bladder, and rectum. All these veins ultimately drain into the internal iliac vein.

Nerve Supply of the Vagina (Fig. 14.23)

BAQ: Write a note on the nerve supply of the vagina.

Ans: The nerve supply of the upper vagina is provided by the sympathetic and parasympathetic nerves of the pelvic plexus. The lower vagina is supplied by the pudendal nerve.

Uterus (Womb) (Fig. 14.24)

LAQ: Describe the uterus (womb) with respect to the following heads: (1) Introduction, (2) Applied anatomy and related functions

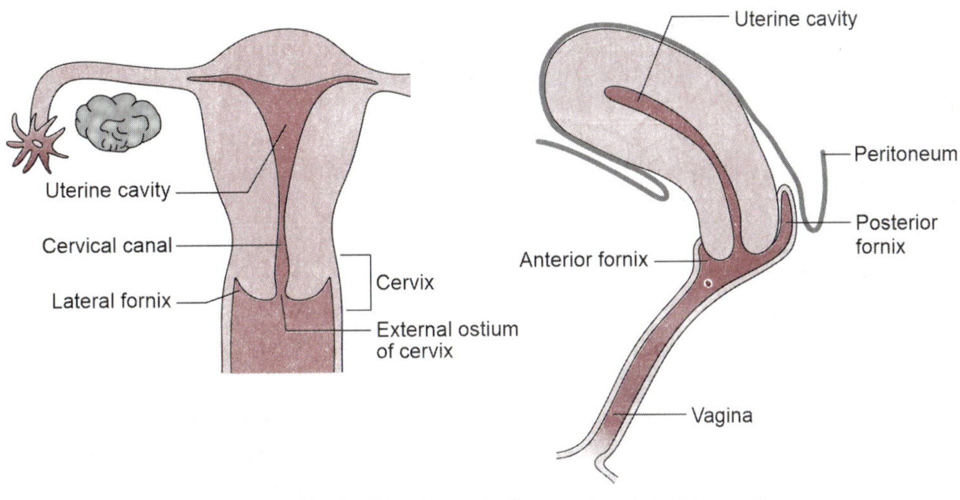

Fig. 14.19: Vaginal fornix and other parts related to vagina

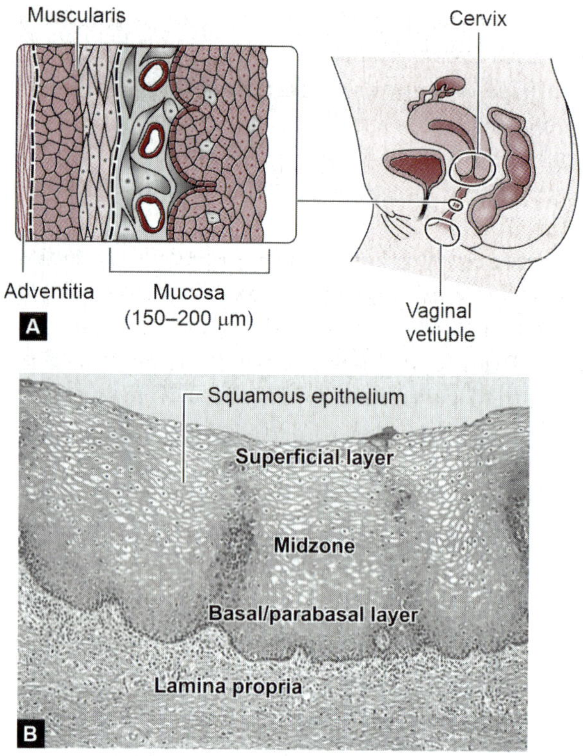

Figs 14.20A and B: Histological layers of vagina

Ans:

1. **Introduction:** The uterus is a secondary sex organ. Secondary sex organs are components of the reproductive system that mature during puberty under the influence of sex hormones produced from primary sex organs like the ovaries in females (and the testes in males).

   The uterus is a hollow muscular organ. It is located in the female pelvis between the bladder and rectum. When the egg leaves the ovary; it can get fertilized and implanted in the lining of the uterus. The main function of the uterus is to nourish the developing fetus till birth of a child.

2. **Applied anatomy and related functions** (Fig. 14.24): The uterus is a hollow thick-walled muscular organ.

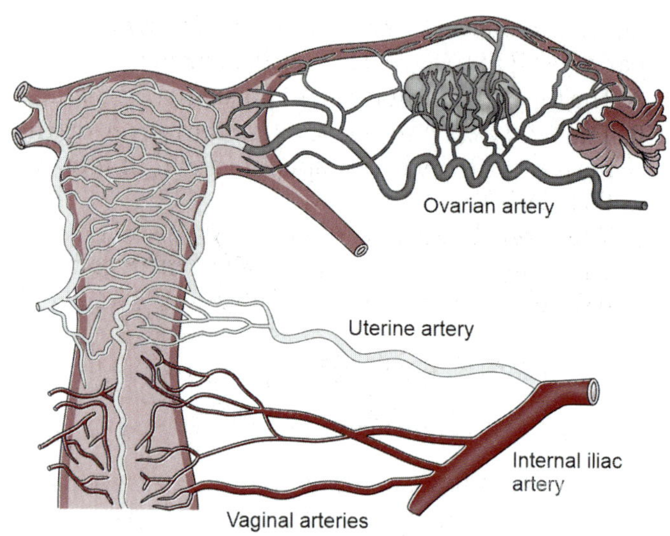

Fig. 14.21: Arterial blood supply of female reproductive system

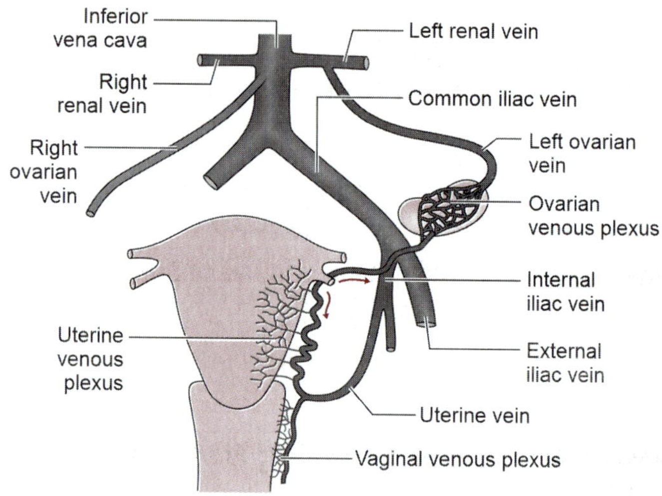

Fig. 14.22: Venous blood supply of female reproductive system

It is located in the female pelvis between the bladder and the rectum. It is connected laterally to the uterine tubes and distally to the vagina. The uterus is capable of expansion so that it could accommodate a growing

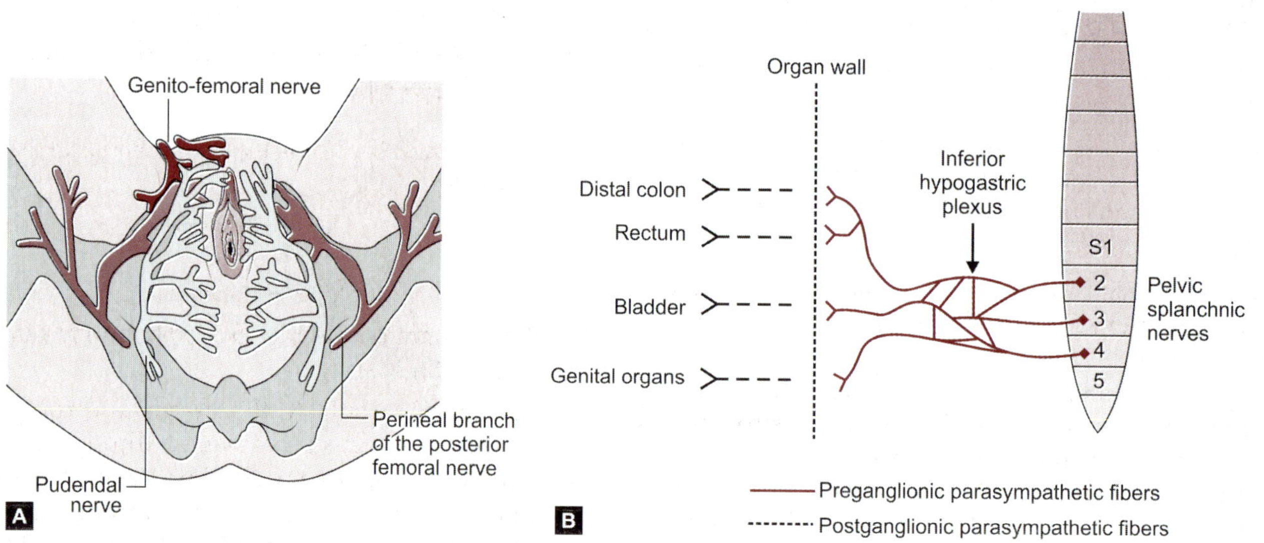

Figs 14.23A and B: Nerve supply of vagina

fetus. The uterus is made up of the following three parts: (A) Fundus, (B) body and (C) cervix.

A. The fundus is the top part of the uterus (Fig. 14.24).

B. The body is the site for implantation of the blastocyst, which is a specific stage of embryo (Fig. 14.24).

C. The cervix is the lower part of uterus linked with the vagina. This part is structurally and functionally different from the rest of the uterus (Fig. 14.24).

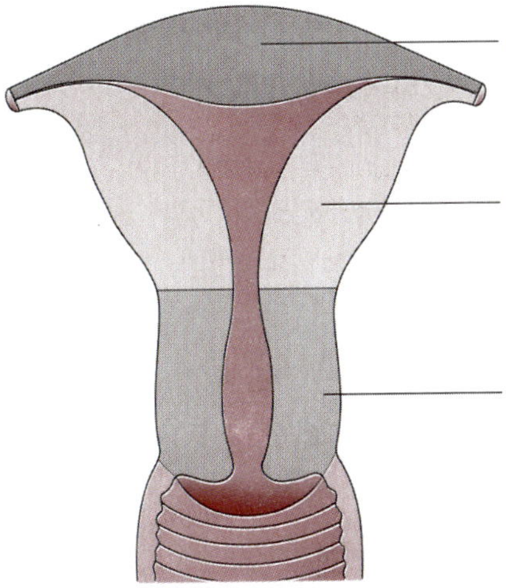

Fig. 14.24: Uterus

BAQ: Draw neat and labelled figure of the uterus.

Ans: Refer to Figs 14.14 and 14.17.

Microanatomical Structure of the Uterus

(Figs 14.25 and 14.26)

BAQ: Write a note on the microanatomical structure of the uterus.

Ans: The fundus and body of the uterus are composed of following three tissue layers (Figs 14.25 and 14.26):

1. Perimetrium: It is a double layered membrane, continuous with the abdominal peritoneum.
2. Myometrium is a thick and smooth muscle layer. The cells of myometrium layer increase in size (hypertrophy) and increase in number (hyperplasia) during pregnancy.
3. Endometrium is an inner mucous membrane lining the uterus. It can be further subdivided into deep stratum basalis and superficial stratum functionalis (Fig. 14.25).

Deep stratum basalis does not change significantly during the menstrual cycle and it does not shed at menstruation.

Superficial stratum functionalis cells increase significantly in response to the action of estrogen and secrete mucous in response to progesterone hormone. Superficial stratum functionalis layer is shed during menstruation and regenerates again from the cells in the stratum basalis layer.

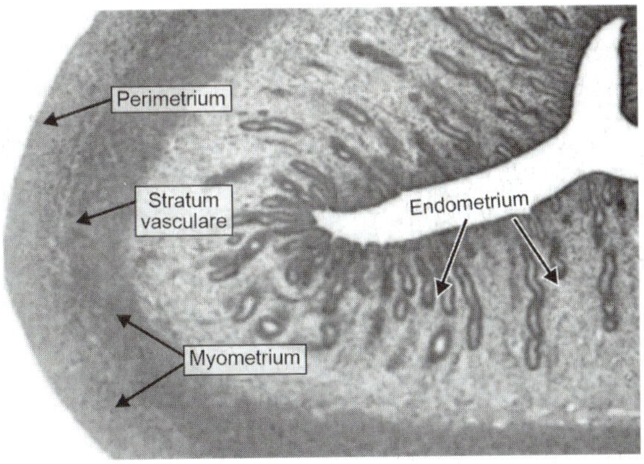

Fig.14.25: Microanatomical structure of the uterus

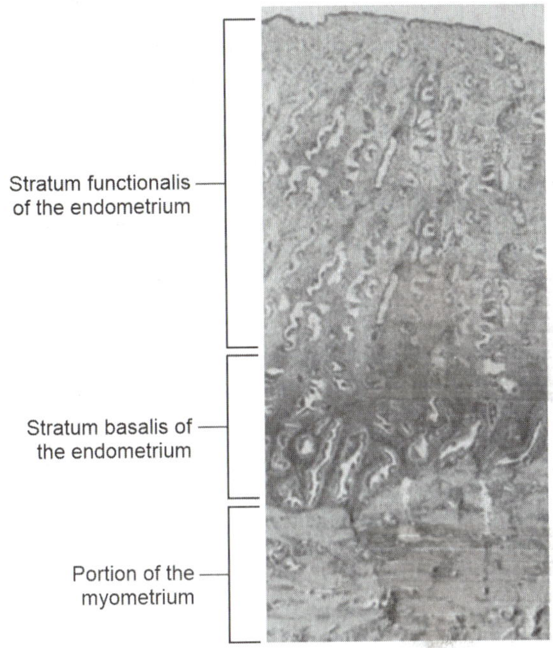

Fig. 14.26: Histological structure of the endometrium

Ligaments of the Uterus

SAQ: Write a note on the ligaments of the uterus.

Ans: The following ligaments provide support to securing the uterus in place: Broad ligament, round ligament, ovarian ligament, cardinal ligament and uterosacral ligament (Fig. 14.27).

Objective: To describe blood supply and innervation of the female sex organs.

Blood Supply and Lymphatics of Uterus

(Figs 14.21, 14.22 and 14.28)

BAQ: Write a note on the blood supply and lymphatic drainage of the uterus.

Ans: The blood supply to the uterus is through the uterine artery. The venous drainage is through a plexus in the broad ligament that drains into the uterine veins.

Lymphatic drainage of the uterus is through the iliac, sacral, aortic and inguinal lymph nodes (Fig. 14.28).

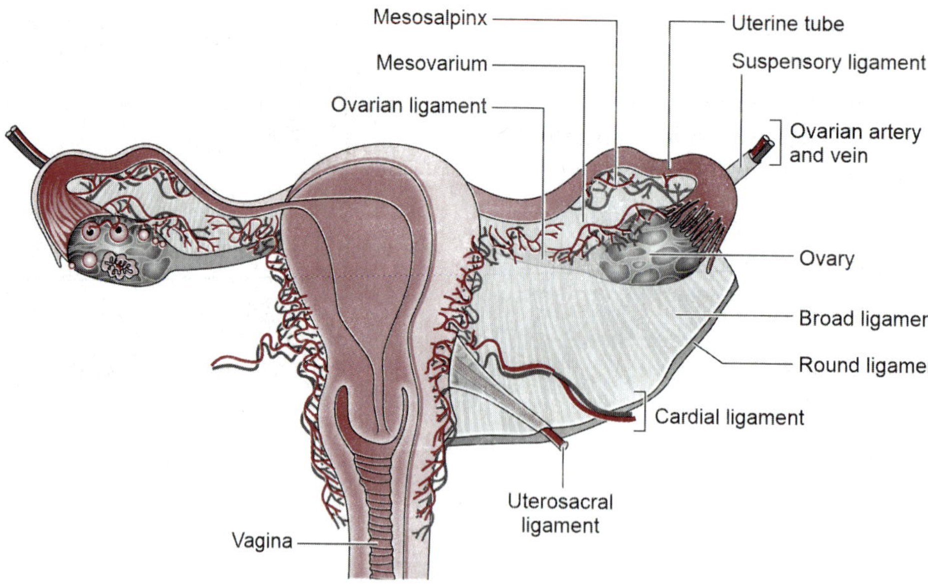

Fig. 14.27: Ligaments of the uterus

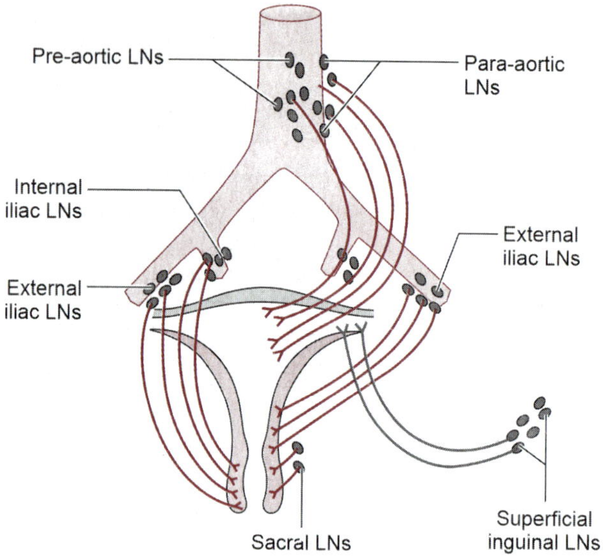

Fig. 14.28: Lymphatic drainage of uterus

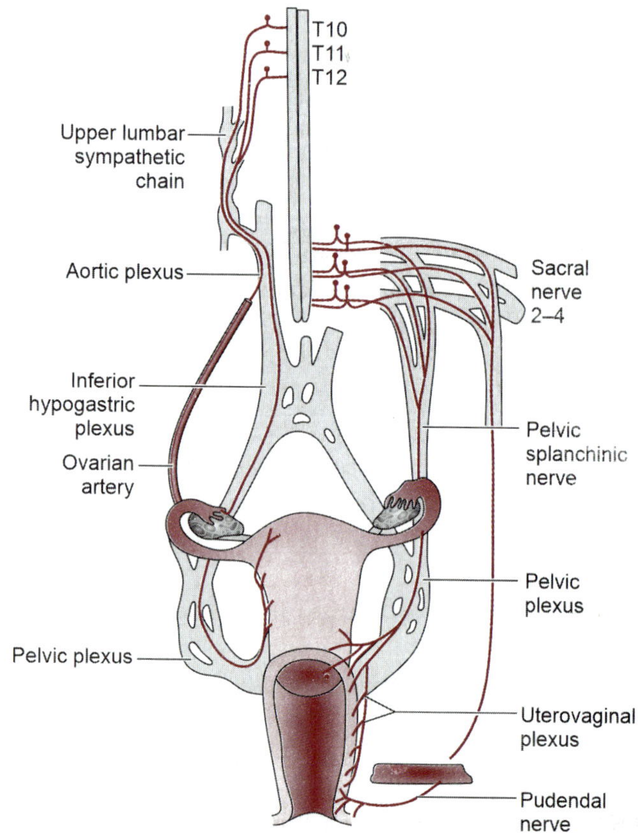

Fig. 14.29: Nerve supply of the uterus

Nerve Supply of the Uterus (Fig. 14.29)

BAQ: Write a note on the blood supply and lymphatic drainage of the uterus.

Ans: The sympathetic nerve fibres of the uterus arise from the uterovaginal plexus. This largely comprises the anterior and intermediate parts of the inferior hypogastric plexus. Parasympathetic fibres of the uterus are derived from the pelvic splanchnic nerves (S2–S4).

> **Objectives:** To describe various anatomical positions of the uterus.

Anatomical Position of the Uterus

SAQ: What is the normal anatomical position of the uterus?

Ans: The uterus normally lies immediately postero-superior (posterior and lateral) to the bladder, and anterior to the rectum (Fig. 14.30).

SAQ: What is an anteverted uterus?

Ans: An anteverted uterus, means the uterus tilts forward at the cervix, toward the abdomen (Fig. 14.30).

SAQ: What is a retroverted (retroflexed or tipped) uterus?

Ans: A retroverted (retroflexed or tipped) uterus means; that tilts backward at the cervix (Fig. 14.30).

SAQ: What is an anteflexed uterus?

Ans: An anteflexed uterus means that bends towards the anterior surface of the body (Fig. 14.30).

SAQ: Which are the three most common abnormal positions of the uterus?

Ans: The three most common abnormal positions of the uterus are as follows: (1) Excessively anteflexed, (2) anteflexed and retroverted and (3) retroflexed and retroverted (Fig. 14.30).

SAQ: What is prolapse of the uterus?

Ans: Due to increased abdominal pressure, the uterus is more likely to prolapse into the vagina. Prolapse of uterus is observed in patients with history of pelvic floor damage.

SAQ: What is hysterectomy?

Ans: Hysterectomy means, surgical removal of the uterus. In the case of suspected cervical or uterine cancer, hysterectomy is performed.

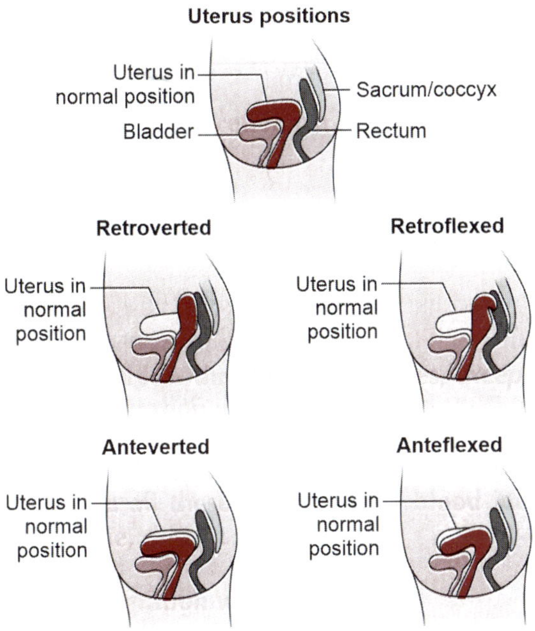

Fig. 14.30: Various positions of the uterus

> **Objective:** To describe the anatomical features and functions of ovaries and Fallopian tube and related disorders.

Ovaries (Figs 14.17 and 14.31)

LAQ: Describe ovaries with respect to the following heads: (1) Introduction; (2) applied anatomical features and (3) functions.

Ans:

1. Introduction: The two ovaries (gonads) are the primary female reproductive organs. The ovaries are located in a shallow depression known as ovarian fossae, one on each side of the uterus (Fig. 14.17). These are present in the lateral walls of the pelvic cavity. The ovaries are held in place by the peritoneal ligaments (Fig. 14.31).
2. Applies microanatomical feature of the ovary (Fig. 14.32A): The ovary has following three main histological features:

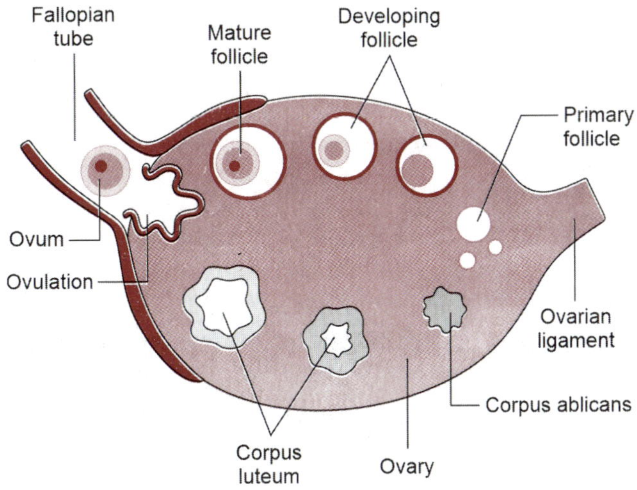

Fig. 14.31A: Overy

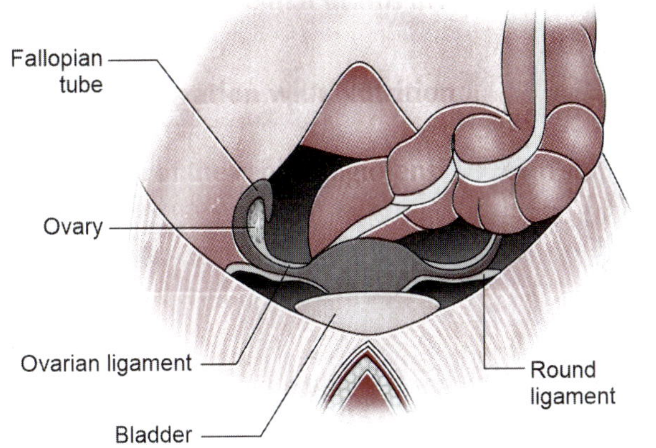

Fig. 14.31B: Ligaments of the female reproductive system

   i. Surface: It is formed of simple cuboidal epithelium (germinal epithelium). Below this layer is a dense connective tissue capsule.
   ii. Cortex: It is comprised of a connective tissue stroma and numerous ovarian follicles. Each follicle contains an oocyte, which is surrounded by a single layer of follicular cells. An oocyte is a cell in an ovary which may undergo meiotic division to form an ovum (Fig. 14.32B).
   iii. Medulla: It is formed by loose connective tissue and a rich neurovascular network, which enters through the hilum of the ovary.
3. Functions: Following are the main functions of the ovaries:
   1. To produce female gametes for fertilisation.
   2. To produce the sex steroid hormones oestrogen and progesterone, in response to stimulated pituitary gland, which releases, gonadotrophins such as FSH and LH.

BAQ: What are ovarian cysts?

Ans: Due to hormonal imbalance and also due to severe pelvic infections, fluid-filled ovarian cysts may develop in the ovary. Most ovarian cysts are benign (not dangerous), do not cause symptoms and may disappear

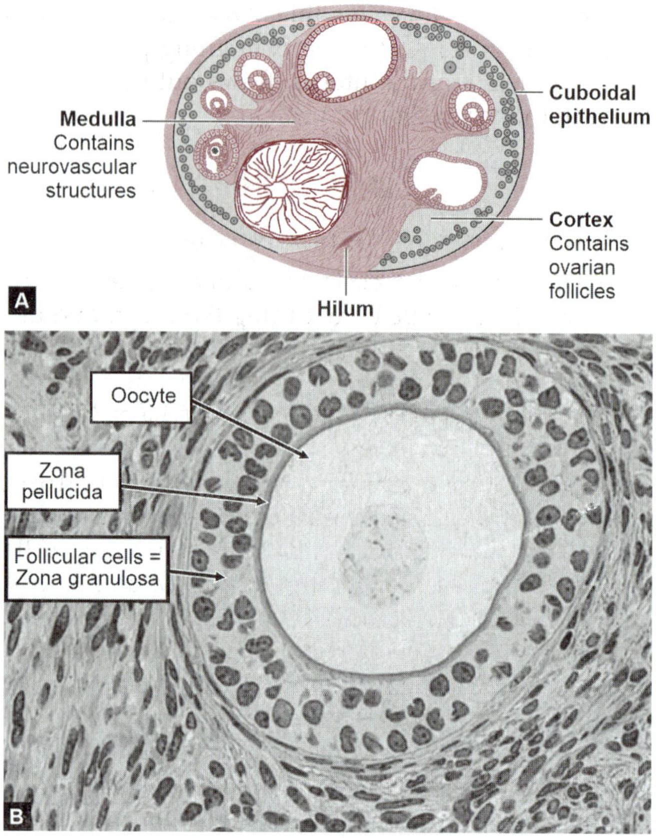

Figs 14.32A and B: Microanatomical features of the ovaries

later on. The ovarian cysts develop during child-bearing years of a women (Fig. 14.33).

In some cases, ovarian cysts may lead to pain during intercourse, menstrual irregularities, and irregular bowel movements. It is then necessary to seek advice and appropriate treatment of a specialist physician.

BAQ: What is polycystic ovary syndrome (PCOS) (or disease (PCOD)?

Ans: In the case of a women suffering from polycystic ovary syndrome (PCOS, or PCOD) many small cysts are seen on their ovaries (Fig. 14.33). Irregular menstrual cycles are observed in PCOS, due to imbalance in reproductive hormones, particularly due to increase in testosterone hormone. The specific characteristic features of PCOS are excessive hair growth and acne on face, back, and chest of a women. PCOS is one of the leading causes of infertility.

SAQ: Write a note on ovarian cancers.

Ans: Ovarian cancers arise from epithelial germ cells. Age, obesity, reproductive history, and genetic factors are the main risk factors for the development of ovarian cancers. Epithelial ovarian tumors develop in the outer surface of the ovaries. These tumors can be benign (not dangerous), with low malignant potential, or malignant (cancerous).

Fallopian Tubes (Fig. 14.34)

LAQ: Describe the Fallopian tubes under the following heads: (1) Introduction, (2) applied anatomical features with related functions.

Ans:

Introduction: The Fallopian tube is a long and slender tube that connect the ovary to the uterus. There is one ovary and one fallopian tube on each side of the uterus. Eggs pass from the ovaries, through the Fallopian tubes, to the uterus. Normally, fertilization of an egg by a sperm takes place in the Fallopian tubes. The fertilized egg then passes to the uterus, where it implants to the uterine lining.

Anatomy of the Fallopian Tube (Fig. 14.34)

Anatomy and related functions: Following are the four main parts of the Fallopian tube (lateral to medial):

1. Fimbriae: These are finger-like, ciliated projections. The fimbriae capture the ovum from the surface of the ovary.
2. Infundibulum: It is a funnel-shaped opening near the ovary to which fimbriae are attached. It catches and channels the released ovum.
3. Ampulla: It is the widest section of the uterine tubes. Fertilization usually takes place in this part.
4. Isthmus: It is the narrow section of the uterine tubes connecting the ampulla to the uterine cavity. The sperms adhere in this part transiently.

The inner mucosa of Fallopian tube is lined with ciliated columnar epithelial cells and non-ciliated secretory cells (peg cells). The peg cells secret lubricating substance and are responsible for the passage of the

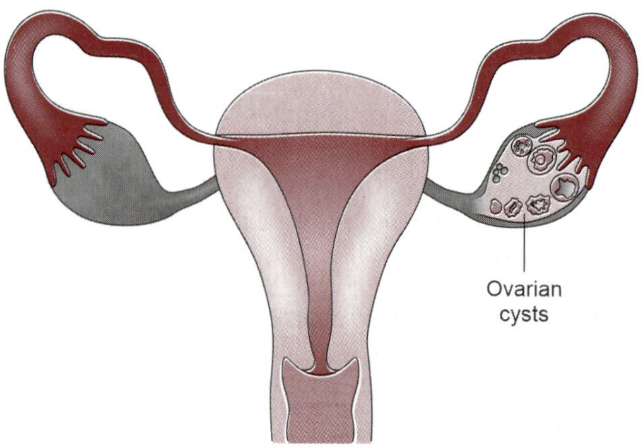

Fig. 14.33: Ovarian cysts

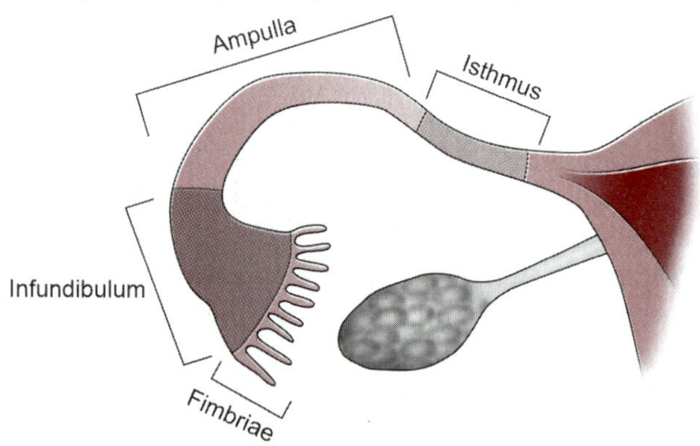

Fig. 14.34: Anatomy of the Fallopian tube

ovum towards the uterus. The peg cells also provide nutrients to the ovum.

Smooth muscle layer contracts to assist with transportation of the ova and sperm. Muscle of ovum is sensitive to sex steroid hormones. Hence, peristalsis is the greatest when estrogen levels are high.

SAQ: What is salpingitis?

Ans: Salpingitis is inflammation of the uterine tubes that is usually caused by bacterial infection. It is caused due to the sexually transmitted diseases such as gonorrhoea and chlamydia. Salpingitis causes damage to Fallopian tubes and is a common cause of female infertility.

SAQ: What is ectopic pregnancy?

Ans: An ectopic pregnancy occurs when a fertilized egg implants and grows outside the main cavity of the uterus. An ectopic pregnancy occurs mainly in a Fallopian tube. In ectopic pregnancy, the fertilised egg cannot survive outside the uterus. If the fertilized egg is left to grow outside uterus, it may damage nearby organs and cause severe loss of blood.

Objectives: To describe the female hormonal cycle. To describe the events of menstrual cycle and related clinical conditions.

MENSTRUATION

SAQ: What is menstruation (menses, menstrual period, cycle or period)?

Ans: Menstruation (menses, menstrual period, cycle or period) is the monthly shedding of the lining of a female uterus. The menstrual blood containing partly tissue from the inside of the uterus, flows out of the body; through the cervix and the vagina.

MENSTRUAL CYCLE (Figs 14.35 and 14.36)

LAQ: Write a note on the menstrual cycle.

Ans: The menstrual cycle is the sequence of events that occur within a female body during the preparation for the possibility of pregnancy and the events that follow in the absence of pregnancy, each month. The menstrual cycles occur specifically on a monthly basis between puberty and menopause.

During the menstrual cycle, sexually matured female body develops one or more eggs and releases them during the time of ovulation. The lining of the uterus and the endometrium, builds up at the same time. After ovulation, this lining changes to prepare for implantation of the fertilized egg to establish a pregnancy. If fertilisation and pregnancy do not occur, the uterus sheds the lining and a new menstrual cycle begins. During menstruation, part of the endometrium and blood products pass out of the body through the vagina.

Phases of Menstrual Cycle

The menstrual cycle is under the control of hormones secreted by pituitary gland in the brain and ovaries. The hormones: Follicular stimulating hormone (FSH), luteinizing hormone (LH) are secreted by the pituitary

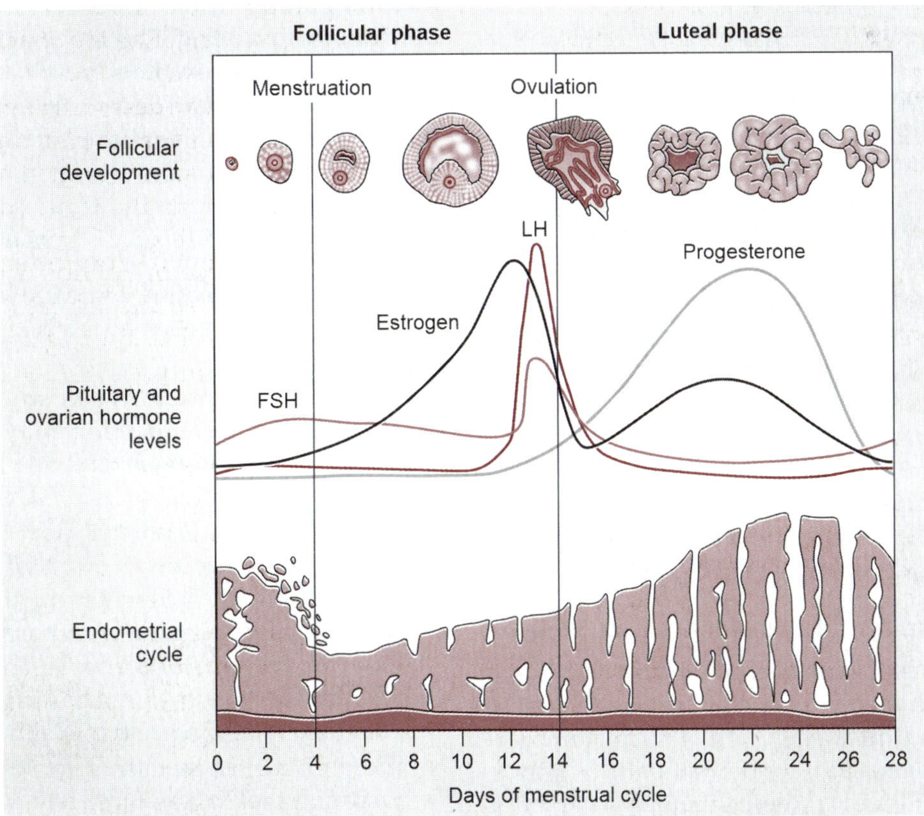

Fig. 14.35: Days of menstrual cycle and the related hormone levels

gland and estrogens, and progesterone are secreted by the ovaries. Menstrual cycle normally varies between 25 to 35 days, with an average of 28 days. The menstrual cycle can be divided into the following phases: (1) Menses phase, (2) follicular phase, (3) ovulation phase and (4) luteal phase

1. **Menses phase:** This phase lasts from day one to day five. During this phase, the lining of the uterus is shed out through the vagina. In most women menses phase lasts for three to five days. However, a period lasting only two days to seven days is considered normal.
2. **Follicular phase:** It begins from day six and lasts up to 14th day. During the early part of the follicular phase, follicular stimulating hormone (FSH) is secreted by the pituitary gland. Rise in FSH causes the development and maturation of ovarian follicles. As the follicles enlarge; these secrete estrogen hormones. The estrogens rise progressively and reaches its peak in 24 hours. The estrogens are necessary for the development of endometrium and maturation of ova (eggs) in the ovaries. The estrogens also initiates rise in luteinizing hormone (LH). High LH levels initiate ovulation and release of ovum from the ruptured follicles and inhibin hormone. Inhibin inhibits secretion of FSH. The levels of progesterone hormone are low during follicular phase.
3. **Ovulation phase:** It occurs roughly at about day 14 in a normal 28-day menstrual cycle. Due to a sudden increase LH, the ovary releases ova (egg). This event is called ovulation.
4. **Luteal phase:** This phase lasts from day 15 to day 28. In this phase, after ovulation, the ruptured follicles from corpus luteum produce progesterone and estrogens. Progesterone prepares the endometrium of uterus for implantation of the fertilized ovum. LH maintains the corpus for few days. The corpus luteum regresses in the absence of fertilization and sheds endometrium, leading to menstruation. The estrogens and progesterone levels decrease significantly and then another new cycle begins.

Increase in the estrogens and progesterone leads to increase in basal body temperature during the luteal phase. If body temperature is recorded daily, it is possible to find out luteal phase by increased body temperature, up to 0.7°C around 14th day of menstrual cycle. Increase in body temperature may remain up to 2–3 days. Similarly, very high levels of LH also indicate beginning of luteal phase (Fig. 14.36).

SAQ: What are the symptoms of menstrual cycle?

Ans: In many women, various unpleasant symptoms are caused due to the specific levels of hormones secreted during menstrual bleeding. These symptoms are, uterine cramps, headache, abdominal pain, irritability and depression. However, these symptoms vary from person to person.

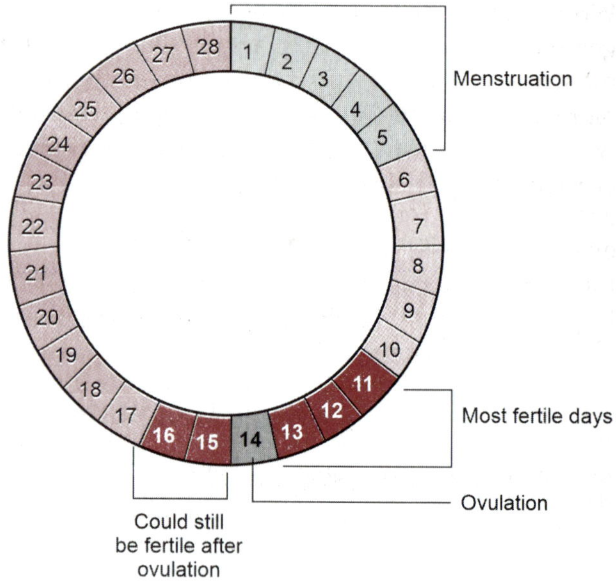

Fig. 14.36: Menstrual cycle: Days of average menstrual cycle (it may vary in different individuals within normal levels)

SAQ: What is amenorrhea?

Ans: Amenorrhea refers to a prolonged absence of menses during the reproductive years of a woman for which the reasons are other than pregnancy.

BAQ: What is the role of estrogens and progestin (synthetic progesterone) as the components of birth control pills?

Ans: The estrogens and progestin (synthetic progesterone) hormones form the main active ingredients of birth control pills. They specifically suppress the ovulation by inhibiting FSH and LH. They also change the nature of cervical mucus so that it becomes difficult for the sperm to go through the cervix and reach an ovum (egg).

Normally, a woman takes hormone pills for 21 days, followed by 7 days of non-functional placebo sugar pills. The cycle thereafter starts again.

General Information Related to the Menstrual Cycle

1. Period is a common word refers to menstruation and menses. Bleeding, typically lasts for 2 to 5 days in women. It serves as a sign that pregnancy has not taken place.
2. During the reproductive years, failure to receive an expected menstruation may provide the first indication to a woman that she may have become pregnant.
3. Menstruation is a normal part of a natural cyclic process that occurs in normal women between puberty and end of the reproductive years. The onset of menstruation, known as menarche, normally occurs between the ages of 8 and 16 and the menopause, between the ages of 45 and 55. Any significant change from this pattern require medical attention.
4. The presence of menstruation does not prove that ovulation took place. Similarly, women who do not ovulate may have menstrual cycles.

5. While menstrual cycle length may vary, 28 days are generally considered as representative of the normal menstrual cycle in women.
6. Normal menstruation lasts for 3–4 days and many women experience uterine cramps during this phase. Normal menstruation involves the loss of average about 50 ml of blood (including shed lining). The enzyme plasmin contained in the endometrium inhibits the blood from clotting. Due to this blood loss, women have higher dietary requirements for iron compared to males to prevent iron deficiency.

Objectives: To understand the path of sperms through the female reproductive tract. To describe the changes occur in hormonal levels during pregnancy. To describe the mechanism of labor and child birth (parturition).

Fertilization (Fig. 14.37)

BAQ: Write a note on fertilization.

Ans: Fertilization takes place, when a sperm cell successfully meets an ovum (egg cells) in the Fallopian tube (Fig. 14.37). Once fertilization takes place, fertilized cell is called a zygote. The zygote moves down the Fallopian tube into the uterus. The zygote then implants into the uterus lining.

After implantation, as the embryo grows, the surrounding trophoblast cells stimulate significant increase in levels of human chorionic gonadotropin (hCG) hormone. hCG interacts with the ovary and promotes the maintenance of the corpus luteum. It stimulates corpus luteum to secrete the hormone progesterone; during the first trimester. Progesterone facilitates formation of specific blood vessels for proper nourishment of the growing fetus.

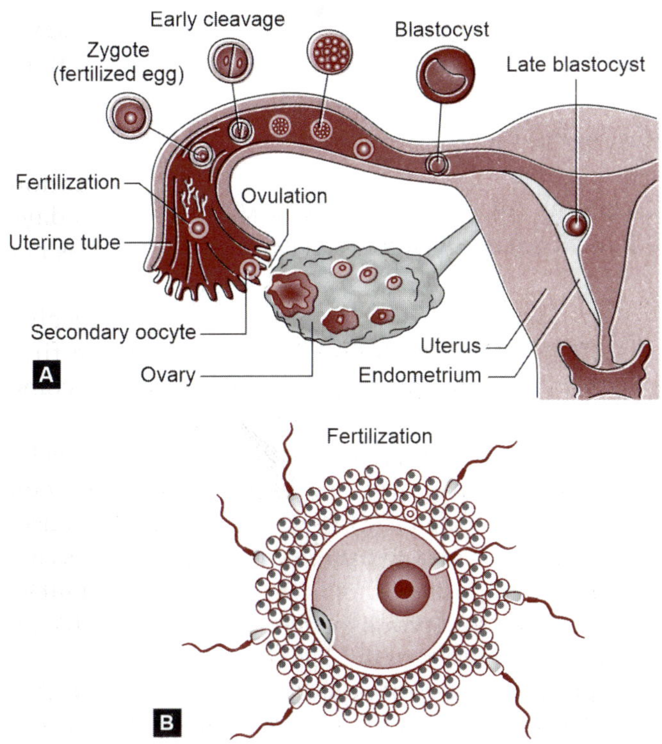

Figs 14.37A and B: Fertilization

Human Chorionic Gonadotropin (hCG) (Fig. 14.38)

BAQ: Write a note on human chorionic gonadotropin (hCG).

Ans: hCG is a hormone produced by the placenta in pregnant females. The hormone stimulates the corpus luteum to produce progesterone to maintain the pregnancy. The hormone appears soon after nine days of conception and reaches a peak between 7th and 12th week of gestation, after which it decreases. hCG is then found in blood, urine, milk and fetal tissues.

hCG interacts with the ovary and promotes the maintenance of the corpus luteum. It stimulates corpus luteum to secrete the hormone progesterone; during the first trimester. Progesterone facilitates formation of specific blood vessels for proper nourishment of the growing fetus.

The following points are important with relation to hCG:

1. High levels of hCG in blood and urine indicate pregnancy. Urine hCG test is used to detect pregnancy.
2. In the absence of a pregnancy and in the absence of hCG, the corpus luteum demises and inhibin and progesterone levels decrease considerably; leading to menstrual bleeding.
3. Due to decreased inhibin levels; FSH levels rise to maintain newly formed follicles.

Ovulation (Fig. 14.39)

BAQ: Write a note on ovulation.

Ans: Ovulation is the release of ovum from the ovaries. In this event, the ovarian follicles rupture and release the mature ovum. After ovulation, during the luteal phase, the ovum remains available for the fertilized by a sperm. The endometrium becomes thick to receive a fertilized egg. If fertilization fails to occur, the uterine lining as well as the ovum degenerate and shed during the menstruation.

The following are the important points about the ovulation:

1. Each women is born with millions of immature ova (eggs) that await ovulation to begin.
2. An ovum (egg) lives 12–24 hours after leaving the ovary and normally only one egg is released each time of ovulation.
3. Ovulation can be affected by stress, illness or disruption of normal routines. Some women may experience; light blood spotting during ovulation.
4. Implantation of a fertilized egg normally takes place 6–12 days after the ovulation.
5. A menstrual period can occur even if ovulation has not occurred and ovulation can occur even if a menstrual period has not occurred.
6. Some women can feel a bit of pain or aching, near the ovaries during ovulation. This is called 'mittleschmerz', which is a German medical term meaning ovulation pain, or midcycle pain.

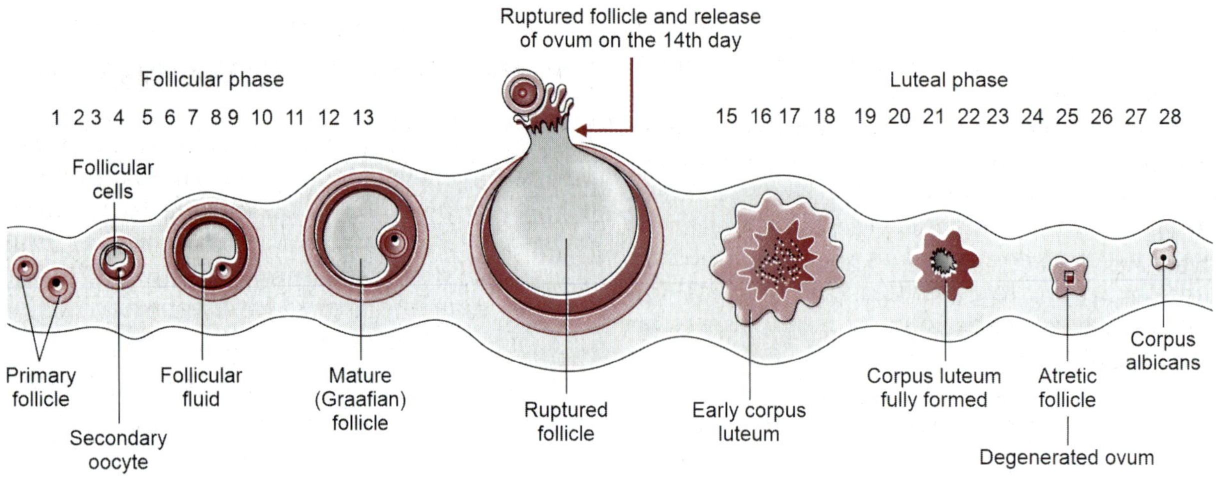

Fig. 14.38: Phases of ovulation

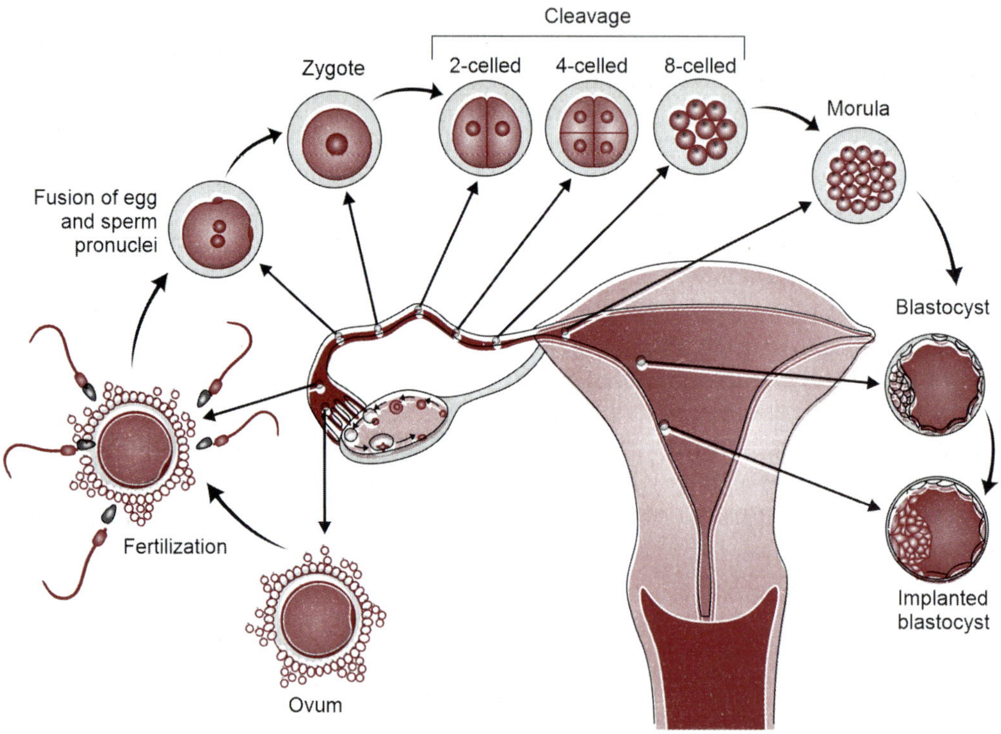

Fig. 14.39: Ovulation, fertilization, and implantation of the blastocyte

7. If an egg is not fertilized, it disintegrates and is absorbed into the uterine lining.
8. Sperm can live in a woman's body up to 5 days after intercourse.
9. Pregnancy is most likely; if intercourse occurs 3 days before ovulation, until 2–3 days after ovulation.

SAQ: What are the fundamental aspects of the pregnancy?

Ans: The following are the fundamental aspects of the pregnancy:

1. Conception
2. Embryo development
3. Fetal growth
4. Role of the placenta
5. Importance of amniotic fluid
6. Maternal adaptation to pregnancy, and
7. Functional maturation of the fetus

Normal Human Pregnancy (Fig. 14.40)

LAQ: Write a note on normal human pregnancy.

Ans: When conception occurs, the ovum is usually fertilized in the Fallopian tube. It becomes a zygote and carries down the tube into the uterus. The zygote divides and becomes a morula, which develops a cavity (the primitive yolk sack) and becomes a blastocyte, which implants into the uterine wall about five days after fertilization. The trophoblast cells on the exterior wall of blastocyte; invade the uterine endometrium and develop into chorionic villi. The chorionic villi gives rise to the placenta. The product of conception at this stage is called an embryo in which a cavity (amnion) forms with the accumulation of amniotic fluid.

The embryo undergoes rapid cell division, differentiation and growth by nourishment obtained from the placenta and the support from amniotic fluid. Organs begin to form in a process called organogenesis from combination of three types of primary cells—the ectoderm, the mesoderm and the endoderm.

At ten weeks, a fetus forms with development of major structures. Rapid fetal growth occurs during the second trimester (13–26 weeks). Many fetal organs begin to mature by the end of second trimester and the fetus weighs approximately 700 g and it is average 30 cm long. Fetal organs complete their prenatal maturation in third trimester (26–40 weeks). The fetus weighs approximately 3200 g and grows to about 50 cm long at the end of the third trimester. Normal labor, rhythmic uterine contractions and birth of a child takes place during a 'term', which is the interval from 37 to 42 weeks.

Objective: To describe the composition and functions of amniotic fluid.

Amniotic Fluid (Fig. 14.41)

BAQ: Write a note on the amniotic fluid.

Ans: The composition of the amniotic fluid resembles a dialysate of the serum of the blood of the mother. During the early years of pregnancy, the amniotic fluid conains mainly water with electrolytes. However, by about the 12–14th week it contains, carbohydrates, proteins, lipids and extracellular matrix (ECM) components.

As the fetus grows, sodium concentration and osmolality of the amniotic fluid decrease and the concentration of excretory substances of the fetus, such as urea, uric acid and creatinine increases.

The amniotic fluid acts as a cushion to the fetus, in which it freely moves in this fluid medium. It prevents the fetus from a possible injury and helps to maintain a constant normal temperature. The volume of amniotic fluid is about 200–300 ml at 16th weeks, 400–1400 ml at 26 weeks, 300–2000 ml at 34 weeks and 300–1400 ml at 40 weeks of the pregnancy.

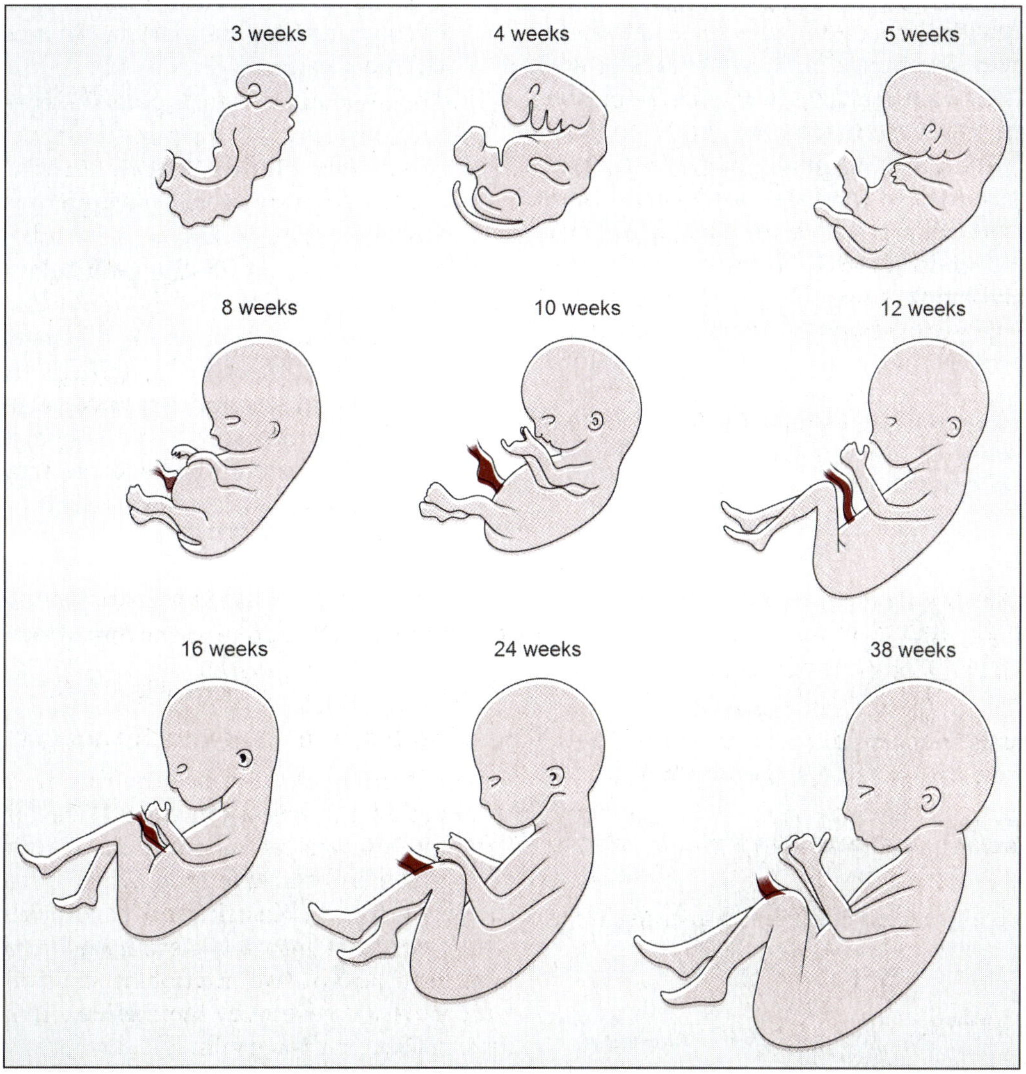

Fig. 14.40: Fetal growth

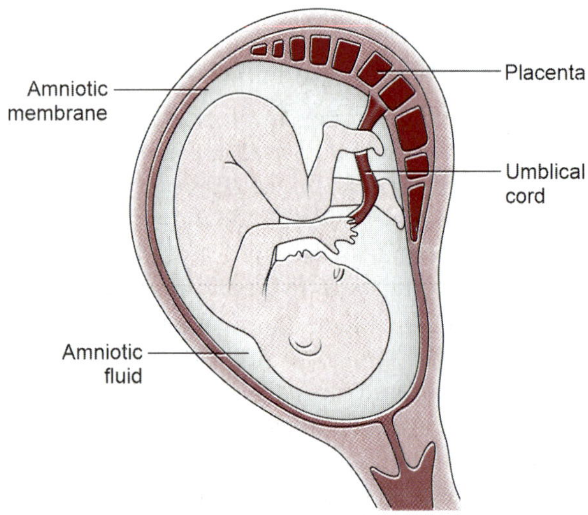

Fig. 14.41: Fetus in amniotic fluid

Functional Maturation of the Fetus

BAQ: Write a note on the functional maturation of the fetus.

Ans: The fetal organs such as lungs, liver, kidneys, etc. mature during the third trimester. The amniotic fluid is required for the proper lung development. Hematopoisis occurs in the liver during the first two trimester and transfers to the fetal bone marrow during first trimester. The fetal blood is produced first by the embryonic yolk sac and then by the liver and finally by the fetal bone marrow. HbA production increases as the fetal bone marrow begins red cell production. At birth, fetal blood contains 75% HbF and 25% HbA. At the end of the first trimester the fetal kidneys begin to produce urine and it becomes the main component of the amniotic fluid.

Objectives: To describe the anatomical features and related functions of female breasts and the role of hormones in the development of mammary glands and lactation. To describe blood supply to the female breasts.

Female Breasts (Fig. 14.42)

LAQ: Write a note on the female breasts with respect to: (1) Introduction and (2) the applied anatomy with related functions.

Ans:

1. Introduction: The female breasts are found at the anterior thoracic wall, anterior to the deep fascia and pectoral muscles. Each breast consists of mammary glands, which are surrounded by connective tissue.
   Both males and females have glandular tissue within the breasts; however, in females the glandular tissue begins to develop after puberty; due to estrogen hormone response. A female mammary gland is a modified exocrine gland that produces milk to feed young child.
2. Applied anatomy with related functions: The mammary gland structure is divided into the following three parts: (A) Skin, (B) parenchyma, and (C) stroma.
   A. The skin of mammary gland consists of a nipple and a areola (Fig. 14.42).
   The nipple is a conical eminent part. It contains circular and longitudinal smooth muscle fibers and rich nerve supply (Fig. 14.42).
   B. The areola is the dark pinkish-brown pigmented area around the nipple. It is rich in modified sebaceous glands. These glands secrete oily secretion that prevents cracking of the nipple and the areola (Fig. 14.42).
   C. The parenchyma is the glandular tissue of the mammary gland. The glandular tissue is part of the breast that makes milk. It is made up of about 15–20 lobes. A lobe of glandular tissue contains branching ducts and terminal secretory lobules. The lactiferous ducts open separately into the nipple. The lactiferous ducts are arranged radially in the nipple. The lactiferous ducts enlarge to form

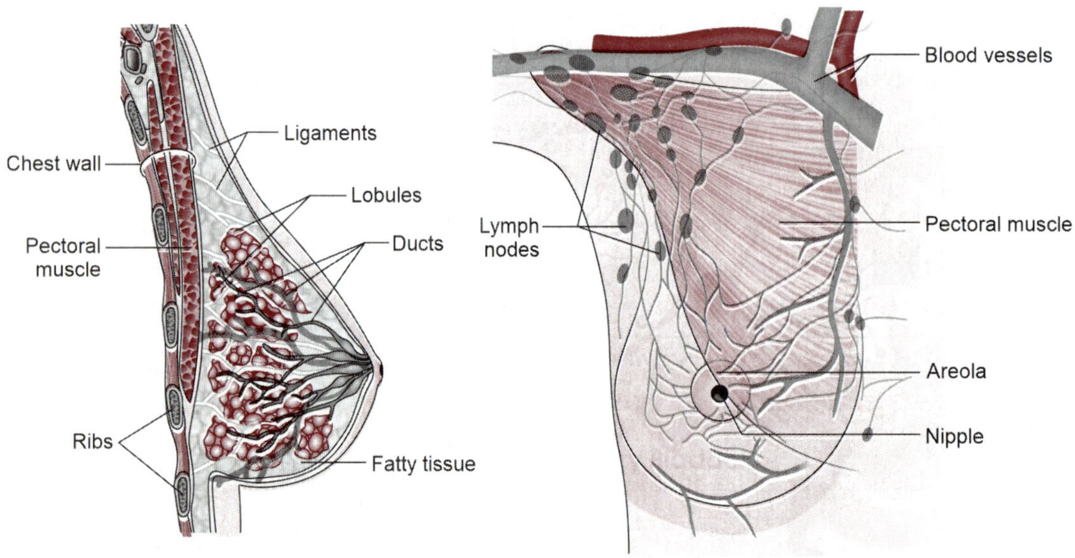

Fig. 14.42: Female breast and mammary gland

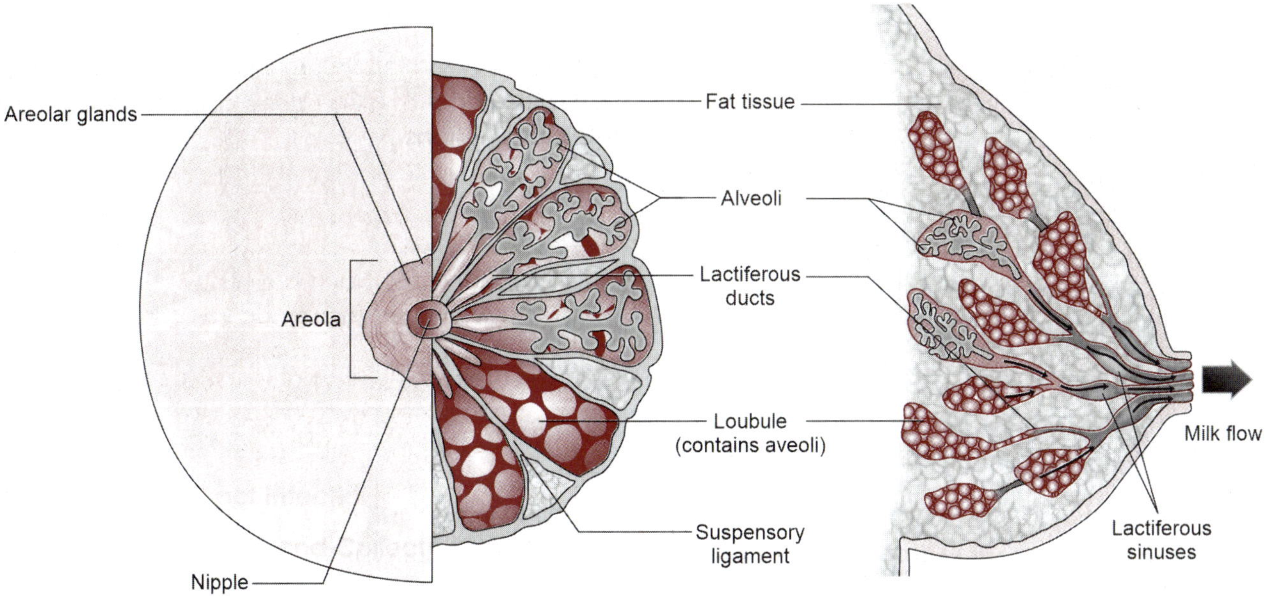

Fig. 14.43: Anatomy of female mammary gland

the lactiferous sinus. The milk is collected in the lactiferous sinuses and it comes out on the suckling by the baby.

The stroma is the supporting framework of the breast around the parenchyma.

The basic components of a mature mammary gland are the alveoli (hollow cavities), (Fig. 14.43), which are lined with milk-secreting cuboidal cells and surrounded by myoepithelial cells (Fig. 14.44). The alveoli join to form lobules. Each lobule has a lactiferous duct that drains into openings in the nipple (Fig. 14.43). Fat tissue is present between the alveoli. The mammary fat tissue is necessary for development of the mammary epithelium.

The myoepithelial cells excrete milk, when stimulated by oxytocin hormone. Milk is excreted in the lobule lumen toward the nipple.

The anatomic changes in the mammary glands depend on the age of a woman, menstrual cycle phase and reproductive status. The mammary glands become active in adult women after childbirth. In this period, prolactin hormone secreted by pituitary gland, stimulates the mammary glands to produce milk. Oxytocin hormone secreted by the hypothalamic stimulates the ejection of milk through the nipple.

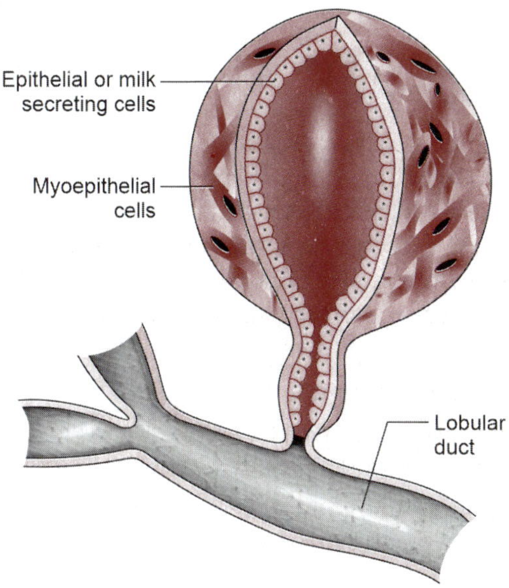

Fig. 14.44: Myoepithelial cells

BAQ: Explain the role of hormones in the development of female breasts and in lactation.

Ans: The estrogen hormones are responsible for the growth of breast tissue ducts and the progesterone stimulate alveolar proliferation. Some growth of breast glandular tissue occurs during puberty, along with deposition of adipose tissue.

During pregnancy, high concentrations of the estrogens and progesterone lead to extensive development of the mammary glandular tissue. The progesterone prevents the mammary glands from lactating. After childbirth, progesterone levels decrease and the levels of prolactin remain raised. The prolactin stimulates the mammary glands to begin lactation.

Blood Supply to the Female Breasts

BAQ: Write a note on the blood supply to the female breast.

Ans:

Arterial Blood Supply to the Female Breasts

Female breast arterial blood supply is from the following arteries (Fig. 14.45):

Branches of the axillary artery supply the lateral part of the breast. These are the superior thoracic artery, acromiothoracic artery, lateral thoracic artery and subscapular artery (Fig. 14.45).

Branches of the internal thoracic artery, supply arterial blood to the medial part of the breast as the medial mammary arteries. Similarly, perforating branches of second, third and fourth intercostal arteries supply arterial blood to entire breast.

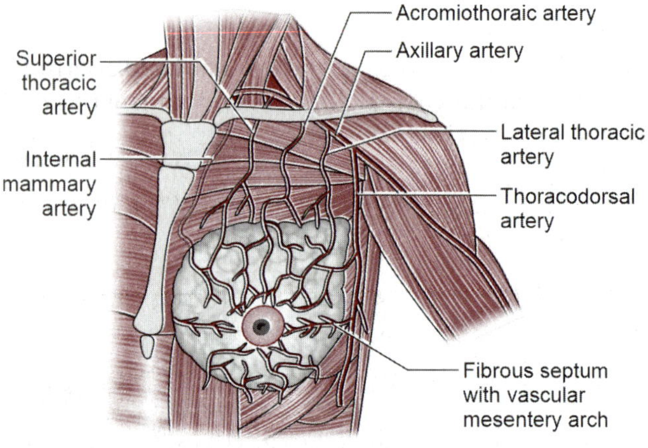

Fig. 14.45: Arterial blood supply to female breast

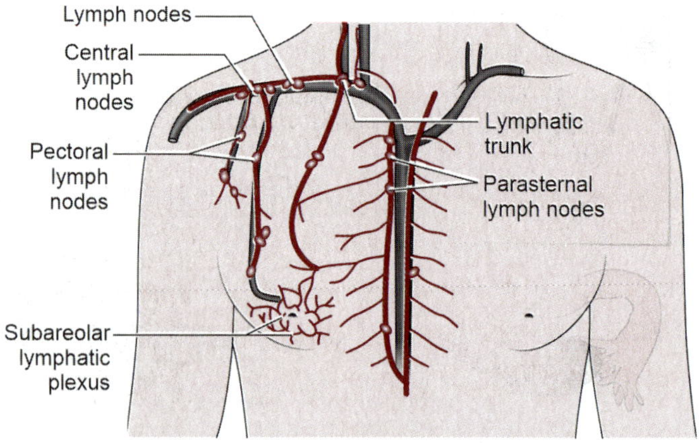

Fig. 14.46B: Female breast lymph drainage

Venous Blood Drainage of the Female Breasts

Venous blood drains through the following veins (Fig. 14.46A):

The breast veins drain into the axillary vein, internal thoracic vein and second to fourth intercostal veins.

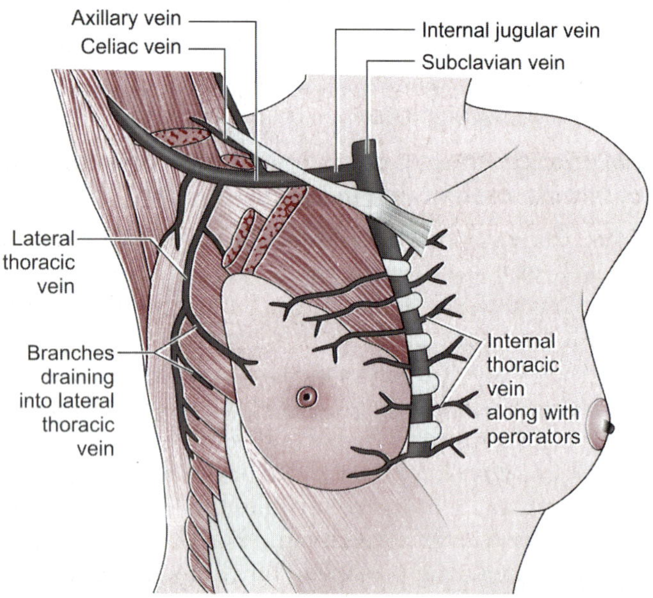

Fig. 14.46A: Venous drainage of female breast

Lymph Drainage from the Female Breast (Fig. 14.46B)

BAQ: Write a note on the lymph drainage from the female breast.

Ans: The lymph from the breast lobules, nipple and areola areas collect into the subareolar lymphatic plexus. About 75% of lymph drains into the pectoral lymph nodes, and then into the axillary lymph nodes. Remaining lymph drains into the parasternal lymph nodes.

SAQ: Why axillary lymph nodes are surgically removed in certain stages of breast cancer?

Ans: Axillary lymph nodes are surgically removed in certain stages of breast cancer to prevent spread of cancer cells in other parts of the body (metastasis).

Objective: To define contraception and describe the common methods of contraception.

CONTRACEPTION

SAQ. Define and explain the term contraception.

Ans: Contraception means the act of preventing pregnancy. In the case of females, the contraception could be achieved by using, contraceptive pills, or by a surgical procedure, that involves blocking or cutting of the Fallopian tubes. In the case of males, the contraception could be achieved by using condoms (thin latex pouches) or by surgical procedure that involves vasectomy, means cutting of the vasa deference.

SAQ: What are oral birth control pills meant for a female?

Ans: The the birth control pills are meant to be taken orally by women (Fig. 14.47B). The pill contains the following two hormones: Progestin (a synthetic form of the hormone progesterone) and estrogen. Proper use of these pills alter the menstrual cycle to eliminate ovulation and prevent pregnancy.

Female Sterilization by Surgical Methods (Fig. 14.47A)

BAQ: Describe briefly the female sterilization by surgical methods.

Ans: Female sterilisation is an operation to permanently prevent pregnancy. A surgical method called tubal ligation is used. It is a surgical procedure for female sterilization in which the Fallopian tubes are permanently clipped, blocked or removed. This prevents the fertilization of eggs by sperms and the implantation of a fertilized egg (Fig. 14.47A).

The following are the two main methods of ligation:

1. **Open abdominal ligation:** It is carried out by means of a surgical incision through the abdominal wall.
2. **Laparoscopic ligation:** It is carried out by means of a fibre optic laparoscope, inserted through a small incision near the umbilicus (the navel).

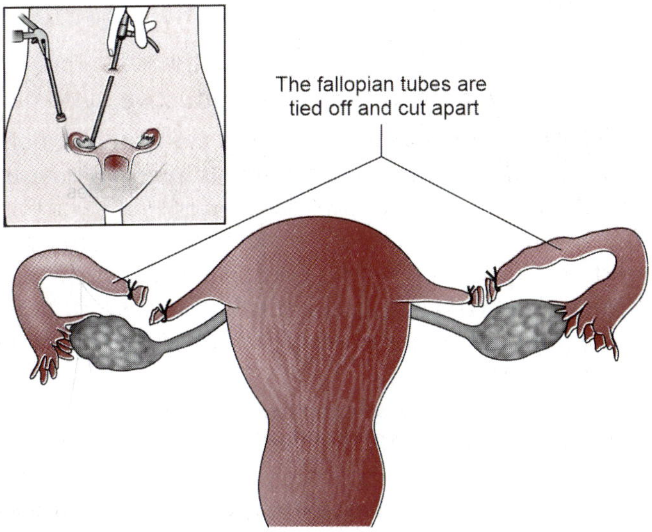

Fig. 14.47A: Ligation of the Fallopian tubes

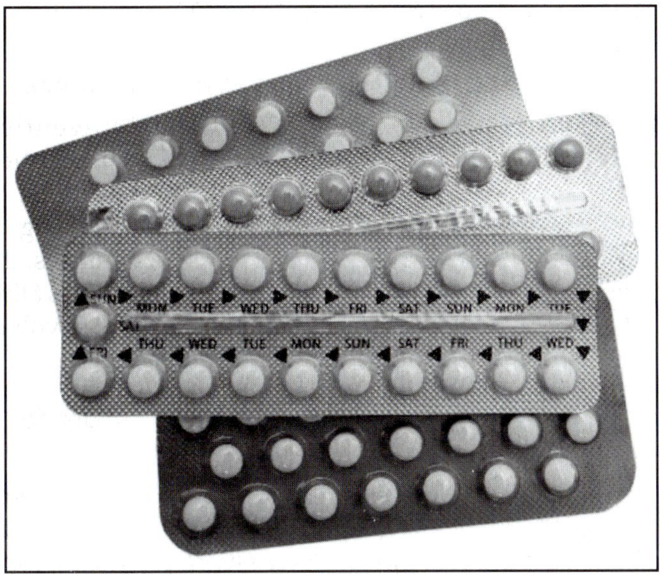

Fig. 14.47B: Female contraceptive pills

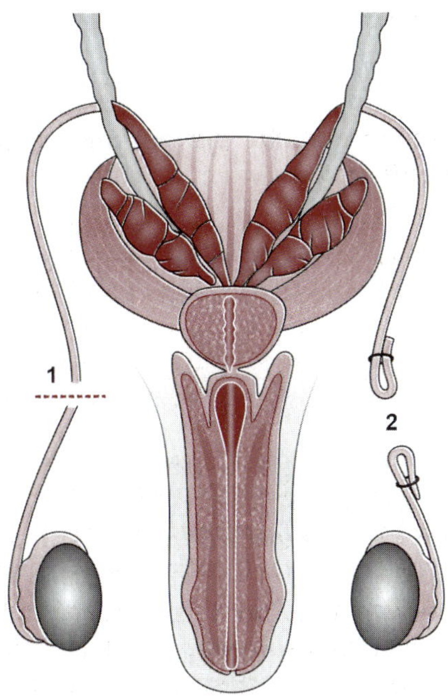

Fig. 14.47C: Cutting off of vas deference

BAQ: Write a note on condoms.

Ans: Condoms are thin pouches that keep sperm from getting into the vagina. A male condom is worn on the penis (Fig. 14.47D). The condoms are usually made of latex (a type of rubber). But some condoms are made of materials that are safe for males with latex allergies, such as polyurethane or polyisoprene.

BAQ: Write a note on sterilization of a male by the surgical method.

Ans: The sterilization of a male is performed by vasectomy (Fig. 14.47C). The vasectomy is a surgical procedure in which the male vasa deference are cut and tied or sealed so as to prevent sperm from entering into the urethra. Vasectomy prevents fertilization of a female through sexual intercourse.

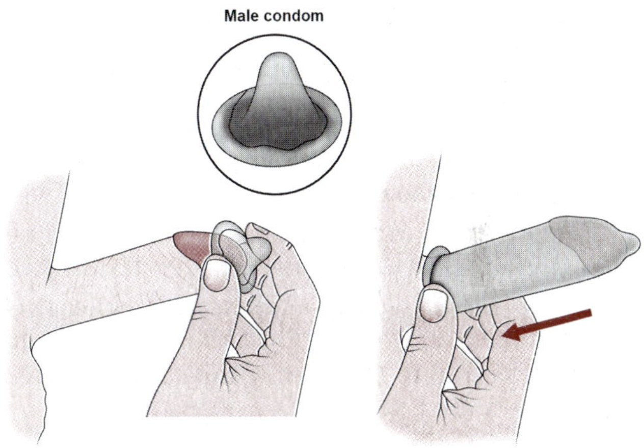

Fig. 14.47D: Condom application

Objective: To discuss the various reasons responsible for delayed puberty.

Delayed Puberty

BAQ: Write a note on delayed puberty.

Ans: Delayed puberty means a boy or a girl lacks or has incomplete development of specific sexual characteristics after the usual age of onset of puberty. The age of onset of puberty depends on normal intake of diet, general health, socioeconomic status, environmental factors and genetics. Boys are considered to have delayed puberty if they lack enlargement of the testicles by age about 14 years. Girls are considered to have delayed puberty if breast development is not observed by age 13 or have not started menstrual cycle by age about 15.

Delayed puberty can be associated with a family history, related to chronic illness (e.g. cystic fibrosis, celiac disease, etc.) or due to hypogonadism (failure of gonads to function normally). Hypogonadism can be primary (due to gonadal disease) or may be secondary (due to hypothalamic or pituitary disease).

Objective: To define menopause and discuss the related post-menopausal symptoms.

Menopause

BAQ: Write a note on menopause.

Ans: Menopause means stoppage of menstrual cycles. The menstrual cycles begin in the women after puberty and continue till the age of 45–50 years. It ceases thereafter with the loss of ovarian functions. The progesterone and estrogen levels decrease considerably; while LH and FSH are elevated due to lack of feedback inhibition by the estrogens.

Before menopause, periods of a woman become irregular. Women often experience hot flashes (warmth on the upper part of the body), during this phase. Hot flashes last from 30 seconds to 10 minutes and may be associated reddish skin, night sweats, shivering, and night sweats. Hot flashes may be observed for four to five years. Other symptoms of menopause observed are mood swings, disturbed sleep, and vaginal dryness. The severity of menopause symptoms may vary among various female.

Postmenopausal women are susceptible to the following two main complications, due to insufficient levels of sex hormones.

1. Atrophy of secondary sex tissues, i.e. mainly of the epithelial tissue of vagina and lower urinary tract.
2. Osteoporosis, which is a major health problem in older women. Decreased density of bones and increased susceptibility to fractures are the main features of osteoporosis.

Objective: To describe the effects of aging on the reproductive systems.

EFFECTS OF AGING ON REPRODUCTIVE SYSTEMS

BAQ: Write a note on the effects of aging on the reproductive systems.

Ans:

Effects of Aging on the Female Reproductive Systems

The menstrual cycles continue till the age of 45–50 years. It ceases thereafter with the loss of ovarian functions. The progesterone and estrogen levels decrease considerably; while LH and FSH are elevated due to lack of feedback inhibition by the estrogens. Due to the hormonal changes the risk for osteoporosis increases. Bones become weak and brittle due to increased tendency for osteoporosis.

Postmenopausal women are susceptible to the atrophy of secondary sex tissues. The epithelial tissue mass of vagina and lower urinary tract decreases. The vaginal wall decreases elasticity, and becomes thin, and dry. Decrease in the breast tissue is also observed. Sex may become painful due to the vaginal changes. The risk of vaginal infections increases. The loss of tone in the pubic muscles results in the increased tendency of prolapse of vagina, uterus, or urinary bladder.

The following specific menopause symptoms are observed: Hot flashes, headaches, sleeping problems, libido (low sex drive), increase in the frequency of urination, lower sex drive (libido).

Effects of Aging on the Male Reproductive Systems

Due to the ageing, testosterone, the male sex hormone decreases significantly. Blood flow to the penis decreases. The elderly male may suffer from erectile dysfunction. The frequency, duration, sensitivity and rigidity of erection gradually decline. Decrease in the volume of semen released during ejaculation is observed. Decrease in libido (sex drive) is observed in the elderly with the advancing age.

Various physiological changes occur with advancing age are related to the decline in the levels of male hormones. These changes are, the loss of bone mass, muscle mass hair loss and increase in the fat mass.

Climacteric

BAQ: Write a note on the climacteric.

Ans: The climacteric is a period of life characterized by physiological and psychic change that marks the end of the reproductive capacity of women and terminates with the completion of menopause. During the climacteric, progressive ovarian failure is responsible for a decline in ovarian estrogen secretion and eventually menstruation ceases. During this period, pituitary gonadotropins are elevated with FSH tending to increase first. This change is more reliable indicator of ovarian failure. Estrogen deficiency is the main cause contributing to the development of post-menopausal osteoporosis.

Objective: To describe the common disorders and diseases related to male and female sex organs.

COMMON DISORDERS OF MALE GONADAL FUNCTION

Prostatic Enlargement

BAQ: Write a note on the prostatic enlargement.

Ans: Prostatic enlargement means the abnormal increase in the size of the prostate gland. Prostate enlargement takes place in most of the men as they get older than 50 years. An enlarged prostate is called benign prostatic hyperplasia (BPH).

Two main prostate growth periods are observed as a man ages. The first occurs early in puberty. The second phase of prostate growth begins around age of 25 and continues during most of life of a man. Benign prostatic enlargement takes place often with the second growth phase.

Increased prostate presses on the bladder and urethra and blocks the flow of urine (Fig. 14.48). The urinary bladder may become weak and lose its ability to empty urine completely. Some urine remains in the bladder. Initially, patient may have trouble passing urine and frequency of urination may increase considerably. Surgical removal of prostate gland becomes necessary, if a patient is not able to pass urine (anuria).

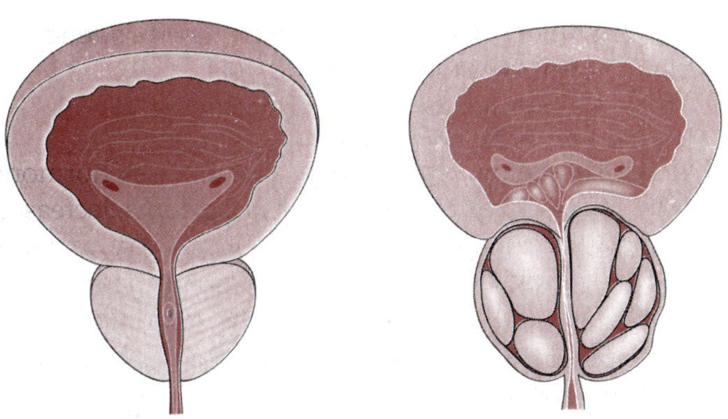

Fig. 14.48: Normal prostate (left) and enlarged prostate (right)

Diagnosis is typically based on symptoms, medical examination, clinical laboratory tests and ultrasound examination.

Although most benign prostate hyperplasia are harmless, it is necessary to rule out prostatic cancer, by histopathological examination of prostate tissue.

Gynecomastia

BAQ: Write a note on gynecomastia.

Ans: Gynecomastia is the development of abnormally large mammary glands in males resulting in breast enlargement.

In neonates gynecomastia may occur physiologically as a result of exposure to maternal estrogens. 50% of normal boys develop gynecomastia due to temporarily increased secretion of estrogens relative to androgens. In neonates and also in boys, gynecomastia resolves spontaneously. In elderly, mild type of gynecomastia may develop due to a decrease in the testosterone secretion.

Other various clinical conditions related to gynecomastia are, chronic liver disease, end-stage renal disease, decreased androgens, androgen insensitivity, etc.

Hydrocele (Fig. 14.49)

BAQ: Write a note on hydrocele.

Ans: A hydrocele is swelling in the scrotum that occurs when fluid collects in the thin sheath surrounding a testicle (Fig. 14.49). Injury, inflammation due to infection, or growth of tumour in testicle may cause fluid formation in the scrotum; that leads to hydrocele formation. A hydrocele is often caused by fluid collecting within the tunica vaginalis; a layer wrapped around the testicle, which derived from peritoneum (Fig. 14.49).

Hydrocele is common in new born children. It usually disappears during first year of age, without treatment. Older boys and adult men can develop a hydrocele due to inflammation or injury within the scrotum and require treatment.

COMMON DISORDERS OF FEMALE GONADAL FUNCTION

Delayed Puberty

BAQ: Write a note on delayed puberty.

Ans: Majority of girls enter puberty by about 13 years of age. Girls with delayed puberty are usually observed due to absence of menstrual period (amenorrhea) or due to the absence of breast development. Girls with amenorrhea or no breast development after the age of 15; require further medical investigations. The pathological causes for the delayed puberty can be due to hypogonadism (the primary ovarian failure), hypogonadotrophic (secondary reason) in hypothalamic

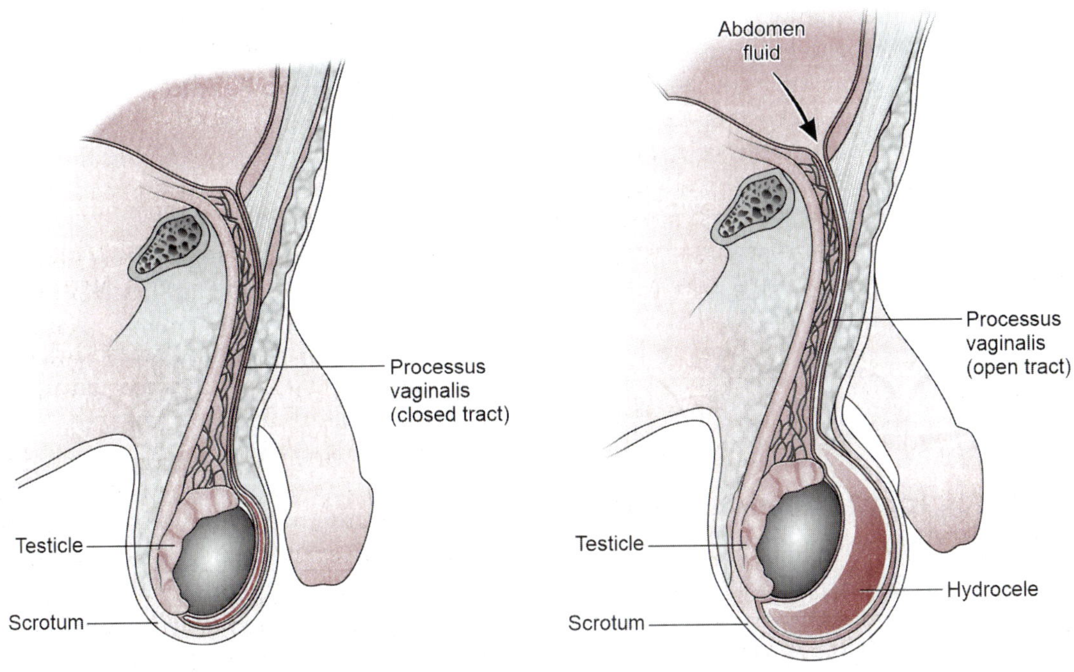

Fig. 14.49: Normal scrotum (left) and scrotum in hydrocele (right)

or pituitary failure, and due to the chronic diseases such as chronic renal disease, celiac disease, etc.

Amenorrhea

BAQ: Write a note on amenorrhea.

Ans: Amenorrhea is the absence of a menstrual period in a woman of reproductive age. It can be primary or secondary. Oligomenorrhea is infrequent menstruation. In women of child-bearing age, the commonest cause of amenorrhea is pregnancy. Apart from pregnancy, amenorrhea is most frequently observed due to hormonal disturbances resulting in the failure of ovulation. Various causes of amenorrhea include, hyperprolactinemia, disordered function of hypothalamus and pituitary coordination, increased androgen production (polycystic ovary syndrome, PCOS), ovarian dysfunction (autoimmune disorder). Intensive exercise regimens, as seen in the case of gymnasts, long-distance runners, ballet dancers and also severe stress can lead to amenorrhea.

Hirsutism

BAQ: Write a note on hirsutism.

Ans: Hirsutism is a clinical condition in women that results in excessive growth of coarse hair on face, chest and back. Extra hair growth arises; mainly due to the excess secretion of the male hormone, testosterone. The commonest cause of hirsutism is polycystic ovary syndrome (PCOS). In PCOS, multiple cysts are present in the ovaries, that are responsible for high levels of tetosterone (Fig. 14.33). Tumors of the ovary and adrenal gland also may lead to increased levels of androgens (male hormones), which may cause hirsutism.

Virilism

BAQ: Write a note on virilism.

Ans: Virilism is a condition in which women develop male sexual characteristics due to androgen (mainly testosterone) producing ovaries, adrenal glands or pituitary glands. Virilization is more extensive than hirsutism and abnormal development of male sexual characteristics are observed such as male-like hair growth on face, chest, back with masculine body features. The use of anabolic steroids can also lead to virilism. Anabolic steroids are synthetic substances that act like testosterone.

SEXUALLY TRANSMITTED DISEASES (STDs) (VENEREAL DISEASES)

Introduction

BAQ: Write a note on sexually transmitted diseases (STDs) (venereal diseases).

Ans: Sexually transmitted diseases (STDs, venereal diseases) are caused by infections that are passed from one person to another during sexual contact. The organisms that cause sexually transmitted diseases may transmit from person to person in blood, semen, or vaginal and other body fluids.

Sexually transmitted infections can be caused by bacteria (syphilis, gonorrhea, chlamydia), parasites (trichomoniasis), fungi (candidiasis) and viruses (HIV, human papillomavirus, genital herpes). STDs may also get transmitted non-sexually from mother to infant during pregnancy or childbirth, or through blood transfusions or shared needles. STIs may cause congenital disorders or death of the developing fetus, following stillbirth or abortion.

Many STIs are transmitted mostly through the mucous membranes of the penis, vulva, rectum, urinary tract and less commonly by the mucous membranes of mouth, throat, respiratory tract and eyes.

Gonorrhea

BAQ: Write a note on gonorrhea.

Ans: Gonorrhea is caused by the *Neisseria gonorrhoeae* bacteria. Gonorrhea is a highly contagious sexually transmitted disease. In men *Neisseria gonorrhoeae* bacteria infect the urethra; leading to acute urethritis with purulent discharge. The bacteria may spread to prostate, bladder and epididymis; ultimately, leading to sterility. In women the bacteria may infect cervix, leading to cervicitis with purulent discharge. Bacteria may then spread to urethra, vulva Fallopian tube and rectum. Infants born of mothers with gonorrhea also may get infected and suffer from acute conjunctivitis and vulvovaginitis.

Syphilis

BAQ: Write a note on syphilis.

Ans: Syphilis is a sexually transmitted infection (STI) caused by *Treponema pallidum* bacteria. The first sign of syphilis is appearance of a small, painless sore called chancre (Fig. 14.50). It can appear on the sexual organs, inside the mouth or inside the rectum. Syphilis spreads through only direct contact with syphilitic chancres. Following are four stages of syphilis: (1) Primary syphilis, (2) secondary syphilis, (3) latent syphilis and (4) tertiary syphilis.

The primary stage of syphilis occurs about three to four weeks after a person gets infected by *Treponema pallidum* bacteria. It begins with appearance of chancre (Fig. 14.50).

In secondary syphilis stage, skin rashes and a sore throat may develop. The rash is usually found on the palms and soles, however, it also may occur on any part of the body (Fig. 14.51).

Latent syphilis stage appears, if syphilis is not treated, which does not indicate any symptoms. Latent syphilis could last for several years before progressing to tertiary syphilis.

Tertiary syphilis occurs after several years or decades; if the initial infection is not treated. Tertiary syphilis can be life-threatening. Some significant clinical conditions related to tertiary syphilis include, stroke, meningitis, blindness, deafness, memory loss, destruction of soft tissue and bone.

First two stages of syphilis are highly infective. A mother infected with syphilis infection can pass this disease to her child; and there is high risk of still birth. If left untreated, syphilis infection can spread in he body and can damage heart, brain, eyes and bones. In neurosyphilis, central nervous system is affected.

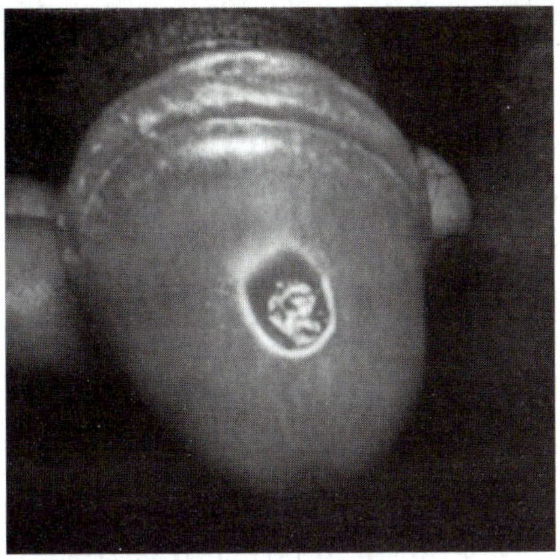

Fig. 14.50: Primary syphilis chancre

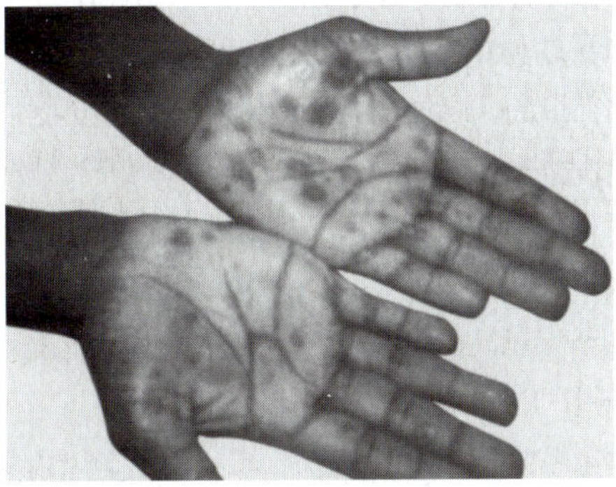

Fig. 14.51: Secondary syphilis sores

Chlamydia (Fig. 14.52)

BAQ: Write a note on chlamydia.

Ans: Chlamydia is a sexually transmitted disease caused by bacteria *Chlamydia trachomatis*. It is transmitted through semen or vaginal discharge by vaginal, oral or anal sex.

In men, chlamydia can spread to the testicles and epididymis, causing epididymitis.

Epididymitis is an inflammation of epididymis; which leads to pain and tenderness of testicles and swollen scrotum.

In women, chlamydia can spread to the womb, and ovaries; leading to pelvic inflammatory disease (PID).

Pregnant woman can pass the chlamydia infection to her baby, which may suffer from conjunctivitis and lung infection.

Trichomoniasis (Fig. 14.53)

BAQ: Write a note on trichomoniasis.

Ans: Trichomoniasis is a sexually transmitted disease caused by a protozoan parasite, *Trichomonas vaginalis*. These protozoal parasites are generally present in female genital and urinary tract and also in urinary tract of men. *Trichomonas vaginalis* cannot persist for long period in the environment and infection occurs by direct contact with trophozoites (growing stage) of the protozoa. Trichomoniasis spreads through vaginal, oral, or anal sex. Men usually have asymptomatic infections. In the case of infected women, the symptoms are redness of vagina, vulvovaginal irritation, vaginal soreness, with frothy and green-yellow vaginal discharge.

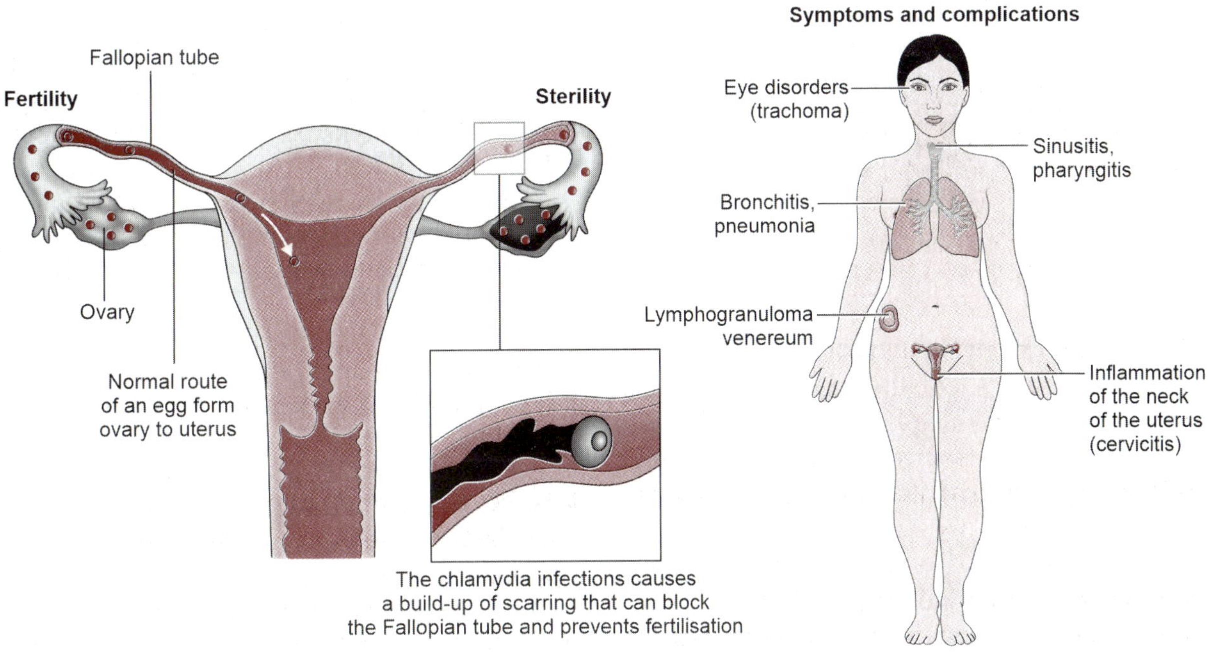

Fig. 14.52: Chlamydia infection

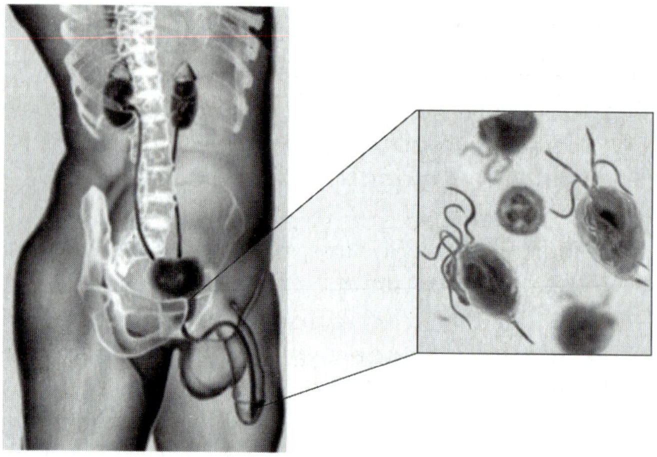

Fig. 14.53: *Trichomonas vaginalis* and infection sites

Acquired Immunodeficiency Syndrome (AIDS)

BAQ: Write a note on Acquired immunodeficiency syndrome (AIDS).

Ans: Acquired immunodeficiency syndrome (AIDS) is caused by the human immunodeficiency virus (HIV) (Fig. 14.54). The four major routes of HIV transmission are, unsafe sex, contaminated needles, breast milk and transmission from an infected mother to her baby at birth. HIV infects T4 lymphocytes. A marked decrease in circulating T4 lymphocytes lead to immunodepression. Immunocompromised patient may suffer from bacterial, fungal and other viral infections. AIDS patients also may develop cancers like Non-Hodgkin's lymphoma and Kaposi's sarcoma. Symptoms of AIDS include fever, weight loss, fatigue, and night sweats. AIDS patient suffers from recurrent infections.

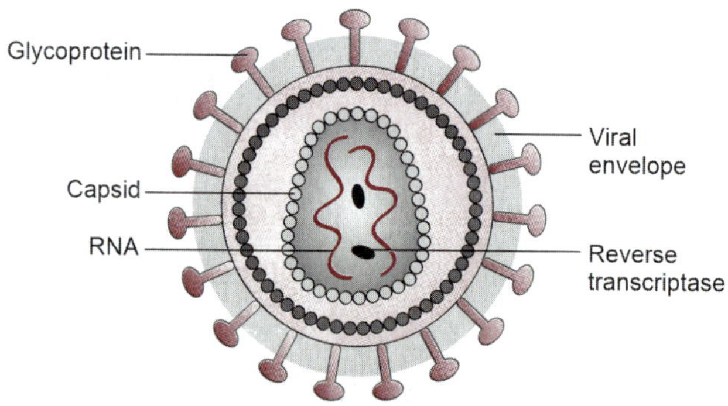

Fig. 14.54: HIV virus

Genital Herpes

BAQ: Write a note on genital herpes.

Ans: Genital herpes is a sexually transmitted disease. It is caused by the herpes simplex virus. Genital herpes can affect both men and women. Genital herpes causes sores; which are painful and itchy blisters.

Uterine Fibroids (Fig. 14.55)

BAQ: Write a note on uterine fibroids.

Ans: Uterine fibroids are abnormal growth of muscle tissue that form in the walls of the uterus. These fibroids mostly are non-cancerous and treatable. Imbalance of estrogen and progesterone lead to growth of the fibroids. Patient with uterine fibroids suffer from irregular bleeding between periods with pelvic pain.

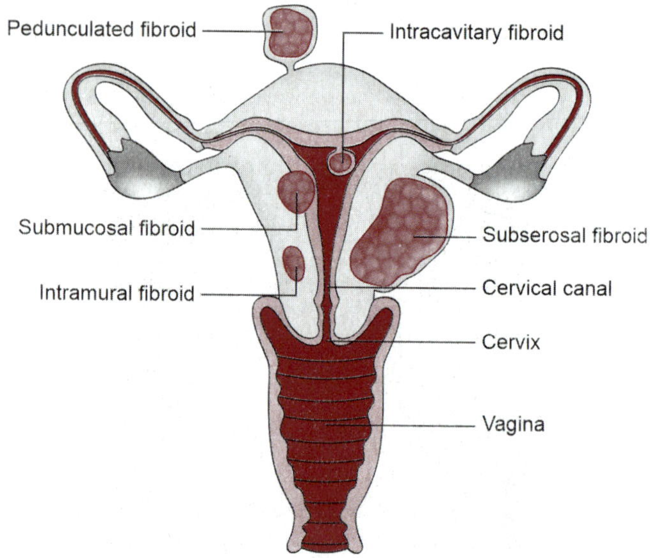

Fig. 14.55: Female uterine fibroids

Testicular Cancer (Fig. 14.56)

BAQ: Write a note on testicular cancer.

Ans: Testicular cancer occurs in the testicles. Testicular cancer is rare and treatable. It appears as a lump or enlargement of tissue in the testis. A feeling of heaviness in the scrotum, pain in the abdomen and back are some of the symptoms of testicular cancer. The survival rate of testicular cancer is higher for patients diagnosed with early-stage cancer.

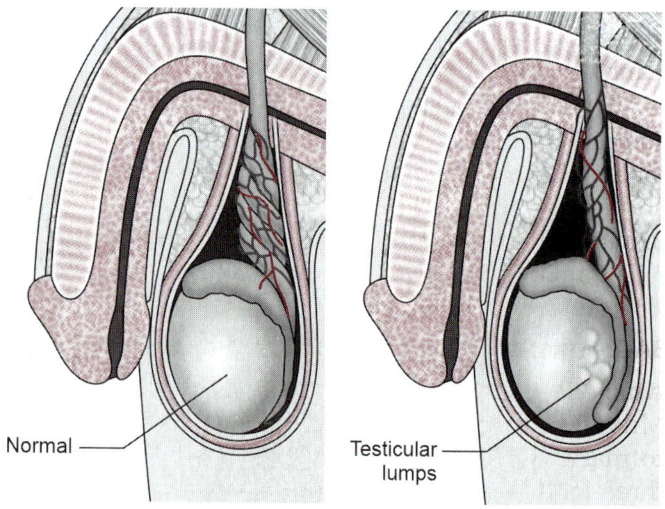

Fig. 14.56: Normal testis and with testicular cancer growth

Cervical Cancer (Fig. 14.57)

BAQ: Write a note on cervical cancer.

Ans: Cervical cancer is abnormal growth of tissue in a woman's cervix. Almost all cervical cancer cases are linked to infection with human papillomaviruses (HPV), a virus transmitted through sexual contact. Most infections with HPV resolve spontaneously and cause no

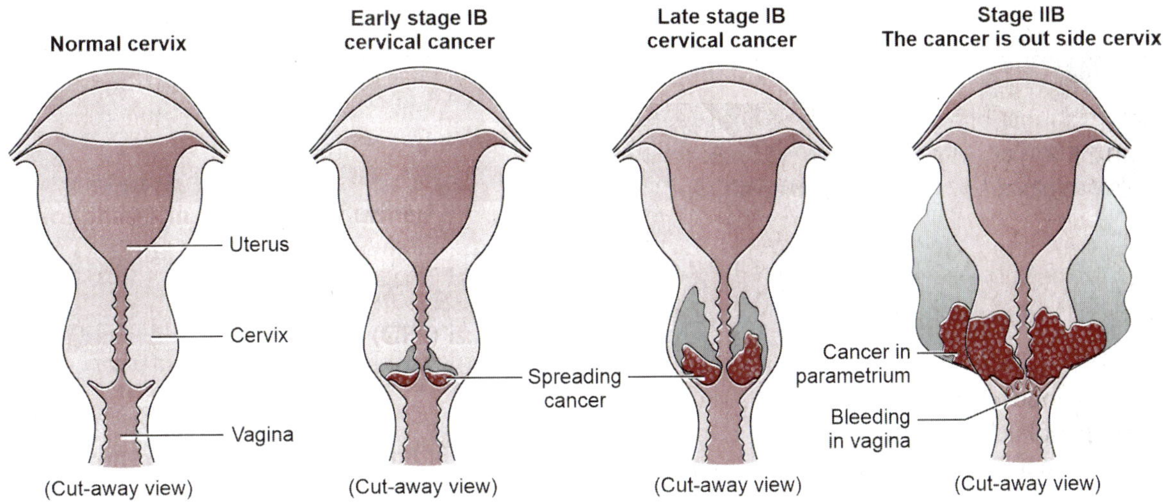

Fig. 14.57: Normal cervix and various stages of cervical cancer

symptoms. However, persistent cervical HPV infection can cause cervical cancer in women.

Cervical cancer is the fourth most common cancer in women. It is treatable during early stage of the disease. Vaginal discharge, cervical bleeding, pelvic pain, fatigue and weight loss are some of the symptoms of cervical cancer.

Candidiasis

BAQ: Write a note on candidiasis.

Ans: Candidiasis is caused by infection of genital tract by the yeast, *Candida albicans*, which are generally present in the normal microflora in the body, including the respiratory tract, skin, gastrointestinal tract, and female urogenital system. Disruptions in the normal vaginal bacterial flora may take place, due to inappropriate use of antibiotics, which can lead to an overgrowth of Candida, causing vaginal candidiasis.

Vaginal candidiasis is also observed in immunocompromised patients. Various symptoms of candidiasis include, purulent vaginal discharge, vaginal soreness and itching, pain during sexual intercourse and while urinating.

Mastitis

BAQ: Write a note on mastitis.

Ans: Mastitis is an inflammation of breast tissue. Milk duct blockage and bacterial infection may lead to mastitis. Mastitis usually occurs during the first three months of breastfeeding. However, it can occur in women who are not on breastfeeding. In mastitis, inflammation of breast tissue lead to swelling, redness, breast pain and fever.

Endometriosis (Fig. 14.58)

BAQ: Write a note on endometriosis.

Ans: Endometriosis is a disorder in which tissue that normally lines the uterus grows outside the uterus. With endometriosis, the tissue can be found on the ovaries, Fallopian tubes, inside the pelvis and in the abdominal cavity (Fig. 14.58). The most common symptoms are pain, menstrual irregularities, pain during intercourse, and sometimes pain during urination and during bowl movements.

During menstruation, if some of the tissue backs up through the Fallopian tubes into the abdomen; it may attach there and grow. Endometriosis can also occur as a result of direct transplantation of tissue in the abdominal wall after a cesarean section. Endometriosis may be genetic in certain families.

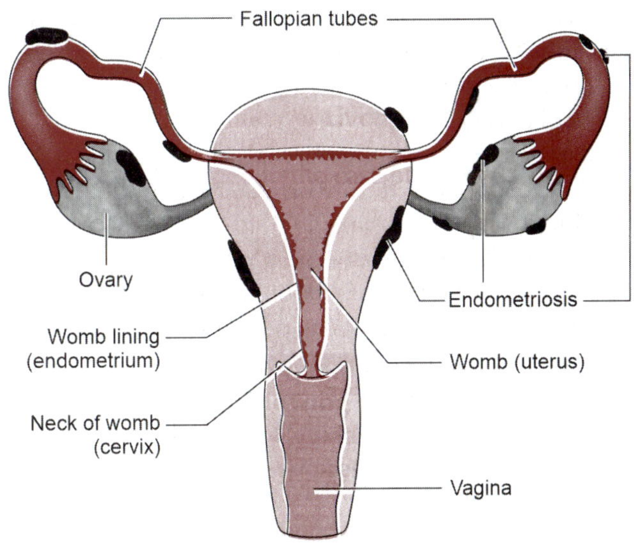

Fig. 14.58: Endometriosis

Objective: To understand and explain the central theme of competency-based medical and paramedical education (CBME): Horizontal and vertical integration of subjects.

BAQ: Show horizontal integration of physiology and biochemistry with the following anatomical change: Destruction of Sertoli cell of the testes.

Ans:

Horizontal Integration with Physiology

Loss of generation of spermatogenesis.

Horizontal Integration with Biochemistry

Absence of the sperms in the seminal fluid composition.

BAQ: Show horizontal integration of physiology, biochemistry and nutrition with the following anatomical change: Development of ovarian cysts (PCOS).

Ans:

Horizontal Integration with Physiology

Increase in the blood circulation of testosterone.

Horizontal Integration with Biochemistry

Increase in the blood circulation of testosterone leads to expression of male characteristics such as increase in the musculature, facial hair and irregular menstruation (as seen in PCOS).

BAQ: Show horizontal integration of physiology, and biochemistry with the following anatomical change: increase in male breasts (gynecomastia).

Ans:

Horizontal Integration with Physiology

Loss of sexual interest (libido).

Horizontal Integration with Biochemistry

Increase in the blood circulation of estrogens, that leads to expression of female characteristic features such as increase in the breast and decrease in the musculature.

BIBLIOGRAPHY

1. Medical Biochemistry, 1st Edition (2023). Godkar PB, Godkar DP, CBS Publishers, New Delhi, India.
2. Text book of Medical Laboratory Technology, 4th Edition, (2024). Godkar PB, Godkar DP, Bhalani Publishing House, Mumbai, India.
3. Anatomy of the Human Body. 42nd Edition. Henry Gray, Editor-in-chief: Susan Standring, Elsevier (2020).
4. Ross and Wilson Anatomy and Physiology in Health and Illness, 13th Edition, by Allison Wynn Grant, Anne Waugh, and Kathleen J. W. Wilson (2018).
5. Schaum's outline of theory and problems of Human anatomy and Physiology, 2nd Edition (1997), Tata MaGraw-Hill Publishing Company Limited, New Delhi, India.

MULTIPLE CHOICE QUESTIONS (MCQs)

Select the correct option.

1. The following is not a reason for erectile dysfunction:
(A) Psychological problems
(B) Uncontrolled diabetes mellitus
(C) Trauma
(D) Priapism

2. This is not an accessory male reproductive gland:
(A) Glans penis (B) Seminal vesicle
(C) Prostate gland (D) Bulbourethral gland

3. Ejaculation of semen is the main function of this part of the male reproductive system:
(A) Glans penis
(B) Seminal vesicle
(C) Prostate gland
(D) Bulbouretal gland

4. The fluid of semen forms in this part of the male reproductive system:
(A) Glans penis (B) Seminal vesicle
(C) Prostate gland (D) Bulbourethral gland

5. Mucus forms in this part of the male reproductive system:
(A) Glans penis
(B) Seminal vesicle
(C) Prostate gland
(D) Bulbourethral gland

6. One of the following statements about the testes is not correct:
(A) The testis are male gonads
(B) These are contained in the scrotum
(C) The average length of testes is about 7 cm
(D) The testis contains several looped tubules

7. This pituitary hormone acts on the leydig cells of the testes to stimulate the production of testosterone:
(A) FSH (B) LH
(C) GH (D) ACTH

8. This pituitary hormone acts on the sertoli cells of testes to stimulate the production of spermatozoa:
(A) FSH (B) LH
(C) GH (D) ACTH

9. The main function of the epididymis is:
(A) To store the sperms for maturation and transport these to the vas deferens.
(B) Transport these to the vas deferens.
(C) Production of spermatozoa
(D) Both (A) and (B)

10. One of the following statements is only correct; regarding the observation of spermatozoa under electron microscope:
(A) Each normal human spermatozoan is made up of four main parts.
(B) The sperm head is flat and measures approximately 7.5 micrometer in length.
(C) The head of a sperm consists of only the acrosome.
(D) The nucleus of a sperm holds whole of the chromatin.

11. One of the following statements is not correct:
(A) The tail of a sperm measures about 50 micrometers
(B) The tail of a sperm consists of five parts
(C) The tail contains a central contractile unit known as the axoneme
(D) By means of the tail, the sperm moves

12. One of this is not a part of the main female reproductive system:

(A) The bulbourethral gland
(B) The uterus
(C) The bilateral Fallopian tubes
(D) The ovaries

13. These are responsible for the supply of mucus for the lubrication of the entrance to the vagina during sexual excitement:

(A) Fallopian tubes
(B) The ovaries
(C) The Bartholin's glands
(D) Both (A) and (B)

14. The following one statement is not correct:

(A) The uterus is made up of the following two parts: (i) Fundus, (ii) cervix
(B) The uterus is a hollow thick-walled muscular organ
(C) The uterus is located in the female pelvis between the bladder and the rectum
(D) The uterus is connected laterally to the uterine tubes and distally to the vagina

15. Secretion of androgens is increased by:

(A) FSH
(B) ACTH
(C) LH
(D) Growth hormone

16. The major source of progesterone during late pregnancy is:

(A) Corpus luteum
(B) Graafian follicles
(C) Adrenal cortex
(D) Placenta

17. Women become susceptible to osteoporosis after menopause due to the decrease in:

(A) hCG (B) Secretion of estrogen
(C) Secretion of LH (D) Secretion of progesterone
(E) Both (C) and (D)

18. Placenta secretes all of the following, *except*:

(A) hCG (B) Estrogen
(C) Progesterone (D) FSH

19. The secondary sexual characters in females are influenced by:

(A) Progesteron (B) Epinephrine
(C) Glucocorticoids (D) Estrogens

20. Testosterone plays important role in the maintenance of:

(A) Regular ovulation
(B) Endometrium
(C) Normal male reproductive system
(D) Both (B) and (C)

21. Weight gain, amenorrhea, hirsutism and hypertension are the most likely cause of:

(A) Polycystic ovary disease (PCOD)
(B) Diabetes mellitus
(C) Disordered hypothalamus
(D) All of the above

22. Normally, fertilization takes place in:

(A) The vagina
(B) The Fallopian tube
(C) The ovary
(D) The uterus

23. The function of male secondary sex organs is:

(A) Fomation of spermatozoa
(B) Maturation of spermatozoa
(C) Transportation of spermatozoa
(D) All of the above

24. The following is not a function of the female secondary sex organs:

(A) Production of gamets
(B) Secretion of estrogens, and progesterone
(C) Secretion of FSH
(D) Secretion of hCG

25. Fetal organs complete their prenatal maturation in:

(A) Third trimester (B) First trimester
(C) Second trimester (D) In the first month of second trimester

26. A retroverted uterus means that tilts:

(A) Forward at the cervix, toward the abdomen
(B) Backward at the cervix
(C) Posterosuperior (posterior and lateral) to the bladder
(D) Towards the anterior surface of the body

27. An anteverted uterus means that tilts:

(A) Forward at the cervix, toward the abdomen
(B) Backward at the cervix
(C) Posterosuperior (posterior and lateral) to the bladder
(D) Towards the anterior surface of the body

28. An anteflexed uterus means that bends:

(A) Forward at the cervix, toward the abdomen
(B) Backward at the cervix
(C) Posterosuperior (posterior and lateral) to the bladder
(D) Towards the anterior surface of the body

29. The following one statement about the ectopic pregnancy is not correct:

(A) An ectopic pregnancy occurs when a fertilized egg implants and grows outside the main cavity of the uterus
(B) In ectopic pregnancy, the fertilised egg cannot survive outside the uterus
(C) An ectopic pregnancy occurs mainly in a Fallopian tube
(D) In ectopic pregnancy, the fertilised egg can survive outside the uterus

30. The following one statement about the menstrual cycle is not correct:

(A) The menstrual cycle is under the control of hormones secreted by pituitary gland and ovaries.
(B) The hormones FSH and LH are secreted by the adrenal cortex
(C) Estrogens and progesterone are secreted by the ovaries
(D) Rise in FSH causes the development and maturation of ovarian follicles

31. This hormone prepares the endometrium of uterus for implantation of the fertilized ovum:

(A) FSH
(B) hCG
(C) Progesterone
(D) LH

32. After missed period, presence of this hormone in the urine indicates pregnancy:

(A) FSH
(B) hCG
(C) Progesterone
(D) LH

33. Menarche, normally occurs between the ages:

(A) 8 and 16 (B) 14–18
(C) 15–17 (D) 8–10

34. The menopause occurs between the ages:

(A) 35 and 45 (B) 55 and 65
(C) 45 and 55 (D) 40 and 45

35. This hormone influences the development of ovarian follicles:

(A) FSH (B) Prolactin
(C) LH (D) Estrogens

36. Body temperature of a women:

(A) Rises after ovulation for about 2–3 days
(B) Decreases after ovulation for about 3–4 days
(C) Does not change after ovulation
(D) None of the above

37. These hormones are responsible for stimulation of milk ejection reflex:

(A) Progesterone–LH
(B) Prolactin and oxytocin
(C) Estrogen–progesterone
(D) LH–FSH

38. These hormones are responsible for the growth of breast tissue ducts and the stimulation of alveolar proliferation:

(A) Progesterone–LH
(B) Prolactin and oxytocin
(C) Estrogen–progesterone
(D) LH–FSH

ANSWERS

1. D	2. A	3. B	4. D	5. D	6. C	7. A
8. A	9. D	10. D	11. B	12. A	13. C	14. A
15. C	16. D	17. B	18. D	19. D	20. C	21. D
22. B	23. D	24. C	25. A	26. B	27. A	28. D
29. D	30. B	31. C	32. B	33. A	34. C	35. A
36. A	37. B	38. C				

MATCH THE COLUMNS

I	II
1. Labia majora	A. Large male mammory glands
2. Bartholin's glands	B. Absence of manstruation
3. Menarche	C. Oliguria
4. Prepuce	D. Scrotum swelling
5. Epididymis	E. External female sex organ
6. Menopause	F. Lubricating mucus
7. Prostate enlargement	G. Hot flushes
8. Gynecomastia	H. Foreskin
9. Hydrocele	I. Storage of sperms
10. Amenorrhea	J. First period

ANSWERS

1. E	2. F	3. J	4. H	5. I	6. G	7. C
8. A	9. D	10. B				

CHAPTER

15

Endocrine System

SAQ: Short answer question: Marks: 2
BAQ: Brief answer question: Marks: 4 or 5
LAQ: Long answer question: Marks: 9 or 10
MCQs: Multiple choice questions: Marks: 0.5 each
Match the columns: Marks: 0.5 each
Draw a labelled diagram: Marks: 5

Objectives: To identify endocrine glands and their secretions. To describe the endocrine system.

INTRODUCTION (Fig. 15.1)

BAQ: Write a note on the endocrine system.

Ans: The endocrine system is made up of specific glands located throughout the body, which synthesize and release hormones directly into blood circulation (Fig. 15.1). The hormones are chemicals that pass through blood circulation and act like catalysts to help various cells in the body to perform different functions. The hormones attach to the specific receptors on the cells, which initiate and control series of chemical reactions needed to carry out normal metabolic reactions. The hypothalamus in the brain is the neural control center; for the functioning of all endocrine glands.

The amount of hormones released by various glands and timing of hormone release is regulated by a mechanism called feedback mechanism, which is build up within the body systems. For example, by feedback mechanism, pancreases produce more insulin; when blood glucose level rises. Similarly, when calcium and inorganic phosphorus increase in blood, parathyroid glands secret parathyroid hormone so that; calcium and inorganic phosphorus could be used for the maintenance of bone integrity, and also for other metabolic reactions requiring calcium and inorganic phosphorus. Various body procedures are controlled by hormones are, respiration, reproduction, growth, sensory perception, movement, sexual development, etc.

The following are major glands of the endocrine system: Hypothalamus, pituitary gland, thyroid gland, parathyroid glands, adrenal glands, pineal body, ovaries and testes.

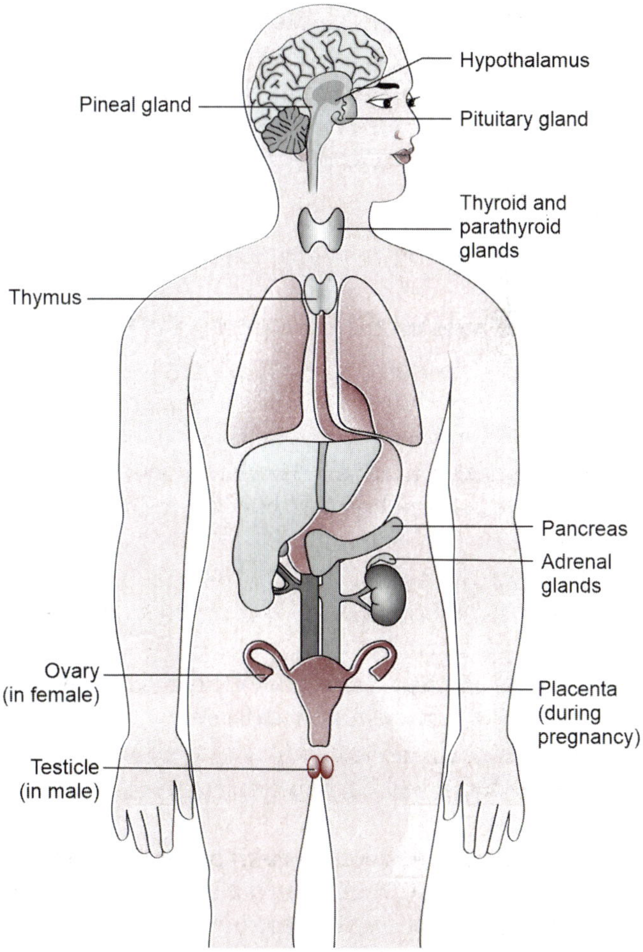

Fig. 15.1: Endocrine systems

Objectives: To describe the endocrine responses. To describe negative feedback and positive feedback mechanisms.

SAQ: What are the feedback mechanisms?

Ans: There are two types of feedback mechanism loops: Positive feedback mechanisms and negative feedback mechanisms. Positive feedback amplifies system output mechanisms and negative feedback decreases output. By this means the system stabilizes around an equilibrium point.

BAQ. Write a note on the feedback mechanisms.

Ans: Refer Chapter 1, page 16.

> **Objective:** To describe the similarities and the differences between enzymes and hormones.

BAQ: What are the similarities and differences between hormones and enzymes?

Ans:

Similarities

Enzymes as well as hormones act as catalysts.

Differences

1. All the enzymes are protein in nature, however all hormones are not protein in nature, only some hormones are protein in nature.
2. The enzymes are secreted by specific cells and act at the site, where these are produced. However, hormones are secreted by endocrine gland and these function at specific target organ, away from the endocrine gland.

> **Objective:** To define and classify the hormones.

LAQ: Write a note on the classification of hormones.

Ans: The hormones can be classified as follows: (1) Classification based on the chemical nature and (2) Classification based on the mechanism of action.

1. **Classification based on the chemical nature:** The hormones can be classified into the following three groups:
   a. Protein or peptide hormones, e.g. insulin, antidiuretic hormone (ADH), oxytocin, glucagon, etc.
   b. Steroid hormones, e.g. sex hormones, glucocorticoids, mineralocorticoids, etc.
   c. Amino acid derivatives, e.g. thyroxine (T_4), triiodothyronine (T_3), epinephrine, norepinephrine, etc.
2. **Classification based on the mechanism of action:** The hormones can also be classified into two broad groups based on the location of receptors to which they bind and the signals used to mediate their action.
   a. *Group 1 hormones:* These hormones bind to intracellular receptors to form receptor–hormone complexes, through which their biochemical functions are mediated. Except for T_3 and T_4, group 1 hormones are derivatives of cholesterol, e.g. estrogens, androgens, glucocorticoids, etc.
   These hormones act through the intracellular receptors located either in the cytosol or the nucleus. The hormone receptor complex binds to specific regions on the DNA (hormone-responsive element) and causes increased expression of specific genes. The ultimate outcome is the production of specific proteins in response to the hormonal action.
   b. *Group 2 hormones:* These hormones bind to cell surface (plasma membrane) receptors and stimulate the release of second messengers (certain molecules). These messengers perform biochemical functions. These hormones are hydrophilic in nature and usually transported in free form, and possess short half-lives. The hormones ACTH, FSH, LH, PTH, glucagon and calcitonin stimulate release of cAMP as the second messenger. The hormones TRH, gastrin, etc. stimulate the release of phosphatidyl inositol/calcium as the second messengers.

SAQ: Give examples of hormones that are protein in nature.

Ans: Insulin, antidiuretic hormone (ADH), oxytocin, glucagon, etc.

SAQ: Give examples of hormones that are steroids in nature.

Ans: Sex hormones, glucocorticoids, mineralocorticoids, etc.

SAQ: Give examples of hormones that are amino acid derivatives.

Ans: Thyroxine (T_4), triiodothyronine (T_3), epinephrine, norepinephrine, etc.

> **Objectives:** To describe anatomical structure of the hypothalamus gland and its functions. To enumerate the hormones secreted by the hypothalamus. To describe the effects and functions of the hormones secreted by the hypothalamus. To describe blood supply and innervation of the hypothalamus.

HYPOTHALAMUS (Fig. 15.2)

LAQ: Write a note on the hypothalamus with respect to the following points: (1) Introduction, (2) applied anatomy and related functions.

Ans:

1. **Introduction:** The hypothalamus is located at the base of the brain, near the pituitary gland of the brain (Fig. 15.2). It controls the other glands of the endocrine system. It works by information received from the nervous system to determine when to inform other glands, to produce hormones; which can control specific functions. The hypothalamus controls many processes in the body, such as control of mood, hunger, thirst, sexual functions, sleep patterns, and moods.

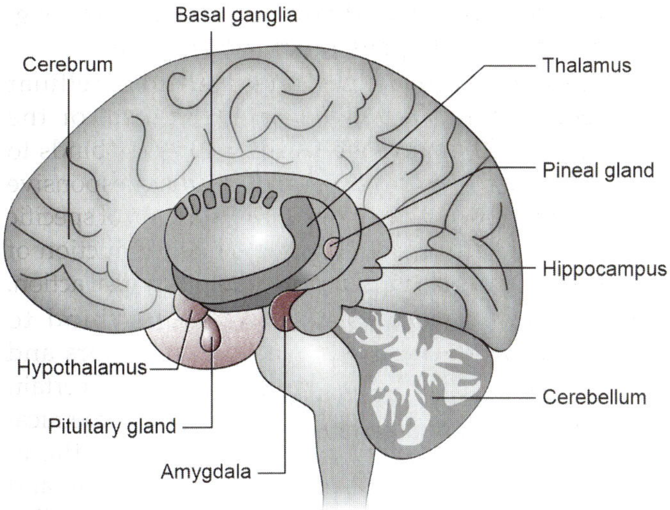

Fig. 15.2: Hypothalamus

Anatomy of Hypothalamus (Fig. 15.3)

2. **Applied anatomy with the related functions:** The hypothalamus has three main regions: The anterior region, the middle region and the posterior region. Each region contains different nuclei, which are clusters of neurons that stimulate release of specific hormones.

Anterior Region of Hypothalamus (Supraoptic Region) (Fig. 15.3)

The following are the main nuclei of anterior region of the hypothalamus: (A) The supraoptic nuclei and (B) the paraventricular nuclei. These nuclei are mainly involved in the secretion of various hormones and some of these hormones also interact with the pituitary gland situated near the hypothalamus (Fig. 15.4) to produce additional hormones, described below. The following

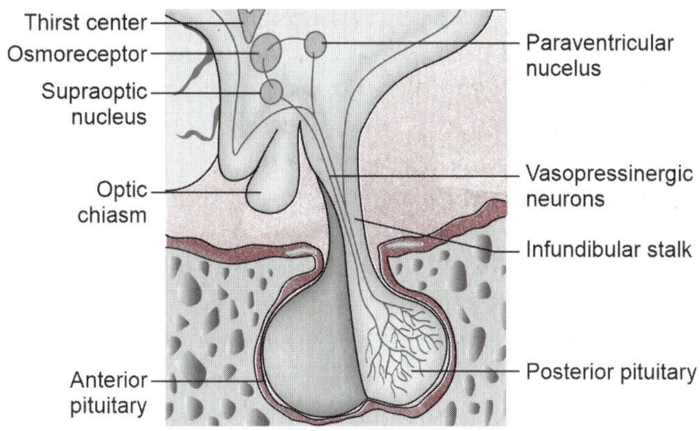

Fig. 15.3: Main nuclei of hypothalamus

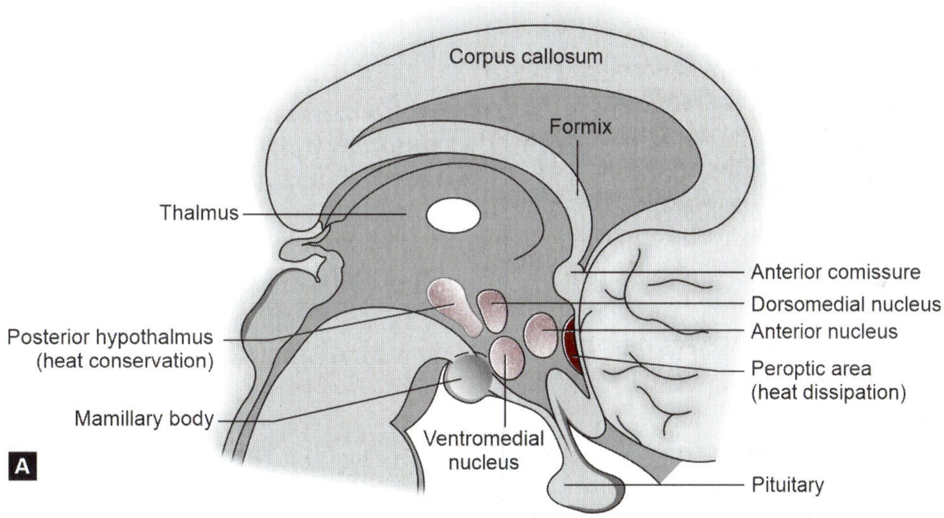

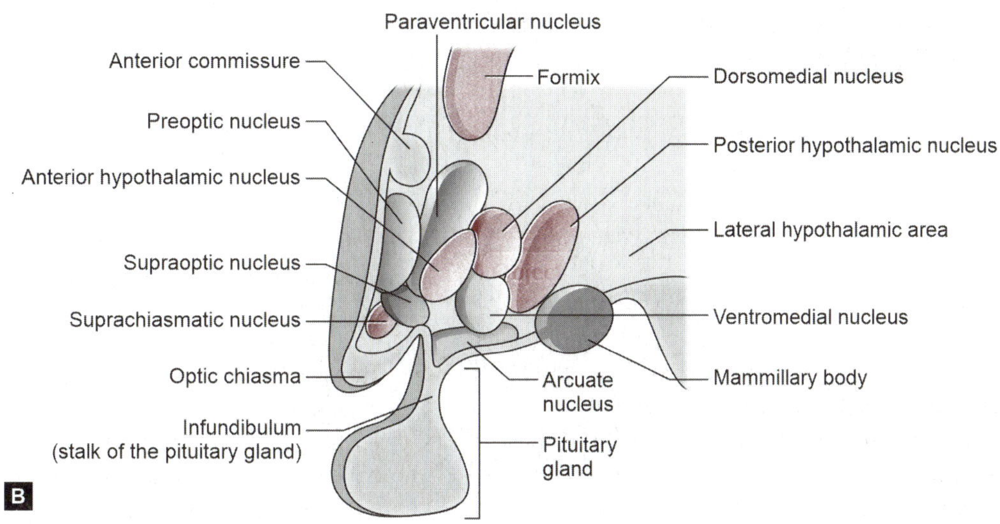

Figs 15.4A and B: Middle region of hypothalamus with dorsomedial and ventromedial nuclei

are very important hormones produced in the anterior region of the hypothalamus: Corticotropin-releasing hormone (CRH), thyrotropin-releasing hormone (TRH), gonadotropin-releasing hormone (GnRH), oxytocin, vasopressin, and somatostatin.

Functions of the Hormones Secreted by Hypothalamus

- **Corticotropin-releasing hormone (CRH):** It is secreted in the response to emotional stress and physical stress. It signals the pituitary gland to produce, adrenocorticotropic hormone (ACTH), which triggers the production of the stress hormone, cortisol. The function of cortisol is to prepare the body for action in response to stress. Cortisol release effects are an increase in blood pressure, blood sugar, and suppression of the immune system.
- **Thyrotropin-releasing hormone (TRH):** It stimulates the pituitary gland to produce thyroid-stimulating hormone (TSH). TSH in turn controls the secretions of triiodothyronine (T_3) and throxine (T_4) hormones released by thyroid gland, which are needed for the normal metabolic reactions of the cells.
- **Gonadotropin-releasing hormone (GnRH):** It stimulates the pituitary gland to produce important reproductive hormones, such as follicle-stimulating hormone (FSH) and luteinizing hormone (LH).
- **Oxytocin:** It acts as a neurotransmitter in the brain. It exerts driving force behind attraction, caregiving, and controls important aspects of the reproductive system, including childbirth and lactation.
- **Vasopressin [antidiuretic hormone (ADH)]:** It plays very important role in regulation of water levels in the body. ADH acts on the distal part of the tubule of the nephrons to reabsorb water.
- **Somatostatin:** It acts on pituitary gland to control release of hormones, such as growth hormone and thyroid-stimulating hormone (TSH). TSH then acts on the thyroid gland to release thyroid hormones.

The anterior region of the hypothalamus also plays important role in the regulation of body temperature through production of sweat. It also maintains the circadian rhythms. A circadian rhythm or circadian cycle, is a natural, internal process that regulates the sleep–wake cycle and repeats approximately after every 24 hours.

Middle Region of Hypothalamus (Tuberal Region) (Figs 15.4A and B)

The major nuclei of middle region of hypothalamus are the ventromedial and arcuate nuclei. The ventromedial nucleus plays important role in the control of appetite, while the arcuate nucleus is involved in release of growth hormone-releasing hormone (GHRH). GHRH stimulates the pituitary gland to produce growth hormone (GH), which is responsible for the growth and development of the body. The dorsomedial hypothalamic nucleus is involved in body-weight regulation, drinking, feeding and circadian activity.

Posterior Region of Hypothalamus (Fig. 15.4B)

The posterior region nuclei are, the posterior hypothalamic nucleus and the mammillary nuclei. The posterior hypothalamic nucleus plays important role in the regulation of body temperature. The role of the mammillary nuclei is involved in the memory consolidation and storage. Hence, damage to the mammillary bodies results in loss of memory (amnesia).

Nerve Supply of Hypothalamus (Fig. 15.5)

BAQ: Write a note on the innervation of hypothalamus.

Ans: The posterior portion of the hypothalamus, called the median eminence, contains the nerve endings of

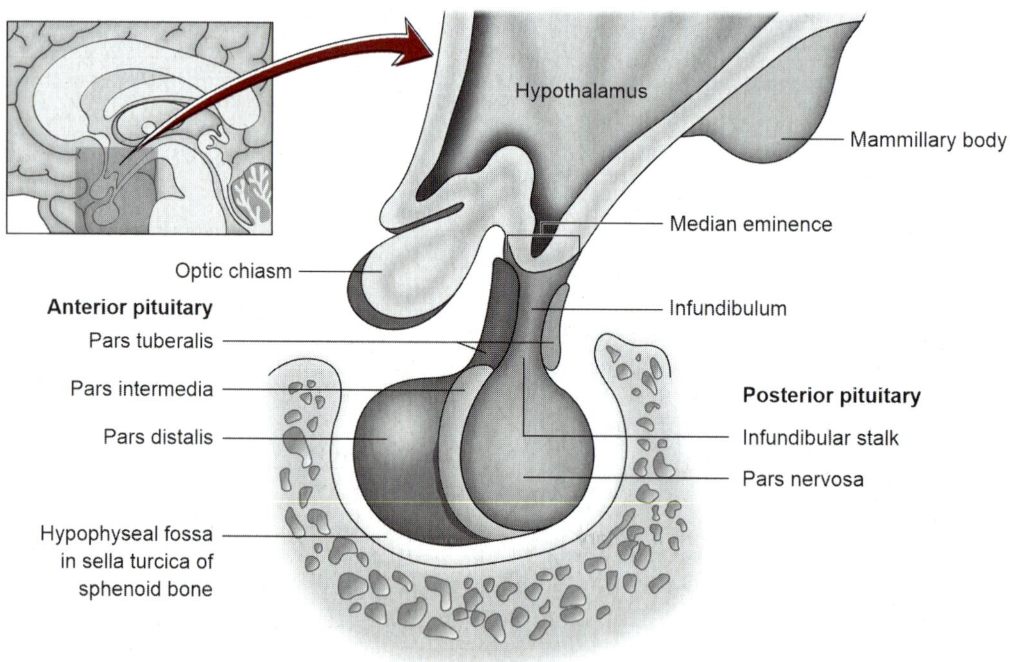

Fig. 15.5: Hypothalamic nerve connections through median eminence to pituitary gland

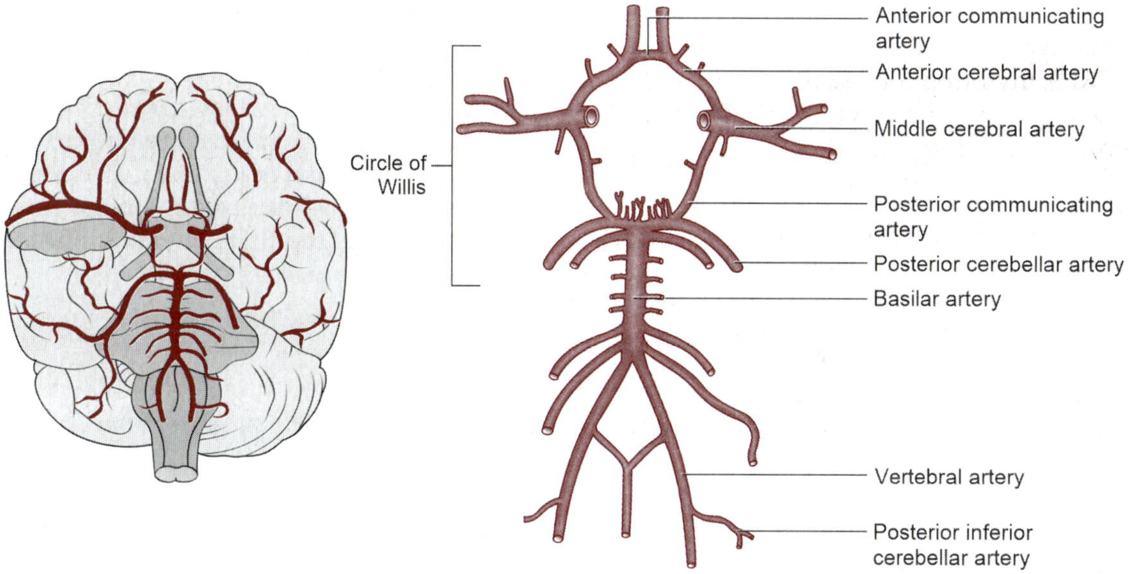

Fig. 15.6: Arterial blood supply to hypothalamus by the circle of Willis

many neurosecretory cells, which run down through the infundibular stalk into the pituitary gland.

Arterial Blood Supply of Hypothalamus (Fig. 15.6)

BAQ: Write a note on the blood supply of hypothalamus.

Ans: The hypothalamus gets arterial blood from the circle of Willis (Fig. 15.6); which surrounds it inferiorly. The anteromedial branches of the anterior cerebral artery, the branches of the posterior communicating artery, and the branches of the posterior cerebral artery supply arterial blood to hypothalamus.

Hypothalamic-hypophyseal Portal System (Fig. 15.7)

BAQ: Write a note on the hypothalamic-hypophyseal portal system.

Ans: The hypothalamic-hypophyseal portal system is a micro-blood capillary system present at the base of the brain. It connects the hypothalamus with the anterior pituitary. Main function of the hypothalamic-hypophyseal portal system is to transport and exchange hormones secreted by hypothalamus and pituitary gland between the hypothalamus arcuate nucleus and anterior part of pituitary gland.

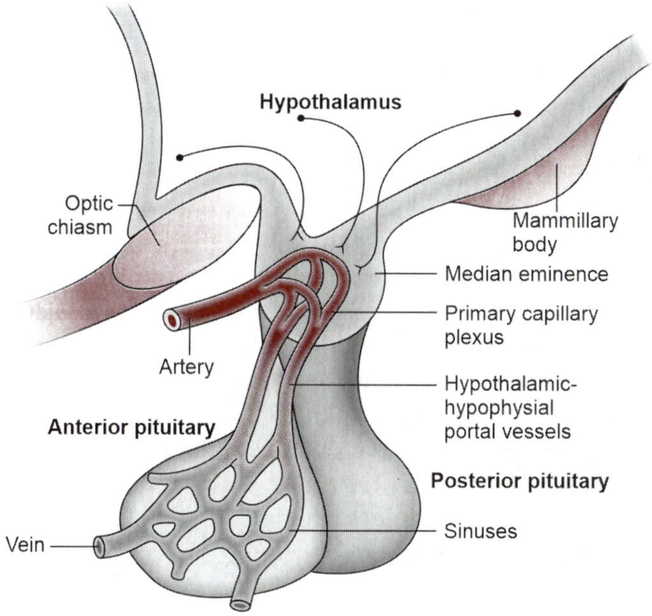

Fig. 15.7A: Hypothalamic-hypophyseal portal system

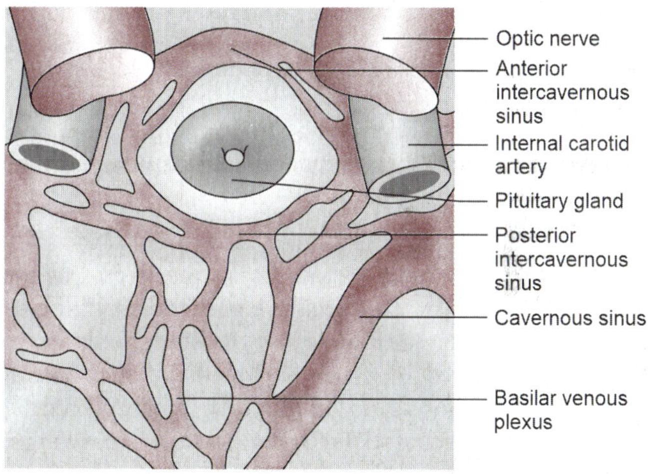

Fig. 15.7B: Intercavernous sinuses

Venous Blood Drainage of Hypothalamus (Figs 15.6–15.8)

BAQ: Write a note on the venous blood drainage of hypothalamus.

Ans: The venous drainage is mainly through the circle of intercavernous sinuses. The anterior intercavernous plexuses drain venous blood to the cavernous sinus (Fig. 15.8B), which then drains to the superior and inferior petrosal sinuses. The superior petrosal sinus joins the transverse sinus to form the sigmoid sinus (Fig. 15.8C). The sigmoid sinus is later joined by the inferior petrosal sinus and becomes the internal jugular vein (Fig. 15.8). Venous blood from the internal jugular vein passes to the right atrium of the heart.

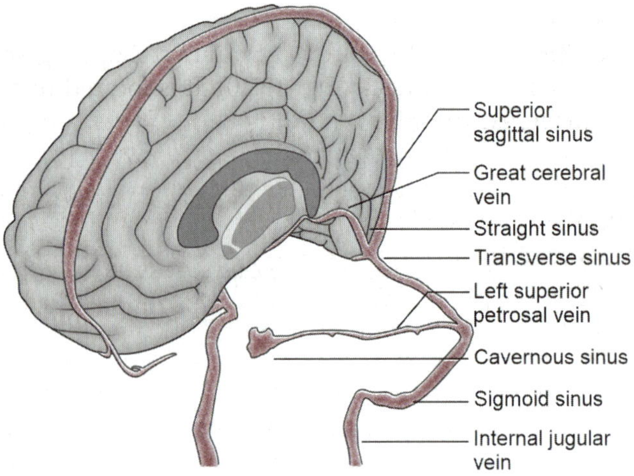

Fig. 15.8: Venous drainage of hypothalamus

> **Objective:** To describe the difference between diabetes mellitus and diabetes insipidus.

BAQ: Write a short note on diabetes insipidus.

Ans: Diabetes insipidus is a clinical condition caused by the deficiency of antidiuretic hormone (ADH). The function of ADH is to reabsorb water from the filtrate formed at the glomeruli, by its action on the distal part of the tubule of the nephron. Due to the deficiency of ADH, water is not reabsorbed and large amount of water is excreted in urine, leading to polyuria. Normal average urine excretion per day is about 1.5–2.0 liters. In diabetes insipidus, urine excretion per day can be up to 20 liters. The treatment on ADH deficiency is usually supportive.

SAQ: What is the difference between diabetes mellitus and diabetes insipidus?

Ans: Diabetes mellitus is caused due to the deficiency of insulin and diabetes insipidus is caused due to the deficiency of ADH. Polyurea is observed in diabetes insipidus and large amount of urine, sometimes up to 20 liters is excreted. In uncontrolled diabetes mellitus, due to high levels of glucose in blood (hyperglycemia) also the patient may suffer from polyuria. However, excretion of urine may be about 4–5 liters per day.

> **Objectives:** To describe anatomical structure of the pituitary gland and its functions. To enumerate the hormones secreted by the pituitary gland. To describe the effects and functions of the hormones secreted by the pituitary gland. To describe the blood supply and innervation of the pituitary gland.

PITUITARY GLAND (Fig. 15.4)

LAQ: Describe the pituitary gland with respect to the following heads: (1) Introduction, (2) applied anatomy and related functions.

Ans:

1. The pituitary gland is small-sized endocrine gland located at the base of the brain.

   The pituitary gland is connected to the hypothalamus through a stalk of blood vessels and nerves called the pituitary stalk (Figs 15.3, 15.5 and 15.7). Hormones secreted by the hypothalamus travel to the pituitary gland through the hypothalamic-pituitary axis, which stimulate pituitary gland to secret specific hormones. These hormones control the other glands in the various parts of the body. The pituitary gland synthesizes hormones that control several other glands such as the thyroid gland, adrenal glands, ovaries and the testicles (Fig. 15.9).

Anatomy of Pituitary Gland (Fig. 15.9)

2. Applied anatomy and related functions: The pituitary gland can be divided into two different parts: The anterior lobe and the posterior lobe.

Anterior Lobe of Pituitary Gland

The anterior lobe of the pituitary gland can be divided into the pars tuberalis and pars distalis. Anterior lobe constitutes about 80% of the pituitary gland.

The anterior pituitary contains several different types of cells that synthesize and secrete the following hormones:

- **Growth hormone (GH):** It regulates growth and physical development of an individual. It stimulates growth in almost all of the tissues. The primary targets of GH are bones and muscles.
- **Thyroid-stimulating hormone (TSH):** This hormone activates thyroid gland to release thyroid hormones, thyroxine (T_4) and triiodothyronine (T_3). The function of the thyroid gland is to convert inorganic iodine present in many foods, and convert it into thyroid hormones: Thyroxine (T_4) and triiodothyronine (T_3). T_4 and T_3 are released into the blood stream and these are then transported to the body cells. T_4 and T_3, control various metabolic reactions and the oxidative metabolic reactions, which produce energy in the form of ATP molecules.
- **Adrenocorticotropic hormone:** This hormone stimulates adrenal glands to produce cortisol.
- **Follicle-stimulating hormone (FHS):** It is responsible for the growth of ovarian follicles, which produce estrogens and progesterone in the ovaries and maintain the menstrual cycles in women. It also plays an important role in males in the production of sperms.
- **Luteinizing hormone (LH):** In females, an acute rise of LH triggers ovulation and development of the corpus luteum. It plays important role in the production of estrogens in women and testosterone in men.
- **Prolactin:** It stimulates growth of breasts and synthesis of milk during pregnancy and after birth of a child.
- **Endorphins:** These are neurotransmitters and these have pain-relieving properties.
- **Beta-melanocyte-stimulating hormone:** It stimulates increase in pigmentation of skin in response to exposure to ultraviolet radiation.

Posterior Lobe of Pituitary Gland

The posterior lobe of the pituitary gland consists mainly of extensions of axons from two pairs of large clusters of nerve cell bodies (paraventricular nuclei, supraoptic nuclei) in the hypothalamus (Fig. 15.4).

The following two hormones are synthesized in the hypothalamus and released in the posterior pituitary: ADH (vasopressin) and oxytocin. These hormones are usually stored in the posterior lobe of pituitary gland until these are released in blood circulation. These hormones are released when the hypothalamus sends messages to the pituitary gland through nerve cell stimulation.

- **ADH:** Antidiuretic hormone acts on the distal part of tubules of nephrons in kidney and promotes reabsorption of water back into the blood circulation. Deficiency of ADH leads to excessive formation and excretion of urine (polyurea).
- **Oxytocin:** It stimulates the release of breast milk. It also stimulates contractions of the uterus during labour and child birth. Oxytocin plays important role in lactation, and human behaviour aspects.

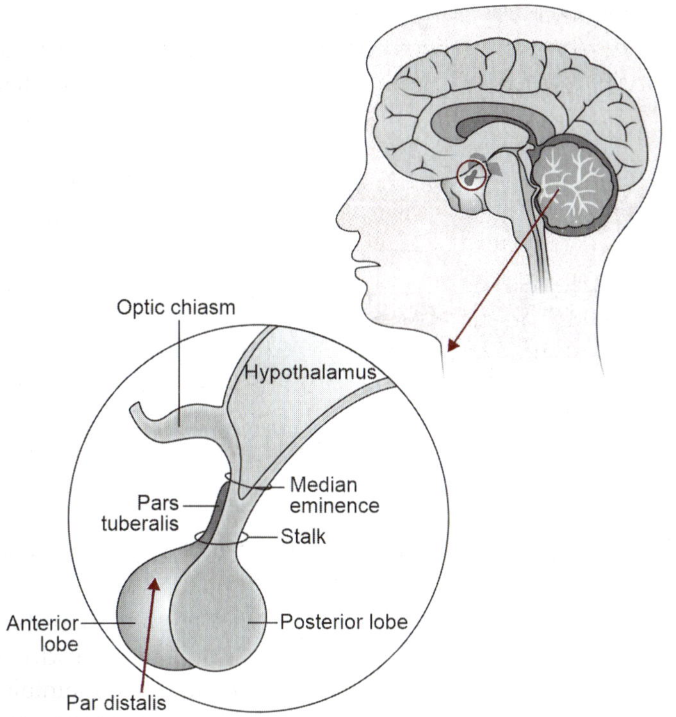

Fig.15.9: Pituitary gland

BAQ: Draw a labelled diagram of the pituitary gland.

Ans: Refer to Fig. 15.9.

> **Objectives:** To describe anatomical structure of the thyroid gland and its functions. To describe the effects and functions of the hormones secreted by the thyroid. To describe blood supply and innervation of the hypothalamus. To describe the various disorders of the thyroid gland.

THYROID GLAND (Figs 15.11 and 15.12)

LAQ: Describe the thyroid gland with respect to the following heads: (1) Introduction, (2) applied anatomy and related functions.

Ans:

Introduction: The thyroid is a butterfly-shaped gland in the front side of neck (Fig. 15.10). It is located under the laryngeal prominence (Adam's apple), a lump of cartilage. In adults it weighs about 25 grams. It is made up of two main lobes. Each lobe of thyroid is about 5 cm long, 3 cm wide, and 2 cm thick. These lobes are connected by a bridge of tissues called the isthmus, which is about 1.25 cm in height and width. The gland is usually larger in women than in men.

The thyroid gland plays very important role in the general metabolism, growth and development of the human body. It regulates many body functions by controlled release of thyroid hormones into the blood circulation.

Anatomy of Thyroid Gland (Fig. 15.12)

Applied anatomy with related functions: The thyroid gland is composed of two lobes, left and right, which are connected by a narrow tissue band, called an 'isthmus' (Fig. 15.13).

The following are the three primary microscopic features of the thyroid gland: (A) Follicles, (B) follicular cells, and (C) parafollicular cells (Fig. 15.12).

A. **Follicles:** Thyroid follicles are small spherical groups of cells. They consist of a rim that has supply of blood, nerves and lymphatics. The rim is surrounded by a specific colloidal space consisting mainly of thyroid hormone precursor proteins known as thyroglobulin, which contains iodine.
B. **Follicular cells:** The core of a follicle is surrounded by a single layer of follicular cells. These cells secret T_3 and T_4, using thyroglobulin present in the core space of follicles; when stimulated by thyroid stimulating hormone (TSH).
C. **Parafollicular cells:** Parafollicular cells are scattered among follicular cells and in spaces between the spherical follicles. These cells secrete the hormone, calcitonin.

Functions of hormones of thyroid gland: The thyroid secretes two hormones, thyroxine (T_4) and triiodothyronine (T_3). Thyroid hormones play important role in maintaining normal carbohydrate metabolism, protein synthesis, cholesterol and triglyceride metabolism. Thyroid hormones play important role in the development of body and body temperature. During infancy and childhood, adequate quamtity thyroid hormone is crucial for brain development. Thyroid hormones are essential for the development of nervous system and sexual maturation. Thyroid hormone increase uptake of oxygen and play important role in the production of ATP molecules by mitochondria. ATP molecules are required for the cellular activities.

Blood, Lymph and Nerve Supply of Thyroid Gland

Thyroid is supplied with arterial blood from the superior thyroid artery, which is a branch of the external carotid artery, and the inferior thyroid artery, which is a branch of the thyrocervical trunk.

The venous blood is drained through superior and middle thyroid veins, which drain into the internal jugular vein, and through the inferior thyroid veins. Arteries and veins form a plexus between the two layers of the capsule of the thyroid gland.

SAQ: What is Adam's apple?

Ans: The Adam's apple or laryngeal prominence is a lump of cartilage. It is more prominent in males compared to that in females. Laryngeal prominence develops during puberty. It protects the vocal cords behind it (Fig. 15.10).

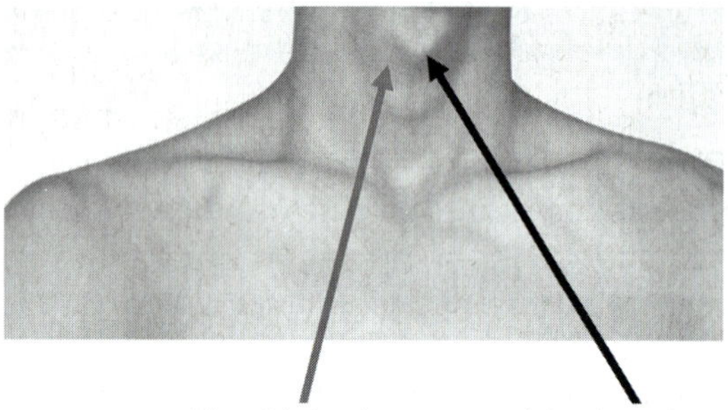

Fig. 15.10: Thyroid gland and Adam's apple

BAQ: Draw a labelled diagram of the anatomy of the thyroid gland.

Ans: Refer to Fig. 15.11.

BAQ: Write a note on the arterial blood supply and venous drainage of the thyroid gland.

Ans: The superior thyroid artery (STA) branching from the external carotid artery (ECA), and the inferior thyroid artery (ITA) branching from the thyrocervical trunk supply the blood to the thyroid gland (Fig. 15.12).

The superior thyroid veins and middle thyroid veins drain into the internal jugular vein. The left and right inferior thyroid veins drain into left and right brachiocephalic veins, which pass venous blood to superior vena cava, which opens in the right atrium of the heart (Fig. 15.15).

Thyroid Gland Lymphatic Drainage (Fig. 15.13)

Lymphatic drainage passes the prelaryngeal lymph nodes (located just above the isthmus) and the pretracheal and paratracheal lymph nodes.

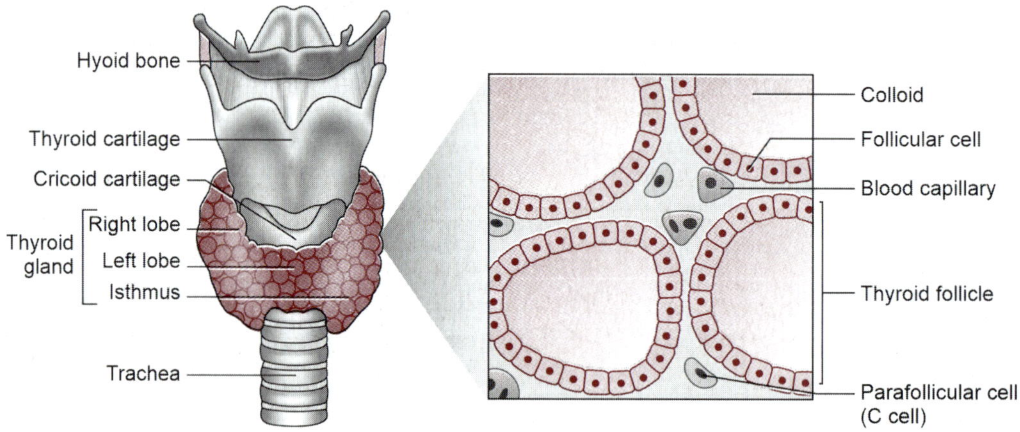

Fig. 15.11: Anatomy of thyroid gland

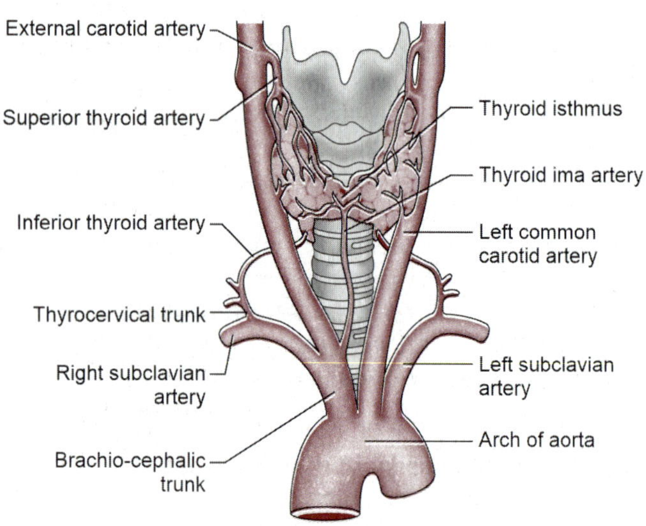

Fig. 15.12: Arterial supply of thyroid gland

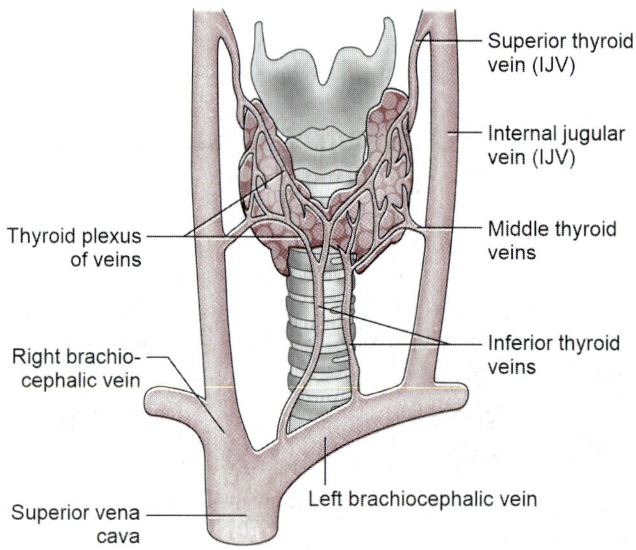

Fig. 15.13: Venous drainage of thyroid gland

Thyroid Gland Nerve Supply (Fig. 15.14)

SAQ: Write a note on the nerve supply of the thyroid gland.

Ans: The thyroid gland receives sympathetic nerves from the superior, middle and inferior cervical ganglion of the sympathetic trunk. The gland receives parasympathetic nerves from the superior laryngeal nerve and the recurrent laryngeal nerve.

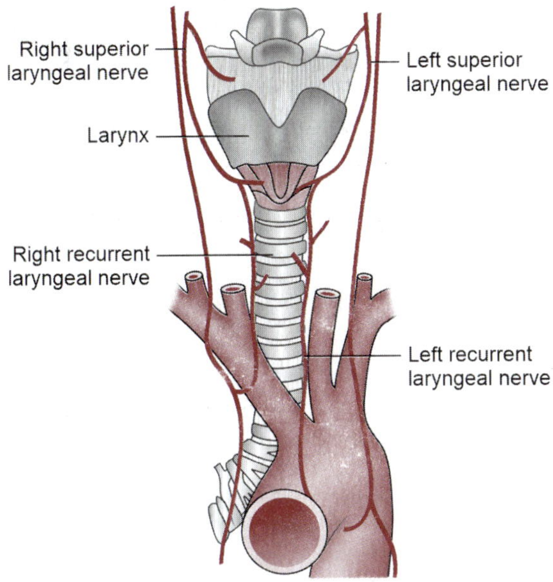

Fig. 15.14: Nerve supply of thyroid gland

THYROID DISEASES

Goiter (Fig. 15.15)

BAQ: Write a note on goiter.

Ans: Goiter is abnormal enlargement of thyroid gland (Fig. 15.17). Goiter can be simple or toxic.

Simple goiter: This clinical condition is caused due to hypothyroidism. In this clinical condition, low levels of thyroid hormones (T_3 and T_4) are observed, with the enlargement of thyroid gland. The following are the underlying causes of simple goiter: Persistent iodine deficiency, genetic abnormality or due to the action of certain drugs.

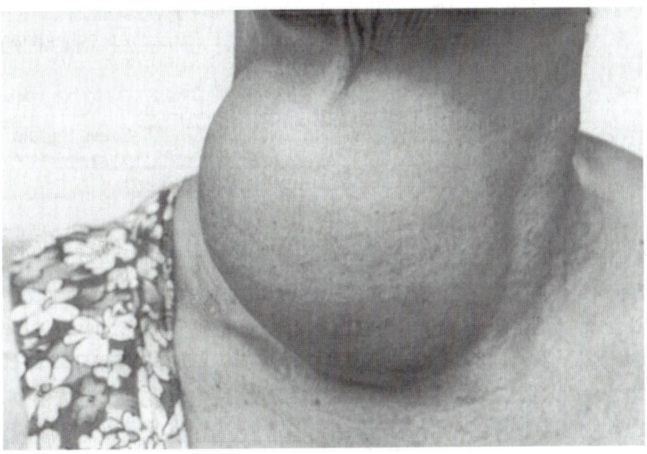

Fig. 15.15: Goiter

Toxic goiter: It is caused due to hyperthyroidism. In this clinical condition high levels of thyroid hormones (T_3 and T_4) are observed. The most common cause of toxic goiter is Graves' disease, in which autoantibodies against the TSH receptors are responsible for the high levels of thyroid hormones.

Thyroiditis

BAQ: Write a note on thyroiditis.

Ans: Thyroiditis is an inflammation of the thyroid gland. It may be caused due to bacterial or viral infection or autoimmune condition such as Hashimoto's disease. Thyroiditis also may be drug-induced or caused due to radiation therapy. Depending upon a specific type of thyroiditis, there may not be symptoms or the symptoms are like hypothyroidism or hyperthyroidism.

Hyperthyroidism

BAQ: Write a note on hyperthyroidism.

Ans: Excessive thyroid hormone production leads to Hyperthyroidism. It is most often caused by Graves' disease, which is an autoimmune disease. Abnormal growth thyroid gland due to nodule formation also leads to overproduction of thyroid hormones. The following are the common symptoms of hyperthyroidism: Loss of weight loss, irregular heartbeat, irritability and sweating.

Hypothyroidism

BAQ: Write a note on hypothyroidism.

Ans: Low production of thyroid hormone leads to hypothyroidism. It may be caused due to damage of thyroid gland caused by autoimmune disease, bacterial or viral disease. Hypothyroidism also may be caused due to hypothalamic or pituitary disease. The following are the common symptoms of hypothyroidism: Depression, decreased heart rate, increase in heart pressure, constipation, fluid retention, increase in weight, and irregularities in menstrual cycles.

BAQ: Write a note on myxedema.

Ans: Myxedema is a severe form of hypothyroidism, as well as in hyperthyroidism. It leads to the accumulation of mucopolysaccharides in the skin and other tissues, leading to the increased thickness of the skin and the thickening of facial features.

BAQ: Write a note on Hashimoto's disease.

Ans: Hashimoto's disease is an autoimmune disorder, in which, the immune system creates antibodies that attack thyroid cells, leading to significant decrease in secretions of thyroid hormones (T_3 and T_4). The following factors are responsible to the onset of Hashimoto's disease: Genetic factors, stress, thyroid infections, radiation exposure, etc.

BAQ: Write a note on Graves' disease.

Ans: It is caused by an autoimmune reaction to thyroid tissue and thyroglobulin, resulting in the development of autoantibodies that mimic the action of TSH, by releasing high levels of thyroid hormones (T_3 and T_4), which depress secretion of TRH (from the hypothalamus) and TSH (from the anterior pituitary gland). Graves' disease has been observed more commonly in women compared to men.

Thyroid Cancer

SAQ: What is thyroid cancer?

Ans: Abnormal growth in thyroid tissue leads to thyroid cancer. Thyroid cancer may lead to changes in voice, difficulty in swallowing, pain in the neck and throat enlargement. Thyroid cancers can be detected by CT scans and MRI scans. Early stage thyroid cancers respond well to radiation and chemotherapy treatments.

Objectives: To describe anatomical structure of the parathyroid gland and its functions. To describe the effects and functions of the hormones secreted by the parathyroid gland. To describe the various disorders of the parathyroid gland.

PARATHYROID GLANDS (Fig. 15.16)

LAQ: Describe the parathyroid gland with respect to the following heads: (1) Introduction, (2) applied anatomy and related functions.

Ans:

Introduction: The parathyroid glands are two pairs of small pea-sized, oval-shaped glands, which are located next to the two thyroid gland lobes in the neck. (Fig. 15.16). The parathyroid glands synthesize and secret parathyroid hormone, which plays an important role in the regulation of calcium levels in the blood.

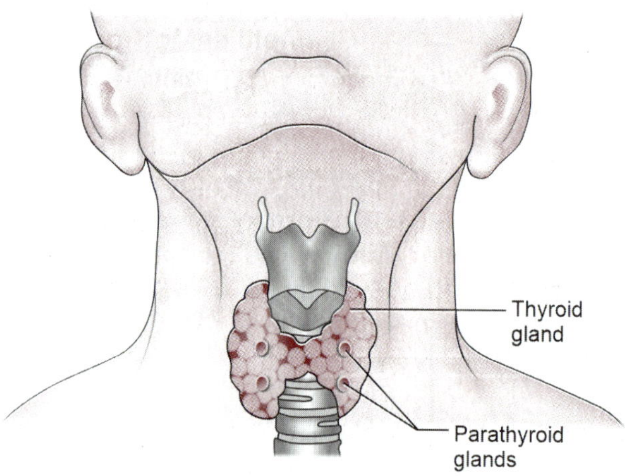

Fig. 15.16: Parathyroid glands

Anatomy of Parathyroid Glands (Fig. 15.17)

Applied anatomy and related functions: The parathyroid glands are separated by a thick connective tissue capsule from the thyroid tissue. Tissue of parathyroid gland contains oxyphil cells and chief cells (Fig. 15.17). The function of the oxyphil cells is not significant, when parathyroid glands are in normal condition. However, oxyphil cells secrete parathyroid hormones, when parathyroid tissue mass increases. The chief cells are epithelial cells, which produce and secrete the parathyroid hormone (PTH), the main hormone involved in the regulation of blood calcium levels.

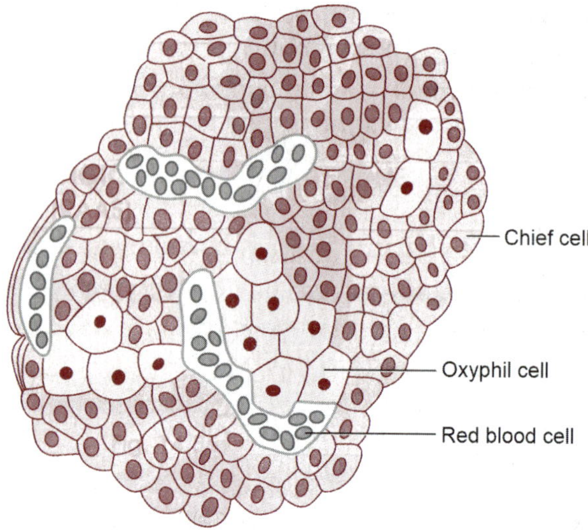

Fig. 15.17: Chief cells and oxyphil cells of parathyroid gland

Functions of parathyroid hormone (PTH): The body needs calcium to mainly maintain strong bones and teeth and also to carry out many important functions like movement of muscles, normal nerves functioning and clotting of blood. When the blood passes through the parathyroid glands, they detect the amount of calcium present in the blood and react by synthesizing appropriate quantity of pathyroid hormone (PTH).

Parathyroid hormone maintains calcium levels in the blood, by increasing the blood calcium levels by its actions on the kidneys, bones and intestine.

Parathyroid hormone stimulates the release of calcium in blood circulation by activating osteocyte cells in the bone. Similarly, PTH acts on renal tubules for increased absorption of calcium from blood filtrate. PTH also acts on small intestine to absorb more calcium. When blood calcium levels are normal, PTH secretions are low.

DISEASES OF PARATHYROID GLANDS

Hyperparathyroidism

BAQ: Write a note on hyperparathyroidism.

Ans: Hyperparathyroidism is caused due to increase in parathyroid hormones in blood circulation. It may be primary hyperparathyroidism or secondary hyperparathyroidism. Following are the common symptoms seen in hyperparathyroidism: Depression, confusion, bone pain, weakness and increased urination. Both primary and secondary hyperparathyroidism may result in osteoporosis.

Primary hyperparathyroidism is caused due to adenoma (abnormal growth of parathyroid cells) present in the tissue of parathyroid gland. Secondary hyperparathyroidism is observed in vitamin D deficiency and when calcium levels are low.

Symptoms of hyperparathyroidism are, weakness, abdominal pain, depression, formation of kidney stones, osteoporosis, etc.

BAQ: Why does person suffering from hyperparathyroidism suffer from osteoporosis?

Ans: In hyperparathyroidism person suffers from hyperactivity of parathyroid glands. Due to excessive secretions of parathyroid hormones; the bones release excessive amounts of calcium ions into the blood circulation. The loss of calcium from the bones leads to osteoporosis. In osteoporosis, the bones develop more internal pores leading to decreased bone mass. Due to osteoporosis, bone become brittle and prone to fractures (Fig. 15.18).

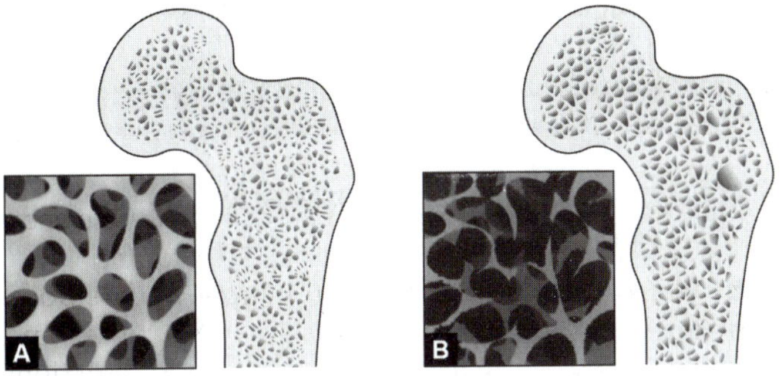

Figs 15.18A and B: (A) Healthy bone; (B) bone in osteoporosis

Hypoparathyroidism

SAQ: Write a note on hypoparathyroidism.

Ans: Hypoparathyroidism is a clinical condition caused mainly due to the following reasons: The damage to the parathyroid glands during surgery of thyroid gland, due to autoimmune disorder or due to radiation therapy. Very low serum calcium and very high inorganic phosphorus are observed in hypoparathyroidism. The most common symptoms of hypoparathyroidism are related to significantly low serum calcium. These symptoms are muscular cramps, tingling sensations in fingers, lips, and toes.

> **Objectives:** To describe anatomical structure of the adrenal gland and its functions. To describe the effects and functions of the hormones secreted by the adrenal gland. To describe blood supply and innervation of the adrenal gland. To describe the various disorders of the adrenal gland.

ADRENAL GLANDS (SUPRARENAL GLANDS) (Fig. 15.19)

BAQ: Write a note on the adrenal gland with respect to the following points: (1) Introduction, (2) applied anatomy and names of the secreted hormones.

Ans:

1. **Introduction:** Adrenal glands (suprarenal glands), are yellow coloured, small, triangular-shaped glands located on top of both the kidneys. There are two adrenal glands (Fig. 15.19). A weak septum of connective tissue separates the glands from the kidneys. The adrenal glands are directly below the diaphragm, and are attached to the diaphragm by the renal fascia, a connective tissue.

The adrenal glands approximately measure 3 cm in width, 5.0 cm in length, and about 1.0 cm in thickness. Average combined weight of adrenal glands is about 11.8 g.

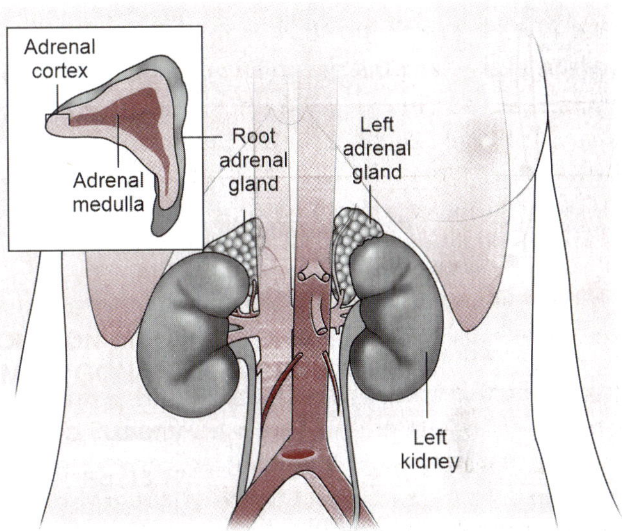

Fig. 15.19: Adrenal glands

Anatomy of Adrenal Glands

2. **Applied anatomy and names of the secreted hormones:** Each adrenal gland has an outer part known as cortex and an inner part known as medulla. The adrenal cortex is divided into the following three main zones: 1. The zona glomerulosa, 2. the zona fasciculata and 3. the zona reticularis.

The adrenal cortex produces three main types of steroid hormones: mineralocorticoids, glucocorticoids, and androgens.

The adrenal medulla part is at the centre of each adrenal gland. It is surrounded by the adrenal cortex. The adrenal medulla contain the chromaffin cells, which synthesize the hormones, catecholamines, such as adrenaline, noradrenaline and dopamine.

BAQ: Draw a labelled diagram of anatomy of the adrenal cortex.

Ans: Refer to Fig. 15.20.

Adrenal Cortex (Fig. 15.20)

BAQ: Write a note on the adrenal cortex.

Ans: The adrenal cortex is the outer region of adrenal glands. It is the largest part of an adrenal gland. It is divided into following three zones: (1) Zona glomerulosa, (2) zona fasciculata and (3) zona reticularis. Each zone is responsible for producing specific hormones (Fig. 15.20).

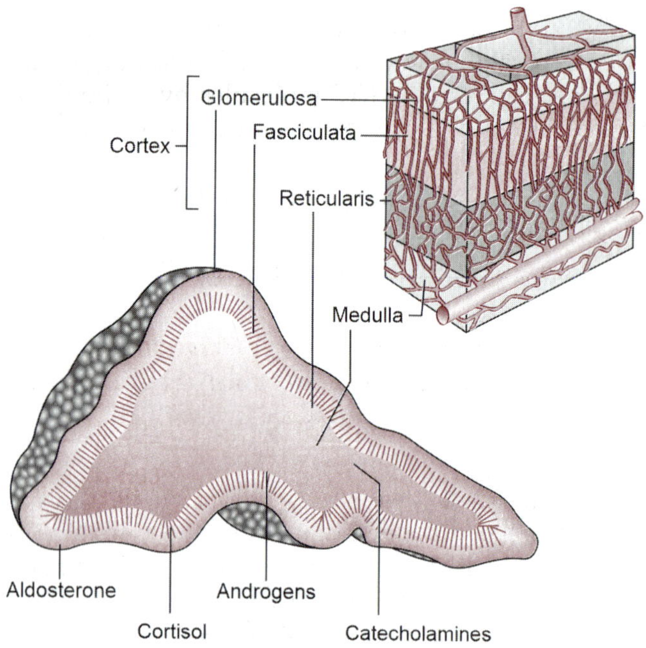

Fig. 15.20: Anatomy of the adrenal cortex

Zona Glomerulosa (Fig. 15.20)

This outermost layer is the main site for synthesis of hormone aldosterone, also known as mineralocorticoid. Aldosterone plays an important role in the normal maintenance of serum sodium and potassium and the regulation of blood pressure.

Zona Fasciculata (Fig. 15.20)

Zona fasciculata is the largest region located between the zona glomerulosa and zona reticularis. The cells in zona fasciculata are responsible for the synthesis of cortisol hormone, which is a major glucocorticoid. It plays important role in the maintenance of blood glucose during fasting state.

Zona Reticularis (Fig. 15.20)

Zona reticularis is the innermost cortical layer. Cell of zona reticularis produce androgens hormones, mainly dehydroepiandrosterone (DHEA), and androstenedione (the precursor to testosterone). These androgens also play important role in the development of male and female characteristic features like the main androgens secreted by the reproductive systems.

Adrenal Medulla (Fig. 15.20)

BAQ: Write a note on the adrenal medulla.

Ans: The adrenal medulla part is at the centre of each adrenal gland (Figs 15.21 and 15.22). It is surrounded by the adrenal cortex. The adrenal medulla secretes mainly the hormones epinephrine (adrenaline) and norepinephrine (noradrenaline). These are secreted in response to stress by the sympathetic-adrenomedullary axis. The adrenaline and noradrenaline act as hormones and neurotransmitters necessary for the maintenance of homeostasis through the autonomic nervous system.

Under the effect of the nervous impulses created by the stress, the sympathetic terminations activate the adrenal medulla to releases epinephrine and norepinephrine. This release is carried out by exocytosis, and breakage of storage vesicles in contact with the cellular membrane. Epinephrine and norepinephrine released by the adrenal medulla pass directly into the blood.

The epinephrine is associated with the conditions needed for 'fight or flight' situations; after the initial sympathetic stimulation. It acts by facilitating the following actions: Constriction of skin blood vessels, increase in metabolic rate, dilation of blood vessels of muscle, heart, and brain, and dilation of the bronchioles, to increase air intake (oxygen).

The main function of norepinephrine is to maintain blood pressure by causing general vasoconstriction (except the coronary arteries).

SAQ: What are catecholamines and their functions?

Ans: The main catecholamines are epinephrine and norepinephrine with small percentage of dopamine. These are secreated by adrenal medulla with response to stress. The catecholamines act as hormones and neurotransmitters necessary for the maintenance of homeostasis through the autonomic nervous system.

Blood Supply of and Venous Drainage of Adrenal Glands (Fig. 15.21)

BAQ: Write a note on the blood supply and venous drainage of the adrenal glands.

Ans: The following three arteries supply blood to each adrenal gland:

1. The superior suprarenal artery. It is a branch of the inferior phrenic artery.
2. The middle suprarenal artery. It is a direct branch of the abdominal aorta.
3. The inferior suprarenal artery. It is a branch of the renal artery.

These blood vessels provide a network of small arteries within the adrenal glands.

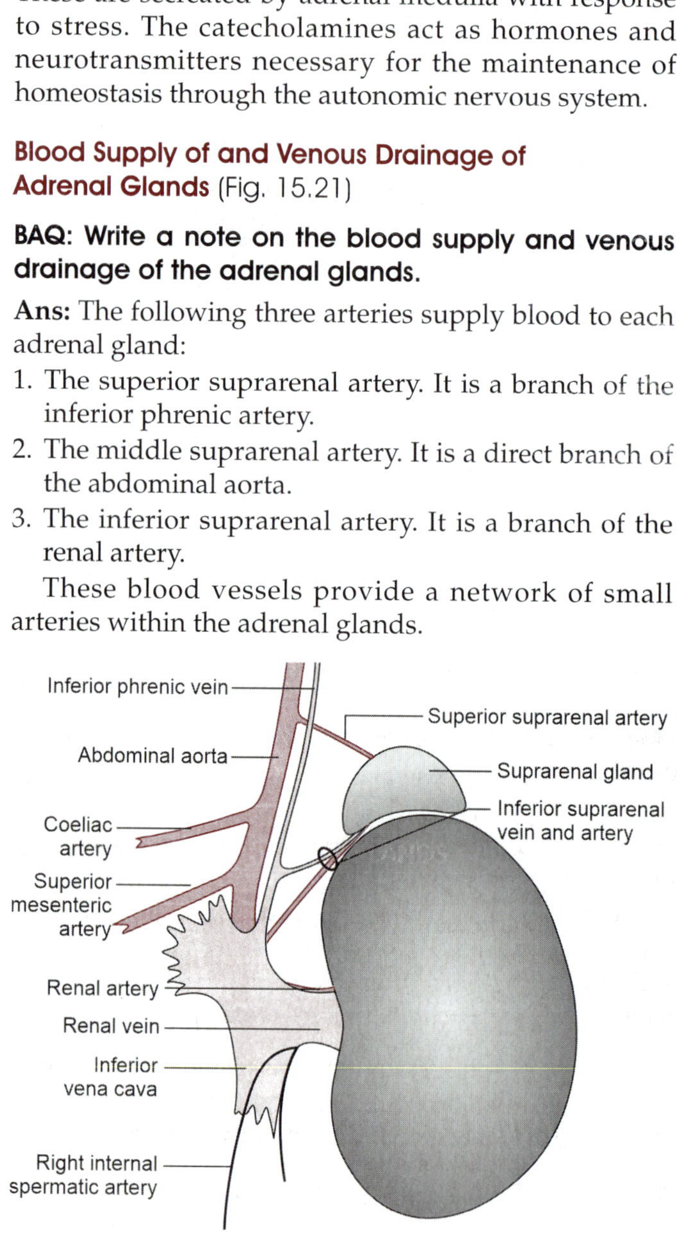

Fig. 15.21: Blood circulation of adrenal gland

Venous blood is drained from the glands by the suprarenal veins. The right suprarenal vein drains into the inferior vena cava. The left suprarenal vein drains into the left inferior phrenic vein (Fig. 15.21). The right inferior phrenic vein drains directly into the inferior vena cava, which drains into the right atrium of the heart.

Innervation of Adrenal Glands (Fig. 15.22)

SAQ: Write a note on the innervation of the adrenal glands.

Ans: The adrenal medulla is innervated by the sympathetic nervous system through preganglionic fibers originating in the thoracic spinal cord, from vertebrae T5–T11.

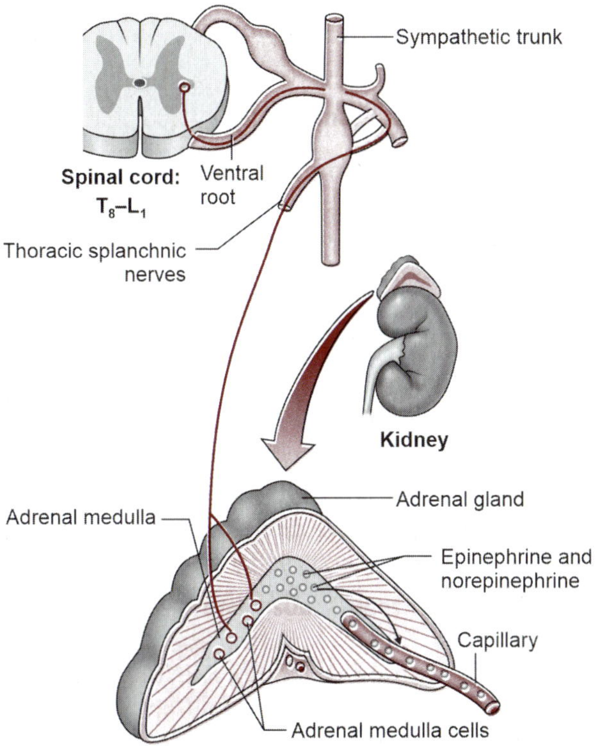

Fig. 15.22: Innervation of adrenal gland

HORMONES OF THE ADRENAL GLANDS

LAQ: Write a note on the hormones of the adrenal gland.

Ans: The hypothalamus secretes corticotropin-releasing hormone (CRH) that stimulates the pituitary gland to secrete adrenocorticotropin hormone (ACTH).

ACTH then stimulates the adrenal cortex to synthesize and release glucocorticoids, mineralocorticoids and androgens (sex hormones) into the blood circulation. Main glucocorticoids are cortisol and corticosterone.

Cortisol

The cortisol is a glucocorticoid hormone. It controls the metabolism of carbohydrates, fats, and proteins. It increases blood sugar, suppresses inflammation, regulates blood pressure and also decrease bone formation.

The cortisol also controls the circadian rhythm. It is released during stress to help cells of the body to get extra energy in the form of ATP molecules by maintaining normal blood glucose levels and by promoting the oxidation of glucose.

Excess cortisol production may take place from nodules in the adrenal gland or excess production of ACTH from a tumor in the pituitary gland.

Corticosterone

The corticosterone has very low glucocorticoid activities. It plays important role as a precursor molecule for the synthesis of mineralocorticoids.

Aldosterone (Mineralocorticoid)

The aldosterone (mineralocorticoid) hormone plays an important role in the homeostasis by the regulation of the main electrolytes; sodium and potassium and blood pressure. Aldosterone acts on kidneys and facilitate the absorption of more sodium into the bloodstream and release potassium into the urine. It plays important role in the regulation of the normal blood pH.

Androgenic Steroids

The quantities of androgens produced by the adrenal gland are very low compared to the total amount of these steroids produced by male and female sex organs.

Epinephrine (Adrenaline) and Norepinephrine (Noradrenaline)

The adrenal medulla secretes the hormones, epinephrine (adrenaline) and norepinephrine (noradrenaline). These hormones also act as neurotransmitters. These are secreted in response to stress. The adrenal medulla hormones initiate the flight or fight responses which are the physiological reactions that occur in response to a harmful event, attack, or threat to an individual for survival. Strong emotions such as anger or fear also leads to the secretion of epinephrine and norepinephrine into the bloodstream.

The epinephrine acts after the initial sympathetic stimulation in response to stress. It acts by facilitating the following actions: Constriction of skin blood vessels, increase in metabolic rate, dilation of blood vessels of muscle, heart, and brain, and dilation of the bronchioles, to increase intake of air (oxygen).

The main function of norepinephrine is to maintain blood pressure by causing general vasoconstriction (except the coronary arteries).

ADRENAL GLAND DISORDERS

Addison's Disease (Adrenal Insufficiency)

BAQ: Write a note on Addison's disease (adrenal insufficiency).

Ans: Addison's disease is a disorder in which the adrenal glands do not produce sufficient hormones (primary adrenal insufficiency). It may be caused due to adrenal gland disease. It is an example of primary adrenal insufficiency. Addison's disease also may be caused due to diseases that damage the hypothalamus or the pituitary gland (secondary adrenal insufficiency).

The primary adrenal insufficiency may cause due to the following various reasons: Autoimmune antibodies against adrenal gland, bacterial or fungal infections, cancer of adrenal gland or genetic disorders of the adrenal gland.

In Addison's disease, due to hormonal insufficiency, very low values of serum sodium, chlorides, bicarbonate and very high values of serum potassium are observed.

The symptoms of Addison's disease include; poor appetite, nausea, vomiting, fatigue, weight loss, darkening of skin (in primary condition), abdominal pain, etc.

Cushing's Disease (Syndrome)

BAQ: Write a note on Cushing's disease (syndrome).

Ans: Cushing disease (syndrome) is primarily caused by adrenal adenoma, which secrete excessive amounts of adrenal hormones. Similarly, secondary cause of Cushing's disease is due to adenomas or excess growth (hyperplasia) of the pituitary gland. The adenomas, secrete excessive ACTH, which in turn stimulates adrenal cortex to secrete excessive amounts of adrenal hormones. Small cell lung tumors also secrete excessive ACTH secretions, which stimulate the adrenal gland to secret high levels of adrenal hormones.

The specific feature of Cushing's disease is high levels of circulating adrenal hormones, leading to very high levels of serum sodium and chlorides and very low levels of serum potassium.

The following are the specific symptoms of Cushing's disease: Appearance of round face, central obesity, muscle weakness, excessive hair growth (hirsutism) on face, chest, abdomen and thighs, generalized weakness, blur vision, decreased fertility, hypertension, poor wound healing, increase in blood sugar, severe depression and extreme mood swings.

Conn's Syndrome

BAQ: Write a note on Conn's syndrome.

Ans: Conn's syndrome (primary hyperaldosteronism) is caused due to adrenal tumors, which secret excessive amounts of aldosterone (mineralocorticoid) hormone. Very high levels of aldosterone lead to very high levels of serum sodium and chlorides and very low levels of serum potassium with increase in rennin.

The symptoms associated with Conn's syndrome are: Increase in blood pressure, muscle weakness, anxiety, fatigue, headache, depression with low serum potassium values.

In secondary hyperaldosteronism, various events such as sudden blood loss, decreased blood flow to the kidneys, due to congestive heart failure, severe liver disease, etc., lead to increase in renin hormone. Increased renin initiates increase in angiotensin I and angiotensin II and increase production of aldosterone by the adrenal glands. This results in the retention of water and sodium, an increase in extracellular volume, and a decrease in serum potassium.

Congenital Adrenal Hyperplasia

SAQ: What is congenital adrenal hyperplacia?

Ans: Adrenal insufficiency may result from congenital adrenal hyperplasia (a genetic disorder). Adrenal cortex in children born with this disease is unable to produce cortisol and (or) aldosterone. Affected children may experience excess secretions of androgens, which may lead to male characteristics in girls and early puberty in boys.

Pheochromocytoma

SAQ: Write a note on pheochromocytoma.

Ans: Pheochromocytoma is caused due to a rare tumor of the chromaffin cells of the adrenal medulla. The symptoms of pheochromocytoma are headache, hypertension, heart palpitations, excessive sweating, tremors, etc. Nearly ninety percent of patients suffering from pheochromocytoma can be cured by the removal of the tumors by surgery.

PINEAL GLAND (Fig. 15.23)

SAQ: Describe the pineal gland under the following heads: (1) Introduction and functions (2) applied anatomy, (3) blood supply and (4) nerve supply.

Ans:

1. **Introduction and functions:** The pineal gland is situated in the middle of the brain. It has size similar to a rice-grain (Fig. 15.23). The pineal gland is reddish-grey coloured gland. It controls circadian rhythm. It secrets melatonin hormone which modulates sleep patterns in both circadian and seasonal cycles.

Anatomy of the Pineal Gland

2. **Applied anatomy:** The pineal gland consists of a functional tissue (lobular parenchyma) mostly made up of specific cells known as pinealocytes. These cells are surrounded by connective tissue spaces. The surface of pineal gland is covered by a capsule. The primary function of the pinealocytes is secretion of the melatonin, which plays important role in the regulation of circadian rhythms.
3. **Blood supply of pineal gland:** Blood is supplied to pineal gland from the choroidal branches of the posterior cerebral artery.
4. **Nerve supply of pineal gland:** The pineal gland receives a sympathetic nerves from the superior cervical ganglion. Parasympathetic nerves from the pterygopalatine and otic ganglia are also present in the pineal gland.

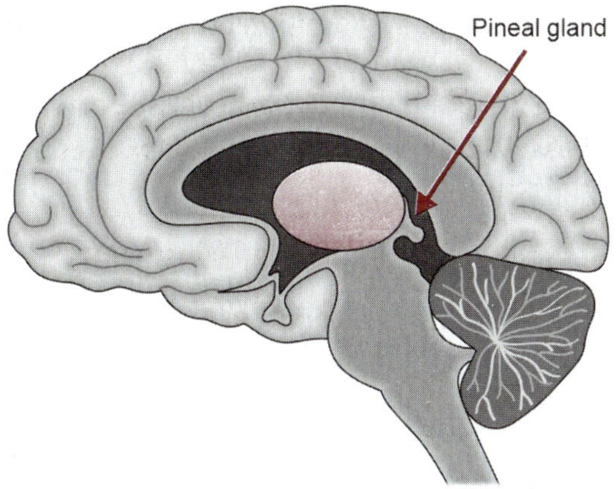

Fig. 15.23: Pineal gland

Ans:

Hormones of the Reproductive System

Refer to Chapter 14, pages 308, 309, 319, 320, 321, 325.

Hormones of the Gastrointestinal Tract

Refer to Chapter 12, page 279.

BAQ: Write a note on testosterone.

Ans: Testosterone is a steroid hormone. It is primarily secreted in the testes of males and the ovaries of females. Small amounts of testosterone are also secreted by the adrenal glands. It is the principal male sex hormone and an anabolic steroid. LH stimulates testosterone production by binding to the receptors on the plasma membrane of Leydig cells of the testes. The testosterone is produced in greater amounts by males, and less by females.

Testosterone stimulates and controls the development and maintenance of male characteristics by binding to androgen receptors. It maintains the activity of the accessory male sex organs and the development of male secondary sex characteristics. Spermatogenesis is regulated by FSH and testosterone.

BAQ: Write a note on estrogens.

Ans: In the ovaries, follicle-stimulating hormone (FSH) and luteinizing hormone (LH) stimulate the production of estrogen. The three major naturally occurring estrogens in women are estrone (E1), estradiol (E2), and estriol (E3). The predominant form is estradiol (E2) in nonpregnant females.

Estrogens are present in both men and women. They are usually present at significantly higher levels in women of reproductive age. They promote the development of female secondary sexual characteristics, such as breasts, and are also involved in the thickening of the endometrium and regulating the menstrual cycle. In males, estrogen regulates the maturation of sperm and necessary for a healthy libido. Estrogens are also responsible for reducing muscle mass, increase vaginal lubrication, increase bone formation, and increase platelet adhesiveness.

Objective: To understand and explain the central theme of competency based medical and paramedical education (CBME): Horizontal and vertical integration of subjects.

BAQ: Show horizontal integration of physiology, biochemistry and nutrition with the following anatomical change: Enlarged thyroid gland (goiter).

Ans:

Horizontal Integration with Physiology

Decrease in the blood circulation of thyroid hormones (T_3, T_4). Decrease in basal metabolic rate (BMR)

Horizontal Integration with Biochemistry

Decrease in the synthesis of thyroid hormones and related decreased metabolism of lipids, carbohydrates, proteins and oxidative pathways.

Horizontal Integration with Nutrition

Suggestion of diet and salt to meet required RDA of iodine (if iodine deficiency is suspected).

BAQ: Show horizontal integration of physiology, and Biochemistry with the following anatomical change: Nodular growth in the thyroid gland (thyrotoxicosis).

Ans:

Horizontal Integration with Physiology

Increase in the blood circulation of T_3 and T_4 and basal metabolic rate (BMR).

Horizontal Integration with Biochemistry

Increased synthesis of thyroid hormones and related increased metabolism of lipids, carbohydrates, proteins and oxidative pathways.

BAQ: Show horizontal integration of physiology and biochemistry with the following anatomical change: Damaged adrenal gland.

Ans:

Horizontal Integration with Physiology

Decrease in the blood circulation of adrenal hormones.

Horizontal Integration with Biochemistry

Decrease in serum sodium and chlorides and increase in serum potassium, due to deficiency of mineralocorticoids secreted by the adrenal gland.

BIBLIOGRAPHY

1. Medical Biochemistry, 1st Edition (2023). Godkar PB, Godkar DP, CBS Publishers, New Delhi, India.
2. Text book of Medical Laboratory Technology, 4th Edition, (2024). Godkar PB, Godkar DP, Bhalani Publishing House, Mumbai, India.
3. Anatomy of the Human Body. 42nd Edition. Henry Gray, Editor-in-chief: Susan Standring, Elsevier (2020).
4. Ross and Wilson Anatomy and Physiology in Health and Illness, 13th Edition, by Allison Wynn Grant, Anne Waugh, and Kathleen J. W. Wilson (2018).
5. Schaum's Outline of Theory and Problems of Human Anatomy and Physiology, 2nd Edition (1997), Tata MaGraw-Hill Publishing Company Limited, New Delhi, India.

MULTIPLE CHOICE QUESTIONS (MCQs)

Select the correct option.

1. **The hypothalamus does not control this process in the body:**
   (A) Mood (B) Hunger
   (C) Sexual functions (D) Thinking
2. **The following statement regarding the hypothalamus is not correct:**
   (A) The hypothalamus has two main regions.
   (B) One of the hormones secreted by the anterior region of hypothalamus is oxytocin.
   (C) Each hypothalamic region contains different nuclei.
   (D) The nuclei are clusters of neurons that stimulate release of specific hormones.
3. **The following statement regarding the hypothalamus is not correct:**
   (A) The posterior region nuclei are, the posterior hypothalamic nucleus and the mammillary nuclei
   (B) The posterior hypothalamic nucleus plays important role in the regulation of body temperature
   (C) The role of the mammillary nuclei is involved in the control of glucose metabolism
   (D) The damage to the mammillary bodies results in the loss of memory (amnesia)
4. **One of the following statements is not correct:**
   (A) The pituitary gland can be divided into two different parts
   (B) The anterior lobe of the pituitary gland can be divided into the pars tuberalis and pars distalis
   (C) Anterior lobe constitutes about 20% of the pituitary gland
   (D) The anterior pituitary contains several different types of cells
5. **The following two hormones are synthesized in the hypothalamus and released in the posterior pituitary:**
   (A) LH and FSH
   (B) ADH and oxytocin
   (C) TSH and T4
   (D) T_3 and T_4
6. **One of the following statements is not correct regarding the thyroid gland:**
   (A) It is located under the laryngeal prominence (Adam's apple)
   (B) In adults, it weighs about 25 grams
   (C) The two lobes of the thyroid gland are connected by a bridge of tissues called the isthmus
   (D) The gland is usually larger in men than in women
7. **The following are the primary microscopic features of the thyroid gland:**
   (A) Follicles (B) Follicular cells
   (C) Parafollicular cells (D) All of the above
8. **This part (or these parts) of the thyroid gland contains iodine:**
   (A) Follicles (B) Follicular cells
   (C) Parafollicular cells (D) Both (A) and (B)
9. **T_3 and T_4 are secreted by:**
   (A) Follicles (B) Follicular cells
   (C) Parafollicular cells (D) Both (A) and (B)
10. **Calcitonin is secreted by:**
    (A) Follicles (B) Follicular cells
    (C) Parafollicular cells (D) Both (A) and (B)
11. **One of the following sentences only is correct:**
    (A) Thyroid follicles are very large spherical groups of cells
    (B) The follicles consist of a rim that does not have supply of blood and lymphatics
    (C) The rim is surrounded by a specific colloidal space consisting mainly, the thyroglobulin protein
    (D) Thyroglobulin mainly contains zinc
12. **Following is the main underlying cause of simple goiter:**
    (A) Persistent iodine deficiency
    (B) Adrenal adenoma
    (C) Thyroid cancer
    (D) Zinc deficiency
13. **Toxic goiter is caused due to:**
    (A) High levels of T_3 and T_4
    (B) High levels of calcitonin
    (C) Autoantibodies against the TSH receptors
    (D) Both (A) and (C)
14. **These cells of parathyroid gland secretes parathyroid hormones:**
    (A) Oxyphil cells (B) Chief cells
    (C) Alpha cells (D) Beta cells
15. **Aldosterone plays an important role in the normal maintenance of serum:**
    (A) Calcium and inorganic phosphorus
    (B) Sodium and potassium
    (C) Chlorides and bicarbonate
    (D) Both (B) and (C)
16. **Excess cortisol production may take place from:**
    (A) Nodules in the adrenal gland
    (B) Excess production of ACTH from a tumor in the pituitary gland.
    (C) Increased mass of thyroid gland
    (D) Both (A) and (B)
17. **One of the following statements related to the hormones is *not* correct:**
    (A) Hormones act as catalysts
    (B) Hormones are chemical messengers
    (C) Hormones are secreted by endocrine glands
    (D) Hormones act only at a site, where they are synthesized

18. Following is one hormone that binds to intracellular receptor:

(A) Thyroxine (B) LH
(C) FSH (D) Glucagon

19. The hormone that binds to cell surface receptor and requires the second messenger action is:

(A) Thyroxine (B) Estrogen
(C) FSH (D) Glucocorticoids

20. Following is a hormone secreted from anterior pituitary:

(A) Glucagon (B) Epinephrine
(C) Oxytocin (D) Growth hormone

21. This hormone is secreted from posterior pituitary gland:

(A) Oxytocin (B) LH
(C) Prolactin (D) Renin

22. Acromegaly results due to excessive release of:

(A) GH (B) ACTH
(C) Thyroxine (D) Glucagon

23. ACTH stimulates the secretion of:

(A) Thyroxine (B) Luteinizing hormone
(C) Glucocorticoids (D) Epinephrine

24. Excessive secretion of ACTH causes:

(A) Addison's disease (B) Myxedema
(C) Cushing's syndrome (D) Thyrotoxicosis

25. Cushing's syndrome leads to:

(A) Excessive cortisol secretion
(B) Excessive thyroxine secretion
(C) Decreased epinephrine secretion
(D) Decreased cortisol secretion

26. All steroid hormones are formed from:

(A) Cholesterol (B) Pyrimidine
(C) Glycerol (D) Purine

27. The significant effect of aldosterone is to:

(A) Decrease the renal reabsorption of sodium
(B) Decrease the reabsorption of chloride
(C) Decrease the rate of tubular reabsorption of potassium
(D) Increase the rate of tubular reabsorption of sodium

28. Following one is the potent stimulator of aldosterone secretion:

(A) Increased potassium concentration
(B) Increased sodium concentration
(C) Decreased potassium concentration
(D) Increased ECF volume

29. Release of aldosterone is stimulated by:

(A) Renin (B) Insulin
(C) Thyroxine (D) Angiotensin II

30. Catecholamine hormones are synthesized in the:

(A) Zona fasciculata of adrenal cortex
(B) Chromaffin cells of adrenal medulla
(C) Zona glomerulosa of adrenal cortex
(D) Zona reticularis of adrenal cortex

31. Following is the hormone required for uterine muscle contraction for childbirth:

(A) Estrogen (B) Progesterone
(C) ADH (D) Oxytocin

32. Action of antidiuretic hormone (ADH) leads to:

(A) Reabsorption of potassium from renal tubules
(B) Excretion of hypotonic urine
(C) Absorption of water from renal tubules
(D) Decrease specific gravity urine

33. An increase in the osmolality of extracellular compartment will lead to:

(A) Stimulation of ADH secretion
(B) Stimulation of oxytocin secretion
(C) Inhibition of ADH secretion
(D) stimulation of secretion of thyroxine

34. Action of parathyroid hormone leads to:

(A) Absorption of calcium at the tubular level
(B) Increase in urinary excretion of phosphates
(C) Increase in absorption of phosphates
(D) Both (A) and (B)

35. Action of calcitonin causes:

(A) Urinary excretion of sodium
(B) Increase in urinary calcium
(C) Urinary excretion of calcium and inorganic phosphorus
(D) Increase in urine potassium

36. Following is the characteristic feature of hyper-parathyroidism:

(A) Low serum phosphorus
(B) High serum phosphorus
(C) High serum calcium
(D) Both (A) and (C)

37. Beta cells of islet of Langerhans of pancreas produce:

(A) Insulin (B) Somatostatin
(C) Thyroxine (D) Glucagon

38. The alpha cells of pancreas islets produce:

(A) Somatostatin (B) Glucagon
(C) Insulin (D) lipase

39. The production of progesterone by corpus luteum cell is stimulated by:

(A) T_3 (B) LH
(C) ACTH (D) TSH

40. Melatonin is synthesized in:

(A) Anterior pituitary gland
(B) Hypothalamus
(C) Adrenal cortex
(D) Pineal gland

41. Melatonin is synthesized from:

(A) Tryptophan (B) Phenylalanine
(C) Valine (D) None of these

42. Posterior pituitary gland secretes following hormone:

(A) TRH (B) LH
(C) Follicle stimulating hormone (D) Oxytocin

43. Diabetes insipidus is caused by the deficiency of:

(A) Insulin (B) T_4
(C) ADH (D) Glucagon

44. Regulation of ACTH secretion occurs by:

(A) Corticotropin releasing hormone
(B) Feedback inhibition by cortisol
(C) CRH
(D) Both (A) and (B)

45. In males, luteinising hormone acts on:

(A) Sertoli cells (B) Prostate gland
(C) Leydig cells (D) All of these

46. All the following statements about FSH are true, *except*:

(A) It increases the synthesis of testosterone
(B) Its secretion is increased by gonadotropin releasing hormone
(C) It is secreted by anterior pituitary
(D) It acts on Sertoli cells

47. In males, secretion of luteinising hormone is inhibited by:

(A) Thyroxine
(B) High blood level of testosterone
(C) FSH
(D) ACTH

48. Secretion of luteinising hormone is increased by:

(A) hCG (B) Testosterone
(C) FSH (D) GnRH

49. Overproduction of growth hormone during childhood causes:

(A) Addison's disease (B) Myxedema
(C) Acromegaly (D) Gigantism

50. Decreased secretion of growth hormone during childhood causes:

(A) Dwarfism (B) Cushing's disease
(C) Acromegaly (D) Wilson's disease

51. PTH causes all of the following, *except*:

(A) Increased intestinal absorption of phosphate
(B) Increased tubular reabsorption of phosphate
(C) Increased tubular reabsorption of calcium
(D) Increased intestinal absorption of calcium

52. Steroid hormones are synthesized from:

(A) Calcitriol (B) Cholesterol
(C) DOPA (D) 7-Hydroxycholesterol

53. Mineralocorticoids regulate the metabolism of all of the following, *except*:

(A) Sodium (B) Potassium
(C) Calcium (D) Chloride

54. Mineralocorticoids increase the tubular reabsorption of:

(A) Potassium (B) Sodium
(C) Chloride (D) Both (B) and (C)

55. The major source of progesterone during late pregnancy is:

(A) Corpus luteum (B) Graafian follicles
(C) Adrenal cortex (D) Placenta

56. Women become susceptible to osteoporosis after menopause due to the decrease in:

(A) hCG
(B) Secretion of estrogen
(C) Secretion of LH
(D) Secretion of progesterone
(E) Both (C) and (D)

57. Placenta secretes all of the following, *except*:

(A) hCG (B) Estrogen
(C) Progesterone (D) FSH

ANSWERS

1. D 2. A 3. C 4. C 5. B 6. D 7. D
8. D 9. B 10. C 11. C 12. A 13. D 14. B
15. B 16. D 17. D 18. A 19. C 20. D 21. A
22. A 23. C 24. C 25. A 26. A 27. D 28. A
29. D 30. B 31. D 32. C 33. A 34. D 35. C
36. D 37. A 38. B 39. B 40. D 41. A 42. D
43. C 44. D 45. C 46. A 47. B 48. D 49. D
50. A 51. A 52. B 53. C 54. D 55. B 56. B
57.D

MATCH THE COLUMNS

I	II
1. Pheochromocytoma	A. Very high levels of GH
2. Diabetes insipidus	B. Very high serum T_3, T_4
3. Diabetes mellitus	C. Pituitary adenomas
4. Acromegali	D. Overproduction of aldosterone
5. Tetany	E. Adrenal medulla chromaffin cell tumors
6. Graves disease	F. Very low adrenocorticosteroids
7. Hashimoto's disease	G. Hyperglycemia
8. Addison's disease	H. Very low serum calcium
9. Cushing's syndrome	I. Very low T_3, T_4
10. Conn's disease	J. Deficiency of ADH

ANSWERS

1. E 2. J 3. G 4. A 5. H 6. B 7. I
8. F 9. C 10. D

CHAPTER

16

Practicals

SAQ: Short answer question: Marks: 2
BAQ: Brief answer question: Marks: 4 or 5
LAQ: Long answer question: Marks: 9 or 10
MCQs: Multiple choice questions: Marks: 0.5 each
Match the columns: Marks: 0.5 each
Draw a labelled diagram: Marks: 5

Note: All the SAQs could be used in the theory examination as well as in practical examination for table viva voce purposes.

COMPOUND MICROSCOPE (Fig. 16.1)

EXPERIMENT 1: Study of a compound microscope.

Introduction

A microscope is used to produce an enlarged and well-defined images of objects. The degree of enlargement is called magnification or magnifying power of the microscope, and it is expressed as the number of times the length, breadth (or diameter) of the object is multiplied. Micro means small and scope means to view.

The light microscope is operated by using the white light of the sun or the light obtained from a tungsten lamp. The laboratory microscope provides a magnification of X40 (scanner), X100 (low power), X400 (high power), and X1000 (oil immersion). The total magnification is obtained by multiplying the magnification of the objective with that of the eyepiece.

Components (Fig. 16.1)

1. Supporting system: It consists of—

a. Foot
b. Limb
c. Revolving nosepiece (objective changer)
d. Stage
e. Mechanical stage (this component gives controlled movement to the object on the slide)

2. Magnification system: It consists of—

The lenses of the microscope. These are mounted in the following two groups (one at each end of the body tube):

a. *Eyepiece:* Here, the microscopist applies his eye.
b. *Objectives:* These are just above the preparation (object) under examination.

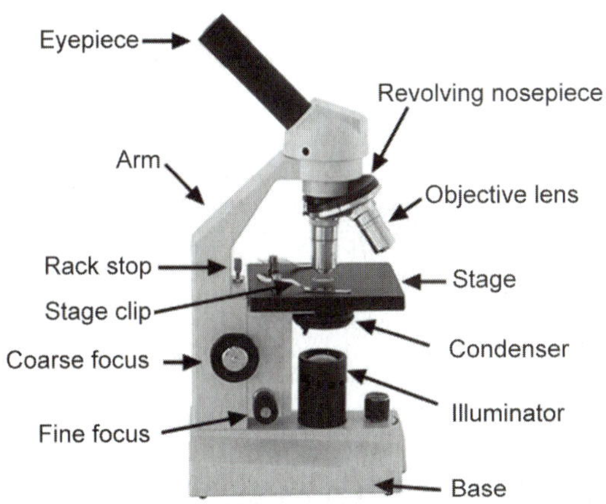

Fig. 16.1A: Monocular microscope

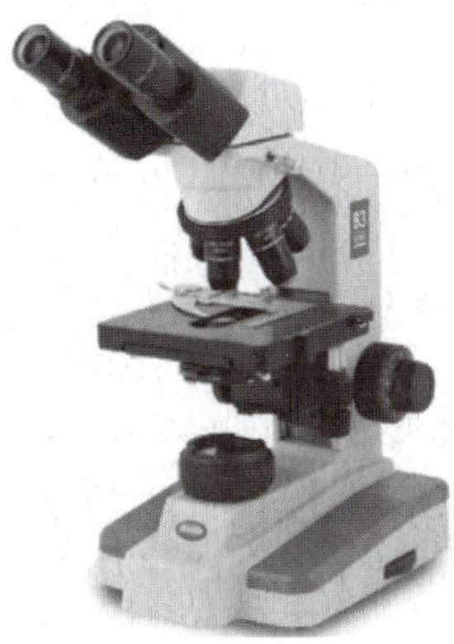

Fig. 16.1B: Binocular microscope

A. Eyepiece (Fig. 16.1)

It is made up of two lenses, the upper eye lens, and the lower field lens. The magnifying power of the eyepiece is marked on it, and the magnification of the image produced is as shown below:

Magnifying power	*Magnification*
X5	5 times
X10	10 times

> ***Note:*** To calculate the total magnification of the object observed, multiply the magnification power of the objective by that of the eyepiece.

Example:

Magnifying power

Objective	*Eyepiece*	*Total magnification*
X40	X5	200
X100	X10	1000

B. Objectives (Fig. 16.2)

- The magnifying power of each objective is shown by a figure engraved on the sleeve of the lens as follows:

Magnifying power	*Magnification*
X10	10 times
X40	40 times
X100	100 times

The third objective (with magnifying power: X100) is called oil immersion objective.

It is marked with a red ring. It must be used with immersion oil.

- The numerical aperture (NA) is also engraved on the sleeve, next to the magnification, e.g.:

NA	*Objective*
0.30	X10
0.65	X40
1.30	X100

Note:

- The greater the NA, the greater the resolving power.
- The recommended length between the objective and the eyepiece is usually 160 mm.
- The recommended thickness of a coverslip = 0.17 mm

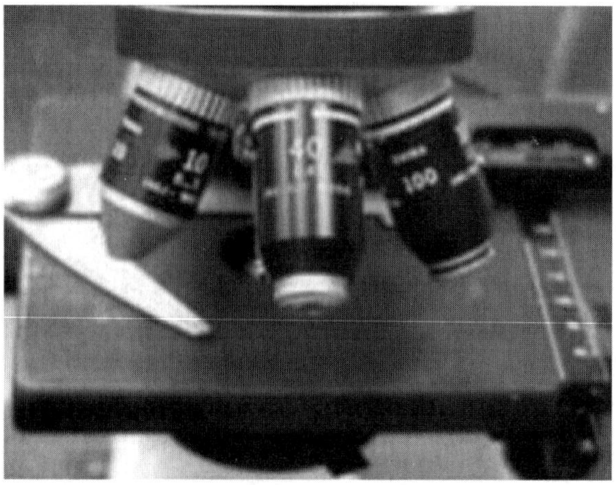

Fig. 16.2: Various objective lenses of a microscope

- Usually, the distance between the front lens of the objective and the object slide (when the image is in focus) is as follows:

Objectives	*Working distance*
X10	5.0–6.0 mm
X40	0.5–1.5 mm
X100	1.5–0.20 mm

- Resolving power

The maximum resolving power of a good medical laboratory microscope is about 0.25 µm. The greater the resolving power of the objective, the clearer the image.

> ***Note:*** The oil immersion objective increases the resolving power by conserving many light rays that would be lost by refraction if a dry objective was used.

3. Illumination System

- **Source of light:**
  a. *Daylight:* The microscope should not be placed in direct sunlight. It should be kept on a table near a window. Light is adjusted by a concave mirror and by the diaphragm (Fig. 16.1).
  b. *Electric light:* It is provided by a lamp built into the microscope beneath the stage. An external lamp also can be used.
- **Mirror:** The mirror reflects rays from the light source onto the object. One side has a concave surface, and the other a plane mirror. In the absence of a condenser, the concave surface of the mirror should be used since the concave surface forms a low-power condenser. In the presence of a condenser, the plain surface of the mirror should be used.
- **Condenser:** It is situated between the mirror and the stage. For maximum illumination, it is raised, and for minimum illumination, it is lowered. The function of the condenser is to bring the rays of light to a common focus on the object to be examined (Fig. 16.2).
- **Diaphragm:** It is within the condenser. It is used to reduce or increase the amount of light by reducing or increasing the angle and, therefore, also the amount of light that passes into the condenser.
- **Filters:** In some microscopes, these are fitted below the condenser. These can be left in place or removed according to the type of object preparation being examined.
- **Adjustment system:** This system is comprised of the following components:
  a. Coarse adjustment screw: It is used to achieve an approximate focus.
  b. Fine adjustment screw: It is used to bring the object into perfect focus. It moves the objective very slowly.
  c. Condenser adjustment screw: This is to adjust the condenser.

d. Condenser centering screws: There are about three screws that are used to center the condenser exactly in relation to the objective.

e. Iris diaphragm lever: This is a small lever fixed on the condenser. It is used to close or open the diaphragm.

f. Mechanical stage controls: Mechanical stage is controlled by two screws. One screw is meant to move it backward and forward and the second screw is meant to move it left or right.

SETTING UP OF THE MICROSCOPE

Position of the Microscope

1. It should be placed on a firm level bench on a square felt pad or on a piece of heavy cloth. The ideal height of the platform is 2′8″.
2. If daylight is to be used, the bench should be placed near the window.
3. If electric illumination is to be used, place the microscope away from the window.

Fitting the Accessories

1. Screw the objectives into the revolving nosepiece in a clockwise direction.
2. Put the eyepiece(s) in place.
3. Fix the condenser under the stage.
4. Fix the mirror on foot.

Positioning the Lamp

(if electrical illumination is to be used)

1. Place the lamp about 20 centimeters in front of the microscope, facing the mirror.
2. Fix the angle of the mirror at about 45°.

Preliminary Adjustment of the Mirror

1. Use the plain side of the mirror.
2. Open the iris diaphragm to the maximum.
3. Raise the condenser.
4. Place a piece of thin white paper on top of the condenser.
5. Adjust the mirror to get the image of the bulb in the exact center of the circle of light.

Centring the Condenser

1. Place a slide preparation on the stage.
2. Lower the condenser and open the iris diaphragm.
3. Examine through the eyepiece; examine with the lowest power objective. Bring the object into focus.
4. Close the diaphragm and raise the condenser slowly until the edges of the circle of the light ring are in sharp focus.
5. Adjust the position of the mirror (if necessary) so that the circle of light is in the exact center of the bright area surrounded by the dark zone.
6. Adjust the centering screws of the condenser accordingly.

Adjustment of the Diaphragm

1. Open the diaphragm completely.
2. Remove the eyepiece and look down the tube.
3. Close the diaphragm slowly until the circle of light on the objective takes up only two-thirds of the surface.
4. Repeat this procedure for each objective.

Adjustment of Eyepieces

1. First, select the eyepiece (X5 or X6)
2. If binocular is used, the distance between the pupils should be adjusted as follows.
3. One of the eyepiece holders has a focusing collar.
4. If the collar is on the left-hand side, then by using the X40 objective, bring the image into focus for the right eye with the right eyepiece.
5. Close the right eye and look through the left eyepiece. If the image is in focus, adjustment is not necessary. If an image is unclear, turn the focusing collar until it is in focus. The microscope is now adjusted for binocular vision.

Focussing the Object (Fig. 16.3)

- **Use of low power objective (X5 or X10)**
  1. Adjust the condenser to the lowest position.
  2. Lower the objective until it is just above the slide preparation.
  3. Raise the objective by using the coarse adjustment screw until a clear image is seen in the eyepiece.
- **Use of high power objective (X40)**
  1. Adjust the condenser about halfway down.
  2. When the object is already adjusted on a low-power objective, by using coarse adjustment, raise the objective very slowly until a blurred image appears on the field.
  3. Bring the image into focus using the fine adjustment. Raise the condenser for sufficient illumination.
- **Use of oil immersion objective (X100)**
  1. Adjust the condenser to the uppermost position. Open the iris diaphragm fully.

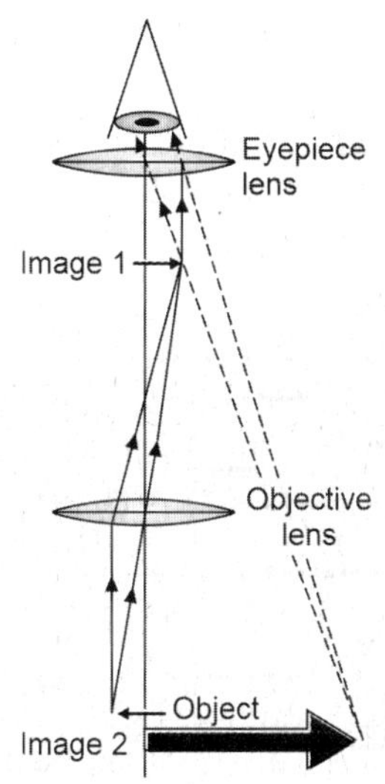

Fig. 16.3: Magnification of the image of an object by a microscope

2. Place a tiny drop of immersion oil on the dry, stained preparation of the slide.
3. Lower the objective until it is in contact with the oil.

> ***Note:*** It is necessary to avoid pressure on the preparation to prevent the breakage of the slide. Look through the eyepiece and turn the fine adjustment very slowly upwards until the image is in focus.

SAQ: What are the magnifying powers of low power, high power and oil immersion lenses?

Ans: Refer to the components of Experiment No. 1.

Care and Maintenance of the Microscope

- Requirements
  1. Clean a fine piece of linen cloth
  2. White absorbent tissue paper
  3. Xylene
  4. Soft cloth
  5. Petroleum jelly
  6. Plastic cover
  7. A fine paintbrush
- Cleaning the objectives
  1. Dry objectives
     Wipe the objectives by using a soft cloth by moving the cloth across (and not circularly).
  2. Oil immersion objectives
     a. Remove the oil with absorbent paper or a dry piece of cloth.
     b. Moisten the cloth with xylene and wipe the lens carefully.
     c. Wipe again with a dry piece of cloth.

Care and Maintenance

At the end of the microscopic examination, remove dust particles by using a fine paintbrush.

- Cleaning the eyepieces
  1. Clean the upper surface of the eyepiece (eye contact) with a soft cloth (or tissue paper).
  2. Clean the lower surface of the eyepiece (inside the microscope tube) with a fine paintbrush.
- Cleaning the condenser and mirror.
  1. The condenser is cleaned with a soft cloth moistened with xylene.
  2. The mirror is cleaned with a soft cloth moistened with alcohol.
- Cleaning the support and the stage
  1. Clean with chamois leather or a soft piece of cloth (xylene should not be used, which may remove the black paint).
  2. The stage can be cleaned thoroughly well by using a piece of cloth impregnated with petroleum jelly.

Precautions

1. Cedarwood oil is widely used when the microscopic examination is carried out under an oil immersion lens; since the refractive index of cedarwood oil is the same as that of glass, i.e. 1.515. This oil dries and cakes in its container on the objective and the condenser. Hence, the oil should be carefully and completely wiped off the objective after use. The oil should not get on the X40 high dry objective.
2. Paraffin oil or mineral oil should not be preferred since its refractive index is not correct, and it often penetrates inside the objective.
3. Never touch the lenses, and never leave a slide on the microscope when it is not in use.
4. When the microscope is not in use, put the low-power objective in the focussing position and keep it covered.

EXPERIMENT 2A: Use of low and high power objectives of a microscope (Fig. 16.4).

Requirements:

1. A urine specimen containing pus cells, epithelial cells, bacteria, and yeast cells, etc.
2. Microscope slides and coverslips
3. Centrifuge tubes
4. Centrifuge
5. Microscope

Procedure:

1. Centrifuge the urine. Decant supernatant.
2. Put a small drop of the sediment on a glass slide and place a coverslip over it (avoid air bubbles between the coverslip preparation and slide).
3. Observe it under low power objective.
4. Observe under high power objective and note down the observations (Fig. 16.4).

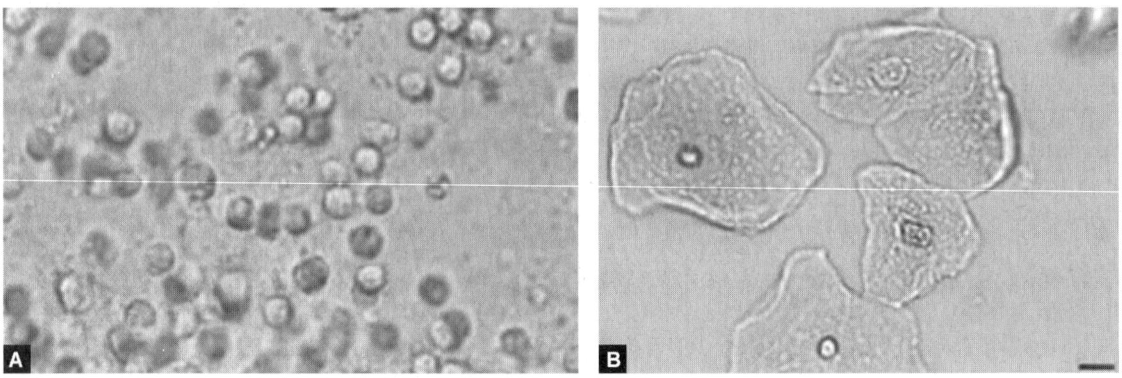

Figs 16.4A, B: (A) Pus cells (X400), (B) epithelial cells (X400)

5. Observations: Large number of pus cells per high power field (HPF) (Fig. 16.4A). About 4–5 epithelial cells per HPF (Fig. 16.4B).

EXPERIMENT 2B: Use of oil immersion objective of a microscope (Fig. 16.5).

Requirements:

1. Gram-stained smear containing
    a. Gram negative bacilli and cocci
    b. Gram positive bacilli
2. Cedarwood oil
3. Microscope

Procedure:

1. Place a small drop of cedar wood oil on the stained smear.
2. Observe the stained smears under an oil immersion lens and write the observations.
3. *Observations:* Gram-positive bacteria appear purple in colour. Gram-negative bacteria appear red in colour.

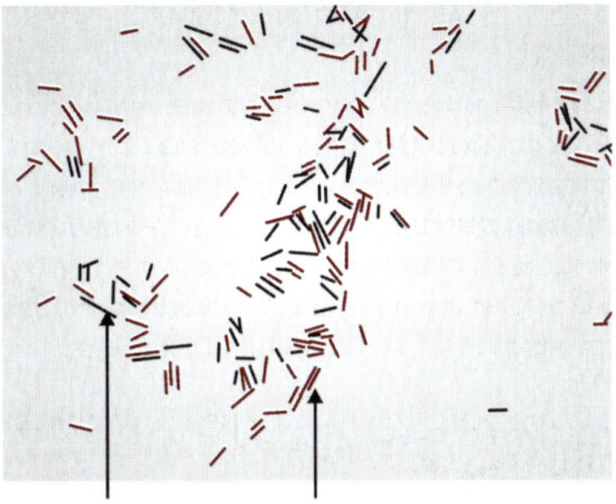

Fig. 16.5: Gram stained observations under oil immersion lens

SAQ: Describe care and maintenance of a microscope.

Ans: Refer to page 358 for care and maintenance of a microscope.

EXPERIMENT 3: Microscopic study of epithelial and nervous tissue.

Refer Chapter 2, Page 33–43 for description of various tissues.

Results of stained tissue sections (staining by hematoxylin and eosin staining method).

1. Cell nuclei: Blue colour.
2. Erythrocytes: Red colour.
3. Muscle, connective tissue, cytoplasm: Varying shades of pink.

Microscopic Observation of Stained Epithelial Tissue (Figs 16.6 and 16.7)

Under a microscope, epithelial cells are distinguished by the following features:

1. The cells have the three basic cell shapes: Squamous, cuboidal, or columnar.
2. The cells are seen closely attached to one another, in either a single layer or in multiple layers. No extracellular material is seen between the attached cells.
3. The epithelial layer on one side face an empty space (or, it will face a secreted substance like mucus) and on the other side may be attached to connective tissue proper (Fig. 16.7).

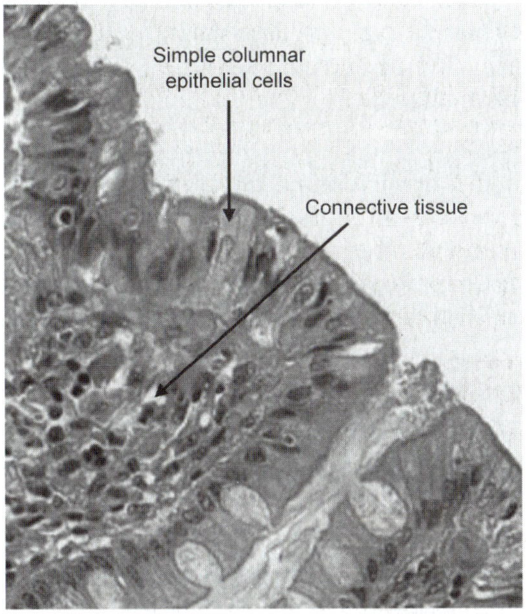

Fig. 16.6A: Simple columnar epithelial tissue

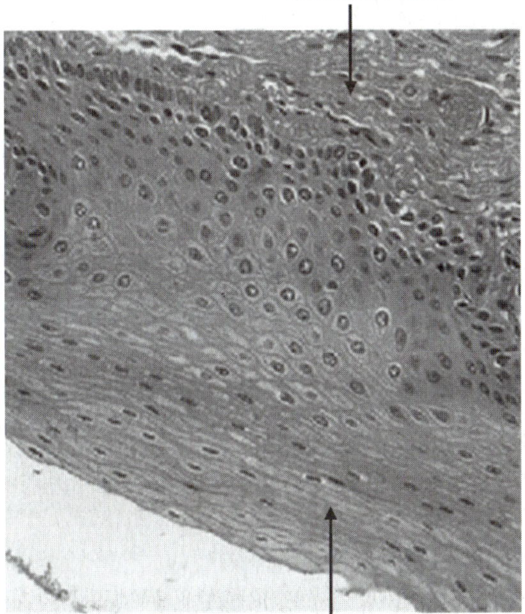

Fig. 16.6B: Stratified squamous epithelial cells

AREOLAR CONNECTIVE TISSUE (Fig. 16.8)

Areolar connective tissue is the most widespread connective tissue of the body. It is present under the skin as subcutaneous tissue in between and around muscles, blood vessels, and nerves. These are also present in bone marrow, submucosa of gastrointestinal tract and respiratory tract.

Microscopic Observation of Areolar Connective Tissue (Figs 16.7A–C)

The fibres of areolar connective tissue are not arranged in a particular pattern. These run in all directions and form a loose network in the intercellular material. Collagen fibres are predominant in this tissue. Collagen fibers usually appear as broad pink bands. Elastic fibres, appear as thin, dark fibres. The mast cells are visible. They have course, dark staining granules in their cytoplasm. The nucleus of mast cells is small, oval and with light staining.

Microscopic Observation of Skeletal Muscle (Fig. 16.7D)

Under the light microscope, muscle cells appear striated with many nuclei squeezed along the membranes. Skeletal muscles are long and cylindrical in appearance. The striations are caused by the regular arrangement of contractile proteins (actin and myosin).

Microscopic Observation of Stained Nervous Tissue (Fig. 16.8)

The cytoplasm of cells is acidophilic and is stained red, and the nuclei and nucleoli are basophilic and are stained blue. Nissl bodies, which are the rough endoplasmic reticulum of neurons, are basophilic, while other cytoplasmic structures are mostly eosinophilic. Axons and dendrites cannot be distinguished.

Nissl bodies are discrete granular bodies of variable size that occur in the cell body and dendrites but not in the axon of neurons.

EXPERIMENT 4A: Identification of axial bones.

Procedure: For the identification of axial bones and related questions, refer to Chapter 4, Figs 4.7–4.19, and respective information.

EXPERIMENT 4B: Identification of appendicular bones.

Procedure: For the identification of appendicular bones and related questions, refer to Chapter 4, Figs 4.23–4.34 and respective information.

SAQ: What is hemocytometry? What are the components of a hemocytometer?

Ans: Hemocytometry means counting of red blood cells, white blood cells and platelets using a standard glass chamber called Neubauer chamber (Fig. 16.10A).

A standard hemocytometer box contains the following components: A Neubauer chamber, hemoglobin (Hb) pipette, RBC pipette, WBC pipette and a glass-plated comparator for Hb determination (Figs 16.9–16.12).

EXPERIMENT 5: Determination of blood hemoglobin by Sahli method

Clinical significance: A decrease in hemoglobin below the normal range is an indication of anemia. It is necessary to find out the type of anemia. A clinical laboratory report of blood complete count may indicate, whether anemia is of iron deficiency type or of hemolytic type or due to any other reason. Hemoglobin concentration decreases during pregnancy also due to hemodilution.

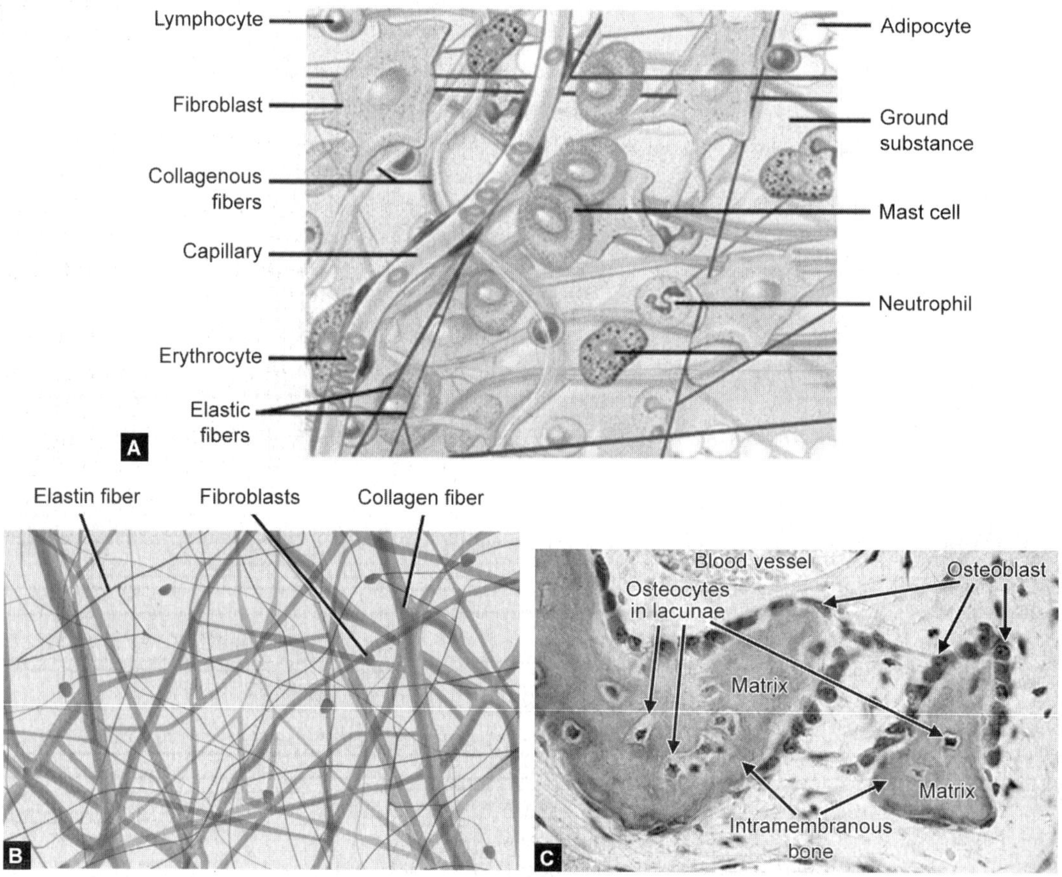

Figs 16.7A–C: (A and B) Areolar connective tissue; (C) stained section of bone

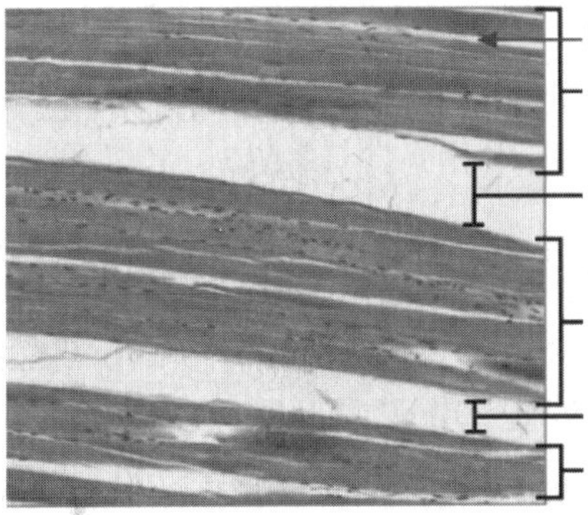

Fig. 16.7D: Skeletal muscle

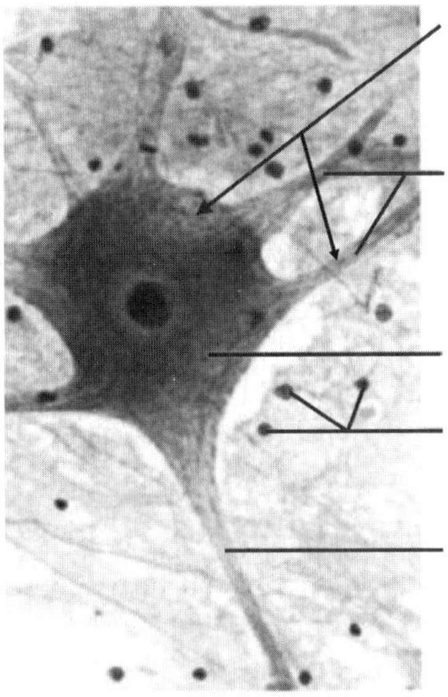

Fig. 16.8: Neuronal tissue

An increase in hemoglobin concentration above the normal range may be seen in clinical conditions such as polycythemia, congenital heart disease, emphysema (due to reduced oxygen supply) and also in severe diarrhea and vomiting (due to loss of body fluids).

Normal values Hb, g/dl (grams per 100 ml blood)

- Men 13–18
- Women 12–16.5
- Children (up to 1 year) 11.0–13.0
- Children (10–12 years) 11.5–14.5
- Infants (full term cord blood) 13.5–19.5

Method: Sahli (acid hematin) method

Principle: When blood is added to 0.1 N hydrochloric acid, hemoglobin is converted to brown-coloured acid hematin. The resulting colour after dilution is compared with a standard brown glass reference blocks of a Sahli hemoglobinometer (Fig. 16.8).

Specimen: Capillary blood or thoroughly mixed anti-coagulated (EDTA) venous blood. The specimen need not be a fasting sample.

Blood storage temperature: If test is not performed immediately, EDTE-blood should be stored in the refrigerator (2–8°C). It should be mixed well before testing.

Requirements (Fig. 16.9):

1. Sahli hemoglobinometer: It consists of:
   a. A standard brown glass mounted on a comparator
   b. A graduated tube (Hellige tube)
   c. Hb pipette (0.02 ml)
2. 0.1N hydrochloric acid
3. Distilled water
4. Pasteur pipettes

> ***Note:*** The graduations on the currently used Hellige tube give 14.5 g as 100%. These are square tubes with graduations in percent on one side and grams per 100 ml (dl) on the other side.

Procedure (Figs 16.10A and B):

1. By using a Pasteur pipette, add 0.1 N hydrochloric acid in the Hellige tube up to the lowest mark (20% mark).
2. Draw blood up to 20 µl mark in the Hb pipette. Adjust the blood column, carefully without bubbles. Wipe excess of the blood on the sides of the pipette by using a dry piece of cotton (or gauze) (Fig. 16.10A).
3. Transfer blood to the acid in the graduated tube, rinse the pipette well, mix the reaction mixture, and allow the tube to stand for at least 10 minutes.
4. Dilute the solution with distilled water by adding a few drops at a time carefully and by mixing the reaction mixture, until the colour matches with the glass plate in the comparator.
5. The matching should be done only against natural light. The level of the fluid is noted at its lower meniscus, and the reading corresponding to this level on the scale is recorded (blood hemoglobin, g/dl) (Fig. 16.10B).

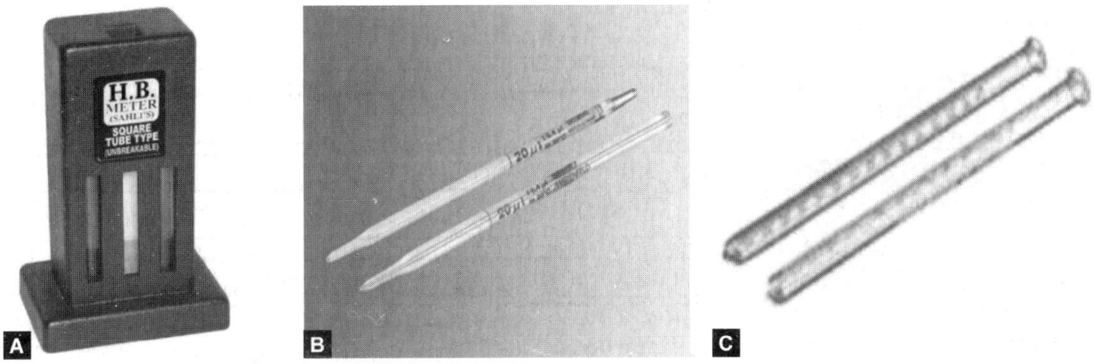

Figs 16.9A–C: The Sahli comparator; (B) Hb pipettes; (C) Hellige tubes

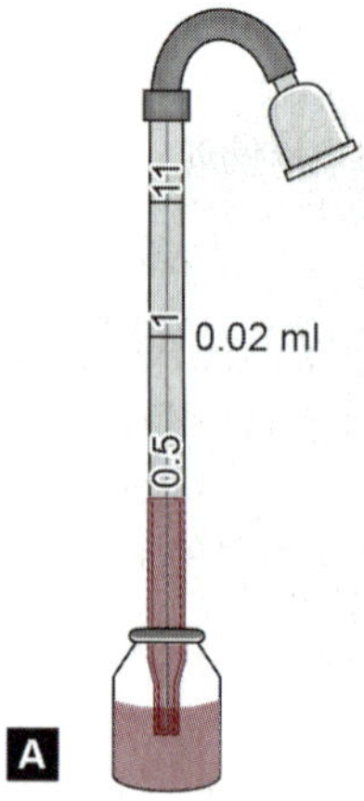

Fig. 16.10A: Drawing blood up to the mark in Hb pipette

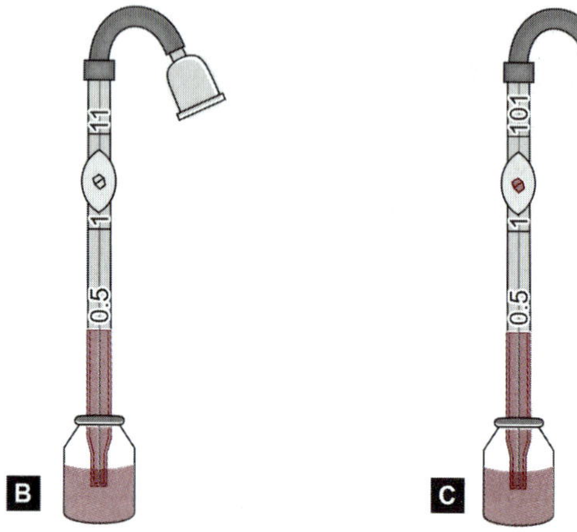

Figs 16.10B and C: (B) Drawing blood up to the mark in a RBC pipette; (C) Drawing blood up to the mark in a WBC pipette

> *Note:*
> 1. This method is useful for places where a photometer is not available.
> 2. It can give an error of up to 1 g/dl.

Precaution: Immediately after use, rinse the Hb pipette by using tap water in a beaker. This prevents the blocking of the pipette.

SAQ: What is the clinical significance of blood hemoglobin determination by Sahli method?

SAQ: What is the normal range of hemoglobin?

SAQ: What is the principle of blood hemoglobin determination by Sahli method?

SAQ: Which anticoagulant is used for Hb determination?

Ans: For the answers of all above questions, Refer to Experiment. 5.

EXPERIMENT 6: Determination of blood hemoglobin by Drabkin test.

Principle: When blood is mixed with Drabkin's reagent containing potassium cyanide and potassium ferricyanide, hemoglobin reacts with ferricyanide to form methemoglobin which is converted to stable cyanmethemoglobin (HiCN) by the cyanide present in the reagent. The intensity of the colour is proportional to hemoglobin concentration in blood, and it is compared with a known cyanmethemoglobin standard a, 540 nm (green filter).

Requirements:

1. *Drabkin's reagent*

   It contains the following components in 1000 ml of distilled water:

   a. Potassium ferricyanide: 400 mg
   b. Potassium dihydrogen phosphate: 280 mg
   c. Potassium cyanide: 100 mg
   d. Nonidet: 1 ml

   This reagent is stable in a polythene container at 2–8°C.
2. *Cyanmethemoglobin (HiCN) standard (Hb standard):* It is commercially available. This standard is directly pipetted in a cuvette, and optical density is measured at 540 nm (green filter): The reading obtained, corresponds to 15 g/dl, hemoglobin.
3. Hb pipette [20 µl (0.02 ml), calibrated]
4. Test tubes (15 × 125 mm)
5. Photometer or spectrophotometer.

Note:

- It is necessary to store Hb standard at 2–8°C.
- Bring this standard to room temperature (25°C ± 5°C) before recording its OD on a photometer.

Specimen:

Same as for Experiment No. 5.

Procedure:

Pipette in the tubes labeled as follows

	Test	*Blank*
1. Drabkin's reagent, ml	5.0	5.0
2. Blood, ml (mixed well)	0.02	—

Mix the contents in the tube labeled as 'Test' thoroughly and wait for 5 minutes.

1. Read OD reading of the 'Test' by setting blank to 100% T at 540 nm (green filter) on a photometer (Fig. 16.11B). If the reading of blank is equal to distilled water, it is not necessary to keep a blank. In that case, read 'Test' against distilled water.
2. Read OD of standard (15 g/dl) by pipetting it directly in a cuvette.

Calculations:

$$\text{Hemoglobin, g/dl} = \frac{\text{OD test}}{\text{OD STD}} \times 15$$

Precautions:

1 The reagent is poisonous, hence handle it carefully. avoid using cyanide, lauryl sulfate has been proposed as a non-hazardous substitute.

2 Mix anticoagulated blood by swirling properly before pipetting. Carefully adjust the blood column up to the graduation mark and use dry cotton to wipe excess blood on the pipette (Fig. 16.10A).

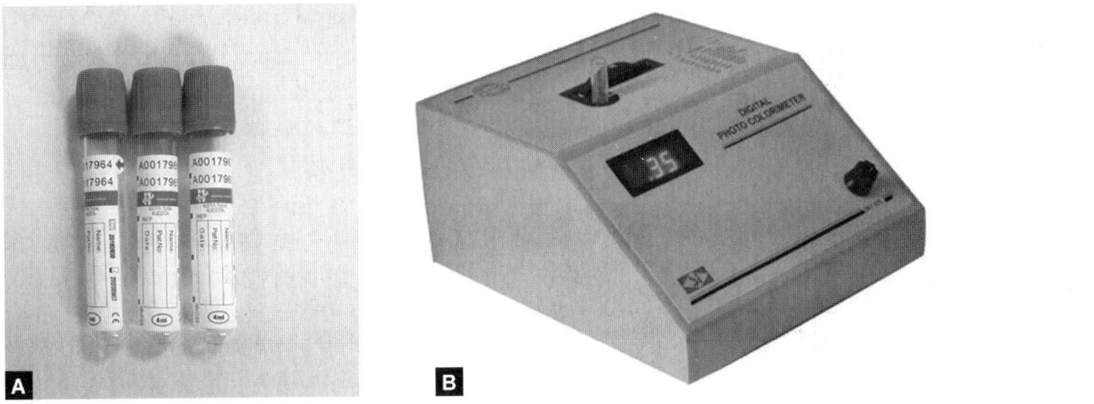

Figs 16.11A and B: (A) EDTA tubes for blood Hb and cell counts, (B) photometer for reading OD and % T readings of solutions

3 Do not discard Drabkin's reagent in the sink. Poisonous cyanide (HCN) gas is released if the sink has an acidic solution. Flush the sink with water and then discard the Drabkin's reagent and continue to flush the water for some time.

4 If capillary blood is used, keep the Drabkin's reagent ready in a test tube. Collect the free-flowing blood into a Hb pipette, wipe the excess blood, and dispense it in the reagent. Mix immediately to avoid clotting of the blood.

SAQ: What is the principle of blood hemoglobin determination by cyanmethemoglobin method?

Ans: Refer to Experiment No. 6.

EXPERIMENT 7: Determination of total red blood cell (RBC) count using a hemocytometer (Fig. 16.12).

Introduction: RBC count is useful for calculating MCV and MCH. The manual method of RBC count is time consuming and imprecise, hence, may not give accurate count of RBCs.

Clinical significance: At birth, the red blood cell count (RBC) varies from 6.5 million to 7.25 million per cubic mm (mm^3 or one microliter)). There is a steady decline after a few hours, and at the end of 15 days to one month, there is a slow rise to normal adult levels. Decrease in RBC count is seen in various types of anemias, pregnancy and old age. An increase in total erythrocyte count is observed in conditions such as polycythemia, and hemoconcentration.

Normal values:

- Male: 4.5–6 × 10^6 cells/mm^3 (µl).
- Female: 4.0–40 × 10^6 cells/mm^3 (µl).

Specimens: 1. EDTA blood or 2. Capillary blood. The specimen need not be a fasting sample.

Principle:

The blood specimen is diluted 1:200 with the RBC diluting fluid, and red cells are counted under high power (40 objective) by using a counting chamber. The number of cells in undiluted blood is calculated and reported as the number of red cells per cu mm (µl) of whole blood.

Requirements:

1. Microscope
2. Improved Neubauer chamber (Fig. 16.12A)
3. RBC pipette
4. RBC diluting fluid

   It is prepared as follows:

   a. Sodium citrate: 3.0 g
   b. Formalin: 1.0 ml
   c. Distilled water: 100 ml

This solution is stable at room temperature (25°C ± 5°C) for at least one year.

Procedure:

1. Mix the anticoagulated blood carefully by swirling the bulb.
2. In the case of capillary blood, the lancet stab should be sufficiently deep to allow the free flow of blood. It is drawn quickly in the RBC pipette.
3. Draw blood up to 0.5 mark in a RBC pipette (Fig. 16.10A).
4. Carefully wipe the excess blood outside the pipette by using cotton or a gauze.
5. Draw diluting fluid up to 101 mark
6. The pipette is rotated rapidly by keeping it horizontal during mixing.
7. After five minutes, by discarding a few drops from the pipette and holding it slightly inclined small volume of the fluid is introduced under the cover slip, which is placed on the counting chamber (Fig. 16.12B).
8. Allow the cells to settle for 2–3 minutes.
9. Place the counting chamber on the stage of the microscope.
10. Switch to low power (10X) objective. Adjust the light and locate the large square in the center with 25 small squares.
11. Now, switch to high power (40X) objective.
12. The red blood cells in the four corner squares and in the center square (marked in the diagram as 'R') are counted (Figs 16.12B and 16.13).

13. Use the following formula for the calculation of red blood cells:

$$\text{Total red blood cells/mm}^3 = \frac{\text{(Number of red cells counted} \times \text{Dilution)}}{\text{Area counted} \times \text{Depth of the diluting fluid}} = \text{Number of red cells counted} \times 10{,}000$$

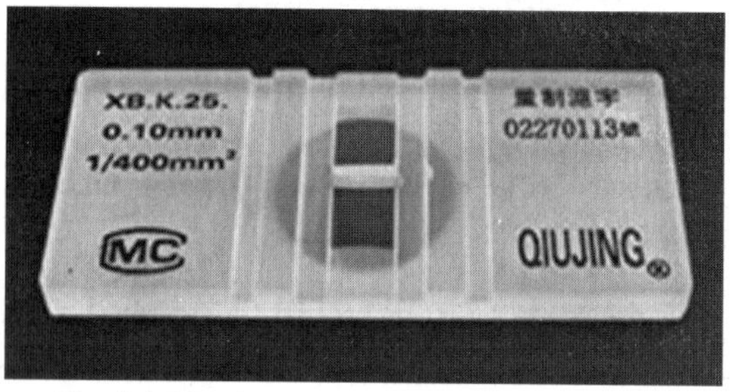

Fig. 16.12A: Improved Neubauer chamber

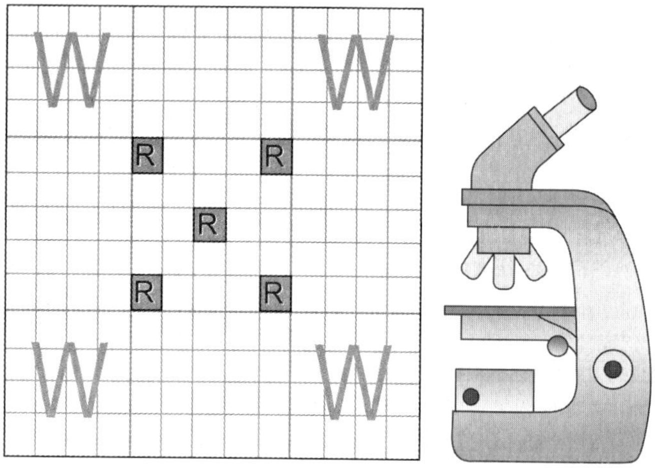

8

Count RBCs in the five 'R' squares of the chamber by using high power objective

Fig. 16.12B: Fields of RBC and WBC count as seen for counting of blood cells under the high power objective

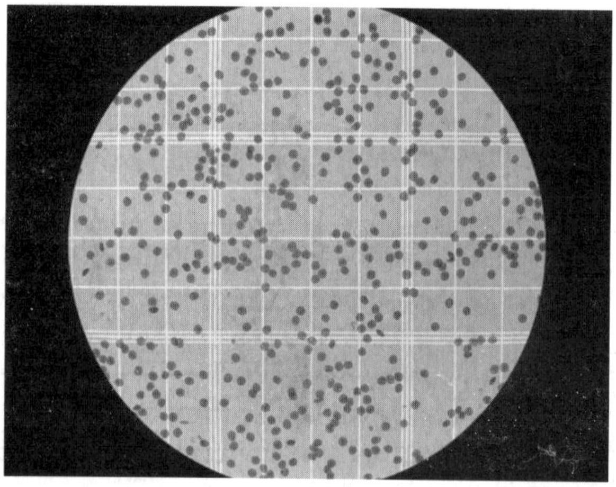

Fig. 16.13: Red blood cells seen under 40 × objective

Sources of error:

A. Falsely high red blood cell counts are obtained due to the following reasons:
   1. Inadequate wiping of the pipette.
   2. Improper pipetting of blood as well as the diluting fluid.
   3. Improper mixing.
   4. Uneven distribution in the counting chamber.

B. Falsely low red blood cell counts are obtained due to the following reasons:
   1. Improper pipetting and dilution (when blood drawn is less and if dilution is above the mark).
   2. Dilution of the contents in the pipette by saliva.
   3. Uneven distribution of the cells in the counting chamber.
   4. Due to a partially clotted blood specimen.

SAQ: What is the clinical significance of RBC count?

SAQ: What is the normal range of RBC count?

SAQ: What anticoagulant is used for RBC count?

Ans: For the answers of all above questions, refer to Experiment No. 7.

EXPERIMENT 8: Determination of total white blood cell (WBC) count using hemocytometer (Fig. 16.12).

Clinical significance: An increase in total white blood cell count of more than 10,000/cu mm (µl) is known as leukocytosis and a decrease of less than 4,000 cu mm (µl) is known as leukopenia.

A. **Causes of leukocytosis:** Increase in WBC count is observed mainly in bacterial infections and in leukemia. In parasitic and viral infections also moderate rise in WBCs is observed. Leukocytosis is also observed in severe hemorrhage. Due to physiological reasons, WBCs also rise moderately in pregnancy and during high temperature.

B. **Causes of leukopenia:** Decrease in WBC count is observed in certain viral and bacterial infections (typhoid), bone marrow depression (specific drug, radiation or chemical reaction) and in certain types of leukemia.

Normal values:

- Adults : 4,000–10,000/mm³ (µl)
- At birth : 10,000–25,000/mm³
- 1 to 3 years : 6,000–18,000/mm³ (µl)
- 4 to 7 years : 6,000–15,000/mm³ (µl)
- 8 to 12 years : 4,500–13,500/mm³ (µl)

Specimens:

1. EDTA blood (blood collected in EDTA anticoagulant)
2. Capillary blood (the specimen need not be a fasting sample).

Requirements:

1. Microscope
2. Improved Neubauer chamber
3. WBC pipette
4. WBC diluting fluid: It is prepared as follows:
   a. Glacial acetic acid: 2.0 ml
   b. 1% (w/v) gentian violet: 1.0 ml
   c. Distilled water: 97 ml

This solution is stable at room temperature (25°C ± 5°C). A pinch of thymol may be added as a preservative.

Principle:

Glacial acetic acid lyses the red cells while the gentian violet slightly stains the nuclei of the leukocytes. Blood specimen is diluted 1:20 in a WBC pipette with the diluting fluid, and the cells are counted under the low power of the microscope by using a counting chamber. The number of cells in undiluted blood is reported per cu mm (µl) of whole blood.

Procedure:

1. Draw blood up to 0.5 mark of a WBC pipette (Fig. 16.10C).
2. Carefully, wipe excess blood outside the pipette by using cotton. Draw diluting fluid up to 11 mark.
3. Mix the contents in the pipette and after five minutes, by discarding few drops, fill the counting chamber and allow the cells to settle for two to three minutes (Fig. 16.12).
4. Focus on one of the "W" marked areas (each having 16 small squares) by turning the objective to low power (10X).
5. Count cells in all four "W" marked corners (Figs 16.12B and 16.14).
6. Calculations:

   Number of white cells/mm^3 (µl) of whole blood =

   $$= \frac{\text{number of white cells counted} \times \text{Dilution}}{\text{Area counted} \times \text{Depth of fluid}}$$

   where dilution = 20

   Area counted = 4 × 1 sq. mm = 4 sq. mm

   Depth of fluid = 0.1 mm (constant)

   Hence, the number of white cells per mm^3 (µl) of whole blood =

   $$\frac{\text{No. of cells counted} \times 20}{4 \times 0.1}$$

   = No. of cells counted × 50

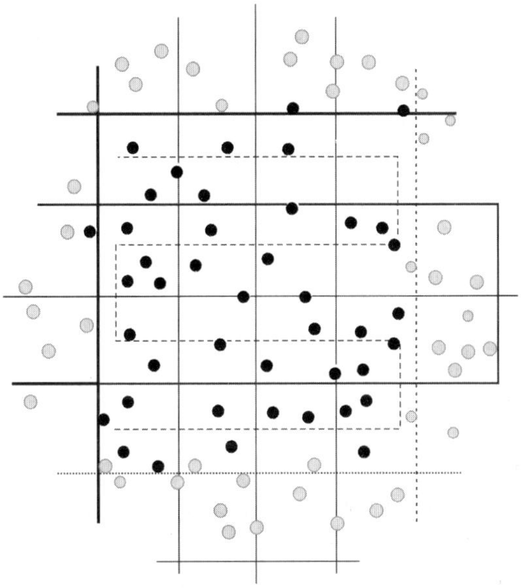

Fig. 16.14: White blood cells seen under 10X objective

SAQ: What is the clinical significance of WBC count?

SAQ: What is the normal range of WBC count?

SAQ: What anticoagulant is used for WBC count?

Ans: For the answers of all above questions, refer to Experiment 8.

EXPERIMENT 9: Determination of differential leukocyte count using a stained blood smear (Fig. 16.15B).

Clinical significance:

The differential count is useful to identify changes in the distribution of white cells, which may be related to specific types of disorders. It also gives an idea regarding the severity of the disease and the degree of response of the body. The following cells are measured in the differential leukocyte count.

1. Neutrophilia: An increase in the percentage of neutrophils is observed in bacterial infection. Decrease in neutrophils is observed in typhoid, measles, influenza, aplastic anemia and in suppression of bone marrow by various drugs and radiation effects.
2. Lymphocytes: An increase in lymphocyte count is seen in certain infections such as mumps, cough, measles, influenza, syphilis, tuberculosis, typhoid, and other chronic infections. Decrease in the lymphocytes may be seen in specific acute stages of infections and in excess irradiation.
3. Eosinophils: An increase in eosinophils is observed in asthma, hypersensitivity reactions, parasitic infestations, and in chronic inflammatory diseases.
4. Monocytes: An increase in monocytes is observed in tuberculosis, malaria, subacute bacterial endocarditis, typhoid, and in kala-azar.
5. Basophils: An increase in basophils usually observed in chronic myeloid leukemia.

Normal values (male or female):

- Neutrophils : 40–75% (mean: 57%)
- Eosinophils : 1–4% (mean: 2%)
- Basophils : 0–1%
- Lymphocytes : 20–45% (mean: 37%)
- Monocytes : 2–8% (mean: 6%)

Note:

1. The blood smear is prepared immediately after skin puncture or venipuncture before mixing with an anticoagulant. If EDTA blood is used, the smear should be prepared within 1–2 hours after the blood draw. The blood smear is stained in Wright's stain, Leishman's stain or in field stain.
2. In this experiment a stained blood smear is used.

Procedure:

1 Choose the portion of the smear where the red cells are beginning to overlap.

2 Place a drop of immersion oil on the smear. Switch to the oil immersion objective and examine the film by moving from one field to the next, systematically.

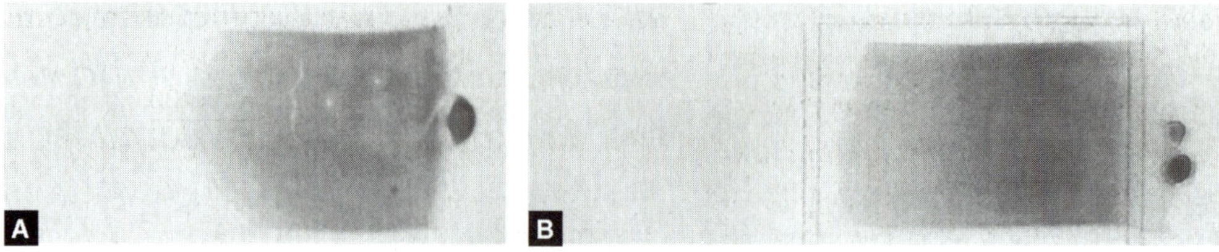

Figs 16.15A and B: (A) Unstained blood smear; (B) stained blood smear

3. Count at least 100 different white blood cells as seen in Chapter 9, Fig. 9.3.

SAQ: What is the clinical significance of WBC differential count?

SAQ: What are the normal ranges of WBC differential count?

SAQ: What anticoagulant is used for WBC differential count?

Ans: For the answers of all above questions, Refer to Experiment No. 9.

EXPERIMENT 10: Determination of packed cell volume (PCV, hematocrit).

Introduction: PCV (packed cell volume, hematocrit) is the amount of packed red blood cells, following centrifugation, expressed as a percentage of the total blood volume.

Clinical significance: Decrease in PCV values are observed in various types of anemias and in hydremia, due to excessive fluid in the blood as occurs in pregnancy. Increase in PCV is observed in polycythemia, severe dehydration, emphysema and congenital heart disease.

Normal values:

- Male: 42–52%
- Female: 36–48% (late pregnancy: 23–37%)

Principle: When anticoagulated blood is centrifuged in a hematocrit tube at high speed, the erythrocytes sediment at the bottom. The red cell column is called packed cell volume (PCV) or hematocrit (Cell volume percent).

Requirements:

1. Specimen
   EDTA blood (the specimen need not be a fasting sample).
2. Wintrobe hematocrit tube (Figs 16.16A and B).
   It is 110 mm long tube with a 3 mm internal bore. It is graduated from 0 up to 100 mm (10 CM). The scale with the descending order is used for PCV determination.
3. Pasteur pipette or a syringe with a needle.
4. Centrifuge.

Procedure:

1. Mix the blood sample carefully.
2. Label a Wintrobe tube (Figs 16.16A and B).
3. Fill the tube by using a Pasteur pipette or a syringe up to the 100 mark (Fig. 16.16A). Avoid trapping of air bubbles.
4. Place the tube in a centrifuge cup (Use another empty Wintrobe tube to fill the opposite cup or a tube filled with another specimen, or water).
5. Centrifuge for 30 minutes at 3000 RPM.
6. Note the reading of PCV (Fig. 16.16B).

Precautions: It is necessary to wash the Wintrobe tube immediately after the test by introducing a thick steel wire repeatedly in the tube under running tap water.

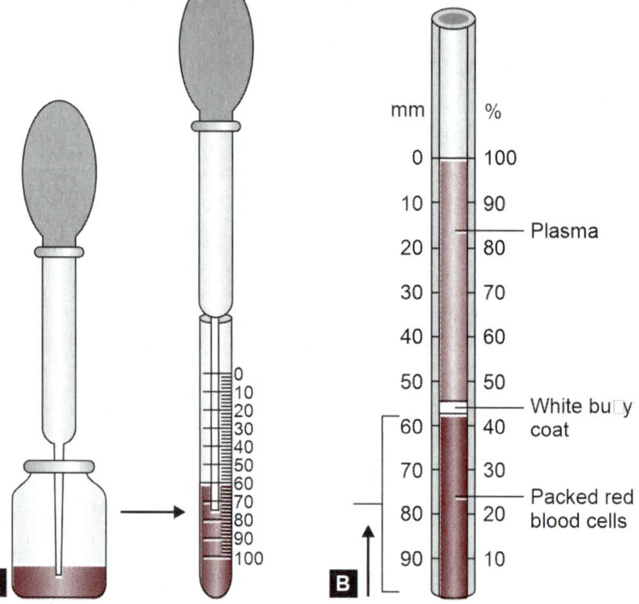

Figs16.16A and B: (A) Introduction of EDTA blood; (B) reading of PCV (40% in this case) in the Wintrobe tube

SAQ: What is the clinical significance of PCV determination?

SAQ: What are the normal ranges of PCV determination?

SAQ: What anticoagulant is used for PCV determination?

Ans: For the answers of all above questions, refer to Experiment No. 10.

EXPERIMENT 11: Determination of erythrocyte indices (Wintrobe constants).

Introduction:

The erythrocyte indices are calculated from: (1) Hemoglobin concentration, (2) PCV, and (3) total erythrocyte count. Three indices commonly calculated are: (a) Mean cell volume (MCV), (b) mean cell hemoglobin (MCH)

and (c) mean corpuscular hemoglobin concentration (MCHC).

MCV value is a measurement of the average size of red blood cells.

MCH value gives mean red cell hemoglobin.

Bigger red blood cells generally contain more hemoglobin, while smaller red blood cells contain less hemoglobin. However, the MCH value indicates, the average concentration of hemoglobin present per red blood cell.

MCHC is a measure of the concentration of hemoglobin per unit volume of red blood cells. MCHC value gives the weight of hemoglobin per 100 ml of packed red blood cells.

Since, hemoglobin is the molecule to which oxygen attaches, MCHC is a measure of the average oxygen-carrying capacity of the red blood cells circulating in the body.

A low MCHC (hypochromia) may mean that there is a lower concentration of hemoglobin within a given volume of red blood cells, hence, a reduced capacity to carry oxygen to the tissues of the body. A high MCHC (hyperchromia) means there is a higher hemoglobin concentration in red blood cells than normal.

MCV does not account for red cell volume. However, MCHC accounts for red cell volume.

Procedure:

1. By using a EDTA blood sample, determine: (a) Hemoglobin, (b) PCV and (c) total erythrocyte count.
2. Determination of mean corpuscular volume (MCV): It is calculated as follows:

$$MCV = \frac{PCV \times 10}{RBC \text{ in millions}}$$

Example:

a. PCV = 45%

b. Erythrocyte count = 5.0 m/mm^3 (µl)

$$MCV = \frac{45 \times 10}{5} = 90$$

- Normal range: 82 to 92 fl
- Increased MCV is observed in macrocytic anemia and decreased MCV is observed in microcytic anemia.

3. Determination of mean corpuscular hemoglobin (MCH): It is calculated as follows:

$$MCH = \frac{Hb \times 10}{RBC \text{ in millions}}$$

Example:

a. Hb = 14.0 g/dl

b. RBC count = 5.0 m/mm^3 (µl)

$$MCH = \frac{45 \times 10}{5} = 28 pg$$

- 1 picogram (pg) 10–12 g
- Normal range 27–32 pg
- Increased values of MCH are observed in macrocytic anemia and decreased values of MCH are observed in microcytic anemia.

4. Mean corpuscular hemoglobin concentration (MCHC): It is calculated as follows:

$$MCHC = \frac{Hb \times 100}{PCV}$$

Example:

a. Hb: 14.0 g/dl

b. PCV: 40%

$$MCHC = \frac{14}{40} \times 100$$

MCHC = 35%

- Normal range: 32–36 g%
- Decreased values are observed in microcytic anemia and increased values are observed in macrocytic anemia.

SAQ: What is complete blood count (CBC) or complete hemogram?

Ans. Complete blood count (CBC) or complete hemogram is a blood report of a patient obtained by using manual methods in a hematology section of a clinical laboratory or by using a hematology autoanalyzer (Fig. 16.17). The following is one example of CBC or complete hemogram of a female patient.

COMPLETE HEMOGRAM

Normal range:

- Hemoglobin: 13.2 g/dl 12–16 g/dl
- Total erythrocyte count: 3.03 × 10^6/mm^3 4.3 ± 0.5 × 10^6/cmm
- Total leukocyte count: 5800/mm^3 5000–10,000/mm^3
- *Differential leukocyte count:*

Neutrophils: 32%	40–75%
Lymphocytes: 62%	20–45 %
Eosinophils: 3%	1–4 %
Monocytes: 1%	2–8%

Stained peripheral blood smear microscopic observations:

- No RBC abnormality seen

• PCV: 37%	36–48%
• MCV: 83.7 fl	82–92 fl
• MCH: 27.1 pg	27–32 pg
• MCHC: 33.0%	32–36%
• Platelet count: 1,77,000	1,50,000–4,00,000/mm^3

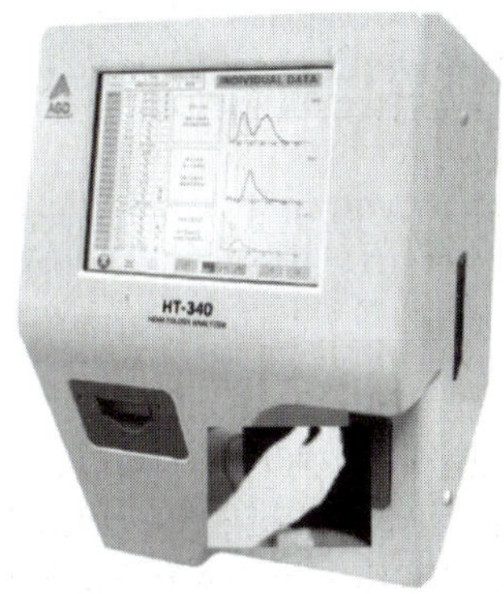

Fig. 16.17: Hematology autoanalyzer (AGD)

SAQ: How complete hemogram is obtained using a hematology autoanalyzer?

Ans: An EDTA mixed blood of a patient is introduced in the hematology autoanalyzer by pressing a specific button as shown in the Fig. 16.16.B. Complete hemogram is displayed on the screen in 2–3 minutes on the screen of an autoanalyzer with a printout.

EXPERIMENT 12: Determination of erythrocyte sedimentation rate.

Clinical significance: Changes in various serum proteins occur in acute infections during active phases of chronic inflammation. In acute infections, tissue injury-related inflammatory response leads to increases in serum proteins such as fibrinogen, globulins, C-reactive protein (CRP) and a decrease in albumin. Determination of acute-phase response is a helpful indicator of the presence and extent of inflammation or tissue damage and also the response to treatment.

Method: Westergren method

Introduction: With reference to Westergren method, diluted blood (in 3.8% sodium citrate solution) is sedimented in an open-ended, dry, and clean glass tube of 30 cm in length and 2.55 mm in diameter, mounted vertically on a stand for one hour. When anticoagulated blood is allowed to stand undisturbed for a period of time, the erythrocytes tend to sink to the bottom. Two layers are formed, the upper plasma layer and the lower one of red blood cells. The rate at which the red cells fall is known as the erythrocyte sedimentation rate.

Normal range:
- Male 0–15 mm after 1 hour
- Female 0–20 mm after 1 hour

Specimens:
1 A small tube (100 × 10 mm) with 2.5 ml mark is used for blood collection (if the tube is not graduated, pipette out 2.5 ml of 3.8% sodium citrate in the tube, and after marking the level of fluid, remove 2.0 ml of the solution leaving 0.5 ml of the anticoagulant in the tube).
2 The tubes with 0.5 ml of 3.8% sodium citrate should be kept ready before blood collection.
3 Patient should be fasting for 12 to 16 hours. Collect blood by venipuncture and add in the tube up to the mark, and mix carefully.

Requirement (Figs 16.18A–C):
1. Westergren ESR tube (Fig. 16.18A)
2. Stand for holding the tube (Fig. 16.18B)
3. Timer or watch

Procedure:
1. Fill the Westergren tube exactly up to the zero mark by means of a rubber bulb (avoid air bubbles).
2. Place the tube upright in the stand. It should fit evenly into the groove of the stand (Fig. 16.18C).
3. Note the time. Allow the tube to stand for exactly one hour.
4. Exactly after one hour, note the level to which the red cell column has fallen (Fig. 16.18B).
5. Report the result in terms of mm/after 1 hour.

Precaution: Wash the tubes as early as possible, under running tap water. Rinse in deionized water and dry in the incubator between 40–50°C.

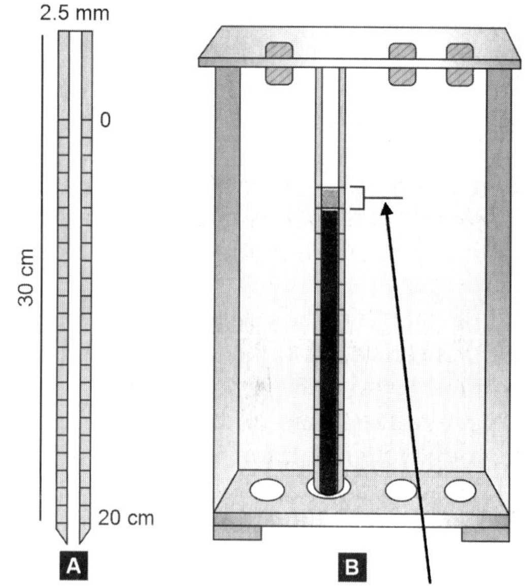

Figs 16.18A and B: (A) Westergren tube, (B) ESR reading

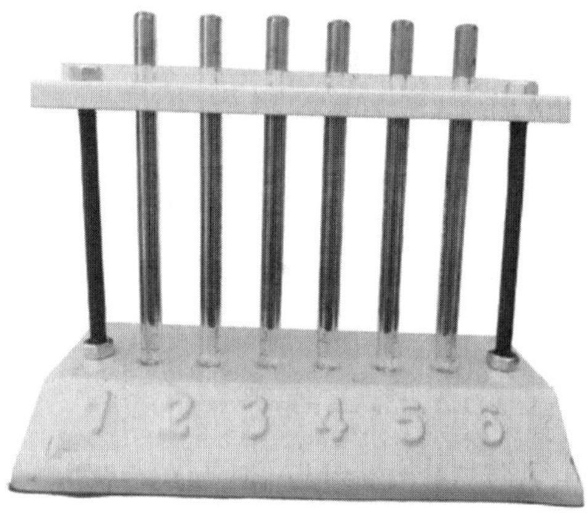

Fig. 16.18C: ESR by Wintrobe method

Note: ESR can also be performed by Wintrobe method. The details of the method are as follows:

Specimen: Fresh fasting EDTA anticoagulated and undiluted blood.

Normal range:
- Male: 0–9 mm/after 1 hour
- Female: 0–20 mm/after 1 hour

Procedure:
1. Mix the blood carefully.
2. Fill the Wintrobe tube to the zero mark by using a Pasteur pipette or by using a syringe (Fig. 16.16A).
3. Place the tube in an exact vertical position on the stand (Fig. 16.18C). Set the timer for one hour.
4. At the end of one hour, note the level of the plasma (in mm) over the erythrocyte column in terms of mm after 1 hour.

> *Note:* This method provides both ESR and PCV values. After noting the ESR value, the same tube can be centrifuged for PCV.

SAQ: What is the clinical significance of ESR determination?

SAQ: What type of blood is used for ESR test by Westergren method?

SAQ: What type of blood is used for ESR test by Wintrobe method?

SAQ: What is the principle of ESR determination?

SAQ: What is the normal range of ESR by Westergren method?

SAQ: What is the normal range of ESR by Wintrobe method?

Ans: For the answers of all above questions, refer to Experiment No. 12.

EXPERIMENT 13: To perform qualitative test for ABO grouping using glass slide method.

Importance: Blood group and Rh typing is very important, since, any individual can safely donate blood or receive a blood transfusion.

Principle: The procedures used with the antisera are based on the principle of agglutination. Normal human red cells possessing antigens will clump in the presence of the corresponding antibody.

Method: Slide method.

Requirements:
1. Glass slides
2. Pasteur pipettes
3. Applicator sticks
4. Centrifuge

Reagents:
1. Anti-A sera (blue colour): Human polyclonal or murine monoclonal.
2. Anti-B sera (yellow colour): Human polyclonal or murine monoclonal.
3. Normal saline (0.85 g/dl sodium chloride in distilled water).

Specimen collection and preparation: No special preparation of the patient is required prior to specimen collection. Blood should be collected by figer prick or in a EDTA tube (or bulb). The test should be performed immediately; otherwise, it is necessary to store the specimen at 2–8°C.

Procedure:
1. Prepare a 10% suspension of red blood cells in normal saline (preparation method as given below):
   a. Mix 5 drops (0.05 ml each) of sedimented red cells with 2 ml of normal saline.
   b. Centrifuge at 1,500 RPM for 1 to 2 minutes. Discard supernatant.
   c. Add 2 ml of normal saline to the sedimented red cells. Mix well. This gives a 10% suspension of red cells.
2. On one half of a glass slide, place 1 drop of anti-A blood grouping serum.
3. On the other half of the slide, place 1 drop of anti-B blood grouping serum.
4. Using a pasteur pipette add 1 drop of the cell suspension to each half of the slide.
5. With separate applicator sticks mix each cell-serum mixture well.
6. Tilt the slide back and forth and observe for agglutination (Fig. 16.19).

> *Note:*
> 1. Tests that show no agglutination within two minutes are considered negative.
> 2. Do not interpret peripheral drying or fibrin strands as agglutination.

Interpretation (Table 16.1, Fig. 16.19):

Table 16.1

Reaction		*Interpretation*
Anti-A	*Anti-B*	*Group*
+	0	A
0	+	B
+	+	AB
0	0	O

Key: 0: No agglutination; +: agglutination

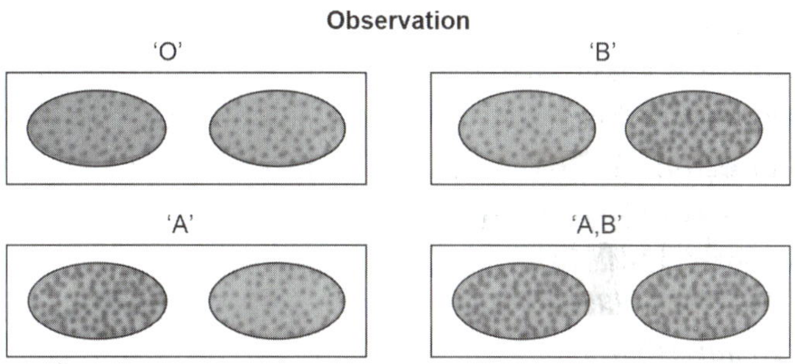

Fig. 16.19: Slide test results of ABO grouping

> *Note:* Blood obtained by finger puncture may be tested directly by the slide method. To avoid clotting the collected blood (on the slide) should be moved quickly with the antisera.

EXPERIMENT 14: Determination of Rho (D) typing using glass slide method.

Requirements:
1. Glass slides
2. Pasteur pipettes

Reagents:
1. Blood typing serum anti-D (human polyclonal or human monoclonal reagents).
2. Normal saline.

Procedure:
1. On a pre-warmed glass slide (40°C to 50°C surface temperature) place one drop of anti-D serum.
2. By using a Pasteur pipette, add one drop of whole blood (in the case of an anemic patient, add one drop of sedimented red blood cells).

3 With an applicator stick, mix the cell-serum mixture well.
4 Tilt the slide back and forth and observe for agglutination. Tests that show no agglutination within two minutes are considered negative.

> *Note:*
> 1. Do not interpret peripheral drying or fibrin strands as agglutination.
> 2. If no agglutination is observed, proceed to Du determination.

SAQ: Why blood group determination and Rh typing is very important?

SAQ: What type of blood is used for ABO group determination?

SAQ: What is the principle of ABO group determination?

Ans: For the answers of all above questions, refer to Experiment No. 13.

EXPERIMENT 15: Determination of bleeding time.

Clinical significance: Determination of bleeding time helps to detect vascular defect and platelet disorders. Prolonged bleeding time is generally associated with thrombocytopenia. In case of von Willebrand's disease, bleeding time is high with a normal platelet count. It is caused by a platelet defect combined with factor VIII deficiency.

Method: Duke's method.

Specimen: Blood collected by earlobe or finger puncture.

Principle: A 1 mm deep incision is made on the earlobe or finger of the patient. The length of time required for bleeding to cease is recorded.

Normal range: 1–5 minutes

Requirements:
1. Sterile lancet
2. Spirit or 70% alcohol
3. Circular filter paper
4. Stopwatch

Procedure (Fig. 16.20A):
1. Clean the earlobe (or finger) with spirit or alcohol by using a piece of cotton. Allow to dry.
2. Puncture the earlobe (or finger) deeply (about 1 mm) by using sterile lancet. Start the stopwatch. The blood should flow freely, without squeezing the ear lobe (or finger).
3. After 30 seconds collect the drop of blood at one corner of the filter paper. Do not touch the skin with the paper.
4. Repeat step no. 3 after every 30 seconds.
5. When bleeding ceases, stop the stopwatch,
6. Note the time on the watch.

> *Note:* If the bleeding is prolonged for more than 10 minutes, discontinue the test and apply pressure to the bleeding spot.

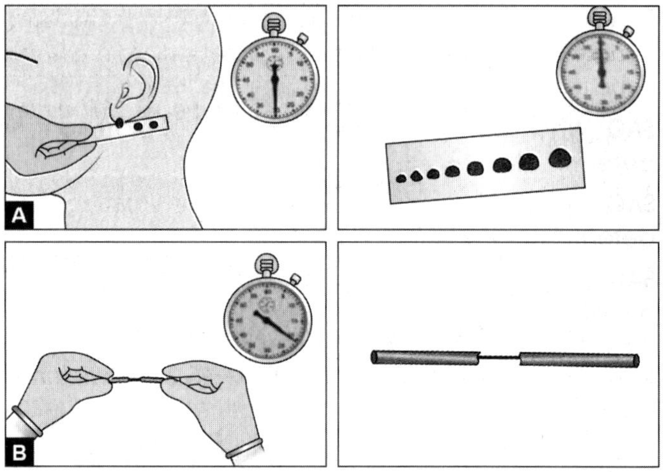

Figs 16.20A and B: (A) Determination of bleeding time; (B) determination of clotting time

SAQ: What is the clinical significance of bleeding time determination?

SAQ: What type of blood is used for bleeding time determination?

SAQ: What is the principle of bleeding time determination?

Ans: For the answers of all above questions, refer to Experiment No. 15.

EXPERIMENT 16: Determination of blood clotting time (Fig. 16.20B).

CLINICAL SIGNIFICANCE

This method is generally useful in severe clotting disorders.

Method: Capillary method

Normal range: 4 to 9 minutes

Specimen: Capillary blood

Principle: Blood is collected in a capillary tube after a finger prick and the stopwatch is started. The formation of fibrin string is noted by breaking the capillary tube at regular intervals. The time is noted at the first appearance of the fibrin string.

Requirements:
1. Sterile lancet
2. Capillary tubes (1.5 mm diameter and 10 to 15 cm length)
3. Cotton
4. Spirit or 70% alcohol
5. Stopwatch

Procedure (Fig. 16.20B):
1. By using a piece of cotton, apply spirit or 70% alcohol to the patient's fingertip.
2. Make a deep (1 mm) incision with a sterile lancet and start the stopwatch.
3. Wipe off the first blood drop and collect blood in the capillary up to two-thirds of its length.
4. After every half minute, break off about 1 cm of the capillary to find out whether fibrin string has formed.

5. When the fibrin string appears, stop the stopwatch and note down the time. Hence, capillary method should be used, when venous blood cannot be obtained.

SAQ: What is the clinical significance of clotting time determination?

SAQ: What type of blood is used for clotting time determination?

SAQ: What is the principle of clotting time determination?

Ans: For the answers of all above questions, refer to Experiment No. 16.

EXPERIMENT 17: Determination of pulse rate.

Introduction: The pulse rate is a measurement of the heart beats per minute, when a person is at rest. When the heart pushes blood through the arteries, the arteries expand and contract with the flow of the blood. Determination of pulse rate indicates heart rhythm.

The pulse may be palpated in an artery that can be compressed near the surface of the body. Following are some prominent areas to feel pulse (Figs 16.21A and B): (1) Neck (carotid artery), (2) the wrist (radial artery), (3) at the groin (femoral artery), (4) behind the knee (popliteal artery), (5) near the ankle joint (posterior tibial artery), and (6) on the foot (dorsalis pedis artery).

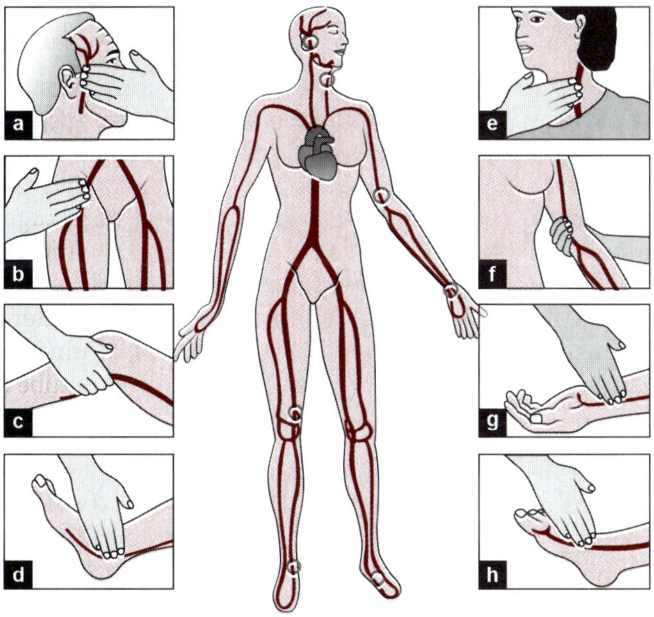

Fig. 16.21A: Pulse rate sites

Normal values (when a person is at rest):

- Babies up to the age of 1 month 100–160 beats per minute.
- Children of the ages 1–10 years 60–120 beats per minute
- Children of the ages 11–17 years 60–100 beats per minute.
- Adults: 60–100 beats per minute.
- Athletes: 40–60 beats per minute.

Clinical significance: Pulse rate may increase or decrease in various clinical conditions. It becomes irregular in arrythmia. Tachycardia is a fast heart. In tachycardia, the resting heart rate is greater than 100 beats a minute. Bradycardia is a slow heartbeat. The resting heart rate is less than 60 beats a minute in bradycardia. A palpitation is a short-lived arrhythmia.

In the case of abnormal heart beats, patient may experience following symptoms: Feeling dizzy, or light-headed, there may be shortness of breath, heart palpitations, chest pain, sweating, pale skin, etc.

A number of clinical conditions may cause an abnormal heartbeat. These include, high blood pressure and coronary heart diseases, etc.

Some medications or substances may lead to increase in pulse rate. These include, caffeine, certain cough medicines, amphetamines, etc.

Other factors that may cause pulse rate to change are stress, smoking, alcohol consumption, etc.

Requirements:

1. *Human volunteer:* A person or patient (on whom pulse rate could be determined)
2. A stopwatch or a watch that has a second hand (that marks seconds).
3. A chart to record the pulse measurement
4. A black pen.

Instructions given to patient:

To get resting pulse rate, person (or patient) should sit still for 10 minutes before checking pulse.

> ***Note:***
> 1. If the patient has walked, climbed stairs, or exerted in the last 20 minutes. Wait for 20 minutes before taking the pulse rate reading.
> 2. Inform the patient about the procedure to be followed for pulse rate determination.

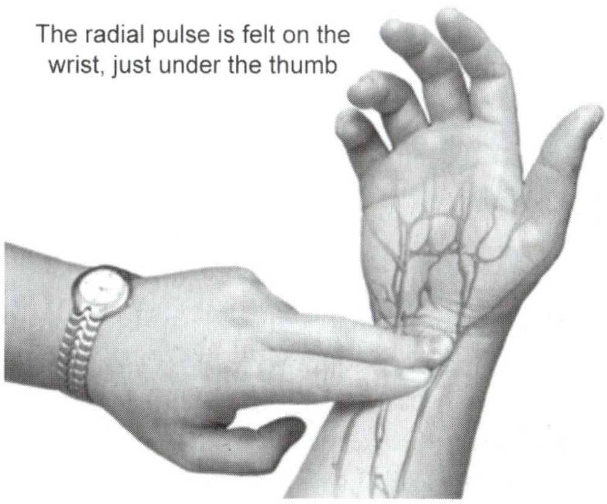

Fig. 16.21B: Determination of pulse rate

Procedure (Fig. 16.21B):

1. Using the first and second fingertips, press firmly but gently on the radial artery, until you feel a pulse.
2. Begin counting the pulse when the clock's second hand is on 12. Or use a stopwatch on mobile phone.

3. Count pulse for 60 seconds (or for 15 seconds and then multiply by four to calculate beats per minute).
4. Note reading in the notebook.
5. Repeat this procedure to confirm first reading of pulse rate.
6. Wash hands.

> ***Note:*** The radial artery is located on the wrist (Fig. 16.21A), just below the base of the thumb.

SAQ: What is the clinical significance of pulse rate determination?

SAQ: What is the normal pulse rate?

SAQ: What are the instruction given to a person, before testing pulse rate?

Ans: For the answers of all above questions, refer to Experiment No. 18.

EXPERIMENT 18: Determination of blood pressure using an automatic blood pressure (BP) equipment (Fig. 16.22).

Introduction: Blood pressure (BP) is the force exerted by the blood on the wall of blood vessels; when the heart contracts and relaxes to circulate blood around entire body. Blood pressure is measured in millimetres of mercury (mmHg). Blood pressure is measured as systolic blood pressure and diastolic blood pressure. Systolic blood pressure is the degree of force when the heart is contracting and the diastolic blood pressure is the degree of force when the heart gets relaxed. Blood pressure is reported as indicating systolic figure first, followed by diastolic figure. For example, when BP of a person is reported as 120–80, means systolic BP is 120 mmHg and diastolic BP is 80 mmHg. The right arm tends to give slightly higher reading of BP, however, it is not significant.

Normal range (reference range):

	Systolic	*Diastolic*
Infants 1–12 months	75–100	50–70
1–5 years	80–110	50–80
6–12 years	85–120	50–80
13–18 years	95–140	60–90
Adults	80–120	60–90

Clinical significance: Hypertension means high blood pressure. It is considered to be higher than the normal values and low blood pressure is considered to be lower than normal values. Usually, hypertension is considered when blood pressure is above 140–90, and it is considered severe if BP is above 180–120.

Following clinical conditions may lead to high blood pressure: Kidney diseases, uncontrolled diabetes mellitus, hormone disorders such as hyperthyroidism, Cushing's syndrome, acromegaly, hyperaldosteronism, and phaeochromocytoma. High blood pressure is often associated with unhealthy lifestyle habits, such as smoking, drinking excessive alcohol. If high BP is not treated, it may increase risk of developing a number of serious long-term health problems such kidney disease, stroke and coronary heart disease.

Following clinical conditions cause low blood pressure: Heart problems, endocrine disorders such as hypoaldosteronism, hypothyroidism, etc. Low BP is also observed in dehydration, excessive blood loss, severe microbial infection (septicemia), severe allergic reaction (anaphylaxis), lack of adequate nutrients in diet and pregnancy.

Method:

Determination of BP using digital BP equipment

Requirements:

1. Digital BP equipment attached with inflatable rubber cuff.
2. Human volunteer: A person (to measure BP).
3. Note book or laptop

Instructions before reading BP:

1. Patient should avoid food, tobacco, caffeine, and alcohol for 30 minutes before taking BP reading measurement.
2. It is advised to pass urine, if bladder is full before taking BP reading
3. In the case of any clinical condition, patient is allowed only life-saving drugs and the list of drugs consumed should be reported to the nurse, pharmacist or doctor.

Preparation of the patient: Make sure the patient is relaxed by allowing 5 minutes to relax before the first reading. The patient should sit upright with their upper arm positioned so it is leveled with their heart and feet flat on the floor. Remove excess clothing that might interfere with the BP cuff or constrict blood flow in the arm. Be sure you and the patient refrain from talking during the reading.

Procedure:

1. Place the blood pressure cuff on upper arm; about one inch above the crease of elbow of the patient (Fig. 16.22).
2. Arrange the cuff over the upper arm with the artery mark positioned directly over the brachial artery. The bottom edge of the cuff should be positioned about one inch (2–3 cm) above the antecubital fossa (Fig. 16.22).
2. Now push the 'on' button on the BP instrument that inflates the cuff (Fig. 16.22).
3. After the cuff fully inflates, air will automatically start flowing back out. Then BP reading will be displayed digitally (Fig. 16.23).
4. See the screen to get your blood pressure reading.
5. Repeat the procedure for one more reading.
6. Note the reading in the note book

EXPERIMENT 19: Determination of blood pressure (BP) using sphygmomanometer equipment (Fig. 16.24).

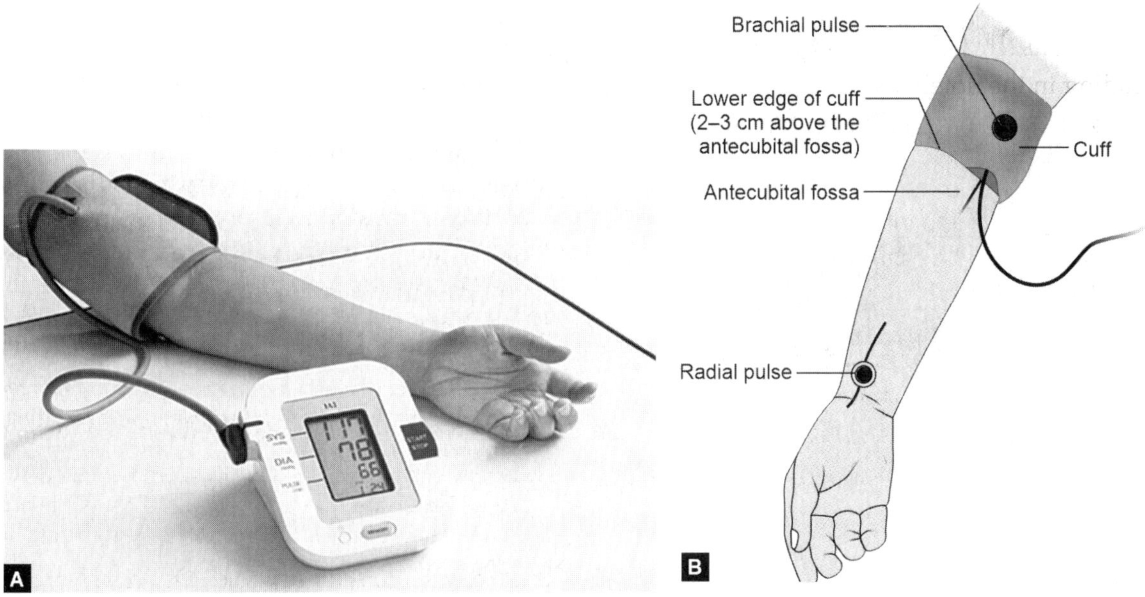

Figs 16.22A and B: Determination of BP

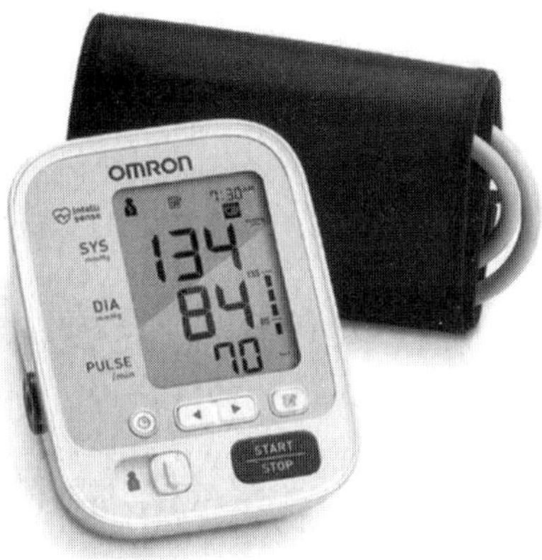

Fig. 16.23: Display of BP reading

Requirements:

1. Sphygmomanometer with inflatable rubber cuff (Fig. 16.24): It consists of an inflatable rubber cuff, which is wrapped around the upper arm of the patient and it is connected to an apparatus that records blood pressure (BP). BP is measured usually in terms of the height of a column of mercury or on a dial (an aneroid manometer) (Fig. 16.24)
2. *Stethoscope* (Fig. 16.25): It is an equipment used to detect low-volume sounds such as a heartbeat (or intestinal, venous, or fetal sounds), when it is connected to ears. A stethoscope may consist of two earpieces connected by means of flexible tubing to a diaphragm that is placed against the skin of the patient.
3. Other requirements are the same as for Experiment No. 20.

Procedure:

A. *Preparation of the patient:*
   1. Instructions given to the patient are the same as for Experiment No. 20.
   2. Allow the patient to relaxed for about 5 minutes.
   3. The patient should sit upright by keeping upper arm positioned in level his position of heart and feet placed flat on the floor.
   4. Remove excess clothing that might interfere with the BP cuff or constrict blood flow in the arm.

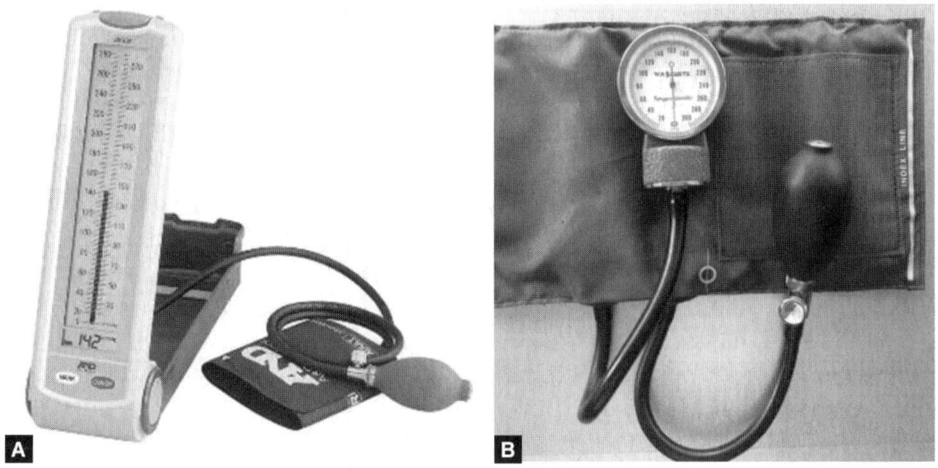

Figs 16.24A and B: (A) Spygmomanometer; (B) inflatable cuff

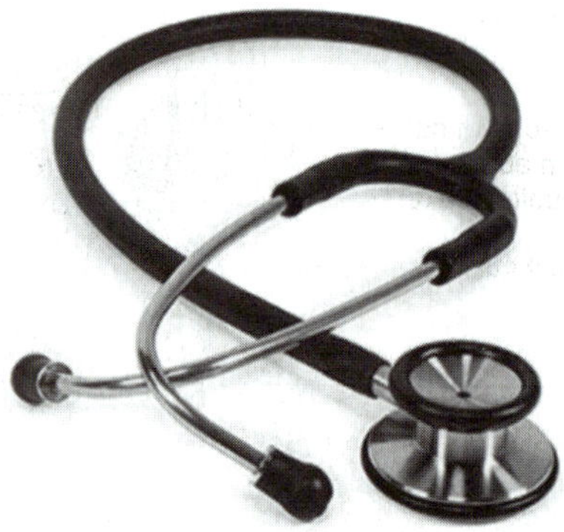

Fig. 16.25: A stethoscope

5. The patient should not talk during the BP reading procedure.

B. *Blood pressure reading:*

1. Choose a proper BP cuff size.
2. Wrap the cuff around the patient's arm (Fig. 16.26).
3. Adjust the BP cuff on the patient's arm.
4. Locate the brachial artery and position the BP cuff so that the artery marker points to the brachial artery.
5. Position the stethoscope on the arm that you have placed the BP cuff.
6. Palpate the arm at the antecubical fossa and locate the strongest pulse sounds and place the bell of the stethoscope over the brachial artery (Fig. 16.25).
7. Inflate the BP cuff. Begin pumping the cuff bulb as you listen to the pulse beats. When the BP cuff has inflated enough, blood flow will stop and you will hear no sounds through the stethoscope. In that case inflate the cuff to 160–180 mmHg.
8. Slowly deflate the BP cuff. The first occurrence of rhythmic sounds heard as blood begins to flow through the artery is the patient's systolic pressure. Note this reading. Now, listen for the diastolic reading as follows:
   i. Continue to listen as the BP cuff pressure drops and the sounds fade
   ii. Note the gauge reading when the rhythmic sounds stop. This is be the diastolic reading.
   iii. Take one more BP reading for confirming the first reading.

> ***Note***
> 1. The American Heart Association (AHA) recommends BP reading using both arms respectively and reporting average reading of BP.
> 2. To check the BP again wait for about five minutes between the two readings.
> 3. Blood pressure is relatively higher in the mornings and lower in the evenings in the normal range.

SAQ: What is the clinical significance of blood pressure (BP) determination?

SAQ: What is the normal BP?

SAQ: What are the instructions given to a patient before BP determination?

SAQ: How a patient is prepared before a BP test?

Ans: For the answers of all above questions, refer to Experiment Nos. 18 and 19.

EXPERIMENT 20: Determination of lung function by using a spirometer.

Introduction: A spirometer is an equipment that is used to measure the volume of air inspired and expired by the lungs (Fig. 26.27).

Spirometry: Spirometry is the most common type of pulmonary function or breathing test. This test measures

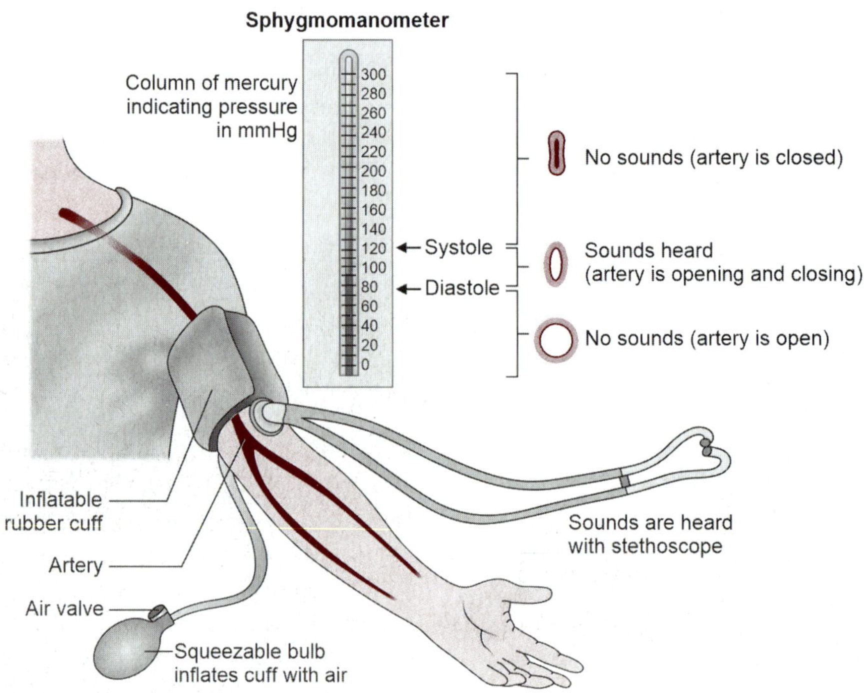

Fig. 16.26: Reading of BP using a spygmomanometer

how much air a patient can breathe in and out of lungs, as well as, how easily and fast the patient can blow the air out of the lungs. Physician may order spirometry if a patient suffers for a long duration from chronic lung disease such as asthma, bronchitis, etc. leading to shortness of breath, wheezing, and cough.

Clinical significance: Spirometry is used to diagnose affected respiratory functions due to asthma, chronic bronchitis, cystic fibrosis, emphysema, pulmonary fibrosis, chronic obstructive pulmonary disease (COPD), COVID-19, etc. Spirometry may also be used to periodically monitor the functions of lungs to evaluate effects of specific prescribed drugs, following treatment on lung ailments.

Requirements:
1. One volunteer or a patient
2. Spirometer

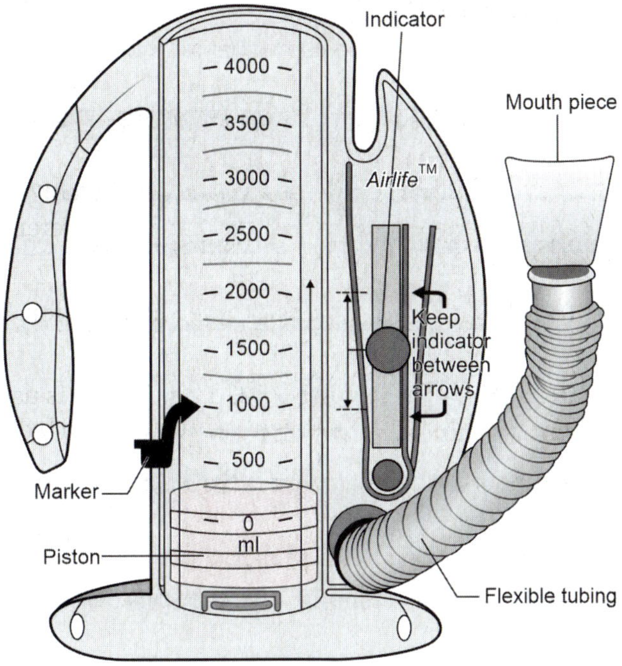

Fig. 16.27: Spirometer

Principle of a spirometer: When the patient breathes air into the tube through the mouthpiece of spirometer, during each cycle of inhalation and exhalation, the jar moves up and down. Piston of the spirometer rises with each deep breath and it is indicated on the scale of the spirometer (Fig. 16.28). Reading depends on the volume of air inhaled or exhaled and the weight attached to the string moves up and down. Percentage of air inhaled or exhales is determined by the goal marker reading on the scale of the spirometer and indicated as Forced Expiratory Volume (FEV) (Fig. 16.28).

> ***Note:*** Ethnicity, age, gender, and body composition are the factors that affect the different ranges of lung capacity among individuals. Hence, setting of normal ranges of FEV among the specific population is necessary.

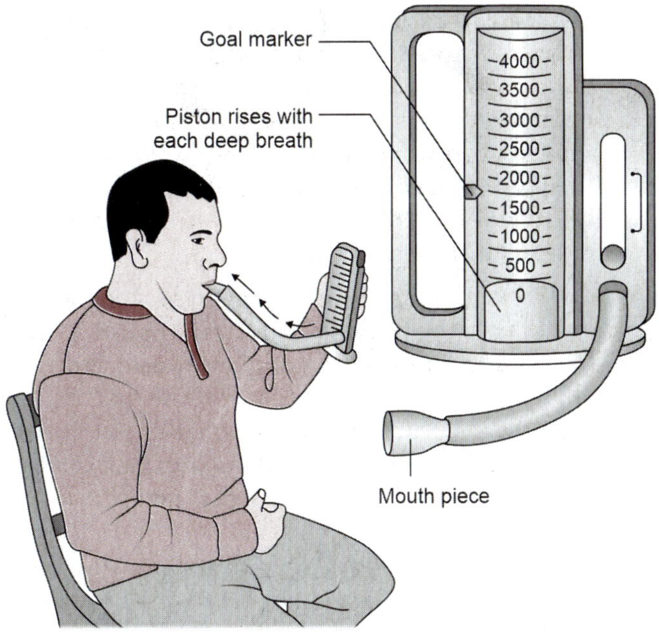

Fig. 16.28: Pulmonary function test using a spirometer

Normal values: Normal results of FEV are 70% or more for adults under 65.

Mild lung condition: FEV: 60–69%

Moderate lung condition: FEV: 50–59%

Procedure:
1. Patient is instructed to exhale (breath out) normally.
2. Put the mouthpiece of spirometer in the mouth of the patient and tell him/her to hold it tightly (Fig. 16.28).
3. Remove the mouthpiece and tell patient to hold breath for 3 seconds.
4. Tell patient to exhale normally and note the reading from the scale of the spirometer.

Calculations:

If patient's reading = 2,500

Goal marker reading = 3000

Percent FEV reading = 83.33

SAQ: What is a spirometer?

SAQ: What is the normal range of forced expiratory volume?

SAQ: What are the instructions given to a patient before testing FEV?

SAQ: What is the clinical significance of FEV test?

Ans: For the answers of all above questions, refer to Experiment No. 20.

EXPERIMENT 21: Determination of blood oxygen saturation using a pulse oximeter.

Introduction: SpO_2 stands for peripheral blood oxygen saturation. It is an estimate of the amount of oxygen in the circulating blood. It is the percentage of oxygenated haemoglobin compared to the total amount of haemoglobin in the blood. In the case of SpO_2, 'S' indicates saturation; 'P' indicates pressure and O_2 is oxygen.

In respiratory distress syndrome, mainly caused by viral and bacterial infections, patient suffers from significantly low levels of blood oxygen (hypoxia). It is necessary to monitor blood oxygen saturation and if hypoxia is present, adequate supply of oxygen and further support of ventilator may save life of a patient. A pulse oximeter is a non-invasive devise used to measure blood oxygen saturation.

Clinical significance: Blood oxygen is very well-regulated within the body. In hypoxemia, when blood oxygen level decreases significantly, it may lead to many adverse effects on individual organ systems such as the brain, heart, and kidneys. In severe respiratory diseases, it is necessary to keep tract of SpO_2 level throughout the sickness phase. Pulse oximetry also may be used in the case of the following matters:

1. During or after surgery, when patient is under sedation. It is necessary to see how medicines are working to treat lungs.
2. To check ability of a patient to handle increased activity levels.
3. To find out, if ventilator support is needed for a patient for breathing.

Pulse oximetry is also used to check blood oxygen level in the following clinical conditions: Heart failure, asthma, lung cancer, chronic obstructive pulmonary disease (COPD), pneumonia, and severe anemia.

Normal value: Blood oxygen saturation: 95 to 100% at or near sea level.

Principle of pulse oximetry: Oximeter works by the principles of spectrophotometry. The relative absorption of red light (absorbed by deoxygenated blood) and infrared light (absorbed by oxygenated blood) correlates to arterial blood oxygen saturation.

A typical pulse oximeter uses an electronic processor and two small light-emitting diodes (LEDs) facing a photodiode through a translucent part of a fingertip or an earlobe. One LED is red, with wavelength of 660 nm, and the other is infrared with a wavelength of 940 nm. Oxygenated hemoglobin absorbs more infrared light and allows more red light to pass through.

Deoxygenated hemoglobin allows more infrared light to pass through and absorbs more red light. The amount of light that is transmitted (that is not absorbed) is measured, which is proportional to SpO_2 (oxygen saturation).

Procedure (Fig. 16.29)

1. Make sure that hand of the patient is relaxed, and below the heart level.
2. Place the oxymeter on index finger of the patient (Fig. 16.29A).
3. Keep the oximeter device on till the reading of oxygen saturation is stable.
4. Note the SpO_2 reading (Fig. 16.29A).
5. Remove oximeter from the finger.

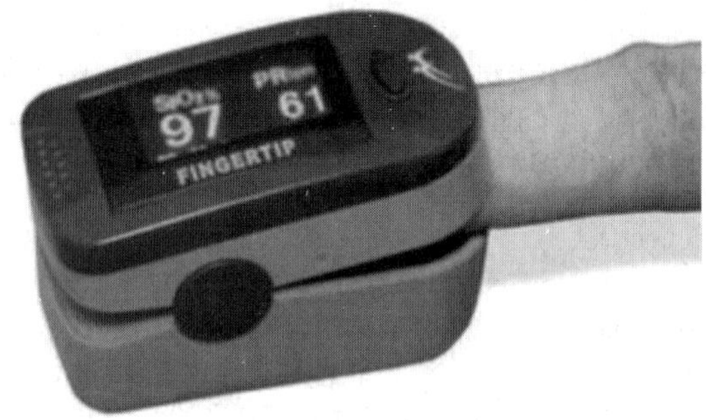

Fig. 16.29A: Working of pulse oximeter

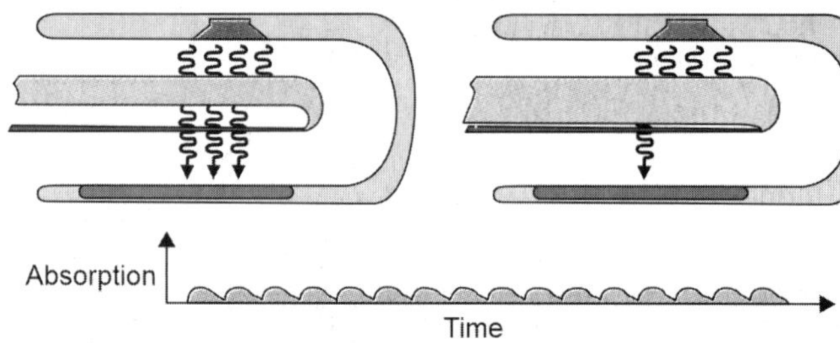

Fig. 16.29B: Principle of pulse oximeter

SAQ: What is the use of a pulse oxymeter?

SAQ: What is the normal range of SpO_2 (blood oxygen saturation)?

SAQ: What is the principle of blood oximeter?

SAQ: What is the clinical significance of blood oxygen saturation?

Ans: For the answers of all above questions, refer to Experiment No. 21.

BIBLIOGRAPHY

1. Medical Biochemistry, 1st Edition (2023). Godkar PB, Godkar DP, CBS Publishers, New Delhi, India.
2. Text Book of Medical Laboratory Technology, 4th Edition, (2024). Godkar PB, Godkar DP, Bhalani Publishing House, Mumbai, India.

Index

B

C

D

E

M

N

O

P

Q

R

S

W

Y

Z